PEDIATRICS for
MEDICAL STUDENTS

Second Edition

PEDIATRICS for MEDICAL STUDENTS

Second Edition

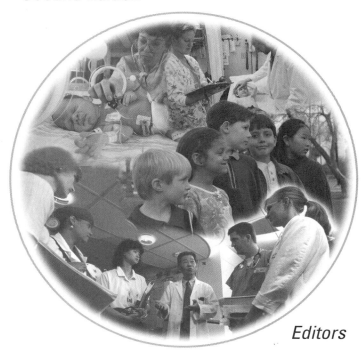

Editors

Daniel Bernstein, M.D.

Professor of Pediatrics
Chief, Division of Pediatric Cardiology
Lucile Salter Packard Children's Hospital
Stanford University School of Medicine
Stanford, California

Steven P. Shelov, M.D., M.S.

Chairman of Pediatrics
Vice President, Infants and Children's
   Hospital
Maimonides Medical Center
Lutheran Medical Center
Brooklyn, N.Y.
Professor of Pediatrics
Mount Sinai School of Medicine
New York, New York

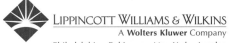
LIPPINCOTT WILLIAMS & WILKINS
A **Wolters Kluwer** Company

Philadelphia • Baltimore • New York • London
Buenos Aires • Hong Kong • Sydney • Tokyo

Editor: Neil Marquardt
Managing Editor: Bridget Hilferty
Marketing Manager: Scott Lavine
Project Editor: Paula C. Williams
Designer: Risa Clow
Compositor: Peirce Graphic Services, Inc.
Printer: Data Reproductions Corp.

Library of Congress Cataloging-in-Publication Data

Pediatrics for medical students / editors, Daniel Bernstein, Steven P. Shelov.
     p. ; cm.
  Includes bibliographical references and index.
  ISBN 0-7817-2941-6
   1. Pediatrics. I. Bernstein, Daniel, 1953- II. Shelov, Steven P.
  [DNLM: 1. Pediatrics. WS 100 P37057 2002]
 RJ45 .P3987 2002
 618.92—dc21

                                                                    2002040637

05 06
2 3 4 5 6 7 8 9 10

We dedicate this book to our present and former students who have always kept us on our toes and our future students who will continue to challenge us to be the best teachers possible. We also dedicate this book to our families: Bonnie, Alissa, and Adam Bernstein; and Marsha, Joshua, Danielle, Eric Shelov, and Jennifer and Owen for their patience and support. We also thank the late Drs. Henry Barnett, and Lewis Fraad and Drs. Michael Cohen, Richard Kravath, Gerald Nathenson, and Abraham Rudolph, as well as Joyce Lavery for her artwork and Elizabeth Nieginski, Bridget Hilferty, Martha Cushman, Paula Williams, and Carol Loyd at Lippincott Williams & Wilkins for their perseverance in seeing this educational adventure through to fruition.

Preface

A revolution is occurring in the world of medicine, one that will have profound effects not only on the way medicine is practiced but also on the way medicine is taught to students at all levels. New terms and phrases such as managed care, health maintenance organization, covered lives, and capitation have filtered into our vocabulary alongside more traditional terms such as tetralogy of Fallot, bronchopulmonary dysplasia, and thrombocytopenic purpura. For health sciences students, perhaps the greatest change will be in the venue in which patients are encountered. There has been a significant shift in health care delivery from the inpatient ward to the outpatient setting, whether a private office or satellite clinic, an ambulatory surgery unit, or a day hospital. The focus of medical care also has shifted more heavily toward prevention, yet the traditional venue for the teaching of health sciences students has too often continued to concentrate on acute and tertiary care. In many settings, roles traditionally carried out by physicians are being performed by other health care providers such as physician assistants, nurse practitioners, and health care technicians.

Pediatrics for Medical Students was written in the midst of this health care revolution to serve as an introductory text for students during their clinical clerkships. It strives to teach students the basics of pediatric clinical practice by concentrating on evaluative skills and logical approaches to both common and uncommon pediatric problems rather than serving as an exhaustive reference. This pediatrics text provides students with insight into the clinical diagnostic skills of some of today's premier pediatric clinicians: To experienced clinicians, the process of developing and refining a differential diagnosis is akin to solving an elegant puzzle. *Pediatrics for Medical Students* also stresses the essentials of modern pediatric medicine with a view toward the challenges of pediatric practice in the 21st century. Finally, it emphasizes the pediatrician's unique developmental perspective and opportunity to actively prevent future illness by altering life habits at an early stage.

Contributors to *Pediatrics for Medical Students* have been chosen from the attending staffs at several major medical schools, based primarily on their communicative skills, teaching abilities, and agreement with the educational philosophy of the text. The contributors have imparted the sense of challenge and accomplishment associated with arriving at a well-conceived differential diagnosis and management plan.

Pediatrics for Medical Students is organized to help students make the transition from the systems-oriented approach of the preclinical years to the problem-oriented approach of the clinical years. Some chapters focus on the general practice of pediatrics; these allow students to appreciate the normal preventive visit, including extensive discussions of preventive strategies and anticipatory guidance. More traditional systems-oriented chapters describe a uniform, systematic approach to developing a differential diagnosis that will serve as a model for assessing all clinical, problem situations. Other chapters focus on emerging areas of health care, including medical ethics, health care economics and managed care, and social and cultural issues in pediatrics.

With the growing complexity of modern pediatric medicine, it is increasingly difficult for beginning students to master all the details of pediatric diseases. *Pediatrics for Medical Students* views pathophysiology as a key to the student's understanding of disease; this approach helps students develop differential diagnoses and logical management. The text also emphasizes differential diagnosis, which goes hand in hand with an appreciation of the appropriate use of diagnostic tests. Medical cost containment issues are interwoven throughout the text. By teaching sound medical practice, students automatically learn cost-effective medical practice. Finally, *Pediatrics for Medical Students* emphasizes, both in a separate chapter and in appropriate context, the medical, epidemiologic, and social implications of our multicultural pediatric population.

Suggested readings at the end of each chapter include several components: one or two recommended textbooks for those desiring a more detailed examination of the subject, several well-written review articles in easy-to-find journals such as *Pediatrics* or *Pediatric Clinics of North America*, and several seminal journal articles in the field. These references are intended for those students whose interest has been piqued and who wish to explore the latest developments in both basic science and clinical research as applied to a particular pediatric illness.

Pediatrics for Medical Students has several unique features, including:

- **Pediatric pearls:** Each chapter contains several key, "take-home" pieces of information that all students should know.
- **USMLE-type questions on CD-ROM:** Questions based on the subject matter in each chapter, with explanations of the answers, both correct and incorrect, are included on the CD-ROM.

- **Updated references, with web site recommendations:** Often additional material on a subject is available on a web site, which is presented in the references.

We hope that students enjoy these important learning tools, find the organization and content of the book useful, and enjoy working with children.

Daniel Bernstein, M.D.
Palo Alto, California

Steven P. Shelov, M.D., M.S.
Brooklyn, New York

Contributors

HARVEY W. AIGES, MD
Vice Chairman and Physician-in-Charge
Department of Pediatrics
North Shore University Hospital
Manhasset, New York

ELIZABETH M. ALDERMAN, MD
Associate Clinical Professor of Pediatrics
Division of Adolescent Medicine
Children's Hospital at Montefiore
Albert Einstein College of Medicine
Bronx, New York

HENRY ANHALT, DO, FAAP, FACOP, FACE
Director, Division of Pediatric Endocrinology
Infants and Children's Hospital of Brooklyn
Maimonides Medical Center
Associate Professor of Clinical Pediatrics
State University of New York Health Science
  Center
Brooklyn, New York

JEFFREY R. AVNER, MD, FAAP
Professor of Clinical Pediatrics
Albert Einstein College of Medicine
Director, Children's Emergency Services
Children's Hospital at Montefiore
Bronx, New York

FATAI BAMGBOLA, MD
Assistant Clinical Instructor
Division of Pediatric Nephrology
Children's Hospital at Montefiore
Albert Einstein College of Medicine
Bronx, New York

PATRICIA CASTANEDA, MD
Assistant Clinical Instructor
Division of Pediatric Nephrology
Children's Hospital at Montefiore
Albert Einstein College of Medicine
Bronx, New York

CAROL CONRAD, MD
Assistant Professor of Pediatrics
Stanford University
Palo Alto, California

GARY V. DAHL, MD
Professor of Pediatrics
Stanford University Medical Center
Stanford, California

JOSEPH V. DICARLO, MD
Assistant Professor of Pediatrics
Stanford University
Palo Alto, California

KATHRYN L. ECKERT, MD
Assistant Professor of Pediatrics
University of Nevada School of Medicine
Reno, Nevada

REBECCA EVANGELISTA, MD
Chief Resident
Department of General Surgery
George Washington University Medical Center
Washington, D.C.

ALAN R. FLEISCHMAN, MD
Senior Vice President
The New York Academy of Medicine
Clinical Professor of Pediatrics
Clinical Professor of Epidemiology and Social
  Medicine
Albert Einstein College of Medicine
New York, New York

LORRY R. FRANKEL, MD
Associate Professor of Pediatrics
Stanford University
Palo Alto, California

KATHLEEN GUTIERREZ, MD
Staff Physician
Clinical Instructor
Department of Pediatrics
Stanford University
Stanford, California

PAUL HARRIS, MD
Professor of Clinical Pediatrics
SUNY–Downstate
Brooklyn, New York

GARY E. HARTMAN, MD
Chief
Department of Pediatric Surgery
Children's National Medical Center
The George Washington School of Medicine
Georgetown University
Washington, D.C.

KIMBERLY A. HORII, MD
Resident in Dermatology
Department of Dermatology
Stanford University School of Medicine
Stanford, California

ELIZABETH K. KACHUR, PhD
Director
Medical Education Development
National and International Consulting
New York, New York

FREDERICK J. KASKEL, MD, PhD
Professor of Pediatrics
Director of Pediatric Nephrology
Children's Hospital at Montefiore
Albert Einstein College of Medicine
Bronx, New York

D. RANI C. KATHIRITHAMBY, MD
Rose F. Kennedy Center
Assistant Professor
Rehabilitation Medicine and Pediatrics
Albert Einstein College of Medicine/
    Montefiore Medical Center
Bronx, New York

JUAN C. KUPFERMAN, MD
Assistant Professor of Pediatrics
Director of Pediatric Nephrology and
    Hypertension
Infants & Children's Hospital of Brooklyn
Maimonides Medical Center
Brooklyn, New York

ALFRED T. LANE, MD
Professor of Dermatology and Pediatrics
Chairman, Department of Dermatology
Director, Pediatric Dermatology
Stanford University School of Medicine
Stanford, California

ROBERT W. MARION, MD
Professor of Pediatrics and Obstetrics/Gynecology
Albert Einstein College of Medicine
Children's Hospital at Montefiore
Bronx, New York

LISA MENASSE-PALMER, MD, FAAP
Attending Pediatrician
Port Washington, New York

FERNANDO S. MENDOZA, MD, MPH
Professor
Division of General Pediatrics
Stanford University
Stanford, California

DAVID M. MERER, MD, FACS, FAAP
Associate Professor of Otolaryngology
New York Medical College
Westchester Medical Center
Valhalla, New York

ANDREW P. MEZEY, MD, MS
Vice Chairman
Department of Pediatrics
Maimonides Medical Center
Brooklyn, New York
Clinical Professor of Pediatrics
Albert Einstein College of Medicine
Bronx, New York

MARIJEAN M. MILLER, MD
Assisting Professor of Ophthalmology and
    Pediatrics
George Washington University
Attending Physician
Children's National Medical Center
Washington, D.C.

LANE S. PALMER, MD, FAAP, FACS
Associate Director
Pediatric Urology
Schneider Children's Hospital
New Hyde Park, New York

WILLIAM D. RHINE, MD
Associate Professor
Department of Pediatrics
Stanford University School of Medicine
Palo Alto, California

MARIS D. ROSENBERG, MD
Rose F. Kennedy Center
Associate Professor of Clinical Pediatrics
Albert Einstein College of Medicine/
    Montefiore Medical Center
Bronx, New York

RON G. ROSENFELD, MD
Chairman and Professor
Department of Pediatrics
School of Medicine
Oregon Health and Science University
Physician-in-Chief
Doernbecher Children's Hospital
Portland, Oregon

CHRISTY SANDBORG, MD
Associate Professor
Department of Pediatrics
Stanford University
Stanford, California

WARREN M. SEIGEL, MD
Chairman, Department of Pediatrics
Director of Adolescent Medicine
Coney Island Hospital
Associate Professor of Clinical Pediatrics
SUNY Health Science Center at Brooklyn
Brooklyn, New York

ALFRED J. SPIRO, MD
Professor of Neurology and Pediatrics
Albert Einstein College of Medicine
Bronx, New York

YOUNG-JIN SUE, MD
Assistant Clinical Professor of Pediatrics
Albert Einstein College of Medicine
Attending Physician, Children's Emergency
  Services
Children's Hospital at Montefiore
Bronx, New York

SUROJ SUPAVEKIN, MD
Assistant Clinical Instructor
Division of Pediatric Nephrology
Children's Hospital at Montefiore
Albert Einstein College of Medicine
Bronx, New York

KAVERI SURYANARAYAN, MD
Assistant Professor
Department of Pediatrics
University of Maryland
Baltimore, Maryland

ELIZABETH C. TEPAS, MD
Department of Pediatrics
Stanford University
Stanford, California

DALE T. UMETSU, MD, PhD
Professor of Pediatrics
Chief, Division of Allergy and Immunology
Director, Center for Asthma and Allergic Diseases
Stanford University
Stanford, California

KRISA P. VAN MEURS, MD
Associate Professor
Department of Pediatrics
Stanford University School of Medicine
Palo Alto, California

ESTHER H. WENDER, MD
Clinical Professor of Pediatrics
Albert Einstein College of Medicine
Bronx, New York

Contents

Introduction

Steven P. Shelov and Daniel Bernstein

Being a medical student or student in the allied health professions nowadays is not easy. Not that it ever was "easy," for surely our selective memory of those years has protected us from remembering the difficult times and has permitted us to glorify the more convivial and rewarding times disproportionately. Nevertheless, we truly believe that current health care students have to contend with elements that did not confront students in the past.

Pediatrics for Medical Students is intended to present a large variety of pediatric "information" in as understandable and usable a fashion as possible, but it would be an error not to take some time to recognize a number of issues relating to education during clinical clerkships that often go unstated and unrecognized. Some of this material is drawn from a landmark article entitled, "The Vulnerability of the Medical Student," published in the journal *Pediatrics* in 1976 by Drs. Edwenna Werner and Barbara Korsch to honor the memory of their mentor, Dr. Lorin L. Stephens. This reference is one we continuously cite to our medical students, residents, and physician assistant students during the course of their training. Other material is drawn from the increasingly important issues of medical issues and accountability for adverse health care outcomes. Still other material is derived from our own cumulative experience of some 50 years of exposure to young trainees in this specialty. Through a combination of these three sources, we hope to bring some context to the material offered in the chapters to follow.

DEALING WITH UNCERTAINTY

The majority of learning and teaching strives toward some sense of achieving certainty. The basic sciences, especially those assembled for your appreciation in preclinical training (i.e., the first 2 years of medical school) have emphasized the need to strive to a level where we are certain about what we do. Whether we are talking about biochemical pathways, the genetic determinants of sickle cell disease, or any of the many facts that you have committed to memory from those years of basic science, your teachers have stressed that there is a great deal of certainty about your evolving knowledge base.

In addition, you learned that the more you applied yourself, the more of these "certain facts" you would know. To be successful in medicine, you are repeatedly told that certainty is always the achievable goal. During the upcoming clinical years, many of your teachers will imply that certainty in clinical medicine is also an achievable goal. Thus, as you jump into that first clinical clerkship, you are no doubt eager to apply your newly mastered knowledge base from the basic sciences to clinical practice. However, you learn that you have not been well prepared for the wall of uncertainty that you encounter as soon as you begin to work up that first patient.

Indeed, you soon learn that clinical medicine is *far from certain* and that any attempt to make it certain quickly leads to a sense of frustration, disappointment, and confusion. Some of this confusion and frustration is avoidable if you recognize that *medicine is often uncertain* and that *in spite of this fact we can still do much for our patients and derive much satisfaction from the careful application of what we have learned.*

We believe that the simple recognition that certainty is not always attainable is an important first step for the beginning clinician. Once you realize that and yet strive to apply all that is known to achieving a more certain state, you will find a more livable sense of balance in your role as a health care provider and no doubt a more satisfying sense of who you are and what you can and cannot do (i.e., you have limitations).

The major reasons for the inability to achieve certainty all of the time (actually, much of the time) are our incomplete knowledge base and the fact that the subjects of our combined art and science are *real people*, not idealized textbook examples. All children with meningitis do not present in the same way; some children with fever are truly more ill than others, yet we may not always know how to spot them. What is the best diagnostic approach? What is the highest yield from a particular test? Parents differ in their ability to recognize developmental delay or aberrances in their child's behavior. How can you best advise them to change their child's behavior?

With those multiple-choice questions we have all spent so much time answering, the answers are *certain;* in clinical medicine, the answers vary. They vary sometimes because of things that may be measurable and other times because of things that are not measurable. The hallmark of a good clinician is the ability to account for these variables. As long as you are systematic in your thinking, eager to embrace alternative explanations, open to suggestions, and *willing to listen at all levels,* you will be successful. Each day you will learn more, experience more, and grow as a clinician, moving a little more from uncertainty to certainty. But be prepared to carry around with you a continued supply of uncertainty, and do not feel you are very different in substance from even the most senior of clinicians you meet; you are different only in degree.

IDENTIFICATION WITH THE PATIENT

Although it may be difficult to remember, you had another life before you became a health care professional. Throughout your past and present life, you witnessed much and incorporated many different experiences and observations into your present persona. You are a function of your parents and friends, your previous life situations, and your original makeup. These parts of you do not disappear when you encounter your first patient; they are, in fact, incorporated into every patient encounter you will have. It is inevitable that you will frequently and often unconsciously compare your present experiences with your previous ones, adapt to them, and allow them to alter your present makeup. Many of these changes occur consciously, but there are many others of which you are not aware.

Some clinical encounters are difficult situations that unconsciously remind you of your own fears, your past or present relationships, or your own family. Those situations, which evoke an overidentification response, are often the most complex. It may be difficult to identify and become conscious of them. Nevertheless, these reminders will play havoc with your sense of stability and create unease and anxiety that you may have difficulty sorting out. Often, overidentification with a patient or family results in a driving need to rectify or fix a problem for which there is no easy solution. To highlight the pitfall of overidentification, we often cite a special quote from the article by Werner and Korsch:

> I believe I would have been a better intern and a better young physician, and that I would have learned more and suffered less, if someone could have told me explicitly,

repeatedly, and patiently that the dying at hand was not my own, that the patient whose death I attended was not, in fact, myself, nor was it my wife, nor my child, nor my parents, nor, fortunately, was it often my friend. And most important, I needed to be told and taught that the dying which I was attending did not, in itself, increase my vulnerability nor the vulnerability of those for whom I cared most deeply. The confusion involved in the sympathetic relationship, wherein identities merge and blur—this is what is intolerable and excruciating and blinding.

You can become aware of when this is happening to you if you are sensitive to your own feelings, realizing that some anxiety should be expected. However, you should recognize that if these feelings begin to affect you in such a way as to influence your satisfaction with your clinical role or your ability to make clear decisions, it may be stronger than you realize and needs to be dealt with in some way. One method that we have found useful is regularly scheduled mentoring groups with students or residents. When discussing overidentification and related issues, other members of the group, including faculty mentors, often share similar experiences and feelings. Once these feelings of anxiety related to overidentification become "fair game" for discussion, the resistance to discussion drops, and each participant is able to contribute his or her own experiences and reactions. The individuals in such a group often come to the realization that their past experiences are inextricably interwoven with their present situations. Because these encounters often deal with life-and-death matters, their relevance becomes highlighted. Recognizing that this is a shared experience with your colleagues is usually the first step in the course of regaining some control over these situations.

SENSE OF RESPONSIBILITY—DEALING WITH LIFE AND DEATH

For medical students, who are protected from the real world by the comfort of the classroom, the basic science years are often just a continuation of the years of college, just more intense and with greater stakes. The clinical years are a different story. Medical students in TV shows embody many of the responses characteristic of new clinicians. At times, bragging and confident, at other times sheepish and lacking confidence, and at still other times frustrated when the role confusion is maddening—all are part of the clinician trainee's mental state.

You, too, are immediately thrust into a "real world" of sick people who may convey signals of helplessness, neediness, illness, anxiety, and uncertainty about their present or future existence, as well as an often overwhelming sense that without your help they will no longer be able to "make it." Much of this has to do with, and is created in response to, the multiple roles and responsibilities demanded of you in dealing with real people undergoing a traumatic loss of who they are because of illness. And you, with all of your newfound wisdom, are expected to make it all better.

The fact of the matter is that there is no way you can possibly do that. You are just at the stage of attempting to integrate your newly learned, although fragile, knowledge base into this whole new world of real patients. Each new clerkship places you in new settings that keep you enough off balance so that you often develop self-doubts. How are you ever going to be able to learn enough, be confident enough in your knowledge and decisions, and just be calm enough to see yourself through successfully in any of these new roles? You will succeed with time. That is why clinical training takes place over years, not months, and why clinical confidence in new roles is a graduated series of responsibilities rather than something you are immediately expected to succeed at in the first few months of clinical experience. Unfortunately, someone forgot to tell your sense of your own expectations about these reservations regarding your level of responsibility. To quote once again from the article by Werner and Korsch:

> The study of medicine is in fact the study of living and dying. No more central nor enormous concern seems to exist: or at least this seems so for the peculiar and puzzling species of men and women who elect to take upon themselves the role of physician. And the innermost mystery of all, the most frightening, the most compellingly interesting, the most inescapable truth encountered in this journey is that one cannot learn about living and dying only in others. One cannot help but make inferences about one's own life and death . . . it seems true beyond doubt that upon one's comprehension of living and dying depends one's ability to serve as a physician.

The solution is for you to feel that you are shouldering a level of responsibility appropriate for your present level of training. You may need some help recognizing this at times, and those more senior to you may also need to be reminded about it. Feeling that you have an overwhelming responsibility for particular patients or their patient outcome will interfere with some of the growth that is essential for your future security as a clinician. This is not to say that you should not eagerly and enthusiastically engage your clinical responsibilities head on. You will gain much more from clinical experiences in which you play an active role. However, being an active participant does not mean you have ultimate responsibility for all of the outcomes, good or bad. The time will come in the future where your level of responsibility will increase; with that will come the increased knowledge and experience and the comfort that is part of that seniority.

TO ERR IS HUMAN . . . (IS ERROR PERMISSIBLE?)

In 1999, the Institute of Medicine issued a report entitled *To Err is Human: Building a Safer Health System*. This highly publicized and critiqued white paper brought the issue of the consequences of medical errors to the forefront. It gives a relatively scathing account of the dire consequences of medical errors in the hospital setting and challenges the universe of the health care setting to develop remedies for these problems. Although many experts have stated the data is poorly drawn from overly high-risk settings and does not pertain to *their* situation, the overwhelming consensus is that much of what the report contains is on target.

As students, you will be thrust into settings in which you have to grapple with health and safety issues as they pertain to a particular setting. Our advice is: learn from the approaches to system change that are taking place around you; apply the principles of critical self-study and change when necessary; and become part of the solution, not part of the problem. Hospitals are complex places, and great care is necessary to ensure that the systems work for the patients, not against them. Reducing medical errors is *everyone's business*. You are in an ideal setting to see the benefits of a positive approach to change. Take advantage of those opportunities to learn and grow.

COMMUNICATION IS THE KEY

> To write prescriptions is easy, but to come to an understanding with people is hard.
>
> *Franz Kafka*

It is not always easy to effectively find out the things you need to know about your patients. Many times it is even harder to tell them about things that are happening to them, especially the difficult things. Nevertheless, good patient communication is the key to becoming a good clinician. In addition, the most difficult and often least clear-cut issues revolve around the psychosocial aspects of their condition. You will quickly discover that diseases are not often explained by one factor alone and that there is much truth in Engel's "unified concept of disease," which holds that every disease has multiple components, a biologic, an emotional, and a social component. These facts are the challenge to clinical medicine, and uncovering them depends on clear communication and the ability to recognize the importance of psychosocial issues. We also recognize that it is often harder to relate to patients who present with a predominance of these issues.

> In a county-type hospital, when everyone's social ills are really in a lot of ways more important than the immediate pneumonia, it is quite a distraction. At County Hospital a patient with terminal cancer is much easier for me to deal with than four or five chronic alcoholics that come in with another pneumonia, and they're starting a decompensate again. You know that no matter what kind of medical treatment you give these people, the society, for them at least, is such that they will be back again. . . . When I have a real patient with real ills that I can handle, I'm very happy.

It is important to combat any resistance that occurs, diminish your skepticism, and realize that the process is a dynamic one. You will come to realize that if you are open to hearing about these "other issues," your patients will feel well served and feel that they have truly made a connection to "their doctor."

Two quotes of Dr. Stephens', from the last two pages of the article by Werner and Korsch, are pivotal and should be required reading for all those who are students or teachers of clinical medicine.

> If the issues described above are disregarded or dealt with only incidentally or accidentally, the students, in large number, will stumble in their desperation into the maladaptive roles seen all around us in graduate physicians. The students will meet these issues by transmuting their patients into abstractions, which offer neither the pain nor gratification of human intimacy. They will take refuge from human responsibility in obsessive attention to detail, to the particular. They will, in futility and panic, resist what they perceive as encroachment on

their territorial imperatives in the form of health-care delivery evaluation, or even physician review processes. They will find other sources of gratification than in professional excellence: the talk in the surgeons' dressing room more often concerns the Dow-Jones averages and the golf course than it does patients, for many reasons, but some of the above pertain. All-gullible, they will accept the force-feeding of the detail man or the latest surgical vogue as the treatment of the lesion. They will avoid the dying patient rather than threaten the protection afford by their illusory defenses. They will continue to get inferior medical care for themselves. They will not allow themselves fascination with the infinite variety of patients' problems and physicians' solutions.

> There are those who will tell you that being a physician is a curse, a life of endless and ambiguous work, where at best we are consumed in a holding action—and all that, without experiencing appropriate appreciation of our sacrifice.

> I do not feel that way. Being a physician I consider the highest privilege I can imagine. Along with the joys from my family, my life as a physician has provided me with moments of epiphany, transcendental moments of lucidity . . . To be a physician—to be permitted, to be invited by another human being into his life in the circumstances of that crucible which is illness—to be a trusted participant in the highest of dramas—for these privileges I am grateful beyond my ability to express . . .

These statements reflect the caution and optimism that occurs as you embark on the long journey of becoming a clinician. It is with these thoughts, encouragements, and reflections that we welcome you to this, your introduction to the world of children's health and disease. Enjoy these times; it is our hope that the material enclosed will help make your journey toward certainty a little bit easier and a great deal more satisfying.

SUGGESTED READINGS

Brennan TA: The Institute of Medicine Report on medical errors—could it do harm? *N Engl J Med* 342: 1123–1125, 2000.

Kohn LT, Corrigan JM, Donaldson MS (eds): *To Err is Human: Building a Safer Health System*. Committee on Quality of Health Care in America, Institute of Medicine, Washington, DC, National Academy Press, 1999.

Werner ER, Korsch BM: The vulnerability of the medical student: Posthumous presentation of L. L. Stephens' ideas. *Pediatrics* 57:321–328, 1976.

General Pediatric Practice

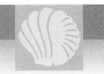

Chapter 1

Approach to the Normal Newborn

Andrew P. Mezey

The arrival of a newborn infant is an extraordinary event for a family. It releases a flood of emotions ranging from great joy and great expectations to great fear. Families feel particularly vulnerable at this time, and all health care providers must be sensitive to this. A careless word or a seeming indifference to a question may cause great pain for the parents. This chapter sets forth an approach to evaluating the newly born infant and communicating with the family.

PRENATAL INTERVIEW

About 4 weeks before the expected date of birth, many pediatric providers offer a prenatal interview to expectant parents whom they have not met. Obstetricians, midwives, leaders of prenatal classes, or friends who have previously enjoyed this experience may refer the parents.

The prenatal interview is an effective way for prospective parents to meet the provider at a relatively unpressured time. It is best to schedule the interview at the end of office hours (i.e., at a time when the office is quieter and the pressure to keep seeing patients is no longer there). Because expectant mothers often work until their due dates, the end of the day is often convenient for both parents.

After the initial introductions and questions relating to how the couple was referred, the interview should take the form of a formal past medical history of both prospective parents. This should include the following topics:

- The length of time the couple has been married
- How easy or difficult it was to achieve conception
- Problems that the parents experienced during this or previous pregnancies
- Medications now being used
- Alcohol and smoking habits
- Problems that they or other family members may have had with their children

- Medical and genetic problems of other family members

Although in many cases the answers to these questions yield relatively little, focusing the discussion in this way helps the pediatrician learn about how the couple interacts, how they deal with apparent tensions, and whether any information elicited from one parent is a surprise to the other. The interview is a good gauge of how well prospective parents communicate. The interview is also a good way for the parents to learn how the physician communicates.

In the average middle class American family, the expectant mother asks most of the questions, with the support of the husband. It is unusual if the man does most of the talking. In such instances, the pediatrician may need to provide the woman with a great deal of support in the first few months of her infant's life. She may be depressed, and this condition may become worse after delivery.

Pediatric Pearl

In some cultural groups, a woman does not speak much in the presence of her husband. This may pose problems in the prenatal interview when questions about parenting issues are discussed.

The next portion of the interview should focus on what the couple plan to do after the baby is born. Although much of this deals with breast-feeding versus bottle-feeding, safety and general care concerns warrant attention. Now is the time to provide information about car seat usage; the risks to the infant of passive exposure to cigarette smoke; fluoride, iron, and vitamin use; and crib safety, including the potential dangers of old cribs and how to determine proper mattress size. Questions about if and when the mother or father plans to return to work, the couple's plans for child care, and the availability of social support from family and friends are all appropriate at this time.

In closing, the pediatrician should ask the parents if there are any issues that have not been covered or are unclear. After that, the pediatrician should explain how he can be reached after the delivery and when and how often the infant will be seen in the hospital. He should also ask the couple to phone him if they have further questions after leaving the office. An interview of this depth takes between 30 and 45 minutes, but it is well worth the investment of time, especially if any problems arise during or after the birth of the infant. **After a successful prenatal interview, the pediatrician has achieved credibility as someone who is concerned about the parents and the unborn child.** This interview makes it easier to discuss issues that may arise at the time of delivery, which occur at an emotionally charged time.

INITIAL EVALUATION OF THE NORMAL NEWBORN

For normal births, it is not necessary for a pediatrician to be present at the delivery. Generally, pediatricians or, in many hospitals, neonatologists attend births when there is more likely to be a need to resuscitate and stabilize the infant. These include cesarean sections, either elective or urgent; multiple births; premature births; or cases in which fetal distress has been noted. The management of the infant in these situations is covered elsewhere in this book.

In most cases, the infant is born without problems, and the hospital staff notify the pediatrician's office of a birth in a routine manner. Hospital personnel call the office and leave a message, and the pediatrician appears at the nursery, usually within 12 hours after the birth, but certainly no longer than 24 hours. After arriving at the nursery, the pediatrician should first review the delivery record and the infant's chart.

Review of the Delivery Record

It is important to note the length of the delivery; the duration of ruptured membranes; the mother's course during labor, particularly temperature elevations that necessitate administration of antibiotics; and the condition of the infant at birth as described by the Apgar score. If a delivery has been long, the mother may be exhausted and perhaps dehydrated, which may interfere with her ability to begin breastfeeding. If the membranes ruptured 24 or more hours before birth, subtle symptoms or signs of infection in the newborn warrant closer attention. If the mother has a history of prolonged rupture of membranes in the presence of fever, it is essential to decide about whether to perform a sepsis workup on the baby, even in the face of a well-appearing infant. The actual management of such infants varies and is covered elsewhere in this book.

The **Apgar score** is the standard, time-honored method for evaluating the well-being of newborn infants at the time of delivery (Table 1.1). In practice, there are usually two Apgar scores, the first done at 1 minute after delivery and the second done at 5 minutes after delivery. Two points are given for each of 5 observations, for a potential total score of 10. Scores of 7–10 at 1 and at 5 minutes are indicative of a stable infant. If the score is less than 7 at 5 minutes, another score is done at 10 and at 20 minutes. If the score remains low, a decision to observe the infant in an intensive care area is appropriate.

Even the most normal infant does not usually have an Apgar score of 10 at 1 minute; most infants have 1 taken off for color. Many parents are familiar with Apgar scoring and will ask about it, so even if the pediatrician is not particularly interested in whether the Apgar score is 8, 9, or 10, the parents will be. The pediatrician should be prepared to discuss it with them (see Table 1.1).

TABLE 1.1 Apgar Score			
Score	**0**	**1**	**2**
Heart rate	Absent	< 100 beats/min	> 100 beats/min
Respiratory effort	Absent	Slow, irregular	Good, crying
Muscle tone	Limp	Some flexion of extremities	Active motion
Reflex irritability (catheter in nose)	Absent	Grimace	Grimace and cough or sneeze
Color	Blue	Body pink, pale, extremities blue	Pink

In addition to noting the Apgar score, it is important to be aware of the resuscitative efforts that have taken place in the delivery room. These may range from routine care to oxygen by face mask to endotracheal intubation. **The more aggressive the intervention, the more concerned the pediatrician should be about the effects of asphyxiation on the infant, even in the face of Apgar scores of 7 or more.**

Review of the Infant's Chart

It is important to review an infant's chart for the blood type and Rh factor of the mother; the infant's blood type and Rh status; the serology and hepatitis B status of the mother; the human immunodeficiency virus (HIV) status of the mother; the infant's vital signs, especially heart rate and respiratory rate; and whether the infant has urinated and passed meconium. If the mother is Rh-negative, the infant is Rh-positive, and the direct Coombs test is negative, the mother should receive RhoGAM within 72 hours of delivery. Comparison of the mother's blood type with that of the infant's determines whether there is a potential ABO incompatibility. The blood bank will report a positive Coombs test, but jaundice associated with non–Coombs-positive ABO incompatibility is possible (see Chapter 10, Neonatology). Therefore, careful observation for the early development of jaundice is necessary in all infants with an ABO setup. [If the mother is O-positive and the infant is type A or B, there is a possibility that the mother's antibodies may cause rapid breakdown of the infant's red blood cells (RBCs).]

If the mother's serology for syphilis is unknown, the test for syphilis should be requested on the cord blood. In many areas, serologic testing of cord blood for syphilis has become routine, even when the mother has been tested during pregnancy. It is also usual in almost all places to determine hepatitis B immune status as part of prenatal care. **The management of the infant of a mother who is a carrier of hepatitis B surface antigen requires the administration of specific immune globulin and hepatitis B vaccine within the first 12 hours after birth.** The American Academy of Pediatrics (AAP) now recommends that *all* infants be immunized against hepatitis B soon after birth. The vaccine is either given in the hospital nursery or deferred until 2 months of age, when the general series of immunizations begins.

Most mothers now receive testing for HIV infection during pregnancy. **If the HIV status of the mother is unknown, it is essential to take a blood sample from the infant (not from the umbilical cord) as soon as possible after birth to determine the presence or absence of HIV antibody.** According to local law, this HIV test may or may not require consent from the parents. If the mother is HIV-negative, no further action is necessary. If the mother is HIV-positive, it is necessary to draw blood from the infant for HIV DNA polymerase chain reaction (PCR) testing and to begin oral zidovudine within the first 8–12 hours of birth. Consultation with a pediatric HIV specialist is mandatory in all children born to HIV-positive mothers.

Examination of the newborn's chart to evaluate its cardiovascular status is also important. The normal range is 120–160 beats/min for the heart rate and 30–40/min for the respiratory rate. Noting deviations from this range helps focus the physical examination. Most infants urinate at or around birth; all should urinate by 12 hours. Failure to do so mandates a careful evaluation of the newborn for renal, bladder, and genital abnormalities, as well as the state of hydration. Most infants pass meconium within 12 hours after birth. Full-term infants who fail to pass meconium by 24 hours and in whom there is evidence of abdominal distention warrant evaluation for anal patency; Hirschsprung disease (congenital megacolon); intestinal obstruction; metabolic problems, including electrolyte abnormalities and hypothyroidism; neuromuscular diseases; and cystic fibrosis.

INITIAL PHYSICAL EXAMINATION

Most infants are born without visible major anomalies. If visible major abnormalities exist, the pediatrician's task is to determine whether any associated disorders such as cardiac or renal malformations are present, and if so, to deal with them as quickly as possible. If no major anomalies are apparent, the task of the pediatrician is to try to rule out any abnormalities by thorough physical examination (Table 1.2). It is important to note any minor problems, point them out to the parents, and explain their implications. Generally, these minor abnormalities are skin-related and obvious even to the casual observer.

General Appearance

Healthy newborns assume a typical position of flexion of the arms and legs when in the supine position because flexor muscle tone is greater than extensor tone. Infants who are not in the

TABLE 1.2	Initial Examination of Newborns: A Checklist
System	**Important Questions**
General appearance	Does the infant appear comfortable?
	Is it pink?
	Are all four extremities flexed?
Skin	Are there any birthmarks?
Head	Is the head circumference normal?
Face	Does the face look normal?
	Are there any stigmata of a recognizable syndrome?
Eyes	Is the red reflex present bilaterally?
	Are the irises round and of the same color?
Nose	Are the external nares symmetrical?
Ears	Are the pinnae symmetrical and normal in shape?
Mouth	Is the palate intact?
	Are there any teeth or masses?
Chest	Are the respirations symmetrical and effortless?
Heart	Is a murmur audible?
	Is the heart rate normal and regular in rhythm?
Abdomen	Is the abdomen convex in shape?
	Are any masses palpable?
Genitalia	
Male	Is the penile meatus in the proper place?
	Are both testes palpable and the same size?
Female	Are the labia majora and minora present?
	Is the vaginal opening present?
Extremities	Does the infant have ten fingers and ten toes?
	Are the arms the same size?
	Are the legs the same size?
	Do the hips abduct fully?
Back	Is the spine straight?
	Are any dimples present in the midline?
Central nervous system	Is flexor tone greater than extensor tone?
	Are both hands fisted?
	Is the infant's cry strong?

flexed position warrant evaluation for hypotonia, which may be a manifestation of many diseases of varying etiology [e.g., progressive spinal muscle atrophy (formerly known as Werdnig-Hoffmann disease), myotonic dystrophy, trisomy 21 (Down syndrome)] or may be related to birth trauma (see EXAMINATION OF THE NERVOUS SYSTEM).

The head of a newborn may not be round because of the molding that occurs as the infant moves through the birth canal. The cranial sutures are not normally fused at birth. A newborn infant with a round head usually signifies that the mother had a cesarean section without a trial of labor. In addition to **molding of the cranium,** there may be swelling over the occiput, or **caput succedaneum,** which is due to accumulation of fluid in the soft tissues above the periosteum, secondary to pressure associated with delivery. It disappears within 24–48 hours (see EXAMINA-

TION OF THE HEAD). Bruises may be visible on the infant's scalp and face if forceps were applied during delivery. These disappear quickly also but, when seen, should prompt the examiner to check carefully for evidence of facial asymmetry secondary to pressure injury to the facial nerve from the forceps. This condition is most often temporary, resolving completely, usually within the first week of life.

In addition, it is important to note an infant's color. Infants are born with hemoglobin levels in the range of 16–17 g/dl; therefore, they are ruddy in appearance when light skinned. Paleness may be secondary to anemia or to poor perfusion. **If a newborn infant appears plethoric (too ruddy), maternal diabetes should be suspected. If the infant is one of twins, twin-to-twin transfusion should be suspected.** Polycythemia in a newborn may be associated with neurologic symptoms, occasionally necessitating a decrease in hemoglobin by removal of some of the RBC mass.

Examination of the Skin

The skin of infants is thinner than that of older children, so blood vessels can easily be seen. The skin may have a mottled appearance known as **cutis marmorata,** a benign condition that will disappear. This condition may develop in older children when they are cold. Many infants have red markings on the upper eyelids, in the area above the nose, sometimes extending onto the forehead, and on the back of the neck. These are known by a variety of names—**nevus flammeus, vascular nevi, salmon patches, "stork bites"** when on the back of the neck, and **"crow's nests"** when above the eyes. These disappear with time or, on the back of the neck, when they become covered with hair.

Sebaceous gland hyperplasia is characterized by small yellow papules that are often seen over the nose and cheek; these disappear spontaneously. **Milia,** which are white papules, smaller than those seen with sebaceous gland hyperplasia, also disappear without treatment. What appears to be acne is sometimes seen in newborns. This is probably related to endocrine influences from the mother and also disappears without treatment.

Strawberry or capillary hemangiomas are elevated strawberry-colored collections of capillaries that have a variable appearance in newborns. They may be flat and look only like a small red dot, or they may be large-sized, elevated lesions. Single or multiple, they may occur anywhere on the skin. These interesting lesions have a life of their own, growing in size for 3–7 months, stabilizing, and then most often involuting completely, with no remaining scar or blemish. The pediatrician should tell parents that the involution most often begins by 1 year of age and is complete by 5 years of age. However, sometimes the lesions may not disappear until after 8 years of age. Leaving them alone, regardless of location, is the best course of action. An exception to this rule is the presence of a strawberry hemangioma on an eyelid, obscuring vision. In this instance, consultation with an ophthalmologist is required.

Cavernous hemangiomas, which are much less common than strawberry hemangiomas, have a less predictable course. These collections of larger blood vessels are often sizable. They may initially appear as bluish masses under the skin, or they may be above and below the skin, or they may be present completely under the skin, occupying an organ such as the liver. When they are very large, they may be associated with thrombocytopenia or, even more rarely, with arteriovenous fistulas, leading to high-output heart failure. Often, they mature by themselves and disappear; at other times, they require treatment with corticosteroids or radiation.

Port-wine stains, also in the nevus flammeus family, are permanent discolorations of the skin that on occasion are associated with arteriovenous malformations in other organs. In **Sturge-Weber syndrome, a port-wine stain is present in the distribution of the first division of the trigeminal nerve,** with vascular anomalies in the brain. In von Hippel-Lindau syndrome, port-wine stain of the face is associated with vascular lesions of the retina and brain. Congenital glaucoma on the side of the lesion may also be present.

Examination of the Head

The head circumference of newborns should always be measured and compared with standards. It should be within two standard deviations of the mean for gestational age. A measurement that is more than two standard deviations from the mean may be a sign of hydrocephalus. A normal, full-term newborn should have a head circumference of approximately 34–35 cm.

Pediatric Pearl

The correct measurement is the largest one that can be obtained when a tape is passed around the parietal bones, just above the ears. The units should be centimeters rather than inches, because almost all pediatricians trained in the United States in the past 35 years have been taught to think of head circumference in terms of centimeters.

The chest circumference should be measured also and compared with the head circumference. In full-term infants, the chest circumference is 1–2.5 cm smaller than the head circumference. If the measurements deviate from these guidelines, consultation with a pediatric neurologist is advisable.

It is important to palpate the scalp for the presence, size, and feel of the anterior and posterior **fontanelles.** The anterior fontanelle is larger, is located at the juncture of the two frontal and two parietal bones, is flat, and sometimes pulsates. Variable in size, it usually measures no less than 1 cm × 1 cm and no larger than 3 cm × 3 cm at birth. If the anterior fontanelle is either larger or smaller, but the head circumference falls in the normal range, nothing more than routine follow-up measurements is necessary. If the head grows normally, the variation in fontanelle size is considered normal. If abnormalities are apparent, either in the newborn period or later, consultation with a pediatric neurologist is recommended. The posterior fontanelle should be present in all newborns, is found at the juncture of the parietal bones and the occipital bones, and is of fingertip size. It is difficult to appreciate fullness, tenseness, or depression over the posterior fontanelle. It is generally closed by 6 weeks of age.

It is also necessary to palpate the head for evidence of **caput succedaneum,** the boggy swelling in subcutaneous tissues (see GENERAL APPEARANCE). Learning to appreciate what a "caput" feels like is worthwhile to differentiate it from more extensive subaponeurotic swellings, swellings that may be associated with significant bleeding. Learning to appreciate closed-space bleeding of the scalp in newborns is essential, because such bleeding may be associated with anemia and significant hyperbilirubinemia. **Cephalohematomas,** which affect between 1 in 10 and 1 in 20 newborns, are not typically seen at the time of the initial examination but are apparent between 24 and 48 after birth. Cephalohematomas are defined as blood below the periosteum; therefore, they are confined to a single bone. In the skull, the various bones have their own periosteum, making it easy to differentiate a cephalohematoma from a subaponeurotic bleed, which can spread over several bones, occurring as it does between the bones and the aponeurosis that covers them. In newborns, cephalohematomas almost always occur over the parietal bone and are associated with a fracture of this bone about 25% of the time. However, when they are found in a newborn, it is unnecessary to obtain a skull radiograph to document the fracture because it is not associated with a depressed skull fracture. These hematomas often last more than 4 weeks, so it is important to document their presence in the newborn period.

☀ Pediatric Pearl

Finding a new cephalohematoma in an older infant who comes in for a routine well-baby visit should make the examiner suspicious of child abuse.

If cephalohematomas are not reported in the newborn nursery but are found only after the infant has gone home, the parents may be falsely accused of child abuse. To avoid unnecessary concern about possible abuse, it is essential to note cephalohematomas at or before discharge.

Skull examination for the presence of symmetry is important. Asymmetric skulls may be associated with abnormalities of the brain or with premature closure of one or more of the sutures between bones. Suture closure in newborns is appreciated by an inability to ballotte the juncture of the two sides of the suture line. Normally, one can feel both sides move up and down in relation to each other. A ridge may also be palpable at the point where the two bones meet, although this finding is not always present when premature suture synostosis is diagnosed in the newborn. **The most common premature suture synostosis in infants is the sagittal suture, the suture separating the two parietal bones;** when pronounced, it is characterized by a lengthening of the skull in the anteroposterior dimension. However, in newborns, this lengthening may not be apparent. Therefore, part of all routine examinations of the skull should include an attempt to detect suture synostosis. It is best to discover this abnormality early, although premature single-suture synostosis is not usually associated with brain abnormalities or progressive damage to the brain. Early diagnosis allows corrective measures, including surgery, to be performed at a time when the best cosmetic results can be achieved.

Finally, it is necessary to examine the skull for bony defects and for tabes of the skull. **Tabes is a ping-pong ball feel of the skull;** depression of the skull by a finger yields this impression. It is a benign condition and disappears over time. Bony defects are usually in this category; they also disappear over time without sequelae. Skull radiographs should be taken to rule out any rare abnormality.

Examination of the Face

In newborns, almost more than at any other time, it is important to look carefully at the face. Look at the face straight on. Is the nose straight? Are the external nares symmetrical? During the birth process the nasal septum can be dislocated from its position in the vomerine notch. Marked asymmetry of the size of the external flares, which are normally of equal size and shape, is a sign of this abnormality. If recognized early, an experienced otolaryngologist can easily return the nasal septum to its normal position.

Look at the eyes. Are they slanting up or down? Do the eyes appear too big or too small? Does one eye appear larger than the other? Do they seem too far apart or too close together? If one eye appears too large or both eyes appear too large, the infant may have congenital glaucoma. **The large eye is called buphthalmos or "ox eye" and is enlarged by the increased pressure in the eye.** The earlier this condition is recognized and treated, the more likely it is that vision will not be impaired. **Eyes that appear too small may be seen with the fetal alcohol syndrome, as a result of narrowing of the palpebral fissures.** In this condition, the eyes may also appear to be too close together. Eyes that appear too far apart may be associated with midfacial abnormalities such as cleft palate syndromes.

Pediatric Pearl

Upward slanting of the eyes is seen in Down syndrome (trisomy 21); downward slanting is seen in Treacher Collins syndrome.

Look at the chin. Infants tend to have small chins, which grow larger as the child grows. However, if the chin is very small (micrognathia), the child may have **Pierre Robin syndrome,** a condition in which the small chin is associated with a small mouth, predisposing the infant to respiratory obstruction by the relatively large tongue. Look in front of the ears for a **preauricular sinus or skin tag.** These are important only from a cosmetic viewpoint in the newborn, but if the examiner fails to see it, the parents surely will. Failure to see these and explain their presence to the parents puts all the other assurances you have given them in doubt. Although preauricular sinuses may become infected later in childhood, they should not be removed in the newborn period. Skin tags can be removed for cosmetic reasons later in the child's life if the child or the parents wish it.

Look at the infant's face while she is crying. Is the face symmetrical? A condition known as **asymmetrical crying facies syndrome** is associated with aortic valve abnormalities. Because a murmur in a newborn may not be appreciated, even when it is associated with serious cardiac malformation, consultation with a pediatric cardiologist is warranted when asymmetry of the face is present. Facial asymmetry may also be associated with facial nerve palsy secondary to pressure on the facial nerve during the birth process. Even when the baby is not crying, this condition can be appreciated and is usually temporary.

Finally, look at the color of the infant's eyes and hair; look at how much hair there is, and look to see whether the face has any bruises or puffy areas. You should mention all these things in your conversation with the parents, reassuring them that any bruises will disappear within a few days and that sparseness of hair now does not mean that the baby will not have a full head of luxuriant hair later. Showing that you have paid attention to this kind of detail as part of your newborn examination assures the parents that you have paid equal attention to the other parts as well.

Examination of the Eyes, Ears, Nose, Mouth, and Throat

A description of a portion of the eye examination appears earlier (see examination of the face). The eyes of newborns may be opened or closed, and it is sometimes difficult to see the infant's opened eyes; this may be possible by holding the infant with one hand on its bottom and the other supporting the head. Slowly raising the infant from a supine to a more upright position may make the infant open its eyes. Further examination of the sclerae, conjunctivae, corneas, irises, and pupils is necessary. **Subconjunctival hemorrhage, either unilateral or bilateral, may be present;** this is not associated with internal damage to the eye, is secondary to the trauma of the delivery process, and disappears by the end of the first week of life. **Conjunctivitis** is not generally appreciated in the first 24 hours after birth. When seen that early it is generally a manifestation of a chemical irritation when silver nitrate has been used for gonorrhea prophylaxis. **Acquired conjunctivitis,** as seen with gonorrhea, does not develop for several days, because infection occurs during the birth process and takes time to become apparent. Conjunctivitis due to *Chlamydia trachomatis* is not usually seen until after the first week of life.

The sclerae in newborns are often blue as a result of their thinness. The **corneas should be clear** and no more than 12 mm in diameter. **Both irises should be the same color.** When they are not, the condition is called **heterochromia iridis** and is associated with **Waardenburg syndrome or rubella embryopathy,** causing atrophy of the iris. Both irises should be present; **aniridia** may be associated with **Wilms tumor** and genital abnormalities in boys. The pupils should be symmetrical, although **unequal pupils (anisocoria) may be seen in up to 25% of normal individuals.** The more severe abnormalities such as colobomas (defects) of the iris warrant the attention of the ophthalmologist.

Examination of both eyes for the presence of a **pupillary red reflex** is necessary. An ophthalmoscope is used, setting the lens at zero, standing at a distance of 12–18 inches, and shining the light first at one pupil and then at the other. A red reflection should be present bilaterally; if it is not, the possibility that something is blocking the passage of light from the cornea to the retina should be a concern. In infants, this is usually the sign of a **cataract.** The absence of a red reflex should be confirmed, and consultation with an ophthalmologist is appropriate. The list of causes of congenital cataract is long and includes congenital infections, metabolic disorders, and chromosomal abnormalities.

Although testing for extraocular muscular movements is not part of a formal examination in newborns, the movements and positions of the eyes are noteworthy. When the infant is looking straight ahead, the eyes are generally in the same position but may not stay that way with motion. This is not unusual. Persistent internal or external deviation is abnormal, although it is unusual to see this in the newborn period except in premature infants.

Examination of the ears for symmetry of size and for normal folding of the external ear is necessary. Abnormalities of the external ear may be associated with renal defects and hearing defects. **A small ear—microtia—is often associated with abnormalities of the middle ear, usually only on the side of the abnormality.** Otolaryngologic referral is appropriate, because the early assessment of hearing is more important than the management of the cosmetic problem. Inspection of the ears for the presence of external auditory canals is warranted, and it is important to make a gentle attempt to visualize the tympanic membranes. This is not easy initially, because the eardrum is in a more horizontal position in newborns. When the membrane is visible, it tends to appear less translucent than in older children.

Examination of the nose should be for symmetry, as described earlier (see EXAMINATION OF THE FACE). Inspection of the philtrum below the nose is necessary. **A flat, inadequately formed philtrum is associated with fetal alcohol syndrome.** In addition, inspection of the nares for patency, secretions, and masses with a nasal speculum is necessary. **With suspected choanal atresia, the clinician should attempt to pass a number 5 French catheter through the nostril.** If this attempt is unsuccessful, an otolaryngologic consult is warranted.

Examination of the mouth and throat is next. The mouth of the newborn should *not* contain teeth. When natal teeth are present, they are usually removed after consultation with a dentist, because they tend to be attached loosely to the gum. When these teeth are not removed, they are usually shed soon after birth; aspiration is a concern. Interesting but usually benign lesions can often be seen in the mouths of newborns. These include small inclusion cysts on the hard palate, generally in the midline, known as **Epstein pearls.** On the alveolar ridges, eruption cysts and mucoceles can sometimes be found; these are benign and disappear spontaneously. Careful inspection of the palate for evidence of a cleft is necessary. Large clefts are difficult to miss, but small ones may go unnoticed. Inspection of the uvula is also important; a bifid uvula may be associated with a submucous cleft of the palate, a condition that predisposes infants to middle ear infections.

The examination of the mouth should include an inspection of the tongue. The tongue generally looks normal, although there are still individuals who insist on making the diagnosis of **tongue-tie** in newborns. The frenulum that attaches the tip of the tongue to the floor of the mouth almost always appears to be short in newborns, compared with that in older individuals. Because of this, a diagnosis of tongue-tie would sometimes be made in the past and the frenulum clipped, without anesthesia, in the newborn nursery, using a small iris scissors. In almost all instances, this procedure is unnecessary. Although instances of actual tongue-tie do exist, they are rare. Before the diagnosis can be made, evidence that the shortening of the frenulum interferes with the functioning of the tongue (e.g., difficulty in sucking) should be present. In older individuals, the shortened frenulum may interfere with the ability to pronounce certain sounds.

A large tongue, **macroglossia,** can sometimes be seen. This condition may be seen in isolation or it can be associated with **Wiedemann-Beckwith syndrome, Down syndrome,** and **Cornelia de Lange syndrome.** Rarely, the tongue can be cleft and, even more rarely, absent; this latter condition is known as congenital aglossia.

At this point, inspection of the neck for evidence of an enlarged thyroid or for any other masses or abnormalities is appropriate. Midline neck masses may be **thyroglossal duct cysts.**

Lateral masses can be **branchial cleft cysts.** Large, soft masses in the neck may be cystic hygromas.

Examination of the Chest

It is important to examine the chest for symmetry. The pattern of respirations should be noted. Most newborns breathe at an average rate of 40 times per minute, but the pattern may not be regular. Breathing should appear effortless, without evidence of nasal flaring; intercostal, subcostal, or supracostal retractions; and without grunting.

Breath sounds should be equal and present on both sides of the chest, although in newborns one can easily be fooled because sounds are transmitted very well from one area of the chest to the other. Therefore, if an abnormality in the pattern of breathing is found, a chest radiograph should be obtained, even in the face of normal breath sounds. It is unusual to hear rales, rhonchi, and wheezes, even in the face of severe respiratory distress.

The average heart rate in newborns is 140 beats/min. At that rate, it is difficult to appreciate the presence of a murmur unless one listens closely and for a period of time. Newborns with cardiac abnormalities, even the most severe such as a hypoplastic left heart may not present with murmurs, or the murmur may be only of a grade 1–2/6 quality. In addition, a murmur audible in a newborn may not be of any clinical significance. Whatever is heard should be described carefully and correlated with other physical and historical findings such as the heart rate, quality of the heart sounds, and quality of pulses in the extremities, especially the femoral pulses.

Coarctation of the aorta or, more broadly, aortic hypoplasia is associated with diminished or absent femoral pulses. However, palpation of femoral pulses in the newborn is not easy. It takes practice before one can be confident that the failure to feel the femoral pulse is because it really is not there. If there is any question of the possibility of coarctation of the aorta, measurement of upper- and lower-extremity blood pressures is warranted. The blood pressure in the legs is lower than that in the arms in most patients with coarctation of the aorta.

A persistent finding of tachycardia or bradycardia should be brought to the attention of a pediatric cardiologist. Loud murmurs, evidence of central cyanosis, heart sounds more easily heard on the right side than on the left side, or difficult-to-hear heart sounds are all reasons to ask for a cardiac consultation, especially if these findings

are appreciated in an infant who is less vigorous than expected.

Examination of the Abdomen

The normal appearance of the abdomen in newborns is full, protruding, and round. It should not be flat or sunken (scaphoid), nor should it appear tense.

Pediatric Pearl

A sunken or scaphoid abdomen is always a cause for concern. Where are the intestines? Is the flat abdomen due to a diaphragmatic hernia? Is it due to poor muscle tone from a neurologic insult or flaccid musculature? In any case, it is a cause for alarm.

A tense abdomen may signify an obstruction in the gastrointestinal tract or a perforation of a viscus, with resultant leakage of gas and the development of peritonitis and ileus. Intestinal malrotation resulting from a defect in development can predispose to volvulus. Intestinal atresias occur with greater frequency in infants with chromosomal abnormalities; these should be suspected in infants with abdomen-related problems who appear to have Down syndrome. **The anus may be imperforate, or there may be a defect in intestinal innervation, as seen in Hirschsprung disease.** Thick meconium may cause a special type of intestinal obstruction, **meconium ileus, which has a strong association with cystic fibrosis.** It is unusual to see a tense abdomen immediately after birth, for it takes some time for the above conditions either to develop or to become manifest.

In addition, the newborn's abdomen has something not found in older individuals—an attached, although cut, clamped or tied umbilical cord. The cut surface of the umbilical cord should be inspected; **two umbilical arteries and one umbilical vein should be present.** The presence of only one umbilical artery is sometimes associated with other anomalies such as renal malformations.

The abdomen should be palpated for the presence of masses. It is best to begin palpating in the right upper quadrant, feeling for the liver. The liver is often palpable up to several centimeters below the right costal margin. This is most often normal and is related to the mobility of the liver rather than to an increase in size. Enlarged livers have a different feel to them, appearing closer to the surface and "fuller" on palpation. Congenital infection resulting from **to**xoplasmo-sis, **r**ubella, **c**ytomegalovirus, **h**erpes simplex, or **s**yphilis (the so-called TORCHS group of diseases) may cause hypertrophy of the liver. Other causes may involve masses within the liver such as cysts, vascular malformations, or tumors.

In the left upper quadrant and laterally, the spleen may also be palpable in newborns, for the same reasons as the liver; it may be normal or enlarged as a result of the presence of a congenital infection. By moving deeper and more distal, it may be possible to feel the kidneys. Although kidneys of normal size may be palpable in some infants, it is difficult for the beginning examiner to appreciate this. However, enlarged kidneys are the most common cause of palpable abdominal masses in the newborn, most often resulting from obstructive lesions of the urinary tract. The presence of an enlarged abdominal mass requires further investigation, which is best accomplished in consultation with a pediatric radiologist and a pediatric surgeon or urologist.

Examination of the Genitalia

The genitalia of female newborns look a bit different from the genitalia of older sexually immature females because of the influence of maternal hormones. At times, **there may even be a bloody vaginal discharge within a few days after birth, resulting from withdrawal bleeding.** The labia majora and labia minora appear full and puffy. The vaginal opening can be seen, as can the hymen, which partially obscures the orifice. The clitoris should be contained within the preputial covering; if it is not, clitoral enlargement should be suspected. This may occur in **congenital adrenal hyperplasia** or, less commonly, in disorders of sexual differentiation. If abnormalities are encountered, consultation with a pediatric endocrinologist is warranted.

Examination of the male genitalia involves checking for the presence of both testes in the scrotum, the shape and size of the penis, the presence of a normal-appearing foreskin, and the position of the urethral meatal opening. The testes may feel enlarged in newborns; this is due to the frequent presence of **small hydroceles** in newborn males. When an enlarged, hard testis is felt, congenital torsion or tumor may be the cause. Consult with a pediatric urologist is necessary.

The penis should be straight. If it appears to be bent downwards (ventrally), a **chordee of the penis** may be present. Chordee of the penis is associated with **hypospadias,** a condition in which the urethral meatal opening is displaced proximally on the ventral aspect of the penis. When a hypospadias is present, the foreskin is incompletely formed, appearing as a "hood" around the glans of the penis. **Epispadias,** a condition much less common than hypospadias, is diagnosed when the urethral opening is displaced to the dorsal aspect of the penis. Rarely, the penis may be very thin and small, a condition known as micropenis. Micropenis can be associated with either a local or a general (e.g., pituitary insufficiency) endocrine disorder. With chordee of the penis, hypospadias, epispadias, and micropenis, consultation with both a pediatric endocrinologist and a pediatric urologist is warranted.

Examination of the Extremities

Careful inspection of the fingers and toes with regard to number, size, and shape is necessary. Parents focus on these areas, and if the examiner fails to find an abnormality that is present, no matter how minor, credibility with the parents is lost. Extra partial digits, connected to a finger, usually the fifth by a pedicle of skin, are not uncommon. Webbing of the toes is often seen and may be familial. Webbing of the fingers is much less common. **Clinodactyly is an inturning of a finger, usually the fifth, may be unassociated with anything else, but can be seen in Down syndrome.** Thumb abnormalities are seen in a number of dysmorphic syndromes.

Abnormalities of the hands are not common, and minor abnormalities of the feet are frequently seen. The most common of these is **forefoot adduction (metatarsus adductus), most likely secondary to intrauterine positioning** during fetal life. If the forefoot adduction is supple, meaning that the foot can be straightened easily, no treatment or consultation is necessary, and the foot will straighten over the succeeding months. If the forefoot adduction is rigid on physical examination, referral to an orthopedist is necessary. **Clubfoot is a combination of forefoot adduction, varus deformity, and shortening of the Achilles tendon.** Treatment of this condition should begin in the newborn nursery. The feet may appear to be convex at the sole, a condition known as rocker-bottom feet; this is usually associated with serious dysmorphic syndromes such as trisomy 18.

Congenital abnormalities of the arms are uncommon, whereas congenital abnormalities of the legs, although usually minor, occur more often. The most common abnormality is **internal**

tibial torsion, often seen in conjunction with forefoot adduction. This condition most likely occurs secondary to intrauterine positioning and is likely to improve without treatment over a period of months, but can take up to 2 years to disappear. **External or internal versions of the hips also occur but are unlikely to be diagnosed in the newborn period. Developmental dysplasia of the hips** (formerly known as congenital dislocation or dysplasia) **occurs more commonly in female infants, particularly in those who have been in a frank breech position during pregnancy.** The condition has a 9:1 female-to-male predominance and is more likely to be seen in firstborn infants.

Pediatric Pearl

Developmental dysplasia of the hips is important to diagnose as early as possible, because early treatment improves the prognosis.

To examine for this condition, the infant is placed in a supine position with the hips and knees flexed, and the middle finger of each hand is placed over the greater trochanter. The thumbs are placed on the inner aspect of the thighs, opposite the lesser trochanter. The hips are flexed and adducted, and a posterior force applied. If the hip is unstable it will dislocate; a clunk or a click may be felt or heard. In case of doubt, the maneuver can be done one side at a time by stabilizing one side of the pelvis and attempting the above maneuver on the other side (Barlow sign). One should also test the range of motion of the hips; 180-degree rotation should be possible. The infant should also be placed in the prone position, and the buttocks should be examined for symmetry. Asymmetry of the buttocks may be due to a dislocated hip. If there is any possibility of the presence of hip dislocation, an immediate orthopedic consult is necessary. Diagnosis of developmental dysplasia of the hip at birth is not always possible; therefore continued assessment during the first few months of life is mandatory. Hemihypertrophy or hemiatrophy of one or more extremities occasionally occurs. **Hemihypertrophy has been associated with Wilms tumor of the kidney.** Other rare skeletal dysplasias such as phocomelia and osteogenesis imperfecta can occur.

Acquired abnormalities of the arms are more common than congenital ones. The most common is a **fractured clavicle,** a condition that occurs in up to 3% of newborns. The diagnosis can be made by feeling for crepitus over the clavicle or by noting an incomplete Moro reflex on the side of the fracture. It is a benign condition, and even if the diagnosis is missed, the clavicle always heals, although it heals with callous formation. If the diagnosis is not made in the newborn nursery, a parent may find the "bump" when the child is several weeks old. When the "bump" is shown to the primary care provider, the question of possible child abuse may arise if the fracture was not documented in the nursery. Therefore, both initial and discharge physical examinations should involve careful searching for the presence of a fracture of the clavicle. **Brachial plexus palsies,** known also by the eponyms Erb and Klumpke palsies, are acquired abnormalities secondary to difficult deliveries. The diagnosis is not difficult to make, because the affected arm is usually flaccid and extended and moves much less well than the unaffected arm. Treatment is supportive, with the arm placed in such a position as to prevent further stress on the brachial plexus. The prognosis depends on how quickly function begins to return. Infants with a good prognosis will regain some muscle tone and begin to move the arm within the first few days after birth. When the diagnosis is made, consultation with a pediatric neurologist is necessary. Some pediatric orthopedists or neurosurgeons are skilled in making operative repairs of brachial plexus injuries.

The rest of the skeletal system, including the spine, is examined at the time the extremities are examined. **Congenital scoliosis** of the spine is rare; when it is seen, it is usually associated with abnormalities of the vertebrae (e.g., hemivertebrae). Neural tube abnormalities such as **meningocele or myelomeningocele** are now often diagnosed prenatally by ultrasound examination or by maternal screening for α-fetoprotein, although supplementation of the diet of pregnant women with folic acid seems to have decreased the incidence of neural tube defects. When present, consultation with a pediatric neurosurgeon is necessary. **Pilonidal sinus,** the most common abnormality of the spine, is found at the very base of the spine. This sinus does not communicate with the spinal canal and does not become infected before adolescence. Therefore, although the parents should be informed of its presence and apprised of its significance, no treatment is necessary. Other abnormalities of the spine such as sinuses, cysts, fatty tumors, or tufts of hair over the thoracic or lumbar areas, are rare. When they are present, consultation with either a pediatric neurologist or neurosurgeon is appropriate.

Examination of the Nervous System

When an infant has had a normal birth and when nothing abnormal has been noted in the delivery room, it is unlikely that any major abnormality of the central nervous system (CNS) will be found on physical examination. In fact, most pediatricians and other providers familiar with newborn examinations can tell at a glance the neurologic status of the newborn. What allows the experienced observer to do that is just that—observation.

Normal newborns, when supine and at rest, hold both upper and lower extremities flexed at the elbows, hips, and knees, because flexor tone is greater than extensor tone (see GENERAL APPEARANCE). If newborns' arms or legs are in extension when the infants are not being stimulated, either extensor tone is increased or all tone is decreased. Infants with decreased tone are "floppy." Investigation of the cause of increased extensor tone or decreased generalized tone is essential, and a quick preliminary judgment is necessary. The cause may be (1) an insult to the CNS such as intracranial bleeding or infection, (2) a congenital disorder of the nervous system or muscles, or (3) sepsis.

It is important to make sure that motor responses are symmetrical. One of the easiest ways to do this is to elicit a **Moro reflex.** This can be done in a variety of ways; the most common is to put one hand below a supine infant's head, raising the head and back, and then to allow the head and back to drop while continuing to support the head and neck with the hand. Infants do not like this and respond by extending their arms and then bringing them back into flexion and into the midline. The legs generally are extended also and then flexed. All these responses should be symmetrical.

The hands of the newborn are kept fisted. The placement of two index fingers in the palms of the hands elicits a grasp reflex. The grasp reflex is so strong and the flexor tone so great that an infant can be lifted off the ground in this manner. When infants are grasped underneath both axillae and lifted up, the shoulder tone is strong enough to support their weight. If the shoulders and arms rise up with this maneuver, decreased muscle tone is present. When placed in a standing position, infants can be induced to "walk" or climb steps, the so-called **stepping reflex.** When the cheeks are stroked on the side of the mouth, the infant will "root," (i.e., demonstrate the **rooting reflex**), a major asset to the infant when placed on the breast of the mother.

The infant can normally handle its secretions; there should be no drooling when the infant is not taking from the breast or bottle. Evidence of an inability to swallow secretions could be due to neurologic problems or to esophageal atresia.

Testing for pain sensation, sight, or hearing is not generally part of the newborn neurologic examination. However, fairly sensitive methods for screening for hearing in the newborn are now available, and this has become part of the routine in some nurseries. Some states have mandated universal hearing testing at birth. The eyes may be open or closed, and it is important to check for the red reflex (see EXAMINATION OF THE EYES, EARS, NOSE, AND THROAT). If infants are willing to keep their eyes open, they may be able to fix on an object or a light by the time of discharge.

MANAGEMENT IN THE HOSPITAL

In most cases, infants now spend no more than 24–48 hours in the hospital when born by vaginal delivery and no more than 72–96 hours in the hospital when born by cesarean section. As recently as 20–25 years ago, a 4-day hospital stay after vaginal delivery and a week-long hospital stay after cesarean section were routine. As a result, the management of issues after the birth of a child has become compressed. It is essential that several issues are discussed with the parents before the mother and infant leave the hospital. The short stay does not allow much time; therefore, organization is important.

Review of the Birth History and the Initial Physical Examination

After finishing the review of the birth record and performing the initial physical examination, discuss the results with the parents. These days, fathers are often present for most of the mother's stay in the hospital, especially if this is the first-born child. If this is the pediatrician's first encounter with the parents, introductions are necessary. The pediatrician should be careful not to appear rushed—this is an important interview, and the parents will "hang on every word" that the physician says. An example of what the pediatrician should say follows:

> The baby is well formed and beautiful (or handsome). All the fingers and toes are present. The arms and legs are normal. The heartbeat is strong and regular. I did not see the color of the baby's eyes. (Or, the baby's eyes are blue, but they may not remain that color.) His hair is black. (If you know the

baby's first name refer to the baby by name.) The bruises on the face will disappear within the next few days. The head will become rounder in the next few days. The marks you see above the eyes and on the back of the neck are very common and will disappear slowly in the course of the next year. The Apgar scores were good. (If necessary, explain what is meant by the Apgar score.) The examination of the reflexes and nervous system is normal . . .

Ask if the parents have any questions about what they have noticed about their infant or about what transpired during delivery or in the labor room. Ask how they plan to feed the baby (see Chapter 4, Principles of Pediatric Nutrition, Fluids, and Electrolytes). Many, if not most, women breastfeed their infants in the hospital, often beginning immediately after delivery. The pediatrician must encourage and be supportive of the mother's decision to breastfeed, must be able to supply information about techniques of nursing, and must make sure that the mother is provided with assistance if necessary. Support by the nursing staff or the hospital's lactation consultant is essential If the mother is breast-feeding for the first time.

Inform the parents about what they can expect to happen in the hospital. Explain that you will make sure to find out the infant's Rh factor if the mother is Rh-negative. Tell where their infant will receive hepatitis B immunization and explain why. When hepatitis B immunization was first introduced, recommendations called for the administration of the first dose in the newborn nursery. Many newborn services and many pediatricians now prefer to give the first hepatitis B immunization in the pediatrician's office in a formulation combined with *Haemophilus influenzae* B immunization. In addition, explain to the parents that if they stay long enough, blood will be drawn for neonatal screening for genetic disorders. If not, arrange for them to come to your office for this procedure. If any problems have come to light, explain how they will be handled.

Be sure to tell the parents how you can he reached if they need to ask you any questions, and tell them when you will return to see them. Sometimes the initial hospital visit is the only visit. Arrangements should be made for them to call you the next day to discuss any problems—there are always problems—and to make arrangements to bring the child in for an office visit. When the infant is discharged from the hospital after only 24 hours, a visit to your office in the next 24–48 hours is appropriate, if only to examine the infant for the presence of jaundice. If the infant stays 48 hours or more and there is no evidence of jaundice, the office visit can be scheduled when the infant is 2–3 weeks old.

Review of the Hospital Stay and the Discharge Examination

Before the mother and infant are discharged from the hospital, it is necessary to review the hospital stay, to discuss the discharge physical examination, and to make plans for seeing the family afterwards. The review of the hospital stay and the discharge physical examination focus on different aspects of care than the initial assessment did. It is a good idea to ask the following questions:

- Is jaundice present?
- How much weight has the baby lost?
- Is the baby taking to the breast or bottle?
- How easy or difficult is the baby to feed?
- Does the baby retain its feeds?
- Is the infant urinating and moving its bowels?
- What is the baby's temperament like? For example, does the baby calm easily, seem regular, and like to be held?
- Are there any new findings on the physical examination, such as the presence of a cardiac murmur, or a rash, or a hip click?

Jaundice is common in newborns. Is the jaundice sufficient to warrant obtaining a bilirubin determination? Any infant with jaundice appearing within the first 24 hours of life requires evaluation. Discharge from the hospital should wait until the evaluation is complete and the bilirubin rise has stopped.

☀ Pediatric Pearl

The appearance of jaundice in the first 24 hours of life can never be diagnosed initially as being physiologic jaundice of the newborn, a condition in which jaundice generally does not appear before the third day of life.

A determination of how far down the body the jaundice extends is an approximate gauge of the level of jaundice. If the jaundice appears after 24 hours of age and is mainly on the face and upper chest, the total bilirubin is probably below 8 mg/dl. If the jaundice extends to the abdomen and upper thighs, the total bilirubin is generally in the range of 12–13 mg/dl. If the infant is over 48 hours old and appears to have only minimal jaundice, it is not necessary to obtain a serum bilirubin determination. Infants with moderate jaundice, corresponding to bilirubin levels in the range of 12–13 mg/dl, require observation to make sure the level stabilizes. In most cases, infants with bilirubin levels at or above 15 mg/dl receive phototherapy.

If the jaundice appears within the first 48 hours of life and if the infant is going home, arrangements for next-day follow-up must be made. Some full-term infants develop jaundice sufficient to require a therapeutic intervention, most commonly phototherapy. The complete differential diagnosis of jaundice and the indications for this treatment are discussed elsewhere in this book (see Chapter 10). **The usual causes are jaundice related to excessive hemolysis, most often resulting from an ABO incompatibility, exaggerated physiologic jaundice, or breast milk jaundice.** Whatever the cause, the presence of jaundice produces great apprehension in the parents. Even if they do not know from previous experience why jaundice is a concern, the fact that tests to discover its etiology and severity are being performed engender great anxiety, much advice from concerned relatives and friends, and many questions as to what harm the jaundice can cause the infant. The clinician should address all of these concerns with a great deal of patience and concern, although the jaundice may be of little actual significance.

It is necessary to ask the mother whether she has any issues concerning breastfeeding; if there are, arrangements must be made to assist her with these concerns after the hospital stay. In many hospitals, a member of the staff is assigned as a breastfeeding coordinator. That individual is responsible for holding breastfeeding classes, making sure that educational literature about breastfeeding is available, and making sure that a member of the nursing staff is available to help the mother in the techniques of breastfeeding her baby.

- How comfortable is the mother with the process?
- Does the baby get on the breast easily?
- Does the baby suck well?
- Has the mother's milk "come in" yet?

In many parts of the United States, "lactation consultants" are available for this purpose, especially for mothers who are breastfeeding for the first time. Some women have significant quantities of milk by the end of the second day, but it often takes about 3–4 days before milk flow becomes established. Prior to that time the mother has a supply of colostrum. The mother should be aware of this.

Regardless of the method of feeding, either breast or bottle, parents want to know how much the baby weighs. There is an obligatory weight loss in almost all infants, because total body water at birth approaches 80% of body weight, dropping to 65%–70% of body weight in the first few days of life. On average, for full-term newborns, this means that the weight loss is about 3–5 oz the first day and another 3–5 oz the second day. The weight then levels off for a few days, after which the baby starts to gain about an ounce per day. It takes about 7–10 days for bottle-fed infants and about 10–14 days for breast-fed infants to regain their birth weight. It is necessary to explain all this to the parents.

Introducing the concept of **infant temperament** to the parents is worthwhile. They grasp this idea easily, for they "see" that their own infant does seem to have his own personality. Some babies appear very calm. When hungry, they cry but not with great intensity. When comforted, they are easy to console. After feeding, they fall asleep quickly, awakening only for their next feeding. Other babies cry with a great deal of intensity, not just when hungry but also with minor disturbances. They are difficult to console and, after feeding, these "difficult" babies may fuss for a while before going to sleep, awakening after a short period of time and crying once again.

Most infants fall in between these two extremes. Recommend to the parents that they purchase a "baby book" that discusses this and other aspects of their child's care. The author recommends *Caring for Your Baby and Young Child: Birth to Age 5* (edited by Steven P. Shelov and published by the AAP). It is important for parents to recognize the aspects of their child's temperament as being innate characteristics. An appreciation of this allows them to respond appropriately to the infant.

Any new findings on physical examination must be discussed with the parents. The examination should include remeasuring the head circumference and comparing it with the original measurement, repeating the entire physical examination, and noting any changes from the initial examination.

In addition, ask the parents to tell you of any new concerns they may have or old ones they feel have not been adequately addressed. If the mother is breastfeeding and requires pain medications or, for that matter, almost any medication other than antimetabolites or radioactive materials, she should be told that the usual doses will not affect her infant. Mention of any tests or procedures that have been performed during the hospital stay is appropriate, including the infant's blood type, the possible administration of hepatitis B vaccine, and the obtaining of blood by heel stick for screening for a variety of genetic disorders.

All states require testing for some genetic disorders, most likely phenylketonuria, galactosemia, and congenital hypothyroidism. For all three conditions, a specific, effective treatment exists, but the diagnosis must be made early in order for the specific treatment to prevent damage to the baby. In order for screening tests for phenylketonuria and galactosemia to be reliable, milk feeds for at least 48 hours are necessary. Because many infants leave the hospital at or before 48 hours and because many infants are breast-fed and the mother's milk supply is usually not established until the third or fourth day after birth, performance of these screening tests may not be accurately completed before the infant leaves the hospital. The parents may need to arrange to have them later in the first week of life.

SUMMARY

In summary, the evaluation of newborn infants at birth requires a knowledge of not only many fields, but also, and perhaps most importantly, a sensitivity for and an understanding of the concerns parents have about the well-being of their own newborn. It is a new start in life, and the parents want it to be a good one for the infant and for themselves. Unlike other situations, in which minor events carry little weight, anything that happens to a newborn infant has great significance. The skillful practitioner recognizes this and incorporates it into all encounters. When this happens, even if difficult situations are encountered, parents will be forever grateful. It is likely that the trust formed between the parents and the pediatrician during this period will make dealing with issues that arise later in childhood easier.

SUGGESTED READINGS

Brazelton TB: Working with families: Opportunities for early intervention. *Pediatr Clin North Am* 42(1):1–10, 1995.

Charlton VE, Phibbs RH: Examination of the newborn. In *Rudolph's Pediatrics*, 20th ed. Edited by Rudolph AM. Stamford, CT, Appleton & Lange, 1996, pp 208–217.

Coleman WL: The first interview with a family. *Pediatr Clin North Am* 42(1):19–30, 1995.

Driscoll IM: Physical examination and care of the newborn. In *Neonatal-Perinatal Medicine: Diseases of the Fetus and Infant*. Edited by Fanaroff AA, Martin RJ. St. Louis, Mosby-Year Book, 1992, pp 325–345.

Kattwinkel J: Perinatal outreach education. In *Neonatal-Perinatal Medicine: Diseases of the Fetus and Infant*. Edited by Fanaroff AA, Martin RJ. St. Louis, Mosby-Year Book, 1992, p 13.

Klaus MH, Kennell JH: Care of the mother, father, and infant. In *Neonatal-Perinatal Medicine: Diseases of the Fetus and Infant*. Edited by Fanaroff AA, Martin RJ. St. Louis, Mosby-Year Book, 1992:465–477.

Shelov SP, Hannemann RE (eds): *Caring for Your Baby and Young Child: Birth to Age 5*. New York, Bantam Books, 1998, pp 3–132.

Thompson GH, Scoles PV: Developmental (congenital) dysplasia of the hip. In *Nelson's Textbook of Pediatrics*, 15th ed. Edited by Behrman RE, Kliegman RM, Arvin AM. Philadelphia, WB Saunders, 1996, pp 1937–1940.

Chapter 2

Health Maintenance Visit

Steven P. Shelov

For the pediatrician, the skills, attitudes, and energy necessary for preventing disease and maintaining health come first. This focus on health maintenance is the centerpiece of a practice unique to the pediatrician, who has strong feelings about this approach, similar to a surgeon's belief in the ability to heal through procedural intervention. For the pediatrician, both physical and emotional factors play roles in preserving health. Recommendations about immunizations, nutrition, and developmental growth help the family cope with psychological setbacks; dysfunction; and problematic emotional periods, in which children make demands on parents. The completeness of the pediatrician's practice is testimony to the deeply held belief that the central, organizing influence for the child is the family; that is, a family that is healthy in all aspects helps ensure a healthy present and future for the child.

This chapter attempts to describe the pediatrician's approach to health maintenance so that the reader can understand the importance of monitoring the growth of the child. The initial regular health maintenance visit, which usually occurs at 2–4 weeks of life, focuses on aspects of physical and behavioral development. It is impossible to summarize all of well-child care in one chapter. Rather, it is intended that the reader apply the principles and outlined guidelines to all subsequent visits, using developmentally appropriate material from the figures, tables, appendix, and the available references identified in the text. The first visit at 2–4 weeks of age sets the stage for the elements for each subsequent visit. Throughout this first, detailed illustrative example of such a visit, summarized questions, topics of potential concern, developmental milestones and physical examination at subsequent ages through age 12, immunizations at different ages, tests and procedures for different ages, and topics in anticipatory guidance are presented.

GENERAL ASPECTS OF A HEALTH MAINTENANCE VISIT

Health maintenance visits are essential anchors for the parents to learn about their infant or child and to achieve an increasingly more satisfied level of competence with each contact. The overall purpose of these visits is for the pediatrician, through education and response to questions, to further empower each and every parent to be as knowledgeable, observant, nurturing, loving, and rewarded as possible. Although this goal may not be attainable at every visit, it should be the object of every encounter.

What better place to begin a discussion of the health maintenance visit than with the newborn infant? The new baby has just returned home. In addition to a number of different emotions and anxieties, family members have questions, which may include:

- Do I know enough to care for this new baby?
- Do I have enough love to go around between my other children and my new baby?
- How will I know if there is something wrong?
- Will I know when I need to call someone for help, and who should I call if I have any questions? It is important to make sure that parents have emergency numbers, especially those of the pediatrician for evenings and weekends.
- How do I know what my baby wants when he cries?

Generally, crying reflects discomfort. The three major causes of this discomfort are hunger, wetness or dampness from soiled diapers, and the need for sleep. However, during the first several months, infants may just cry as they develop the ability to self-regulate varying body states. This irritability, or **colic,** usually subsides by the age of 3 months (see CRYING AND COLIC).

The anxieties of new parents, especially parents of first children, often obscure the intrinsic sense of their own competence and innate abilities. Anxiety often leads to uncertainty and, with that uncertainty, often a sense of being overwhelmed. One of the most important roles of the pediatrician, especially in the first few months of life of the new infant, is to relieve the parents' anxiety, reassure and teach by being available and responsive to the parents' needs and questions, and repeatedly support their own parental capabilities and instincts. The more the pediatrician can strengthen the parents' sense of competence, the more happy and secure parents will be with their parenting role and the more confident they will be with their new baby.

In the early days of parenting, **health maintenance visits** and frequent telephone contacts in between office visits provide support and confidence-building interactions with new parents. The actual process of these important visits is one that the experienced pediatrician repeats so many times that they become second nature to every encounter with children and their families. The first health maintenance visit often serves as the paradigm for teaching in similar visits. Although the details of each visit, specifically the content of information sought and shared with the parents, is targeted to the developmental age and stage of the child, the process remains systematic, comprehensive, and predictable.

Health Assessment at 2–4 Weeks

Setting

As with any person-to-person encounter, making sure the mother and father feel comfortable in their initial visit is essential. This may mean ensuring that there is enough room for everyone, including anticipated baby paraphernalia (e.g., diapers, wipes, water, changing table) and that there are a minimum number of interruptions. There is nothing worse than for a first conversation about a newborn infant to be repeatedly interrupted by a number of telephone calls or door-knocking intrusions. It is essential to ask nursing and clerical staff to hold all but necessary calls.

Different practitioners have different styles, but note taking during the interview is often the expected norm. It indicates to parents the importance of what they are saying and that the pediatrician is really listening to their issues and including them as part of their child's record. The physician should also make clear to parents that if they have a list of prepared questions, they should feel free to consult them at any time during this visit. It is important to reassure the parents that **no questions are silly or unnecessary.**

Interview

Patience is crucial at the very beginning. Getting adjusted, comfortable, and ready to listen while carrying a small, often squirmy bundle sometimes takes time. At every visit during the first 6 months of life, it is necessary to ask some important questions at the beginning of the interview, such as:

- How are you doing with the baby? Are there any things at home that I should know about?
- Do you have any questions or concerns about the past several weeks?
- Are you enjoying your baby at least some of the time?
- Do you feel like you have settled into a routine, and if so, are you comfortable with it? Are you getting some rest at least part of every day?
- Have any things changed since we last saw each other, either with the baby or in your home setting?
- How have you been handling the crying episodes? Is there a pattern to the crying, and what kinds of things seem to make your baby stop crying?
- What is the baby's sleeping pattern like? Does the cycle seem to be reversed?
- (For breastfeeding mothers): Has your milk come in, are you comfortable with breastfeeding, and do you have any excessive soreness, cracking, or discharge at the nipple?
- (For all mothers): Do you think your baby is satisfied after the feeding? How often does she feed?
- Do you have any specific questions about the baby's condition [e.g., bowel movements, skin color (jaundice), eye discharge, umbilical stump granuloma, excessive amounts of crying or fussiness, change in appearance or behavior]?

It is also important to learn about how life at home is proceeding in general. The pediatrician may ask:

- How are things going with the father of the baby? Are other people helping you with some of the house chores? Numerous studies now reinforce the importance of paternal involvement in all aspects of infant and child care. The earlier the involvement, the greater the child's and parents' satisfaction and the greater the positive influence on the child's development. The father's participation in care also allows for some rest time for the mother, which is much needed in the first several months of life, especially if she is breastfeeding.

- How are siblings (if there are siblings at home) handling the presence of the new baby? Are you spending time with your other children, who are probably feeling a little deprived of time with you? Classically, older siblings, especially those who are 2–4 years older than the new infant, regress somewhat when the new baby comes home. It is important for parents to take some separate time with older siblings to show that they have not forgotten their other children and that they are still as important as ever. (It should be noted that some breakdown in toilet training may even occur for a short period of time.)
- Are routine tasks around the house generally being taken care of (e.g., shopping, bill paying, odds and ends)?
- Are the grandparents, if present, too involved and intrusive, or are they helping just to the proper degree?

The overall purpose of these initial questions is to establish a broad foundation for open and honest communication. There are no "unimportant questions." Initial questions are explorative, looking for any sources of additional stress that might be interfering with the initial, important bonding period with the new baby. In the first month, infants are not as easy to relate to as they are later. Their ability to make eye contact, be consoled, and relate to other individuals is usually quite variable, even from day to day. Infants usually do not have a responsive smile at this time (if it were there, it would help), so parents need even the smallest of signs of reassurance that they are doing a good job. Positive comments about how well the infant looks and how well the parents are doing are reassuring statements that pediatricians should repeat to parents during their first visit to the office.

Important issues in the First Month of Life

At the conclusion of the interview part of the visit, it is important to ask again if the parents have any other questions. The questions may be about issues that the pediatrician may have introduced or anything else that may come to mind. Often, during the interview, topics may arise that remind the parents of problems they had not thought of earlier. This is an opportunity to discuss these issues further.

SLEEP. Infants at this age are naturally predisposed to sleep 12–14 hours a day but usually not more than 3–4 hours at a stretch. That means the baby *will **not** sleep through the night during this time,* and this leads to the exhaustion about which parents often complain. Therefore, it is crucial that the mother develops some arrangements that allow her to get some rest during each day. This is especially true if she is breastfeeding.

> ### Pediatric Pearl
> During the first months of life, it is recommended that infants be placed on their backs or sides when going to sleep (see SLEEP PATTERNS).

FEEDING. The feeding schedule during these first several weeks is often erratic. During the first month of life, infants, especially those who are breastfed, may feed as often as every 2 hours or, sometimes every 3–4 hours. Each day may also be different from the one before, which adds to the confusion of the first month. It is important that parents are aware that infants often lose weight until they are 3–4 days old, then regain weight to equal their birth weight by 10 days of age (possibly 2 weeks for breastfed infants), and then start to gain weight predictably and quickly. There may be some days when they are especially hungry and others when they are less so. (See Chapter 4 for more specific information on infant feeding.)

CRYING AND COLIC. Crying is particularly stressful for new parents. During the first month of life, infants often cry for up to 3–5 hours per day. In many cases, this fretting appears to occur for no reason; the parents have checked for soiled diapers, open diaper pins with cloth diapers, the need for additional feeding, or the rare but painful event of a hair getting caught around one of the infant's toes or fingers. Some of the techniques that may console a fussy infant include rocking, swaddling, nestling closely on the shoulder, or the judicious use of a pacifier. Occasionally, fussiness is due to a sensitivity to a specific formula or a food the mother has eaten that is passing into her breast milk. Over the course of the first few months these episodes generally diminish in frequency and intensity, but **occasionally, infants remain extremely fussy. These infants are sometimes referred to as colicky babies.**

The cause of these colicky episodes is not clear, and they appear to be particularly severe during the late afternoon or evening, often lasting 3–4 hours at a stretch. Recently, data derived from a number of carefully controlled studies have reinforced the understanding that colicky infants are simply more difficult to console. Because they appear to lack some ability to self-regulate their own state, they need additional soothing measures such as holding, rocking, and motion to help them self-regulate. Although no measures for handling this problem are guaranteed to be successful, these techniques may help bring both parents and infants through these mutually disruptive episodes. It is reassuring to know that these intense, fussy periods usually subside by the time the infant is 3 months of age.

Interview Questions at Subsequent Visits

It should be noted that the questions listed in this section are only a sample of those that may be appropriate. They relate to developmental milestones of which the parents should be aware. A more complete discussion of age-appropriate developmental milestones appears later in the chapter (see DEVELOPMENTAL AND BEHAVIORAL ASSESSMENT) and in *Guidelines for Health Supervision* (see SUGGESTED READINGS).

Infancy: 1–6 Months

The clinician should ask the usual questions regarding home life with the infant since the last visit and whether there have been any changes that need to be discussed. In addition, some age-specific questions are appropriate, including:

- Is your baby on a more regular sleeping schedule and sleeping through the night? By age 3–4 months, most infants sleep through the night, much to everyone's relief.
- Are you putting your baby to sleep on his back? New American Academy of Pediatrics (AAP) guidelines recommend placing the infant on the back or side during the first months of life unless there are contraindications.
- Is the feeding going all right? Have you been able to stop the middle-of-the-night feeding?
- Is your baby more responsive?
- Is your baby smiling?
- Is your baby making a variety of different sounds?
- Is your baby responding to sounds by quieting or looking at you?
- Are you carefully "baby-proofing" your home as your baby becomes increasingly active and mobile?
- Are you considering going back to work? If

so, what child care arrangements have you worked out?
- Have you noticed your baby has developed more of a personality?

Infancy: 6–12 Months

- How are you handling your baby's increasing mobility? Have you adequately "baby-proofed" your home?

Pediatric Pearl

"Baby-proofing" is mandatory as the infant reaches 6–12 months of age. The kitchen, bathroom, changing table, and play areas are prime targets. For example, it helps to clean undersink cabinets and put the changing table in a corner.

- Is your baby sleeping through the night, or as the baby approaches his first birthday, has he begun to wake up? Sleeping through the night usually takes place around 3 months, but often at 9–10 months of age, infants start to wake up again for a period of time.
- Are you introducing more variety of strained and then junior foods?
- Are you thinking about weaning your baby from the breast or bottle, and have you at least introduced him to the concept of the cup? Weaning usually takes place near the first birthday, although some parents like to continue breastfeeding well into the second year of life and sometimes occasionally beyond.
- Have you noticed your infant becoming more afraid of strangers and also more reluctant to leave you? Stranger anxiety is frequent during the last half of the first year. This normal developmental milestone reflects the increasing ability of the infant to distinguish the mother or other primary caregiver from a nonprimary caregiver. This normal phase may lead to some separation anxiety into the second year as well.
- How are you adjusting to your baby's increasing independence?

Early Childhood: 1–2 Years

- Have you introduced your child to playmates, and how does she interact with them?
- Has your baby taken her first steps? Have walking and running created problems for you or the rest of the family?
- How are things going with the child's brothers and sisters?
- How are the new child care arrangements going (if the parent has returned to work)?

- What personality differences have you noticed?
- How are you handling the "terrible twos," the normal but difficult stage of development (if the child has entered this period)? Parents struggle with the bossiness and increasing independence of these often stormy months. Nevertheless, they are important stages of independence that a toddler must experience.
- Has disciplining your active toddler been a problem?
- What kinds of toys and games does your child now enjoy?
- Does your child enjoy books? It is never too early to read to children. Reading reinforces language, assists in object identification, and promotes attachment.
- How much television does your child watch, and what kinds of shows do you allow her to see? The earlier parents begin to limit television viewing to 1–2 hours per day at a maximum and indicate preferences concerning content, the earlier children start to develop their own appropriate television-watching habits.
- Is your child eating meals with you, and is her diet fairly well balanced ?
- Does your child still take a nap during the day? A morning and afternoon nap during these years is quite normal and expected, although not all children take such naps.
- Does your child sleep in her own room, and has your child "graduated" to a "real bed" from a crib? Sometimes, parents use the second birthday as the time to try a true bed. A junior bed may offer a more secure sleeping environment for the more fearful toddler.

Early Childhood: 2–3 Years

- How are the discipline issues going? These issues are often the most pressing for parents. Several respected parent manuals or developmental texts contain numerous approaches to limit-setting.
- Have you started toilet training, and how is it going? The median age for toilet training is 33 months, with bowel control coming before bladder control.
- Does your child still wet the bed at night, although he is dry during the day? Often nighttime wetting is still a normal finding until 4–5 years of age. (See Chapter 5, BED-WETTING (ENURESIS) IN SCHOOL-AGE CHILDREN.)

Pediatric Pearl

It is important to advise parents to minimize the fuss over bed-wetting. Bed-wetting beyond 6 years of age (primary nocturnal enuresis) often requires a separate approach, which is individualized to the family and *never* involves punishment. A variety of conditioning and positive reinforcement techniques are appropriate.

- Is your child starting to play more nicely with his playmates?
- Is your child starting to show lots of different emotions such as pleasure, anger, joy, protest, warmth, and assertiveness? Children begin to show different types of temperament, which are often displayed through different emotions. Children who are very quiet or very assertive often have different "personalities," and different ways of dealing with stress, anger, happiness, and sadness. Parents recognize this easily and know that they have to respond differently to their children, depending on the specific temperament.
- Is your child recognizing and naming lots of different objects?
- Does your child recognize letters and numbers?
- Is your child showing all of the developmentally active behaviors seen at this age? Running, going up and down stairs, and throwing a ball are three common examples. The Denver II is designed to assist the clinician in identifying children whose rate of development differs significantly from peers of the same age (Figure 2.1).
- Is he talking and using sentences of one, two, or three words?
- Is he beginning to learn how to take turns and to share?
- Are you finding time to just play and have fun with your active child?

Additional questions for the remainder of the preschool period and the school-age years can be found in the useful publication from the AAP, entitled *Guidelines for Health Supervision.** In addition, *Bright Futures in Practice,** published by the AAP, contains many of the recommended developmental questions. Finally, the well-respected book for parents, *Caring for Your Baby and Young Child, Birth to Age Five,** published by

---

*To obtain copies, write the AAP at the following address: 141 N.W. Point Blvd., Elk Grove Village, IL, 60007.

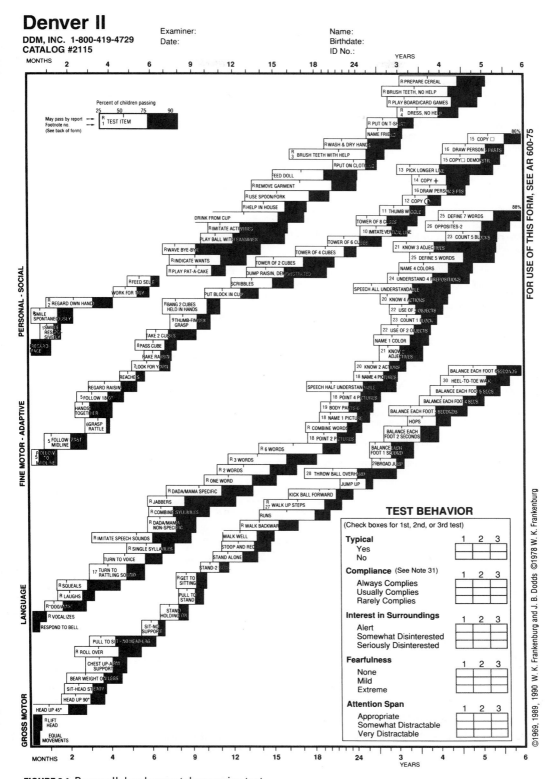

FIGURE 2.1. Denver II developmental screening test.

DIRECTIONS FOR ADMINISTRATION

1. Try to get child to smile by smiling, talking or waving. Do not touch him/her.
2. Child must stare at hand several seconds.
3. Parent may help guide toothbrush and put toothpaste on brush.
4. Child does not have to be able to tie shoes or button/zip in the back.
5. Move yarn slowly in an arc from one side to the other, about 8" above child's face.
6. Pass if child grasps rattle when it is touched to the backs or tips of fingers.
7. Pass if child tries to see where yarn went. Yarn should be dropped quickly from sight from tester's hand without arm movement.
8. Child must transfer cube from hand to hand without help of body, mouth, or table.
9. Pass if child picks up raisin with any part of thumb and finger.
10. Line can vary only 30 degrees or less from tester's line. |/
11. Make a fist with thumb pointing upward and wiggle only the thumb. Pass if child imitates and does not move any fingers other than the thumb.

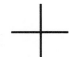

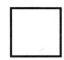

12. Pass any enclosed form. Fail continuous round motions.
13. Which line is longer? (Not bigger.) Turn paper upside down and repeat. (pass 3 of 3 or 5 of 6)
14. Pass any lines crossing near midpoint.
15. Have child copy first. If failed, demonstrate.

When giving items 12, 14, and 15, do not name the forms. Do not demonstrate 12 and 14.

16. When scoring, each pair (2 arms, 2 legs, etc.) counts as one part.
17. Place one cube in cup and shake gently near child's ear, but out of sight. Repeat for other ear.
18. Point to picture and have child name it. (No credit is given for sounds only.)
    If less than 4 pictures are named correctly, have child point to picture as each is named by tester.

 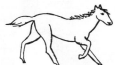

19. Using doll, tell child: Show me the nose, eyes, ears, mouth, hands, feet, tummy, hair. Pass 6 of 8.
20. Using pictures, ask child: Which one flies?... says meow?... talks?... barks?... gallops? Pass 2 of 5, 4 of 5.
21. Ask child: What do you do when you are cold?... tired?... hungry? Pass 2 of 3, 3 of 3.
22. Ask child: What do you do with a cup? What is a chair used for? What is a pencil used for? Action words must be included in answers.
23. Pass if child correctly places <u>and</u> says how many blocks are on paper. (1, 5).
24. Tell child: Put block **on** table; **under** table; **in front of** me, **behind** me. Pass 4 of 4. (Do not help child by pointing, moving head or eyes.)
25. Ask child: What is a ball?... lake?... desk?... house?... banana?... curtain?... fence?... ceiling? Pass if defined in terms of use, shape, what it is made of, or general category (such as banana is fruit, not just yellow). Pass 5 of 8, 7 of 8.
26. Ask child: If a horse is big, a mouse is __? If fire is hot, ice is __? If the sun shines during the day, the moon shines during the __? Pass 2 of 3.
27. Child may use wall or rail only, not person. May not crawl.
28. Child must throw ball overhand 3 feet to within arm's reach of tester.
29. Child must perform standing broad jump over width of test sheet (8 1/2 inches).
30. Tell child to walk forward, ⚭⚭⚭➤ heel within 1 inch of toe. Tester may demonstrate. Child must walk 4 consecutive steps.
31. In the second year, half of normal children are noncompliant.

OBSERVATIONS:

FIGURE 2.1. *(CONTINUED)*

the AAP, is another good source for up-to-date developmental questions and advice (see SUG-GESTED READINGS).

PHYSICAL EXAMINATION AND DEVELOPMENTAL ASSESSMENT

The **health maintenance visit** should focus on careful assessment of the developmental and neurologic status of the infant (less crucial after the preschool period) and a head-to-toe physical examination. The pediatrician often smoothly integrates the physical and developmental components into an overall physical assessment.

Developmental and Behavioral Assessment: First Month of Life

The first question parents have when they see the pediatrician examining their newborn baby is, "Is my baby developing normally?" During the first month of life, neonatal neurologic development is still quite dominated by the presence of normal reflex responses. **The developmental assessment is the cornerstone of health maintenance visits in all children.**

Chapter 1 gives a complete picture of the developmental capabilities of the newborn, including neonatal reflexes. By the end of the first month, the **Moro reflex, stepping reflex,** and **tonic neck reflex** are still present, but it is normal to start to see these become slightly diminished. Each of the neonatal reflexes totally disappears at different ages (Table 2.1) and, for the most part, is rarely in evidence beyond the fourth month of life. Nevertheless, the 1-month-old infant is still quite a tightly wound package. The extremities are in flexed position, a significant degree of head lag is still present when she is pulled up from a supine position, and when lying on her abdomen, she can barely raise her head off the mattress.

In addition, Chapter 1 also discusses the behavior and temperament of the newborn infant. Clearly, no significant new facets of behavior become obvious during the first month of life. Changes, however subtle, often register with parents, who cannot easily verbalize them. It is important and useful for the pediatrician to raise them, because parents are very observant and want to talk about their observations of their baby. Therefore, the first cues to follow are those of the parents. When asked "What is your baby like?" parents have some clear idea, even at this very early age. Some might say that their baby is so quiet, sometimes they wonder if everything is all right. Others might comment that their baby seems "just right." By this they mean the baby cries sometimes, spits up occasionally, seems to sleep several hours at a time and then wakes up,

seems to feed without much fuss, and generally seems to have a good disposition. Still other parents say that their infant seems fretful, fidgety, and bad-tempered, with fits of unexplained crying, erratic feeding patterns, and irregular sleeping patterns. It seems that the baby is tense, restless, and even hyperactive. The parents are also having difficulty relating positively to the infant, because it never seems that they can do anything to make the baby happy.

All these scenarios are not only real but normal. Each reflects a different disposition or "personality" that researchers in child development have often characterized as an infant's **temperament.** No particular one is better than another, although the irritable, fretful infant is certainly more difficult from a day-to-day perspective for all caregivers. What makes the fretful infant even more difficult during this first month is that babies are difficult to "read" at such a young age. They usually are not yet very responsive, and it is often difficult to know whether what the parent is trying to do is really making any difference. The "normal" behavior patterns of new infants become the foundation for the parents' interactions over these first several months, and reassurance, explanation of their normality, and significant support for the more stressed and overwhelmed parents of the more "difficult" baby are the pediatrician's important work at the first health maintenance visit. Discussing temperament, what it means, and how important it is for parents to start building connections to the infant, often despite not feeling responded to, should be a part of every health maintenance visit.

At different stages, different behavioral and personality issues arise. However, each developmental event usually forms on the foundation of the child's underlying temperament. It is important that there be enough time allowed to at least begin the discussion about these issues during this first visit. Once the parents understand that their infant is normal and that their parenting style during the initial month has had little to do with the way their baby is, they can learn to play the crucial role in taking the steps needed to make their baby secure and engaged in his surroundings. At each subsequent visit, especially in the first several years of life, these issues of behavioral development become paramount parental concerns. The child's behavior includes adaptation to the many aspects of growing up in the home and soon in an environment outside the home (child care and formal schooling). These phases of socialization and behavior will be important topics for discussion between pediatri-

TABLE 2.1	Newborn Reflexes*	
Reflex	Age When Reflex Appears	Age When Reflex Disappears
Moro reflex	Birth	2 months
Walking/stepping	Birth	2 months
Rooting	Birth	4 months
Tonic neck reflex	Birth	4–5 months
Palmar grasp	Birth	5–6 months
Plantar grasp	Birth	9–12 months

*These reflexes are some an infant performs during his first weeks. Not all infants acquire and lose these reflexes at exactly the same time, but this table gives a general idea of what to expect.

cian, parent, and eventually the child. Often it is well worth setting aside a specific part of each health maintenance visit to address these issues. Over time, in the experience of pediatricians, parents struggle most with these issues and most need the guidance and advice of the pediatrician.

Developmental and Behavioral Screening in Subsequent Visits

Young Childhood: Infancy and Preschool Years

The developmental stages of infants and children are often the initial focus of every health maintenance visit. Over the past three decades, a useful and efficient developmental screening device known as the Denver II has become standardized (see Figure 2.1). It is used to monitor children's development from the first month of life through school entry at approximately 5 years of age (developmental surveillance). Although there have been several iterations of this tool and the development of a short developmental questionnaire, it is well worth the time spent in learning to be comfortable with this excellent screening procedure. The purpose of developmental surveillance is evaluation of the developmental progress of the infant or child reliably when it is measured in four dimensions: **gross motor, fine motor–adaptive, language,** and **personal–social.** The Denver Developmental chart allows the pediatrician to recall the specific stages of development and to place the child developmentally in some percentile, compared with other children of the same age. Contained within these developmental assessment measures are the specifics for each stage (see Figure 2.1), which serve as reminders for the pediatrician in guiding the evaluation. The physician may share the results of the developmental assessment with the parents at each visit and discuss them in anticipation of the upcoming weeks or months before the next visit.

Middle Childhood: School-Age Years

Although the developmental milestones reached during the school-age years are less significant than those in infancy and the preschool years from a motor or language standpoint, they become increasingly significant with regard to social, cognitive, and emotional factors. It is crucial to discuss these issues at annual health maintenance visits during the school-age years. The emotional and psychologic well-being of the school-age child is often hard to discern during these years. Often, a parent is unable to engage a busy, active, peer-involved 8-year-old child. Nevertheless, there is usually much going on

during this time, and it is important that parents and the pediatrician become aware of any trouble signs that may be building under the surface. Recently, a child psychiatrist and pediatrician at Massachusetts General Hospital developed a measure for screening for psychosocial or emotional problems in the school-age child. This instrument, called the Pediatric Symptom Checklist, is a 30-item self-administered questionnaire that takes about 5 minutes of a parent's time to complete (Figure 2.2). This well-validated questionnaire, which is also currently used for children in the preschool years, is intended to identify children who may be experiencing some interpersonal or emotional difficulties.

Although the Pediatric Symptom Checklist is not designed to allow for a definitive diagnosis of the specific problem or difficulty, **it at least allows for the identification of an "at risk" child and some objective reason for a referral.** Pediatricians who have used it consistently find it has resulted in an increase in the accuracy of their referrals and an enhanced ability to be more aware of potential problem issues with a child or family.

Physical Examination

The complete physical examination focuses on the recording of accurate height, weight, and head circumference as well as the physical findings from head-to-toe, including the infant's **vital signs—temperature, heart rate, respiration rate,** and **blood pressure.** The clinician should plot the infant's measurements graphically [Figures 2.3 and 2.4 (girls), 2.5 and 2.6 (boys), and 2.7]. During the first visit especially, new parents are intensely interested in how their baby is growing, and it is important to show them graphically as well as tell them the specific number. Often, parents have a "baby book" with them in which they write down their baby's "vital statistics." This gives the pediatrician an opportunity to review the concept of growth rate and percentiles in easy-to-understand terms.

Specific Areas of Examination

HEAD. Careful examination of the head should start with a careful measurement of the occiput–frontal circumference with a tape measure. **It is important to measure the circumference at the same place each time to ensure consistency from visit to visit.** At birth, the normal occiput–frontal circumference is 35 cm, and it increases each month, quite rapidly in the first few months, and then more slowly but predictably in the subsequent months of the first year of life.

Pediatric Symptom Checklist

Please mark under the heading that best fits your child:

	(Points 0) Never	(Points 1) Sometimes	(Points 2) Often
1. Complains of aches or pains	_____	_____	_____
2. Spends more time alone	_____	_____	_____
3. Tires easily, little energy	_____	_____	_____
4. Fidgety, unable to sit still	_____	_____	_____
5. Has trouble with a teacher	_____	_____	_____
6. Less interested in school	_____	_____	_____
7. Acts as if driven by a motor	_____	_____	_____
8. Daydreams too much	_____	_____	_____
9. Distracted easily	_____	_____	_____
10. Is afraid of new situations	_____	_____	_____
11. Feels sad, unhappy	_____	_____	_____
12. Is irritable, angry	_____	_____	_____
13. Feels hopeless	_____	_____	_____
14. Has trouble concentrating	_____	_____	_____
15. Less interest in friends	_____	_____	_____
16. Fights with other children	_____	_____	_____
17. Absent from school	_____	_____	_____
18. School grades dropping	_____	_____	_____
19. Is down on himself or herself	_____	_____	_____
20. Visits doctor with doctor finding nothing wrong	_____	_____	_____
21. Has trouble with sleeping	_____	_____	_____
22. Worries a lot	_____	_____	_____
23. Wants to be with you more than before	_____	_____	_____
24. Feels he or she is bad	_____	_____	_____
25. Takes unnecessary risks	_____	_____	_____
26. Gets hurt frequently	_____	_____	_____
27. Seems to be having less fun	_____	_____	_____
28. Acts younger than children his or her age	_____	_____	_____
29. Does not listen to rules	_____	_____	_____
30. Does not show feelings	_____	_____	_____
31. Does not understand other people's feelings	_____	_____	_____
32. Teases others	_____	_____	_____
33. Blames others for his or her troubles	_____	_____	_____
34. Takes things that do not belong to him or her	_____	_____	_____
35. Refuses to share	_____	_____	_____

FIGURE 2.2. Pediatric symptom checklist. For the school-age child, a total of 28 points is suspicious; for the preschool child, a total of 24 points is suspicious.

Pediatric Pearl

A handy method to remember about the occiput–frontal circumference is:

- Increases 2 cm/month for the first 3 months
- Increases 1 cm/month for the next 3 months
- Increases ½ cm/month for the next 6 months

Therefore, the resulting head circumference at 1 year is about 47 cm, which is approximately the 50th percentile for all infants when plotted on the head circumference growth chart.

It is also important to feel the anterior and posterior fontanelles carefully; both should still be open at birth. The anterior should still be about 1–2 × 1–2 cm, but the posterior should, at best, be only a fingertip opening. The posterior fontanelle closes by 4 months of age, and the anterior fontanelle closes between 12 and 18 months of age.

In addition, it is necessary to examine the scalp for any evidence of cephalohematoma or other abnormality. The suture lines should still be quite open and should not have any evidence of fusion or ridging at this age. The skull should be symmetrical. There may not be much hair at this age; some of the newborn hair will have normally disappeared, and reassurance that new, more permanent hair will soon emerge is necessary.

Birth to 36 months: Girls
Length-for-age and Weight-for-age percentiles

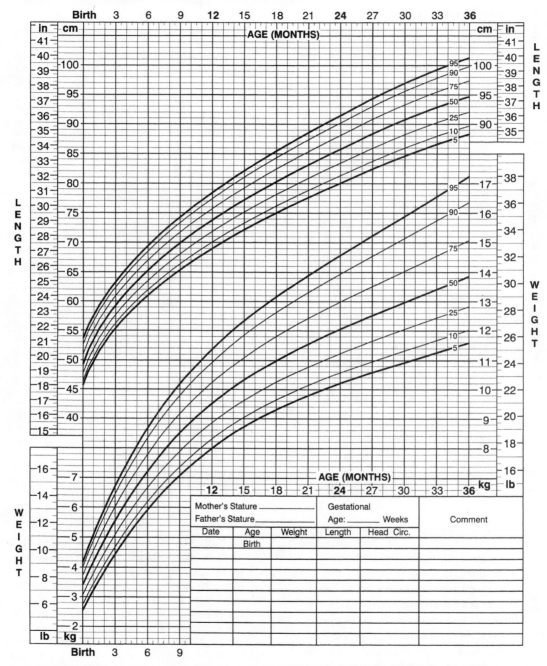

FIGURE 2.3. Length-for-age and weight-for-age percentiles for girls (birth–36 months), Centers for Disease Control and Prevention. Developed by the National Center for Health Statistics in collaboration with the National Center for Chronic Disease Prevention and Health Promotion. http://www.cdc.gov/growthcharts

2 to 20 years: Girls
Stature-for-age and Weight-for-age percentiles

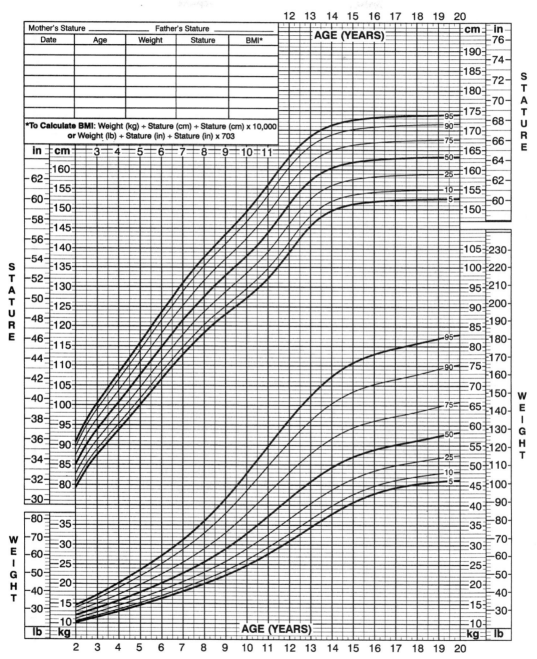

FIGURE 2.4. Stature-for-age and weight-for-age percentiles for girls (2–20 years), Centers for Disease Control and Prevention. Developed by the National Center for Health Statistics in collaboration with the National Center for Chronic Disease Prevention and Health Promotion. http://www.cdc.gov/growthcharts

Birth to 36 months: Boys
Length-for-age and Weight-for-age percentiles

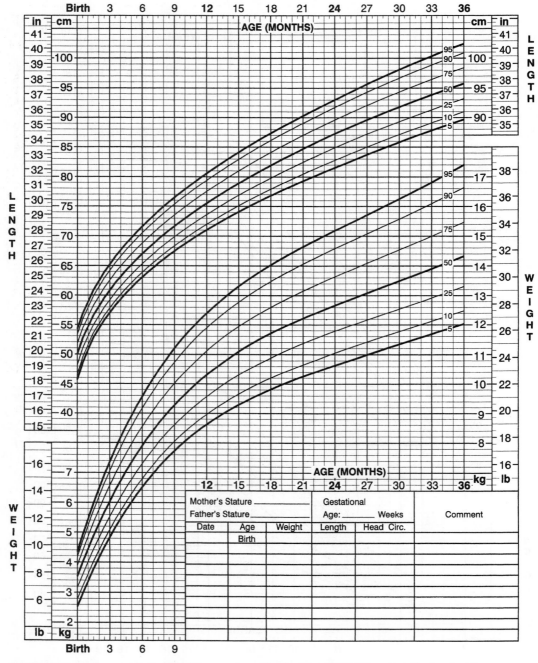

FIGURE 2.5. Length-for-age and weight-for-age percentiles for boys (birth–36 months), Centers for Disease Control and Prevention. Developed by the National Center for Health Statistics in collaboration with the National Center for Chronic Disease Prevention and Health Promotion.

2 to 20 years: Boys
Stature-for-age and Weight-for-age percentiles

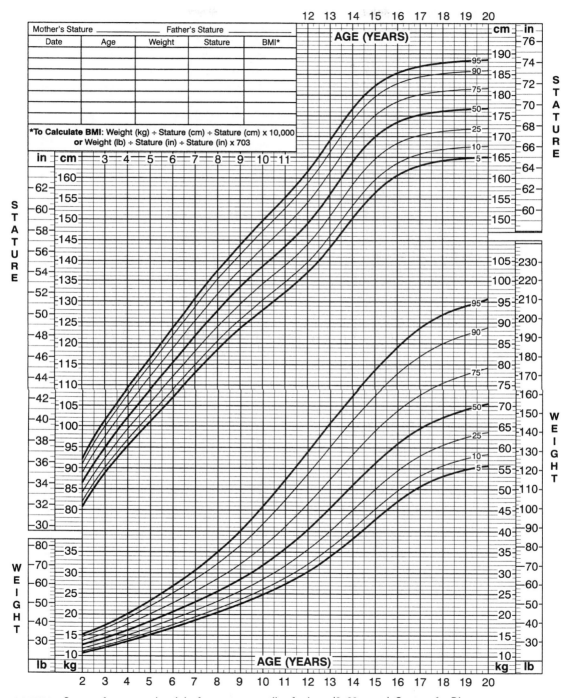

FIGURE 2.6. Stature-for-age and weight-for-age percentiles for boys (2–20 years), Centers for Disease Control and Prevention. Developed by the National Center for Health Statistics in collaboration with the National Center for Chronic Disease Prevention and Health Promotion. http://www.cdc.gov/growthcharts

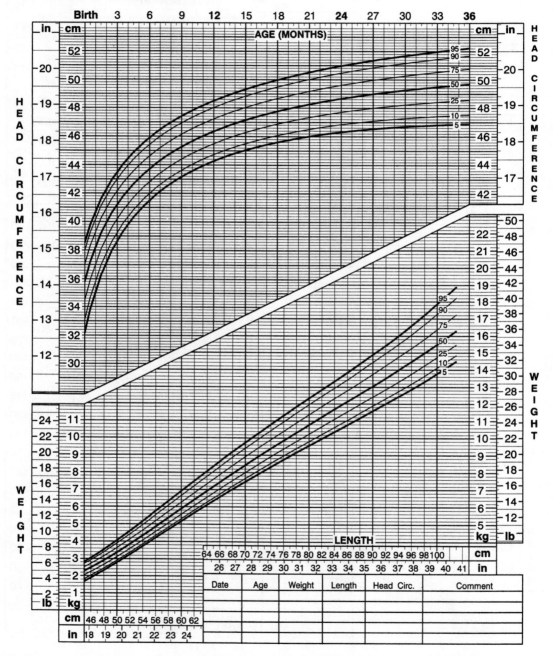

FIGURE 2.7. Head circumference charts for boys and girls (birth–36 months), Centers for Disease Control and Prevention. Developed by the National Center for Health Statistics in collaboration with the National Center for Chronic Disease Prevention and Health Promotion.

Birth to 36 months: Girls
Head circumference-for-age and
Weight-for-length percentiles

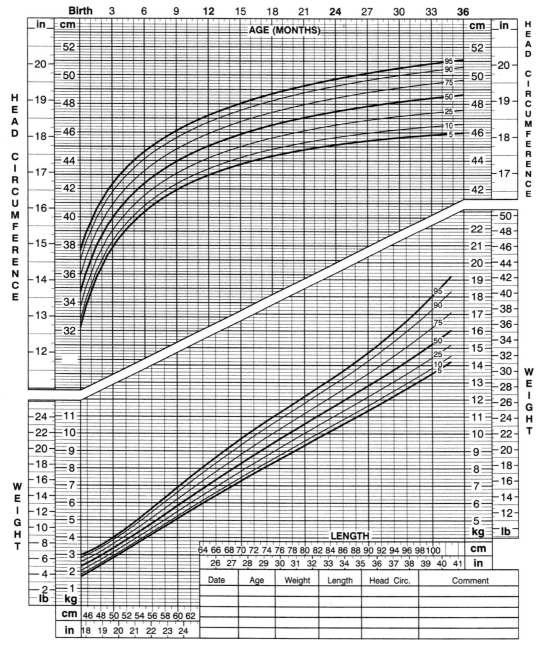

FIGURE 2.7. *(CONTINUED)*

EYES. Examination of the eyes should check for any discharge, either reflective of a **conjunctivitis**, a neonatally acquired *Chlamydia* **infection**, or evidence of a blocked tear duct or **dacryostenosis**. The pediatrician should elicit a **red reflex** to ensure that there are no cataracts. The eyes will normally have a slightly dysconjugate gaze, and the physician may need to reassure that this is normal in the first month or so.

EARS. Examination should look for any evidence of **otitis media**. An otoscope with an air insufflating bulb attached should always be used. After careful examination of the normal landmarks of the tympanic membrane, looking at the ear for normal landmarks (Figure 2.8), the examiner should introduce a slight puff of air into the ear canal with the attached bulb, making sure there

is a good seal between the speculum and the external auditory meatus. This procedure should cause the tympanic membrane to move slightly (like a crinkling sail) and then snap back, provided there is no fluid behind the membrane. If no tympanic membrane movement is apparent, the possibility of otitis media warrants consideration.

MOUTH. It is necessary to examine the throat to check that there are no palatal abnormalities and that the gums are normal. No teeth should be present. Natal teeth should have been removed.

HEART AND LUNGS. The pediatrician should listen carefully to the heart and lungs, both anteriorly and posteriorly. It is important to determine the respiratory rate and heart rate and to listen to the

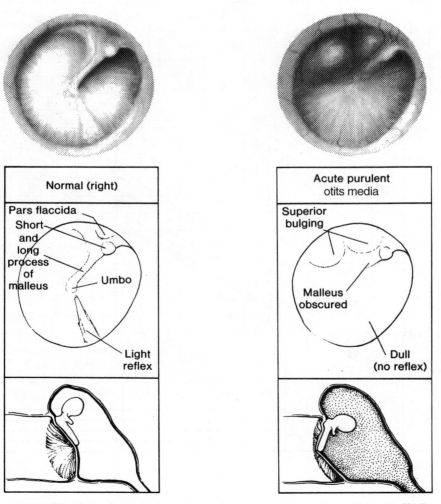

FIGURE 2.8. Drawings of normal tympanic membrane and acute purulent otitis media (OM).

heart carefully for any evidence of murmurs. The normal respiratory rate is 36–40/min, and the heart rate is 120–140 beats/min. With the lungs, there should be evenness of breath sounds through the chest.

Examining the heart from the anterior position, thorough listening over aortic, pulmonary, and sternal borders, midclavicular line, and at the point of maximum impulse is necessary. Occasionally, a murmur that was not appreciated in the newborn nursery may be audible. This often is a small **ventricular septal defect (VSD).** Careful auscultation over the back should also be routine; occasionally a residual **patent ductus arteriosus (PDA)** can be heard there.

ABDOMEN. A thorough abdominal examination should allow for palpation of any abnormal masses. The abdomen is usually quite soft when an infant is not crying, so palpation of the liver and right upper quadrant, the spleen and left upper quadrant, and both kidneys and fairly deep palpation looking for any masses or other abnormalities should be routine. If the infant is crying and uncooperative, try working with the parent to calm the baby, allowing the opportunity for a complete and thorough examination.

Examination of the umbilicus should show a well-healed stump. If there is discharge and the mother states that she often sees blood at the top of diaper, then this may indicate that an **umbilical granuloma** has developed at the site of the umbilical stump. This is easily cauterized in the office.

GENITOURINARY SYSTEM. Careful examination of the genitourinary area is necessary. In boys who have been circumcised, the prepuce should be completely healed with smooth, pink epithelium. In girls, it is necessary to spread the labia to ensure that there are no adhesions. The pediatrician should encourage parents to be sure to use warm water and cotton balls to carefully clean all of the creases and folds in which loose stool can easily become trapped.

EXTREMITIES. Examination of all extremities is necessary, with special note taken of the examination of the hips. It is essential to perform Ortolani and Barlow maneuvers to be sure there is no **congenital hip dysplasia** (formerly known as **congenital dislocation of the hip**) [Figure 2.9]. During a careful and complete examination of the hips, equal abduction should be evident.

SKIN. A careful survey of the skin is necessary. The pediatrician should look for any evidence of

rash or **hemangioma.** Often, a **hemangioma is** *not* **seen at the newborn examination, because it may take a month or so for the abnormal vessels to become tortuous enough to show through the epidermis.** If a hemangioma is discovered, it is most important that the parents know that this will become larger over time and **that the best response is to "do nothing," assuming it is the usual kind of capillary hemangioma.** After enlarging during the first year or two, most capillary hemangiomas gradually involute and become smaller in the next several years.

NEUROLOGIC EXAMINATION. At the first-month visit, there are relatively few specific neurologic findings that do not relate to the developmental and reflex examination (see DEVELOPMENTAL AND BEHAVIORAL ASSESSMENT). Over the subsequent months and years, the neurologic and developmental examination remain intertwined, and certainly abnormalities or deviations from the norm in the developmental assessment would suggest some underlying neurologic concern.

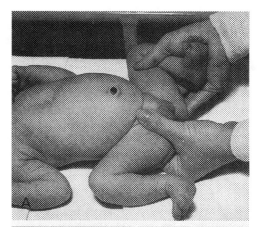

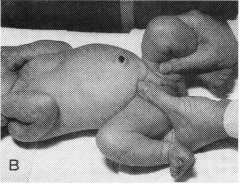

FIGURE 2.9. (*A*) Ortolani and (*B*) Barlow maneuvers.

However, cranial nerve, motor, sensory, and reflex examinations should be routine at every health maintenance visit.

Physical Examination in Future Visits

The actual physical examination changes little over the course of future health maintenance visits. However, the pediatrician should keep some points in mind as the child grows older, such as:

- Develop the ability to perform the physical examination in the mother's arms as much as possible.
- Never start your physical examination too abruptly.

Pediatric Pearl

At appropriate ages, engage children with lots of talk, conversation, puppet play, or whatever creative ideas you may have. Do not be afraid to "ham it up" a little; babies love it, and actually parents do, too.

- Start with the least intrusive part of the examination first. Examine the abdomen first, then listen to the chest (use a warm stethoscope), perform the developmental assessment needed, and examine the head, eyes, skin, genitalia, and extremities carefully.
- Complete the examination with a careful look at the ears, performing tympanoscopy each time, and finally look in the mouth as efficiently as possible. When examining the ears, try having the mother hold the baby on one of her shoulders firmly while holding the head still and then looking at the "outside" ear. When this is complete, ask her to switch shoulders, and you can examine the other ear.
- While conducting the physical examination, ask the parents if they have any questions. Certainly, if you see any abnormalities, point them out with an explanation immediately.

IMMUNIZATIONS

Immunization against several diseases is routine in the United States. Their routes of administration vary. The newborn infant should have received the first immunization in the first days of life while still in the hospital. This first vaccine is the first dose of the **hepatitis B** vaccine, which is important to prevent acquisition of the hepatitis virus. This extremely safe vaccine, a genetically engineered product, is administered in three doses (Figure 2.10). The other recommended immunizations, which are also presented in Figure 2.10, include vaccines against **diphtheria (D), pertussis (whooping cough) [now in a acellular version, aP], and tetanus (T), which are combined as DTaP; polio (inactivated) [IPV];** *Haemophilus influenzae* **(Hib or** *Haemophilus* **conjugate vaccine); measles, mumps, and rubella (usually given as MMR); and varicella (Table 2.2).** Optimally, children should receive each immunization at a particular age (see Figure 2.10; Table 2.3). Certain reportable side effects of standard immunizations may occur (Table 2.4). The AAP recommends that each practitioner consult the specific vaccine insert for specific **contraindications** to a particular vaccine. Whenever a vaccine is administered, it is important to explain carefully to the parent all of the rationale for the vaccine and the potential side effects. The AAP and the Centers for Disease Control and Prevention also require that a written consent be obtained for each vaccine administered.

Detailed information about all the childhood vaccines is lengthy and is beyond the scope of this overview of the health maintenance visit. The pediatrician should consult the complete report known as **"The Red Book,"** a resource published every 3 years by the AAP Committee on Infectious Diseases. This superb publication, which is also available as a CD-ROM to allow greater accessibility, gives details of all specific and current recommendations concerning immunizations and is truly the definitive reference with respect to these issues. Table 2.2 and Figure 2.10 come from the most current edition of that book. However, because many of the specifics change relatively quickly, it is always best to be sure to determine the existence of even more current, up-to-date references.

LABORATORY TESTS AND PROCEDURES

During the first health maintenance visit at 2–4 weeks of age, it is most important to perform follow-up laboratory tests of those **neonatal screening battery of tests done in the nursery. Newborn infants undergo tests for hypothyroidism, phenylketonuria, sickle cell disease (in some states), and a number of other inborn errors of metabolism. If the newborn had been discharged before 24 hours of age, then it is necessary to perform repeat neonatal screening at this visit.** No additional laboratory tests are necessary at this initial visit.

The AAP has a well-established schedule for performing routine laboratory work with infants

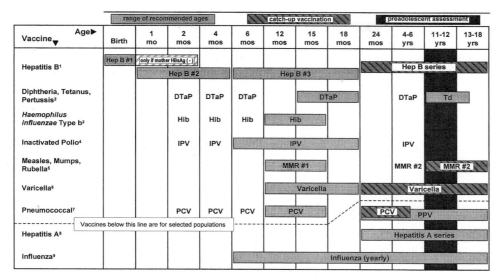

Vaccine ▼	Age ► Birth	1 mo	2 mos	4 mos	6 mos	12 mos	15 mos	18 mos	24 mos	4-6 yrs	11-12 yrs	13-18 yrs
	range of recommended ages				catch-up vaccination				preadolescent assessment			
Hepatitis B[1]	Hep B #1	only if mother HBsAg (-)								Hep B series		
		Hep B #2			Hep B #3							
Diphtheria, Tetanus, Pertussis[2]			DTaP	DTaP	DTaP		DTaP			DTaP	Td	
Haemophilus influenzae Type b[3]			Hib	Hib	Hib	Hib						
Inactivated Polio[4]			IPV	IPV		IPV				IPV		
Measles, Mumps, Rubella[5]						MMR #1				MMR #2	MMR #2	
Varicella[6]						Varicella				Varicella		
Pneumococcal[7]			PCV	PCV	PCV	PCV			PCV	PPV		
Hepatitis A[8]				Vaccines below this line are for selected populations					Hepatitis A series			
Influenza[9]						Influenza (yearly)						

Approved by the Advisory Committee on Immunization Practices (www.cdc.gov/nip/acip), the American Academy of Pediatrics (www.aap.org), and the American Academy of Family Physicians (www.aafp.org).

This schedule indicates the recommended ages for routine administration of currently licensed childhood vaccines, as of December 1, 2001, for children through age 18 years. Any dose not given at the recommended age should be given at any subsequent visit when indicated and feasible. ▓▓▓ Indicates age groups that warrant special effort to administer those vaccines not previously given. Additional vaccines may be licensed and recommended during the year. Licensed combination vaccines may be used whenever any components of the combination are indicated and the vaccine's other components are not contraindicated. Providers should consult the manufacturers' package inserts for detailed recommendations.

1. **Hepatitis B vaccine (Hep B).** All infants should receive the first dose of hepatitis B vaccine soon after birth and before hospital discharge; the first dose may also be given by age 2 months if the infant's mother is HBsAg-negative. Only monovalent hepatitis B vaccine can be used for the birth dose. Monovalent or combination vaccine containing Hep B may be used to complete the series; four doses of vaccine may be administered if combination vaccine is used. The second dose should be given at least 4 weeks after the first dose, except for Hib-containing vaccine which cannot be administered before age 6 weeks. The third dose should be given at least 16 weeks after the first dose and at least 8 weeks after the second dose. The last dose in the vaccination series (third or fourth dose) should not be administered before age 6 months.
    Infants born to HBsAg-positive mothers should receive hepatitis B vaccine and 0.5 mL hepatitis B immune globulin (HBIG) within 12 hours of birth at separate sites. The second dose is recommended at age 1–2 months and the vaccination series should be completed (third or fourth dose) at age 6 months.
    Infants born to mothers whose HBsAg status is unknown should receive the first dose of the hepatitis B vaccine series within 12 hours of birth. Maternal blood should be drawn at the time of delivery to determine the mother's HBsAg status; if the HBsAg test is positive, the infant should receive HBIG as soon as possible (no later than age 1 week).
2. **Diphtheria and tetanus toxoids and acellular pertussis vaccine (DTaP).** The fourth dose of DTaP may be administered as early as age 12 months, provided 6 months have elapsed since the third dose and the child is unlikely to return at age 15–18 months. **Tetanus and diphtheria toxoids (Td)** is recommended at age 11–12 years if at least 5 years have elapsed since the last dose of tetanus and diphtheria toxoid-containing vaccine. Subsequent routine Td boosters are recommended every 10 years.
3. *Haemophilus influenzae* **type b (Hib) conjugate vaccine.** Three Hib conjugate vaccines are licensed for infant use. If PRP-OMP (PedvaxHib® or ComVax® [Merck]) is administered at ages 2 and 4 months, a dose at age 6 months is not required. DTaP/Hib combination products should not be used for primary immunization in infants at ages 2, 4 or 6 months, but can be used as boosters following any Hib vaccine.
4. **Inactivated polio vaccine (IPV).** An all-IPV schedule is recommended for routine childhood polio vaccination in the United States. All children should receive four doses of IPV at ages 2 months, 4 months, 6–18 months, and 4–6 years.
5. **Measles, mumps, and rubella vaccine (MMR).** The second dose of MMR is recommended routinely at age 4–6 years but may be administered during any visit, provided at least 4 weeks have elapsed since the first dose and that both doses are administered beginning at or after age 12 months. Those who have not previously received the second dose should complete the schedule by the 11–12 year old visit.
6. **Varicella vaccine.** Varicella vaccine is recommended at any visit at or after age 12 months for susceptible children, i.e. those who lack a reliable history of chickenpox. Susceptible persons aged ≥13 years should receive two doses, given at least 4 weeks apart.
7. **Pneumococcal vaccine.** The heptavalent **pneumococcal conjugate vaccine (PCV)** is recommended for all children age 2–23 months. It is also recommended for certain children age 24–59 months. **Pneumococcal polysaccharide vaccine (PPV)** is recommended in addition to PCV for certain high-risk groups. See *MMWR* 2000;49(RR-9);1–35.
8. **Hepatitis A vaccine.** Hepatitis A vaccine is recommended for use in selected states and regions, and for certain high-risk groups; consult your local public health authority. See *MMWR* 1999;48(RR-12);1–37.
9. **Influenza vaccine.** Influenza vaccine is recommended annually for children age ≥6 months with certain risk factors (including but not limited to asthma, cardiac disease, sickle cell disease, HIV, diabetes; see *MMWR* 2001;50(RR-4);1–44), and can be administered to all others wishing to obtain immunity. Children aged ≤12 years should receive vaccine in a dosage appropriate for their age (0.25 mL if age 6–35 months or 0.5 mL if aged ≥3 years). Children aged ≤8 years who are receiving influenza vaccine for the first time should receive two doses separated by at least 4 weeks.

For additional information about vaccines, vaccine supply, and contraindications for immunization, please visit the National Immunization Program Website at www.cdc.gov/nip or call the National Immunization Hotline at 800-232-2522 (English) or 800-232-0233 (Spanish).

FIGURE 2.10. Recommended immunization schedule for children (2002) according to the American Academy of Pediatrics (AAP).

TABLE 2.2 Vaccines Licensed in the United States and Their Routes of Administration		
Vaccine*	**Type**	**Route†**
Bacille Calmette-Guérin (tuberculosis)	Live bacteria	ID‡ (preferred) or SC
Cholera	Inactivated bacteria	SC, IM, or ID‡
DTaP	Toxoids and inactivated bacteria (without capsule)	IM
Hepatitis B	Inactivated viral antigen: yeast recombinant-derived, plasma-derived	IM; if risk of hemorrhage, SC
Haemophilus b conjugate (HbCV)	Polysaccharide-protein conjugate	IM
Influenza	Inactivated virus	IM
	Subvirion (split)	IM
Measles	Live virus	SC
Meningococcal	Polysaccharide	SC or IM
MMR	Live viruses	SC
MR	Live viruses	SC
Mumps	Live virus	SC
Plague	Inactivated bacteria	IM
Pneumococcal	Polysaccharide	IM or SC
Poliovirus (trivalent)		
IPV	Inactivated virus	SC
Rabies	Inactivated virus	IM or ID‡,§
Rubella	Live virus	SC
Tetanus and Td, DT (adsorbed)	Toxoids	IM
Tetanus (fluid)	Toxoid	SC
Typhoid		
Parenteral	Inactivated bacteria	SC (boosters may be ID‡)
Oral	Live attenuated bacteria	PO
Varicella	Live attenuated virus	IM
Yellow fever	Live attenuated virus	SC

*DT = diphtheria and tetanus toxoids (for children < 7 years of age); Td = tetanus and diphtheria toxoid (for children = 7 years of age and adults); DTP = diphtheria and tetanus toxoids and pertussis vaccine adsorbed; HBPV = *Haemophilus* b polysaccharide vaccine; HbCV = *Haemophilus* b conjugate vaccine; MMR = measles, mumps, and rubella vaccine; MR = measles and rubella vaccine; IPV = inactivated poliovirus vaccine.
†ID = intradermal; SC = subcutaneous; IM = intramuscular; PO = oral.
‡The intradermal dose is different from the subcutaneous and intramuscular doses.
§Used for prophylaxis only.

and children at regular intervals (Figure 2.11). This chart indicates the need for and the timing of **vision screening, hearing screening, tuberculin testing, hemoglobin and hematocrit determination, urinalysis, and dental referral.** It is important that these guidelines be followed at the indicated times; these recommendations are the consensus of experts in the field.

ANTICIPATORY GUIDANCE

With the completion of the physical examination and any appropriate procedures, tests, or other interventions, this phase of the health maintenance visit involves any concerns or issues the parent might need to deal with over the upcoming weeks before the next visit, which will occur in about 1 month. The issues usually covered in these steps

of anticipatory guidance are **nutrition, injury prevention, sleep patterns, anticipated developmental and behavioral milestones,** and **daily routines and activities.** These categories can serve as the template for all future anticipatory guidance discussions. Chapter 4 contains additional information about nutrition guidance during the first 5 years of life, and Appendix 2.1 presents the specific injury prevention guidelines from the American Academy of Pediatrics/The Injury Prevention Program (TIPP).

Nutrition

Breastfeeding remains the feeding method of choice. During the first month, the establishment of a satisfying breastfeeding experience is an important goal. By this first visit, usually breastfed

TABLE 2.3 Recommended Immunization Schedules for Children Not Immunized in the First Year of Life*

Recommended Time/Age	Immunizations	Comments
Younger than 7 years		
First visit	DTaP, Hib,[†] HBV, MMR	If indicated, tuberculin testing may be done at same visit. If child is 5 years of age, Hib is not indicated in most circumstances.
Interval after first visit		
1 month (4 weeks)	DTaP, IPV, HBV, Var[‡]	The second dose of IPV may be given if accelerated poliomyelitis immunization is necessary, such as for travelers to areas where polio is endemic.
2 months	DTaP, Hib,[†] IPV	Second dose of Hib is indicated only if the first dose was received when younger than 15 months.
≥ 8 months	DTaP, HBV, IPV	IPV and HBV are not given if the third doses were given earlier.
Age 4–6 years (at or before school entry)	DTaP, IPV, MMR[§]	DtaP is not necessary if the fourth dose was given after the fourth birthday; IPV is not necessary if the third dose was given after the fourth birthday.
Age 11–12 years	See Figure 2.10	
7–12 years		
First visit	HBV, MMR, dT, IPV	
Interval after first visit		
2 months (8 weeks)	HBV, MMR,[§] Var,[‡] dT, IPV	IPV may also be given 1 month after the first visit if accelerated poliomyelitis immunization is necessary.
8–14 months	HBV,[∥] dT, IPV	IPV is not given if the third dose was given earlier.
Age 11–12 years	See Figure 2.10	

HBV = hepatitis B virus; Var = varicella; DTaP = diphtheria and tetanus toxoids and acellular pertussis; Hib = *Haemophilus influenzae* type b conjugate; IPV = inactivated poliovirus; MMR = measle-mumps-rubella; dT = adult tetanus toxoid (full dose) and diphtheria toxoid (reduced dose), for children 7 years of age or older and adults.

*Table is not completely consistent with package inserts. For products used, also consult manufacturer's package insert for instructions on storage, handling, dosage, and administration. Biologics prepared by different manufacturers may vary, and package inserts of the same manufacturer may change. Therefore, the physician should be aware of the contents of the current package insert.

[†]If all needed vaccines cannot be administered simultaneously, priority should be given to protecting the child against the diseases that pose the greatest immediate risk. In the United States, these diseases for children younger than 2 years usually are measles and *Haemophilus influenzae* type b infection; for children older than 7 years, they are measles, mumps, and rubella. Before 13 years of age, immunity against hepatitis B and varicella should be ensured. DTaP, HBV, Hib, MMR, and Var can be given simultaneously at separate sites if failure of the patient to return for future immunizations is a concern.

[‡]Varicella vaccine may be administered to susceptible children any time after 12 months of age. Unimmunized children who lack a reliable history of varicella should be immunized before their 13th birthday.

[§]Minimal interval between doses of MMR is 1 month (4 weeks).

[∥]HBV may be given earlier in a 0-, 2-, and 4-month schedule.

babies are nursing every 3 hours or so and feed throughout the night. By now, the mother's milk supply should be well established, although there may have been some days of discomfort or engorgement during the first week at home; infants and mothers are usually quite settled into a routine. The mother should have been able to find several comfortable positions for positioning the infant, and each feeding usually lasts 20–30 minutes, with approximately 10–15 minutes on each breast.

It is important to be very encouraging and supportive of the mother who is beginning to breastfeed her infant, because usually if the

TABLE 2.4	**Reportable Events Following Immunization***	
Vaccine/Toxoid	**Event**	**Interval From Vaccination**
DTaP, aP, DTaP/ poliovirus combined	Anaphylaxis or anaphylactic shock	
	Encephalopathy (or encephalitis)[†]	24 hours
	Shock–collapse or hypotonic–hyporesponsive collapse[†]	7 days
	Residual seizure disorder[†]	
	Any acute complication or sequela (including death)	7 days
	See package insert[††]	No limit (see package insert)
Measles, mumps, and rubella vaccines; DT, Td, T toxoids	Anaphylaxis or anaphylactic shock	24 hours
	Encephalopathy (or encephalitis)[†]	15 days for measles, mumps, and rubella vaccines; 7 days for DT, Td, and T toxoids
	Residual seizure disorder[†]	
	Any acute complication or sequela (including death)	No limit
	See package insert[††]	See package insert
Inactivated poliovirus vaccine	Anaphylaxis or anaphylactic shock	24 hours
	Any acute complication or sequela (including death)	No limit
	See package insert[††]	See package insert

*Events listed are required by law to be reported to the United States Department of Health and Human Services; however, the Vaccine Adverse Events Reporting System (VAERS) will accept *all* reports of suspected adverse events after the administration of *any* vaccine.

[†]Aids to interpretation:
- Shock–collapse or hypotonic–hyporesponsive collapse may be evidenced by signs or symptoms such as decrease in or loss of muscle tone, paralysis (partial or complete), hemiplegia, hemiparesis, loss of color or change of color to pale white or blue, unresponsiveness to environmental stimuli, depression of or loss of consciousness, prolonged sleeping with difficulty arousing, or cardiovascular or respiratory arrest.
- Residual seizure disorder may be considered to have occurred if no other seizure or convulsion unaccompanied by fever or accompanied by a fever of < 102°F occurred before the first seizure or convulsion after the administration of the vaccine involved, AND, if in the case of measles-, mumps-, or rubella-containing vaccines, the first seizure or convulsion occurred within 15 days after vaccination OR in the case of any other vaccine, the first seizure or convulsion occurred within 3 days after vaccination, AND, if two or more seizures or convulsions unaccompanied by fever or accompanied by a fever of < 102°F occurred within 1 year after vaccination.
- The terms seizure and convulsion include grand mal, petit mal, absence, myoclonic, tonic–clonic, and focal motor seizures and signs.
- Encephalopathy means any substantial acquired abnormality of, injury to, or impairment of brain function. Among the frequent manifestations of encephalopathy are focal and diffuse neurologic signs, increased intracranial pressure, or changes lasting ≥ 6 hours in level of consciousness, with or without convulsions. The neurologic signs and symptoms of encephalopathy may be temporary with complete recovery, or they may result in various degrees of permanent impairment. Signs and symptoms such as high-pitched and unusual screaming, persistent inconsolable crying, and bulging fontanelle are compatible with an encephalopathy but in and of themselves are not conclusive evidence of encephalopathy. Encephalopathy usually can be documented by slow-wave activity on an electroencephalogram (EEG).

[††]Refer to the contraindication section of the manufacturer's package insert for each vaccine.

mother can remain relaxed, comfortable, and reassured that the baby is growing and **gaining weight,** then she feels that all of the initial adjustment has been worth it. Usually, after the first month, the feeding process becomes more predictable. Although there may normally be occasional days of sudden "surges in apparent hunger and appetite," infants generally take in approximately 110–150 kcal/kg, which is optimum for growth. This usually translates into 3–4 oz every 3 hours in the first month. At this time, it is a good idea to give mothers some referral material so they may find answers to some of their questions regarding the specifics of breastfeeding. Two excellent sources are *The Womanly Art of Breastfeeding,* a publication of La Leche League, and *Caring for Your Baby and Young Child: Birth to Age 5* (see SUGGESTED READINGS).

Recommendations for Preventive Pediatric Health Care

Committee on Practice and Ambulatory Medicine

Each child and family is unique; therefore, these **Recommendations for Preventive Pediatric Health Care** are designed for the care of children who are receiving competent parenting, have no manifestations of any important health problems, and are growing and developing in satisfactory fashion. **Additional visits may become necessary if** circumstances suggest variations from normal.

These guidelines represent a consensus by the Committee on Practice and Ambulatory Medicine in consultation with national committees and sections of the American Academy of Pediatrics. The Committee emphasizes the great importance of continuity of care in comprehensive health supervision and the need to avoid **fragmentation of care**.

AGE[a]	PRENATAL[1]	NEWBORN[2]	INFANCY 2-4d[3]	By 1mo	2mo	4mo	6mo	9mo	12mo	EARLY CHILDHOOD[b] 15mo	18mo	24mo	3y	4y	MIDDLE CHILDHOOD[c] 5y	6y	8y	10y	ADOLESCENCE[c] 11y	12y	13y	14y	15y	16y	17y	18y	19y	20y	21y
HISTORY Initial/Interval	•	•	•	•	•	•	•	•	•	•	•	•	•	•	•	•	•	•	•	•	•	•	•	•	•	•	•	•	•
MEASUREMENTS Height and Weight		•	•	•	•	•	•	•	•	•	•	•	•	•	•	•	•	•	•	•	•	•	•	•	•	•	•	•	•
Head Circumference		•	•	•	•	•	•	•	•	•	•	•																	
Blood Pressure												•	•	•	•	•	•	•	•	•	•	•	•	•	•	•	•	•	•
SENSORY SCREENING Vision		S	S	S	S	S	S	S	S	S	S	S	O[d]	O	O	O	O	O	S	O	S	S	O	S	S	O	S	S	S
Hearing		O[d]										S	S	S	O	O	O	O	S	O	S	S	O	S	S	O	S	S	S
DEVELOPMENTAL/ BEHAVIORAL ASSESSMENT[e]		•	•	•	•	•	•	•	•	•	•	•	•	•	•	•	•	•	•	•	•	•	•	•	•	•	•	•	•
PHYSICAL EXAMINATION[f]		•	•	•	•	•	•	•	•	•	•	•	•	•	•	•	•	•	•	•	•	•	•	•	•	•	•	•	•
PROCEDURES-GENERAL[g] Hereditary/Metabolic Screening[11]		•																											
Immunization[12]		•	•	•	•	•	•	•		•		•		•	•			•	•				•						
Hematocrit or Hemoglobin[13]					•																								
Urinalysis																													
PROCEDURES-PATIENTS AT RISK Lead Screening[14]							*		*																				
Tuberculin Test[15]																													
Cholesterol Screening[16]																													
STD Screening[17]																				*	*	*	*	*	*	*	*	*	*
Pelvic Exam[18]																													
ANTICIPATORY GUIDANCE[i] Injury Prevention[20]		•	•	•	•	•	•	•	•	•	•	•	•	•	•	•	•	•	•	•	•	•	•	•	•	•	•	•	•
Violence Prevention[21]		•	•	•	•	•	•	•	•	•	•	•	•	•	•	•	•	•	•	•	•	•	•	•	•	•	•	•	•
Sleep Positioning Counseling[24]		•	•	•	•	•	•																						
Nutrition Counseling[25]		•	•	•	•	•	•	•	•	•	•	•	•	•	•	•	•	•	•	•	•	•	•	•	•	•	•	•	•
DENTAL REFERRAL[26]												▼																	

1. A prenatal visit is recommended for parents who are at high risk, for first-time parents, and for those who request a conference. The prenatal visit should include anticipatory guidance, pertinent medical history, and a discussion of benefits of breastfeeding and planned method of feeding per AAP statement "The Prenatal Visit" (1996).
2. Every infant should have a newborn evaluation after birth. Breastfeeding should be encouraged and instruction and support offered. Every breastfeeding infant should have an evaluation 48-72 hours after discharge from the hospital to include weight, formal breastfeeding evaluation, encouragement, and instruction as recommended in the AAP statement "Breastfeeding and the Use of Human Milk" (1997).
3. For newborns discharged in less than 48 hours after delivery per AAP statement "Hospital Stay for Healthy Term Newborns" (1995).
4. Developmental, psychosocial, and chronic disease issues for children and adolescents may require frequent counseling and treatment visits separate from preventive care visits.
5. If a patient comes under care for the first time at any point on the schedule, or if any items are not accomplished at the suggested age, the schedule should be brought up to date at the earliest possible time.
6. If the patient is uncooperative, rescreen within 6 months.
7. All newborns should be screened per the AAP Task Force on Newborn and Infant Hearing statement, "Newborn and Infant Hearing Loss: Detection and Intervention" (1999).
8. By history and appropriate physical examination; if suspicious, by specific objective developmental testing. Parenting skills should be fostered at every visit.
9. At each visit, a complete physical examination is essential, with infant totally unclothed, older child undressed and suitably draped.
10. These may be modified, depending upon entry point into schedule and individual need.
11. Metabolic screening (eg, thyroid, hemoglobinopathies, PKU, galactosemia) should be done according to state law.
12. Schedule(s) per the Committee on Infectious Diseases, published annually in the January edition of Pediatrics. Every visit should be an opportunity to update and complete a child's immunizations.
13. See AAP Pediatric Nutrition Handbook (1998) for a discussion of universal and selective screening options. Consider earlier screening for high-risk infants (eg, premature infants and low birth weight infants). See also "Recommendations to Prevent and Control Iron Deficiency in the United States", MMWR, 1998;47 (RR-3):1-29.
14. All menstruating adolescents should be screened annually.
15. Conduct dipstick urinalysis for leukocytes annually for sexually active male and female adolescents.
16. For children at risk of lead exposure consult the AAP statement "Screening for Elevated Blood Levels" (1998). Additionally, screening should be done in accordance with state law where applicable.
17. TB testing per recommendations of the Committee on Infectious Diseases, published in the current edition of Red Book: Report of the Committee on Infectious Diseases. Testing should be done upon recognition of high-risk factors.
18. Cholesterol screening for high-risk patients per AAP statement "Cholesterol in Childhood" (1998). If family history cannot be ascertained and other risk factors are present, screening should be at the discretion of the physician.
19. All sexually active patients should be screened for sexually transmitted diseases (STDs).
20. All sexually active females should have a pelvic examination. A pelvic examination and routine pap smear should be offered as part of preventive health maintenance between the ages of 18 and 21 years.
21. Age-appropriate discussion and counseling should be an integral part of each visit for care per the AAP Guidelines for Health Supervision III (1998).
22. From birth to age 12, refer to the AAP injury prevention program (TIPP*) as described in A Guide to Safety Counseling in Office Practice (1994).
23. Violence prevention and management for all patients per AAP Statement "The Role of the Pediatrician in Youth Violence Prevention in Clinical Practice and at the Community Level" (1999).
24. Parents and caregivers should be advised to place healthy infants on their backs when putting them to sleep. Side positioning is a reasonable alternative but carries a slightly higher risk of SIDS. Consult the AAP statement "Changing Concepts of Sudden Infant Death Syndrome: Implications for Infant Sleeping Environment and Sleep Position" (2000).
25. Age-appropriate nutrition counseling should be an integral part of each visit per the AAP Handbook of Nutrition (1998).
26. Earlier initial dental examinations may be appropriate for some children. Subsequent examinations as prescribed by dentist.

Key:
- • = to be performed
- S = subjective, by history
- * = to be performed for patients at risk
- O = objective, by a standard testing method
- ← → = the range during which a service may be provided, with the dot indicating the preferred age.

NB: Special chemical, immunologic, and endocrine testing is usually carried out upon specific indications. Testing other than newborn (eg, inborn errors of metabolism, sickle disease, etc) is discretionary with the physician.

The recommendations in this statement do not indicate an exclusive course of treatment or standard of medical care. Variations, taking into account individual circumstances, may be appropriate. Copyright ©2000 by the American Academy of Pediatrics. No part of this statement may be reproduced in any form or by any means without prior written permission from the American Academy of Pediatrics except for one copy for personal use.

FIGURE 2.11. Recommendations for preventive pediatric health care according to the American Academy of Pediatrics (AAP).

If parents have chosen the bottle-feeding method, several excellent **infant formula** preparations are available. These preparations have a cow's milk foundation that has been altered to provide a more suitable casein:whey ratio, a more digestible form of fat, and vitamin fortification. They can be purchased either in a "ready-to-feed" variety, which is quite expensive, or in a concentrate form, which requires reconstitution with water. Some of the formula preparations come in a powder formulation that is also convenient for travel purposes. See Chapter 4 for the types of formula and their specific contents with respect to type of carbohydrate, fat, and protein contained, as well as a more detailed discussion of nutrition.

Injury Prevention

Although this is perhaps not a major issue for all infants at the 1-month visit, a number of issues should be considered even during these relatively immobile first few months.

- When traveling in an automobile, **is the baby in an approved infant restraint or car seat all the time? Until the baby weighs 18 lb (approximate age: 10 months), she should ride facing backwards.** Proper installation of car seats according to manufacturer's recommendations is crucial. It is also necessary, regrettably, to check the car seat safety recall list to be sure parents are not purchasing a car seat that has been recalled. The Consumer Product Safety Commission or Consumers Union usually has an updated recall list.
- Are the parents using seat belts themselves **all the time?**
- Is the changing table in a safe place (preferably, in a corner with two walls on a side)? Are the necessary changing supplies near at hand?
- Is the **hot water heater turned down to 120°F,** especially if the infant bathes in a sink with a swing-out faucet?
- Is the infant never left alone in the house, car, or outside?
- Are pacifiers never attached with a string around the infant's neck? **Choking is a major hazard for infants,** especially those who shave a string around the neck.
- Is the crib safe and approved according to national standards? Modifications made in 1985 include (1) a slat distance of 2⅜ inches or less, (2) no cutouts in headboards, (3) no protruding corner posts, (4) a mattress that fits snugly

against the side rail, and (5) a side-lowering mechanism that is not accessible to the infant.
- Is there a smoke detector in all appropriate places in the home?
- Are small objects kept out of the reach of the infant?

Obviously, as the baby becomes more mobile with increasing age, these child safety measures become increasingly important and need to be discussed at each visit. Appendix 2.1 contains a detailed list of age-appropriate safety measures.

Sleep Patterns

During the second month of life, the sleep pattern of infants usually becomes more regular, but they probably will still not sleep through the night. It is important to remind parents about the recent guidelines that recommend that they put their infants to sleep on the side or on the back, especially in the first several months of life. This recommendation is derived from the review of the research that may implicate the prone sleeping position in sudden infant death syndrome (SIDS) events. Although the research design has some distinct flaws, the expert panel convened at the AAP has concluded that it would be most responsible to advise parents of this possible association and to act accordingly.

Young infants also have two fairly long naps during the day, one in the morning and one in the afternoon. Usually, by 3–4 months of age, the sleep routine changes, and the majority of infants sleep through the night.

Anticipated Developmental and Behavioral Milestones

Patterns in Infants

Consultation of the Denver II or the AAP child care book (*Caring for Your Baby and Young Child: Birth to Age 5*) allows for review of the developmental milestones to look for in the next month or two.

GROSS AND FINE MOTOR DEVELOPMENT. The infant is increasingly able to raise his head off the mattress while in a prone position and, when pulled up, has increasingly better head control; is able to stretch out his legs and kick; and is able to open and shut his hands, bring them to his mouth, swipe at dangling objects, and start to grasp toys and shake them.

VISUAL DEVELOPMENT. The infant watches faces intently and follows moving objects in front more effectively and through a wider arc, appears to recognize familiar objects and people at a distance, and begins to coordinate his hands and eyes.

HEARING AND SPEECH DEVELOPMENT. The infant's hearing should be fully developed, and now the baby smiles at the sound of the parent's voice. He begins to babble vowel-type guttural sounds, may even start to imitate some sounds, and begins to turn toward direction of sound, by the age of 3 months.

EMOTIONAL AND SOCIAL DEVELOPMENT. The infant begins to develop a social smile, increasingly enjoys playing with other people, becomes increasingly expressive with face and body grimaces and movements, and may even imitate some of the movements that he sees. In addition, the infant loves to react to high-contrast books; mobiles; rattles, music, and songs; and, especially, mirrors, by the third month.

Future Developmental Stages

At this time, the pediatrician should share with the parents the developmental expectations for future time periods, using those milestones found in the Denver II scoring and explanation sheet (see Figure 2.1) as well as the information contained in *Bright Futures in Practice* (AAP). However, it is important not to become too specific about the exact timing of developmental milestones. Some infants develop at different rates than others. It is essential to ensure that parents have this perspective so that they do not become overly anxious if their infant is not visibly developing at the *exact* same rate as a friend's child or the parents' other children. It is most important to remember that the infant is acquiring new milestones on a regular basis, even if slightly slower or more rapidly than in written materials or actual experiences. Guidelines for developmental milestones are just that—guidelines. The Denver II is quite clear that there is a "range of expected" for each developmental stage, and it is critical that the pediatrician reinforce that some variability in when children do certain things is perfectly normal.

Daily Routines and Activities

In the midst of the harried first weeks to months of the life of a new infant, with all of the required schedules that the baby forces the parents to fit into to, it is important that the parents find time for their own peace and quiet. Each day the parents should find a way to talk about things other than the infant. Some time for mutual renewal is necessary; often, with all of the excitement and demands of the baby, this is forgotten. The pediatrician can help reinforce the importance of each parent taking some respite time, either together or separately. It is crucial to "recharge the batteries" in order to maintain the energy and perspective it takes to properly care for an infant.

CLOSING THE VISIT

The closing of the health maintenance visit should have several goals, which include:

- To reinforce your appreciation for all the parents have done in the time since the last visit
- To reinforce your recognition of how well the parents have cared for an infant or child, how well they have observed certain factors, and how responsive they have been despite possible fatigue
- To make sure that the parents or children have no additional questions that they would like to have answered
- To be sure they know how to reach the pediatrician or the office if necessary
- To identify any remaining anxieties they may be feeling
- To confirm their next appointment and what to expect at that time

SUGGESTED READINGS

American Academy of Pediatrics: *Bright Futures in Practice: Physical Activity*. http://www.aap.org/advocacy/physicalactivity.htm

American Academy of Pediatrics: *Guidelines for Health Supervision*. Elk Grove Village, IL, American Academy of Pediatrics, 1993.

American Academy of Pediatrics Committee on Infectious Diseases: Report of the Committee on Infectious Diseases ("The Red Book"). Elk Grove Village, IL, American Academy of Pediatrics, 2001.

Shelov SP, Hannemann R (eds): *Caring for your baby and young child: Birth to age 5*. New York, Bantam Books, 1993.

APPENDIX 2.1

Guidelines for Safety Counseling

Early Childhood Safety Counseling Schedule

Preventive Health Visit	Minimal Safety Counseling		
Age	Introduce	Reinforce	Materials
Prenatal/Newborn	Infant Car Seat Smoke Alarm Crib Safety		AAP Family Shopping Guide to Car Seats Infant Furniture TIPP Slip
2 Days To 4 Weeks	Falls	Infant Car Seat	
2 Months	Burns—Hot Liquids	Infant Car Seat Falls	Blue Safety Sheet (Birth–6 Months)
4 Months	Choking/Suffocation	Infant Car Seat Falls Burns—Hot Liquids	Blue Safety Survey Blue Safety Sheet (Birth–6 Months) AAP Choking Brochure
6 Months	Poisonings Burns—Hot Surface	Falls Burns—Hot Liquids Choking	Beige Safety Sheet (6–12 Months) Poison TIPP Slip Syrup of Ipecac Local Poison Center Sticker
9 Months	Water/Pool Safety Convertible Car Seat	Poisonings Falls Burns	AAP Family Shopping Guide to Car Seats Beige Safety Sheet (6–12 Months)
1 Year	Firearm Hazards Car Seat Safety	Water/Pool Safety Falls Burns	Yellow Safety Sheet (1–2 Years) Water/Pool Safety TIPP Slips AAP Firearms Safety Brochure
15 Months		Car Seat Safety Poisonings Falls Burns	Yellow Safety Survey Yellow Safety Sheet (1–2 Years)
18 Months	Car Seat Safety	Poisonings Falls Burns Firearm Hazards	Yellow Safety Sheet (1–2 Years)
2 Years	Falls—Play Equipment, Tricycles/Helmets Pedestrian	Car Seat Safety Water/Pool Safety Burns Firearm Hazards	Green Safety Survey Green Safety Sheet (2–4 Years)
3 Years		Car Seat Safety, Pedestrian Falls Burns Firearm Hazards	Green Safety Sheet (2–4 Years) AAP Firearms Safety Brochure
4 Years	Car Seat Safety or Booster Seat Safety	Pedestrian Falls—Play Equipment Firearm Hazards	AAP Family Shopping Guide to Car Seats Green Safety Sheet (2–4 Years)

Guidelines for Safety Counseling *(Continued)*

Middle Childhood Safety Counseling Schedule

Preventive Health Visit	Minimal Safety Counseling		
Age	Introduce	Reinforce	Materials
5 Years	Water/Pool Safety Bicycle Safety	Firearm Hazards Pedestrian Safety Booster Seat Use	Pink Safety Sheet (5–6 Years)
6 Years	Fire Safety	Bicycle Safety Booster Seat Use Pedestrian Safety Firearm Hazards	Peach Safety Survey Peach Safety Sheet (6–8 Years)
8 Years	Sports Safety	Bicycle Safety Booster Seat/Seat Belt Use	Purple Safety Sheet (8–10 Years)
10 Years	Firearm Hazards	Sports Safety Seat Belt Use Bicycle Safety	Gold Child Survey Gold Safety Sheet (10–12 Years)

Counseling Guidelines
The First Year of Life

Household Hazards	Counseling Guidelines
1. Do you put the crib side up whenever you leave your baby in the crib?	**Keep crib sides raised.** Crib sides need to be kept up and firmly secured to prevent falls. Even if your baby currently can't roll over or pull up, there's always a first time.
2. Do you leave the baby alone on tables or beds, even for a brief moment?	**If you leave, even for a moment, place your baby in a playpen or a crib with the sides up.** Emphasize the necessity of anticipating developmental stages; the baby's first rollover should not lead to a fall.
3. Do you leave the baby alone at home?	**Provide constant supervision.** Never leave your baby alone in the home without a capable baby-sitter, at least 13 years old who can respond to emergency situations. Poisonings may occur in a matter of minutes; choking, falls, fires, and similar emergencies require immediate attention.
4. Do you keep plastic wrappers, plastic bags, and balloons away from your children?	**Keep plastic bags and balloons away from your children.** Plastic wrappers and bags form a tight seal if placed over the nose and mouth. Balloons can be inhaled into the windpipe and may cause death from choking.
5. Does your child wear a pacifier or jewelry around his or her neck?	**Do not put anything around a baby's neck— objects around the neck may strangle the baby.**

(continued)

Guidelines for Safety Counseling *(Continued)*

Counseling Guidelines
The First Year of Life (Continued)

Household Hazards	Counseling Guidelines
	Necklaces, ribbons, or strings around a baby's neck may get caught on parts of furniture or other objects and cause strangulation. Drawstrings also should be removed from all children's clothing.
6. Does your child play with small objects such as beads or nuts?	**Do not allow your child to play with small objects.** Any small objects that can be placed in the mouth (including plant parts) are potential hazards. Even small pieces of food may cause problems; children should not run or play while eating. Parents should be informed about emergency treatment for the choking child. Use the American Academy of Pediatrics (AAP) brochure *Choking Prevention and First Aid for Infants and Children*. Round or cylindrical food or objects are especially hazardous.
7. Are any of your baby-sitters younger than 13 years?	**Select an experienced baby-sitter.** All sitters should be at least 13 years old and mature enough to handle common emergencies. Use the AAP handout *Baby-sitting Reminders*.
8. How frequently is the heating system checked where you live?	**Check heating systems at least once a year.** This annual inspection helps prevent carbon monoxide poisoning, fires, and system malfunction.
9. Are your operable window guards in place?	**Place operable window guards on all windows in your home.** Window guards should be well repaired and inspected regularly. Keep furniture away from windows that can give a climbing toddler access to a window sill. Apartment windows should have guards above the second floor. The spaces above and below window guards should be less than 4 inches to prevent a child from falling through. Children leaning on screens can fall through and be seriously injured.
10. Do you ever place your baby in an infant walker?	**Do not place your child in a walker.** Every year, more than 8,000 injuries occur to children in walkers.

Guidelines for Safety Counseling *(Continued)*

Counseling Guidelines
The First Year of Life (Continued)

Burns	Counseling Guidelines
11. Does anyone in your home ever smoke?	**About one third of home fires involving fatalities are caused by smoking.** Smoking in bed or improper disposal of ashes or butts endangers children sleeping in adjacent rooms who may be trapped in the event of fire.
12. Do you have a plan of escape from your home in the event of a fire?	**Develop an escape plan in the event of a fire in the home.** Identify appropriate exit routes and a family meeting point away from the house.
13. Do you have working fire extinguishers in your home?	**Buy a fire extinguisher for the home.** The most common causes of home fires are cooking and heating equipment. Multipurpose dry chemical extinguishers should be available in the kitchen and in any room with a furnace or fireplace.
14. Do you have working smoke alarms in your home?	**Install a smoke alarm in your home.** Most fire-related deaths occur at night and are the result of inhaling smoke or toxic gas. There is a critical period of 4 minutes to get outside after the alarm sounds. Smoke alarms are recommended for each floor, but particularly for furnace and sleeping areas. Batteries should be checked monthly and replaced yearly.
15. Do you ever drink or carry hot liquids when holding your baby?	**Do not drink or carry hot liquids when holding your child or when children are nearby.** Scalds result from spilled hot food and drink; scalding injuries can be decreased by avoiding use of tablecloths and keeping cups and saucers from the edge of tables.
16. Do you ever use woodstoves or kerosene heaters?	**Erect barriers around space heaters.** The use of space heaters, woodstoves, and kerosene heaters has been associated with severe burns to toddlers. Appropriate barriers should protect children.

Water Safety	Counseling Guidelines
17. Do you leave the baby alone in or near a tub, pail of water, or toilet, even for a brief moment?	**Never leave a child alone in or near a tub, pail, toilet, or pool of water.** The bathtub is a source of severe scalding burns. If the phone or doorbell rings, don't leave an infant or toddler alone even for a moment. Young children can drown in less than 2 inches of water.

(continued)

Counseling Guidelines
The First Year of Life (Continued)

Water Safety	Counseling Guidelines
18. Do you have a pool or hot tub where you live?	**Fence in your pool or hot tub on all 4 sides.** Nationally, drowning is the leading cause of injury-related death in children younger than 1 year.

Auto Safety	Counseling Guidelines
19. Do you use a car safety seat in the car on every trip at all times?	Your child should ride in a car safety seat during every trip, even if you will only be traveling a short distance.
20. Does your car have a passenger air bag?	**NEVER place an infant in front of an air bag.**
21. Where do you place your child's car safety seat in the car?	**Seat a child in the rear seat of the car.** This is the safest place in the car. Infants should ride facing the rear of the car until they are at least 1 year of age AND at least 20 pounds.

Bicycle Safety	Counseling Guidelines
22. Does your child ride on your bicycle with you?	**Do not carry children younger than 12 months on bicycles.** Infants too young to sit in a rear bike seat should never be carried on a bicycle. Children 12 months to 4 years old who can wear a helmet may ride in a rear-mounted seat. Use of backpacks or frontpacks is not recommended. Parents should avoid riding in busy streets. With small children, falls frequently result in head injuries. Children should always wear a helmet that meets Consumer Product Safety Commission (CPSC) or Snell Memorial Foundation standards.

Firearm Hazards	Counseling Guidelines
23. Is there a gun in your home or the home where your child plays or is cared for?	**Remove all guns from places children live and play.** More than 5,000 children and adolescents are killed by gunfire each year—injuries almost always inflicted by themselves, a sibling, or a friend. Handguns are especially dangerous. If you choose to keep a gun at home, store it unloaded in a locked place. Lock and store the ammunition in a separate place.

Guidelines for Safety Counseling *(Continued)*

Counseling Guidelines From 1 to 4 Years (Part 1)

Household Hazards	Counseling Guidelines
1. Do you leave your child alone at home?	**Never leave small children alone in the home.** Parents should be aware of the child's rapid acquisition of new abilities.
2. Are any of your baby-sitters younger than 13 years?	**Select an experienced baby-sitter.** All sitters should be at least 13 years old and mature enough to understand parental instructions and handle common emergencies. Use the American Academy of Pediatrics (AAP) handout *Baby-sitting Reminders.*
3. Do you keep plastic wrappers, plastic bags, and balloons away from your children?	**Keep plastic bags and balloons out of reach.** Plastic wrappers and bags form a tight seal if placed over the mouth and nose and may suffocate the child. Balloons can be inhaled into the windpipe and may result in death from choking.
4. Do you know how to prevent your child from choking?	**Small objects and solid foods such as hot dogs, peanuts, grapes, carrots, or popcorn may block your child's airway.** Any small objects that can be placed in the mouth are potential hazards. Children should not run or play while eating. Parents should learn CPR and emergency treatment for the choking child. Use the AAP brochure *Choking Prevention and First Aid for Infants and Children.*
5. Do you have mechanical garage doors?	**Mechanical garage doors may crush a child.** Install only garage door openers with sensors.
6. Are your operable window guards in place?	**Place operable window guards on all windows in your home.** Window guards should be well repaired and inspected regularly. Keep furniture away from windows that can give a climbing toddler access to a window sill. Apartment windows should have guards above the second floor. Windows should not be able to open more than 4 inches to prevent a child from falling through. Children leaning on screens can fall through and be seriously injured.
7. Is your child in the yard while the lawn mower is in use?	**Keep small children out of the yard while the lawn mower is in use.** Potential injury results from the machine itself and from objects thrown by the blade. Children should not be passengers on ride-on mowers.

(continued)

Counseling Guidelines From 1 to 4 Years (Part 1) (Continued)

Household Hazards	Counseling Guidelines
8. Do you place gates at the entrance to stairways (for children younger than 3 years)?	**Use gates on stairways.** Use gates at the top and bottom of entrances to stairways because young children can quickly crawl or climb up the stairs from the lower level. Accordion-style gates are hazardous and can trap the child's head, causing death.
9. Is your baby's crib near a window or a drapery covering?	**Place your baby's crib away from windows.** Cords from window blinds and draperies can strangle your child. Tie cords high and out of reach.
10. Do you check for safety hazards in the homes of friends or relatives where your child may play?	**Check for hazards in homes your child may visit.** Other homes, especially those with no children or older children, may pose particular hazards from poisonings, falls, pools, and guns.
11. Have any of your children ever had an injury requiring a visit to the doctor or hospital?	**Report any history of injuries to the pediatrician.** The pediatrician is able to explore the causes and discuss preventive measures. It has been shown that stressful family situations can be causally linked to repeated injuries in children (3 or more injuries within 12 months). Also note that once an ingestion has occurred, another incident is likely within a year.

Firearm Hazards	Counseling Guidelines
12. Is there a gun in your home or the home where your child plays or is cared for?	**Remove all guns from places children live and play.** More than 5,000 children and adolescents are killed by gunfire each year—injuries almost always inflicted by themselves, a sibling, or a friend. Handguns are especially dangerous. If you choose to keep a gun at home, store it unloaded in a locked place. Lock and store the bullets in a separate place, and make sure to hide the keys to the locked boxes.

Poisonings	Counseling Guidelines
13. Do you keep household products, medicines (including acetaminophen and iron), and sharp objects out of the reach of your child and in locked cabinets?	**Keep medicines and hazardous products out of the sight and reach of children.** Household products, medicines, and sharp objects should be stored locked in high places out of the child's sight. Keep household products in their original containers and never in food or beverage containers.

Guidelines for Safety Counseling *(Continued)*

Counseling Guidelines From 1 to 4 Years (Part 1) (Continued)

Poisonings	Counseling Guidelines
14. Do you dispose of old medicines?	**Dispose of old medicines.** All old medications should be safely disposed of by flushing them down the toilet.
15. Do you have safety caps on all bottles of medicine?	**Purchase medicines with child-resistant safety caps.** Remember to securely replace the cap and store the medicine out of the child's reach.
16. Does your child chew on paint chips or window sills?	**Inspect walls for peeling paint.** Paint that is peeling and chipped or is on chewable surfaces is a potential lead hazard. Approximately 85% of all homes built in the United States before 1978 have lead-based paint in them. Housing built before the 1950s poses particular risk for exposure to lead.
17. Do you have syrup of Ipecac in the house? 18. Do you know how to use syrup of Ipecac?	**Learn first aid for poisoning.** Parents should be advised about the appropriate action to take when harmful substances have been ingested. Give parents a prescription for syrup of Ipecac and instruct them to consult a Poison Center or physician before using it. Give them the telephone number of the local Poison Center.
19. How frequently is the heating system checked where you live?	**Heating ventilation systems should be checked at least once a year.** This annual inspection helps prevent carbon monoxide poisoning, fires, and system malfunction. Carbon monoxide detectors also are available to provide an early warning before the deadly gas builds up to a dangerous level.

Counseling Guidelines From 1 to 4 Years (Part 2)

Burns	Counseling Guidelines
1. Do you use electrical appliances in the bathroom?	**Do not use electrical appliances within the reach of a child in the bathroom.** Electrical current hazards are increased by wetness. Appliances must be used with extreme caution in the presence of water.
2. Do you keep electrical appliances and cords out of your child's reach?	**Keep electrical cords out of a child's reach.** Mouth burns in children can result from chewing on the end of a live extension cord or on a poorly insulated wire. Cords should not be within reach of a child.
3. Do you keep matches and cigarette lighters out of the reach of your children?	**Keep matches and lighters out of the reach of children.**

(continued)

Guidelines for Safety Counseling *(Continued)*

Counseling Guidelines From 1 to 4 Years (Part 2) (Continued)

Burns	Counseling Guidelines
4. Does anyone in your home ever smoke?	Annually, 5,600 fires are started by children younger than 5 years playing with matches and lighters. These fires cause 150 deaths per year. **Most deaths due to home fires are caused by smoking.** Smoking in bed or improper disposal of ashes or butts endangers children sleeping in adjacent rooms who may be trapped in the event of fire. Twelve percent of residential fires are associated with smoking.
5. Do you have a plan for escape from the home in the event of a fire?	**Develop an escape plan in the event of a fire in the home.** Identify appropriate exit routes and a family meeting point away from the house. Do not use elevators in apartment buildings if there is a fire. Ask your fire department for help in designing an escape plan. Use the American Academy of Pediatrics (AAP) handout, *Protect Your Home Against Fire . . . Planning Saves Lives.*
6. Do you have working fire extinguishers in your home?	**Buy a fire extinguisher for your home.** The most common causes of home fires are cooking and heating equipment. Multipurpose dry chemical fire extinguishers should be available in the kitchen and in any room with a furnace or fireplace.
7. Do you have working smoke alarms in your home?	**Install a smoke alarm in your home.** The majority of fire-related deaths occur at night and are the result of inhaling smoke or toxic gas. There is a critical period of 4 minutes to get outside after the alarm sounds. Smoke alarms are recommended for each floor, but particularly for furnace and sleeping areas. Check the batteries monthly and change them once every year.
8. Have you checked the temperature of the hot water where you live?	**Check hot water temperature.** A third-degree burn can occur in only 6 seconds with a water temperature of 140°F. The temperature of a water heater should be set no higher than 120°F.
9. Do you keep the handles of pots and pans on the stove out of the reach of children?	**Keep hot pots and pans out of the reach of children.** Scalds in the kitchen are common; pot handles should be turned inward from the edge of the stove and be out of your child's reach. The kitchen is the most dangerous room for children. Keep children out of the kitchen when you are cooking, or put them in a playpen or high chair to keep them secure.

Guidelines for Safety Counseling *(Continued)*

Counseling Guidelines From 1 to 4 Years (Part 2) (Continued)

Water Safety	Counseling Guidelines
10. Do you leave your child alone in the bathtub?	**Don't leave your child alone in a tub, even for a moment.** The bathtub is a source of severe scalds and also poses a potential drowning hazard. If the telephone or doorbell rings, don't leave your child alone or in the care of another child, even for a moment.
11. Do you take your child on a boat?	**Always wear a Coast Guard-approved life jacket.** Everyone on the boat should wear a Coast Guard-approved life jacket. At least 1 adult swimmer should be present for each child who cannot swim. Use the AAP handout *Life Jackets and Life Preservers.*
12. Do you have a pool or hot tub where you live?	**Fence in your pool or hot tub on all 4 sides.** Drowning is the second leading cause of death of children nationally in this age group. Children most often drown when they fall into a pool that has not been completely fenced in on all 4 sides. Between 60% and 90% of drownings among children younger than 4 years occur in swimming pools.
13. Do you allow your child to swim unsupervised?	**Do not let children swim without supervision.** Never—not even for a moment—leave your children alone or in the care of another child in wading or swimming pools, spas, or other open standing water.

Bicycle Safety	Counseling Guidelines
14. Does your child ride on your bicycle with you?	**Use an approved child carrier.** Infants too young to sit in a rear bike seat should never be carried on a bicycle. Children 1 to 4 years of age who can wear a helmet may ride in a rear-mounted seat. Use of backpacks or frontpacks is not recommended. Parents should avoid riding in busy streets. With small children, falls frequently result in head injuries. Children should always wear a helmet that meets Consumer Product Safety Commission (CPSC) or Snell Memorial Foundation standards.

Auto Safety	Counseling Guidelines
15. How are your children restrained when they ride in a car?	**Children this age should always be properly restrained in a car safety seat. Select a car**

(continued)

Guidelines for Safety Counseling *(Continued)*

Counseling Guidelines From 1 to 4 Years (Part 2) (Continued)

Auto Safety	Counseling Guidelines
	safety seat that fits your child's size and weight and that can be installed properly in your car. Use it every time you are in the car. Remember that children should ride in car safety seats until they are about 4 years old and weigh about 40 pounds. Children who weigh from 40 pounds up to about 80 pounds (or until they are about 4 feet 9 inches tall) should ride in booster seats with lap/shoulder harnesses. Adults wearing seat belts are effective role models. Use the AAP brochure *Family Shopping Guide to Car Seats* for a list of car safety seats that meet federal standards.
16. Do you leave your child alone in the car?	**NEVER leave a child alone in a car.** Children and car keys should always be removed from the car and the car kept locked. In addition to the many dangers of leaving children alone in the car, death from excess heat may occur in warm weather in a closed car in a short time.
17. Where do you seat your children in the car?	**Seat a child in the rear seat of the car.** This is the safest place in the car. Never allow children to ride in the cargo area of a station wagon or truck.
18. Does your car have a passenger air bag?	**Never put children in front of passenger air bags.**
19. Do you lock the car doors before driving?	**Buckle up and lock up!** Before the car moves, all seat belts or child safety seats should be properly fastened and all doors should be locked.
20. Does your child play in the driveway or in or near the street?	**Young children should not play in driveways or near busy streets.** Parents should always walk behind the car before backing down a driveway. Children may not be seen in the rear view mirror and could be run over.

Toy Safety	Counseling Guidelines
21. Do you check your child's toys for safety hazards?	**Inspect toys for safety hazards.** Repair or discard broken toys. Inspect your child's toys for projectile and sharp parts or small detachable parts. Some toys may pose hazards from electric shock and burns. Toys intended for older children should not be accessible to toddlers and preschoolers. Follow age guidelines on toy packaging.

Guidelines for Safety Counseling *(Continued)*

Counseling Guidelines From 5 to 9 Years (Continued)

Firearm Hazards	Counseling Guidelines
1. Is there a gun in your home or the home where your child plays or is cared for?	**Do not keep guns in your home.** Guns, especially handguns, should be removed from the environments where children live and play. If firearms are in the home, they must be stored unloaded in a locked place and out of the reach of children. Guns are frequently involved in unintentional shootings in this age group, and homicides and suicides also occur. Parents should ask if the homes where their child visits or is cared for have guns and how they are stored.

Household Hazards	Counseling Guidelines
2. Do you let your child operate a power lawn mower?	**Never let children this age operate a lawn mower or ride with you on one.** Potential injury results from the machine itself and from objects thrown by the blade. Ride-on mowers are not recreational vehicles. Refer to the American Academy of Pediatrics (AAP) Safety Slip *Lawn Mower Safety.*
3. Have any of your children ever had any injuries requiring a visit to the doctor or hospital?	**Report any history of injuries to the pediatrician.** The pediatrician is able to explore the causes and discuss preventive measures. It has been shown that stressful family situations can be causally linked to repeated injuries in children (3 or more injuries needing medical attention within 12 months).
4. How frequently is the heating system checked in your home?	**Heating ventilation systems should be checked at least once a year.** This annual inspection helps prevent carbon monoxide poisoning, fires, and system malfunction.

Burns	Counseling Guidelines
5. Do you and your children know how to get out of your home safely in the event of a fire?	**Develop an escape plan in the event of a fire in the home.** Identify appropriate exit routes and a family meeting point away from the house. Do not use elevators in apartment buildings if there is a fire. Use the AAP handout *Protect Your Home Against Fire . . . Planning Saves Lives.*
6. Does anyone in your home ever smoke?	**A third of deaths due to home fires are caused by smoking.**

(continued)

Guidelines for Safety Counseling *(Continued)*

Counseling Guidelines From 5 to 9 Years (Continued)

Burns	Counseling Guidelines
	Smoking in bed or improper disposal of cigarette ashes or butts endangers children sleeping in adjacent rooms who may be trapped in the event of fire. Twelve percent of residential fires are associated with smoking.
7. Does your child play with matches or lighters?	**Do not let children play with fire.** Keep matches and lighters out of the sight and reach of children. They commonly ignite flammable materials, which may result in severe burns and house fires.
8. Do you have working fire extinguishers in your home?	**Buy a fire extinguisher for your home.** Extinguishers should be available in kitchens and in rooms with a furnace or fireplace.
9. Does your child play with firecrackers or sparklers?	**Do not let children play with fireworks.** Firecrackers and sparklers can cause serious burns and injuries and should not be played with by children. Bystanders often are seriously injured by fireworks as well. An estimated 10,000 injuries related to fireworks are reported annually to the U.S. Consumer Product Safety Commission (CPSC).
10. Do you have working smoke alarms in your home?	**Install smoke alarms in your home.** Most fire-related deaths are the result of inhaling smoke or toxic gas. There is a critical period of 4 minutes to get outside the home after the alarm sounds. Smoke detectors are recommended for each floor, but particularly for furnace and sleeping areas. Be sure to test the alarm monthly to be certain that it is working. Change the batteries every year.

Water Safety	Counseling Guidelines
11. Does your child know how to swim?	**Teach children how to swim.** Swimming is an important life skill that all children should acquire. However, even if children know how to swim, there are still hazards. They may not retain their swimming skills in an emergency; even competent young swimmers should not swim unsupervised.
12. Does your child know the rules of water and diving safety?	**Teach and enforce the rules of swimming and diving safety.** Drowning is the second most common cause of death in children of this age. Knowledge of swimming is not enough to prevent drowning. Children should swim in supervised areas only. The "buddy" system is desirable.

Guidelines for Safety Counseling *(Continued)*

Counseling Guidelines From 5 to 9 Years (Continued)

Water Safety	Counseling Guidelines
13. Does your child wear a life jacket when on a boat?	Teach your child to always enter the water feet first. Use the AAP handouts *Life Jackets and Life Preservers, Pool Safety for Children,* and *Water Safety for Your School-aged Child.* **Be sure your child wears a life jacket when on a boat.** Everyone on the boat should use a Coast Guard–approved life jacket. At least 1 adult swimmer should be present for each child who cannot swim.

Auto Safety	Counseling Guidelines
14. Does your child use a booster seat or seat belt when riding in the car?	**A booster seat should be used on every trip by all children who weigh from 40 pounds up to about 80 pounds (or until they are about 4 feet 9 inches tall). Seat belts should not be used until the lap belt can be worn low and flat on the hips and the shoulder belt can be worn across the shoulder rather than the face or neck.** Shoulder belts should be installed in the back seats of cars that do not have them.
15. Does your car have a passenger air bag?	**Never seat a child in front of a passenger air bag.**

Pedestrian Safety	Counseling Guidelines
16. Do your children cross the street by themselves?	**Teach your child pedestrian safety skills.** More than half of motor vehicle-related deaths in school-aged children are caused by pedestrian injuries. All children should learn safe street-crossing skills and should demonstrate those skills to the parent before supervision ends. Children will still require supervision when crossing the street. Parents often think their children are able to handle traffic safety by themselves, but most children don't have the skills to handle these risky situations until at least 10 years of age. Parents should be reminded that children • Often act before thinking and may not do what parents or drivers expect • May assume that if they see the driver, the driver sees them • Can't judge speed like adults • Are shorter than adults and can't see over cars, bushes, and other objects

(continued)

Guidelines for Safety Counseling *(Continued)*

Counseling Guidelines From 5 to 9 Years (Continued)

Pedestrian Safety	Counseling Guidelines
	• Need a place to play away from cars and the street

Bicycle Safety	Counseling Guidelines
17. Has your child learned about bicycle safety?	**Teach and enforce bicycle safety rules.** Bicycle crashes can result in serious injury and death. Children should not ride in the street at this age. They should ride on bike paths, in parks, or in protected areas. They should never ride after dark. Bicycles should be equipped with coaster brakes at this age because the child may not be developmentally ready to use hand brakes appropriately. Use the AAP handout *Safe Bicycling Starts Early.* The size of the bicycle should be appropriate for the child. Use the AAP handout, *Choosing the Right Size Bicycle for Your Child.*
18. Does your child wear a helmet every time he or she rides a bike?	**Wear a bicycle helmet.** All children should wear a bicycle helmet approved by the CPSC. Parents should set an example by wearing helmets when they ride bikes as well.

Recreational Safety	Counseling Guidelines
19. Does your child participate in sports?	**Wear protective gear during sports.** Despite safety measures such as protective padding and helmets, the risk of injury is present in all sports. Children should be made aware of the risks that go with the sports they play. The chance of injury becomes greater with the degree of contact in a sport. Football, wrestling, gymnastics, soccer, ice hockey, and track/running have the highest rates of injury. Lower leg (knee and ankle) injuries are the most common injuries in major sports. Children should not participate in boxing because of the high risk of brain damage. Many serious sports injuries could be prevented if players wore protective equipment, particularly head and eye protection. Parents should encourage the use of such gear and teach their children that wearing protective gear increases the long-term enjoyment of the sport. If your child uses a scooter, skateboard, or rollerblades, a helmet, knee and elbow pads, and wrist guards should be worn. Use the AAP brochure *Sports and Your Child.*

Guidelines for Safety Counseling *(Continued)*

Counseling Guidelines From 5 to 9 Years (Continued)

Recreational Safety	Counseling Guidelines
20. Does your child participate in horseback riding?	**All children should wear an approved equestrian helmet when riding a horse.** All horseback riding activities should be supervised by an adult.

Counseling Guidelines From 10 to 12 Years

Firearm Hazards	Counseling Guidelines
1. Is there a gun in your home or any of your friends' homes?	**Do not play with guns!** More than 300 children die each year of unintentional gunshot wounds. BB guns and paint pellet guns often cause severe eye injuries. Air rifles are dangerous weapons that can kill.

Burns	Counseling Guidelines
2. Do you have working smoke alarms in your home?	**Check to see that your home has a smoke alarm.** Most fire-related deaths are the result of inhaling smoke or toxic gas. There is a critical period of 4 minutes to get outside the home after the alarm sounds. Smoke alarms are recommended for each floor, but particularly for furnace and sleeping areas. You should know appropriate exit routes and a family meeting point away from the house.

Bicycle Safety	Counseling Guidelines
3. Do you ever ride with passengers on your bike?	**Never ride with passengers on your bike.** This may impair your stability and visibility and lead to an injury.
4. Do you wear a helmet when you ride your bike?	**Always wear a helmet when riding a bike.** This protects you from head injury. Use the American Academy of Pediatrics (AAP) handout *Safe Bicycling Starts Early.*

Auto Safety	Counseling Guidelines
5. Do you wear a seat belt in the car?	**Buckle up.** Seat belts save lives and should be used by all children. Remind your parents to buckle up as well.
6. Do you ride in cars that have passenger air bags?	Do not sit in front of a passenger air bag. The safest place for children to ride is in the back seat.
7. Where do you sit in the car?	The safest place for you to ride is in the back seat, buckled up.

(continued)

Guidelines for Safety Counseling *(Continued)*

Counseling Guidelines From 10 to 12 Years (Continued)

Pedestrian Safety	Counseling Guidelines
8. When you want to cross the street, what is the first thing you should always do?	**Follow safety rules when crossing the street.** • Always stop at the curb, roadside, or at the outside edge of a parked car. • Always look left–right–left before entering the area of the road in which cars travel, even if a traffic light says "walk." • If a car is coming, wait until it passes and look left–right–left again. • Proceed to cross the street only when the road is clear.

Water Safety	Counseling Guidelines
9. When playing near water (for example, rivers, ponds, lakes, oceans), is it OK to play alone?	**Never play near water without an adult nearby.** Even if children can swim, they should never play unsupervised near bodies of water into which they may fall because they may not retain their swimming skills in an emergency. Water conditions (rapids, tides) may overwhelm otherwise capable swimmers.

Farm Safety	Counseling Guidelines
10. Do you live or work on a farm?	**Farm equipment is very dangerous to children.** Parents may need to be counseled for this question.

*Safety sheets can be obtained from The Injury Prevention Program (TIPP) of the American Academy of Pediatrics (AAP).

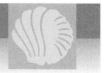

Chapter 3

Adolescent Medicine

Elizabeth M. Alderman and
Warren M. Seigel

Adolescence, from the beginning of puberty until early adulthood, is a time of accelerated physical growth and maturity coincident with significant psychosocial and cognitive development. The chronologic boundaries of adolescence are roughly defined as between the ages of 12 and 21 years. Although most adolescents are healthy, an estimated 6% have chronic illnesses that limit daily activity such as diabetes, cancer or other hematologic disorders, development disabilities, mental retardation, and asthma. However, the leading causes of morbidity and mortality in this age group are not these chronic conditions but rather injuries, homicide, and suicide, as well as the sequelae of early sexual activity and substance use.

This chapter contains a description of the physical and psychologic changes that occur during puberty. Following this is a discussion of several issues of importance during adolescence—violence, suicidal behavior, substance abuse, eating disorders, and sexual activity. The second part of the chapter addresses the special health concerns of adolescent athletes. Participation in sports, both individually, community-based or on school teams, provide young adults with a healthy venue to develop both physical and psychosocial skills.

ADOLESCENT PHYSICAL GROWTH AND DEVELOPMENT

The stages identified by J.M. Tanner are traditionally used to describe physical growth and development of the genitalia and secondary sexual characteristics of adolescents. Tanner stages describe female breast and pubic hair development (Figures 3.1 and 3.2 as well as male genitalia and pubic hair growth (Figure 3.3).

Girls

The earliest sign of puberty in girls is the appearance of the breast bud (thelarche), which may normally occur as young as 8 years of age.

In fact, the average age of breast development has decreased over the past century. In the United States, Tanner 2 breast development occurs at about 9.9 years of age in Caucasian girls and 8.8 years of age in African-American girls. Subsequent breast development involves further enlargement of the areola and breast (Tanner 3), appearance of the secondary mound (Tanner 4), and the mature female breast (Tanner 5). Simultaneous changes in the distribution of pubic hair occur, beginning with a sparse amount of long hair over the labia majora (Tanner 2), and progressing to darker, curlier, coarser hair (Tanner 3). Then, most of the mons pubis is covered with pubic hair (Tanner 4), and finally, an adult pattern of pubic hair (Tanner 5) is apparent. Breast development may take up to 4 years and pubic hair growth up to 2.5 years. Many fully mature women have Tanner 4 breast development or pubic hair.

The average age of menarche, which is approximately 12.8 years for Caucasian girls and 12.16 years for African-American girls, coincides with at least Tanner 4 breast and pubic hair development. In girls, the growth spurt usually occurs approximately 6 months before menarche and is coincident with the end of the Tanner 3 stage, a year after breast development begins. The peak of the growth spurt usually precedes menarche (Figure 3.4).

Boys

Physical maturity usually occurs approximately 6 months later in boys than in girls. The first signs of puberty are testicular and scrotal enlargement (Tanner 1 to Tanner 2), which occur at an average age of 11.5 years. Within a year of these changes, the penile length begins to increase (Tanner 3). Further growth of the testes and scrotum occurs, with increased scrotal rugae and penile diameter (Tanner 4) and eventually adult-size testicles (approximately 22 ml) and

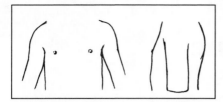

Stage 1 Perpubertal: Elevation of papilla only.

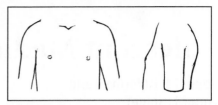

Stage 2 Breast bud: Areola widens. Elevation of small mound of subareolar tissue and erect papilla.

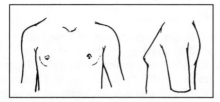

Stage 3 Continued enlargement of breasts and widening of areola, but without separation of contours.

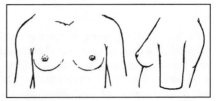

Stage 4 Areola and papilla separate from the contour of the breast forming a secondary mound.

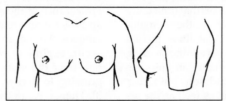

Stage 5 Mature female breast with areola and breast in same plane, erect papilla.

FIGURE 3.1. Tanner stages of female breast development.

Stage 1 No pubic hair.

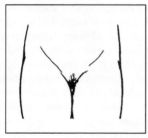

Stage 2 A sparse amount of long, somewhat pigmented hair over labia majora primarily.

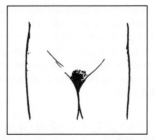

Stage 3 Pubic hair darkens, coarsens and curls, and spreads sparsely over the mons pubis.

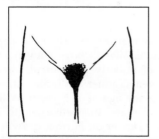

Stage 4 Abundant, coarse, adult-type hair limited to the mons pubis.

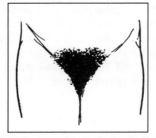

Stage 5 Adult-type and quantity of hair with spread to the medial aspect of the thighs.

FIGURE 3.2. Tanner stages of female pubic hair growth.

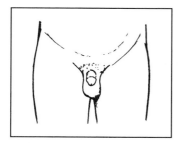

Stage 2 Sparse growth of long, slightly pigmented hair, at and lateral to base of penis. Testes and scrotum begin to enlarge, with pigmentation and thinning of scrotum.

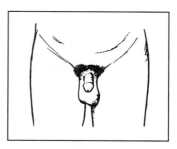

Stage 3 Pubic hair darkens, coarsens and curls, at and lateral to base of penis. Penis lengthens and scrotum further enlarge.

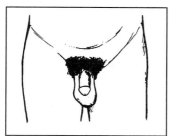

Stage 4 Abundant, coarse, adult-type hair limited to the pubic region with no extension to the thighs. Further growth of testes and scrotum, with increased pigmentation of scrotum, and increase in width and length of penis.

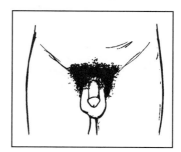

Stage 5 Adult-type and quantity of hair with spread to the medial aspects of the thighs. Adult size and shape of genitalia.

FIGURE 3.3. Tanner stages of male genital development and pubic hair growth.

penis (Tanner 5). Simultaneous changes in the distribution of pubic hair occur, with growth beginning at the base of the penis (Tanner 2) and progressing to darker, coarser hair (Tanner 3). The hair then covers a much larger area (Tanner 4) and finally assumes an adult pattern (Tanner 5), which is usually attained by ages 14–16 (Figure 3.5).

The growth spurt in boys is usually coincident with Tanner 4 development of genitalia. On average, the growth spurt begins at approximately 11.5 years of age and is complete by 13–17 years. Nocturnal emissions or wet dreams are first noticed at Tanner 3. Change of voice usually occurs between Tanner 3 and 4 (see Figure 3.5).

Axillary hair development in boys begins at the same time as Tanner 4 development of pubic hair. One year later, facial hair develops and starts at the corners of the upper lip and spreads medially. Hair growth on the upper cheek, lower lip, and chin follows. Chest hair growth is a post-pubertal event.

ADOLESCENT PSYCHOSOCIAL AND COGNITIVE DEVELOPMENT

Adolescence is a time not only of rapid physical growth and maturational changes but also a period of behavioral metamorphosis; children who once relied solely on their parents and followed their wishes developed into autonomous adults who are now capable of making their own choices. The in-between period is marked by changes in body image, emergence of strong peer group influence, risk-taking behaviors, and the development of an adult pattern of sexuality and personal values. When discussing cognitive and psychosocial development, it is best to divide adolescence into early (12–14 years of age or junior high), middle (15–17 years of age or high school), and late (18–21 years of age or college and/or employment) stages.

Early adolescence is characteristically a period of egocentricity. Experiencing rapid physical changes, adolescents wonder, "Am I normal?" and are very self-conscious. The peer

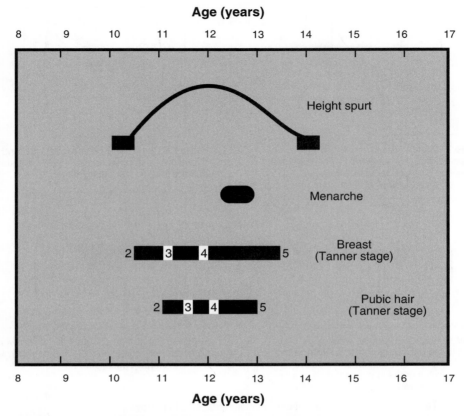

FIGURE 3.4. A summary of physical growth and development in girls, showing the sequence of pubertal events for average American girl.

group is also very important at this stage, with the opinions of friends being just as, if not more important than, those of parents. This is the stage during which adolescents begin to behave independently and require a greater degree of privacy. Risk-taking behavior is likely as young adolescents try to establish independence and ensure peer approval. Cognitively, early adolescents still rely on concrete thinking and have difficulty conceptualizing the future well.

Middle adolescence is the stage of greatest turmoil. At this time, conflicts with parents are often most prevalent. During middle adolescence, teenagers may feel immortal and omnipotent, thus contributing to risk-taking behavior. Dating same or opposite sex and romantic relationships with the opposite sex and the onset of sexual activity often begin at this time. The peer group remains important. Middle adolescents have a greater sense of self and are less preoccupied with pubertal changes. During this stage, adolescents acquire the beginnings of abstract thinking and can make decisions based on formal operational thought. Middle adolescents are frequently able to view global issues intelligently and can relate to the feelings of others.

Late adolescence is marked by separation from parents with an appreciation of parental values but with the distinct emergence of personal values. There is comfort with body image and the development of a full sense of self-identity. Cognitively, late adolescents have the ability to conceptualize and verbalize their thoughts fully, appreciate the ramifications of their actions, weigh alternatives in making decisions, and plan future vocational and educational goals. Issues of emancipation are very important and are the final tasks of adolescence. Older adolescents must learn to live on their own and become emotionally and economically self-sufficient.

MORTALITY IN ADOLESCENTS

The three leading causes of death in adolescence are all **behavioral: injury, homicide,** and **suicide.** Malignancy, the leading physical cause of

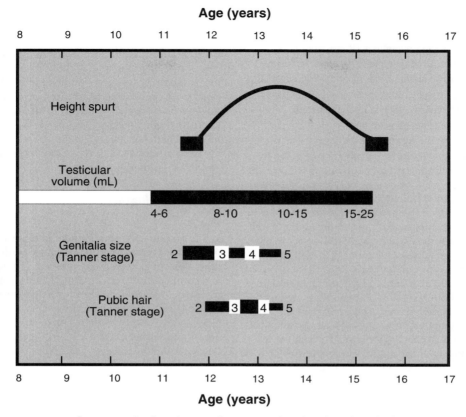

FIGURE 3.5. Sequence of pubertal events for average American boy. A testicular volume of less than 4 ml as determined by an orchidometer (Prader beads) represents the prepubertal stage.

death, finishes a distant fourth to these behavioral issues. Many, if not most, violent deaths are intertwined with issues of personal and family dysfunction and do not occur as isolated events.

INJURY OR HOMICIDE

Accidents are the leading cause of death in adolescents. Nearly 60% of all adolescent deaths are due to accidents and unintentional injuries. Boys are more at risk of accidents and injuries than girls. Older adolescents are more likely to die from motor vehicle injuries, while younger adolescents are at greatest risk for drowning and injurious death with weapons. Many of these injuries occur while teenagers are under the influence of alcohol. The combination of youthful drinking, learning to drive, risk-taking behaviors, and feelings of immortality all contribute to the exceedingly high rate of morbidity and mortality associated with automotive collisions.

Homicide is the second leading cause of death in adolescents. It accounts for 11.6 deaths/100,000 teenagers, with the rate for African Americans 20 times higher than it is for Caucasians. High rates of homicide relate directly to the accessibility of guns; 9% of boys and 1% of girls in high school say they carry a gun. Many more have access to guns on a regular basis. Half of homicide victims know their assailant, and the fatal event usually occurs during an argument.

Clinical Evaluation: History

Taking a comprehensive psychosocial history from adolescents entails assurance of confidentiality in most circumstances. Exceptions involve circumstances in which the life of a particular adolescent or another person may be in danger or reports of alleged physical, sexual, or emotional abuse by a parent or relative.

The **HEADSSS** mnemonic (**H**ome, **E**ducation, **A**ctivities, **D**rugs/alcohol/cigarettes, **S**exuality, **S**uicide, **S**exual/physical/emotional abuse) may be used to help remember the important aspects of the psychosocial history that must be discussed with adolescents.

To evaluate adolescents for risk of death from injury, it is important to inquire about risk-taking behaviors and a history of previous accidents or injuries. Questions about drug and alcohol use, which may put them in jeopardy, are appropriate in younger adolescents, and inquires about substance abuse and driving habits necessary in older adolescents. Questions about seat belt use (i.e., personal and family use) and possession of weapons are also important. The clinician should inquire about access to weapons, and whether the teenager has ever witnessed a murder or a shooting, and whether he belongs to a gang. Again, the key is anticipatory guidance. By asking these questions, while assessing the degree of risk to a particular teenager, the examiner can educate the adolescent about the dangers of weapons and the real possibility of getting caught in the line of fire.

Management

When working with adolescents who are at risk for injuries, **it is important not to scold, lecture, or be judgmental.** The physician should educate teenagers by providing anticipatory guidance about seat belt use and the risks of drinking and driving. Adolescents should realize the importance of assigning a designated driver whenever going out with friends and of providing for a safe ride home. Emphasis of the importance of seat belt use in automobiles and helmet use when riding a bicycle, motorcycle, scooter, or minibike is critical. It is essential to encourage adolescents to steer clear of weapons and discuss alternatives for dealing with violence and confrontation. The health care provider should also speak to the parents of adolescents about the hazards of weapons in the home and emphasize strategies for addressing drinking and driving.

SUICIDE

Suicide is the third leading cause of death in adolescents. In the past 30 years, the rate of suicide among teenagers has tripled. Among high school students, 25% of girls and 14% of boys have seriously considered suicide or made a suicide attempt. Girls are more likely to attempt suicide, but the outcome in boys is five times more likely to be fatal. Girls are more likely to ingest medicines, and boys are more likely to use violent means such as weapons and hanging. Adolescents with preexisting psychiatric problems and those who abuse drugs and alcohol are more likely to attempt suicide. Young adolescents may not be able to conceptualize the consequences of a suicide attempt and may not have other coping strategies for their problems.

Clinical Evaluation

History
When taking a history, **the goal is identification of the risk factors** for suicide. Many adolescents who attempt suicide are depressed. Often, there is a conflict with parents, friends, or a romantic interest. Educational or legal problems may be a cause. If any of these situations exist, the physician should explore them further. Questions about depressive symptoms such as loss of appetite, anhedonia, sleep disturbance (too much or too little), and feelings of hopelessness or helplessness are important. It may be appropriate to ask teenagers whether they have ever thought about hurting themselves, have a suicide plan, or have ever attempted suicide, especially if they required medical attention. When asking adolescents about peers, suicide attempts on the part of friends can be a topic of discussion. Questions about substance abuse, which decreases judgment, increases impulsivity, and affects mood, thus aggravating the risk of attempting suicide, are also necessary.

Family health history is very important. Mental illness or alcohol or substance abuse in the family should alert the clinician to the possibility of depression and suicidal ideation.

Physical Examination
Few signs on physical examination point to the risk of suicide. Weight changes may occur with depression. The physician should look for any scars, especially on the wrists, that may have been due to a previous suicide attempt or physical abuse. Description of the physical signs of various drug ingestions is discussed in Chapter 23.

Management

Prevention is the key to management of suicide. The goal of prevention is identification of those adolescents who are at risk for suicide (see

HISTORY). If a particular adolescent is deemed to be at risk, other health professionals should be consulted—a social worker experienced in working with teenagers and a child psychiatrist or psychologist. The physician needs to involve family and all other significant adults in counseling.

Pediatric Pearl

All adolescents who attempt suicide *must* be hospitalized.

Hospitalization not only provides a "cooling off" period for teenagers but also allows the physician to determine the best course of treatment while the adolescents are in a safe environment where any further suicide attempt can be prevented. When adolescents are admitted to the hospital for attempted suicide, the physician must determine why it happened and decide, in conjunction with mental health professionals, the best course of treatment, whether outpatient counseling (individual, family) or inpatient psychiatric hospitalization. If a particular adolescent requires medication for major depression or psychosis, it will be initiated during the hospitalization. It should be pointed out that adolescents who have survived a suicide attempt have the greatest risk for death from suicide.

CAUSES OF MORBIDITY IN ADOLESCENTS

The major causes of morbidity in adolescents are substance abuse and sexual activity. In addition, eating disorders such as anorexia nervosa and bulimia nervosa, which have their onset during adolescence, are a source of significant psychologic and physical morbidity.

Adolescents experiment with drugs and develop sexual identity as part of their psychosocial and cognitive development. However, these behaviors put teenagers in jeopardy of accidents, injuries, violence, pregnancy, and acquiring sexually transmitted infection (STI), including human immunodeficiency virus (HIV). The physician helps identify those teenagers involved with substance abuse and who are sexually active, which involves exploring why they are putting themselves at risk. Intervention should then occur to prevent the morbidity.

SUBSTANCE ABUSE

The majority of adolescents, who are well adjusted, have experimented with cigarettes and alcohol, the most commonly used substances. Cigarette smoking, which often begins in middle school, is on the rise. In the most recent survey of high school students, over 70% have ever tried cigarettes; 25% smoke one or more cigarettes per day. White girls are the largest group to begin smoking and continue the practice. Surveys of high school seniors demonstrate that approximately 88% have tried alcohol.

Such surveys also indicate that 58% of high school seniors have tried marijuana. Many teenagers use drugs only on an intermittent basis, and drug use interferes with peer and family relationships in only a small minority of adolescents. Younger teenagers do not have the ability to link current behavior to long-term consequences and are more concerned about peer acceptance. Because these adolescents are not cognitively mature, they may make errors in judgment even while merely experimenting. Situations in which intoxication is associated with particular risk include sexual activity, violent behavior, delinquent behavior, transient depression that may lead to a suicide attempt, and, certainly, driving automobiles.

Clinical and Laboratory Evaluation

History

The mainstay of determining whether adolescents are on a collision course with substance use is obtaining a thorough history.

Pediatric Pearl

The clinician who is evaluating adolescents should interview teenagers and parents separately.

The goal of the physician is gaining the trust of both adolescents and parents and ensuring confidentiality of the teenagers. Adolescents respect the physician's knowledge and authority as long as this trusted adult is a good listener who can maintain confidentiality.

Talking to children and parents about drug use should begin at yearly health care maintenance visits at about age 10 years; surveys of high school seniors reveal that 24% had tried alcohol before age 13. Questions about what types of drugs are used and settings of usage are appropriate. The physician should also try to assess the degree of intoxication to determine whether drug use has ever put the teenager at risk. It is important to ask about drug use in friends and parents, because this may be the only way to determine the teenager's risk of beginning drug use.

School progress serves as an important clue to the possibility of drug use. Attendance problems or any decline in grades may suggest substance abuse as an etiology. Changes in family relationships (divorce, death) or disruption of the peer group (new neighborhood, breakup with a romantic interest) may lead to substance use. Questions about sexual activity or delinquent behavior are appropriate. Studies have shown the existence of a problem behavior syndrome (i.e., in many teenagers, risky behaviors are clustered).

As noted previously, it is important to screen for depression. Drug abuse may be a result of depression or a cause of it. Mood swings may also be due to drugs or an underlying psychologic problem that predisposes the adolescent to substance use.

When talking to parents, it is a good idea to ask about family relationships and if the teenager is stealing money, has sold possessions, has undesirable friends, or has had overt signs of drug use or intoxication. However, it is important to weigh the information ascertained from the parent against that obtained from the teenager.

Physical Examination

The findings on physical examination that indicate substance abuse are subtle and are most often only found in seriously addicted teenagers. In general, the physical examination is not of help in detecting previously unsuspected substance abuse. The clinician is most dependent on information gathered by history to suggest potential physiologic consequences of specific drugs.

Laboratory Evaluation

Either urine or blood may be screened for drug metabolites. Urine tests can identify cocaine, methadone, amphetamines, diazepam, opiates, and barbiturates. Blood tests or a breath alcohol test can detect only alcohol.* It is relatively easy to detect illicit substances in body fluids such as blood or urine, but drug testing in adolescents is controversial. At the center of this controversy is the belief that surreptitious testing is unethical and destroys the trusting physician–adolescent relationship. The American Academy of Pediatrics (AAP) condones such drug testing only if the particular adolescent is mentally incompetent to make an informed decision or the life of the adolescent is in danger.

Management

Management of adolescents who use drugs must address not only the drug abuse itself but also the reasons for the abuse. If an individual teenager is merely experimenting with alcohol or marijuana in a social setting and it is not interfering with school, family, peers, or cognitive growth, then anticipatory guidance is important. It is also imperative to point out that even experimentation may place adolescents in risky situations, and the physician should help teenagers modify behavior so they avoid intoxication, do not drink while driving, or use a designated driver. In younger teenagers, the clinician should stress postponement of drug experimentation.

If it is determined that a teenager has a serious drug abuse problem—he is displaying signs of physical or psychologic dependence or that drug use is interfering with normal adolescent development—initiation of treatment is essential. The primary care physician may offer this treatment alone or in consultation with a mental health professional with drug abuse expertise. Alternatively, referral to an ambulatory drug treatment program may be appropriate. Family therapy may be necessary, and peer support such as Alcoholics Anonymous is sometimes of help. However, if a teenager requires medically supervised treatment for an abstinence syndrome, has a less-than-optimal family environment, has an underlying psychiatric illness, or has not responded to outpatient therapy, then inpatient therapy or residential treatment is indicated.

There are two types of residential treatment: (1) an adolescent drug treatment unit in a hospital, and (2) a nonmedical therapeutic community. Selection among these alternatives is usually best left to a clinician with special expertise in drug abuse. The AAP has developed guidelines for assisting in the determination of the most appropriate treatment modality for a particular patient.

SEXUAL ACTIVITY

Close to 50% of high school students have been sexually active; 61% of all male students and 48% of all female students are nonvirgins. The health risks of early sexual activity are unwanted pregnancy and STIs such as syphilis, gonorrhea,

---

Use of alcohol can only be detected in a clinical setting by a blood test. The breathalyzer test is only utilized in a law enforcement setting.

chlamydia, and HIV. In the past 20 years, the morbidities associated with sexual activity have increased in adolescents. Close to 1 million adolescent girls become pregnant each year, and 25% of all sexually active teenagers acquire an STI. The physician must identify those adolescents at risk for the consequences of early sexual activity and, if the adolescent is sexually active, provide options for effective contraception.

Clinical and Laboratory Evaluation

History

Beginning at 8 years of age, the physician should inquire about sexuality and discuss the impending body changes of puberty with children and parents. Not only does this establish a trusting, open relationship between physicians and children, but it also encourages the parents to talk to their children about sex. As children reach adolescence, the physician should ask whether they are attracted to the opposite or the same sex, how this attraction is expressed, and whether they are sexually active. It is also important to ask whether their peers are having sex, because this is a predictor of the teenagers' behavior.

Pediatric Pearl

Young adolescents who abuse drugs, are delinquent, or are having problems in school are more likely to become sexually active.

TABLE 3.1 What to Ask Adolescents Regarding Sexual Activity

Ask adolescents whether they are **sexually active.** If so:
- Ask about the number of current and lifetime partners.
- Ask what they are doing to prevent pregnancy (i.e., if any form of contraception is used).
- Ask girls about the presence of any unusual vaginal discharge, and ask boys about any dysuria or penile discharge.
- Inquire about any lesions in the pubic area.
- Ask whether there has been any previous sexually transmitted infection or pregnancy.

Always ask adolescent girls whether they **menstruate.** If so:
- Ask about the date of their last menses.
- Ask whether the interval between it and the previous menses and the duration were usual.

More detailed questions should follow (Table 3.1). It is also important to ask whether a teenager has ever experienced physical or sexual abuse, because this may predispose her to early sexual activity and promiscuity.

Physical Examination

Sexually active adolescents require a more involved physical examination than non–sexually active teenagers. For all boys, a thorough testicular examination looking for lesions and masses is imperative. Penile lesions or discharge and inguinal adenopathy, if present, must be noted especially in sexually active boys. The physician should provide instructions concerning testicular self-examination. For girls, a complete pelvic examination, including a speculum examination to visualize the cervix and vaginal mucosa for lesions, discharge, and friability, is necessary. Cervical tests for gonorrhea and chlamydia, as well as a Papanicolaou smear, are performed simultaneously. A bimanual examination allows for assessment of uterine size, if pregnancy is suspected, as well as the cervical motion tenderness associated with salpingitis. An abdominal examination reveals a gravid uterus if the pregnancy is over 4 months. It is also important to note the presence of adnexal masses or tenderness.

Laboratory Evaluation

All sexually active adolescents require yearly syphilis screening. Sexually active girls require yearly Papanicolaou smears to detect cervical cancer, evidence of human papillomavirus infection, and cervicitis. Cervical gonorrhea and chlamydia tests should also occur yearly, if girls are symptomatic, or if they have a new partner. In girls with a vaginal discharge, a wet prep (mixture of the discharge with normal saline or potassium hydroxide viewed under a microscope) may help distinguish yeast vaginitis, bacterial vaginosis, trichomoniasis, and cervicitis (Table 3.2). In teenagers with multiple partners, all STI screenings should occur more frequently—certainly if the adolescent is symptomatic.

Boys require a urinalysis. Pyuria or positive test for leukocyte esterase on first-void urine is associated with sexually acquired urethritis. The existence of pyuria or penile discharge requires tests for gonorrhea and chlamydia as well as treatment for presumptive urethritis.

If vaginal or penile lesions are suggestive of herpes infection, performance of a Tzanck test and culture of the lesion is necessary. If pregnancy is suspected, measurement of β-human chorionic gonadotropin (β-HCG) level is important. Serum

TABLE 3.2 Findings on Wet Prep	
Infection	**Appearance**
Monilia (yeast) vaginitis	Hyphae, buds (revealed best by adding KOH)
Bacterial vaginosis	Clue cells (epithelial cells with cytoplasmic studding)
Trichomoniasis	Trichomonads
Cervicitis	Multiple white blood cells

KOH = potassium hydroxide.

β-HCG may be positive even before the occurrence of a missed menstrual period. Testing for HIV may be appropriate for adolescents with risk factors such as male homosexual activity, unprotected sexual intercourse, intravenous drug use, or any symptoms of HIV infection. HIV testing should be available to all adolescents who are diagnosed with STIs. In addition, all sexually active adolescents should receive the immunization series to protect against hepatitis B. If not previously immunized, all adolescents should receive Hepatitis B immunizations.

Management

Sexually Transmitted Infections (STIs)

Most STIs respond to drug therapy (Table 3.3). Making the diagnosis of an STI should be the springboard to talking to the teenager about the risks and consequences of unprotected sex and the need to use condoms for prevention of STIs as well as pregnancy.

Pediatric Pearl

Adolescents who are diagnosed with STIs are legally entitled to confidential care in all 50 states.

Concurrent treatment of the sexual partner is mandatory. The clinician should test for cure for gonorrhea or chlamydia infection 2 weeks after the cessation of therapy. Preferably, adolescent girls who are diagnosed with acute salpingitis should be admitted to the hospital for intravenous antibiotics for two reasons: (1) the risk of noncompliance with medications, and (2) the consequences of partially treated salpingitis, which are tubo-ovarian abscess, adhesions, and future infertility.

Pregnancy

Of the more than 1 million girls who become pregnant yearly in the United States, one-third are younger than 15 years; two-thirds of these pregnancies are unintentional. One-half of these girls continue the pregnancy to term, slightly fewer elect termination, and the rest experience miscar-

riages or stillbirths. Adolescent pregnancy is associated with a greater risk of complications, including low birth weight and maternal health and nutritional problems. The consequences of adolescent parenthood are unstable family formation and decreased chances of completing education.

The clinician should discuss the options available to pregnant girls in a developmentally appropriate way, usually with the assistance of a social worker or options counselor. If teenagers decide to continue the pregnancy, then early initiation of prenatal care, preferably in a teen pregnancy program, is mandatory. After the delivery, or if the pregnancy is terminated, a currently available contraceptive method must be initiated to prevent future pregnancies (Table 3.4). Girls who are sexually active may benefit from the oral contraceptive pill or injectable progestins, which are effective in preventing pregnancy. However, only barrier methods such as condoms prevent STIs, so concurrent condom use is usually recommended. Consideration of hormonal contraceptive options is appropriate when counseling teenagers. Clinicians may prescribe contraception confidentially in most jurisdictions (Table 3.5).

EATING DISORDERS

Eating disorders are another cause of morbidity and, sometimes, mortality in adolescents. Anorexia nervosa, which occurs in 0.5% of adolescent girls, is distinct from bulimia nervosa, which occurs in 1%–3% of this population. Each illness stems from an abnormal body image. The *Diagnostic and Statistical Manual of Mental Disorders*, 4th ed. (DSM-IV) defines the criteria for diagnosis of these two illnesses (Table 3.6).

Pathophysiology

Anorexia nervosa and bulimia nervosa affect almost every organ system. Vomiting, at times induced by ipecac, laxative abuse, or limited intake in order to lose weight causes abnormalities of fluids and electrolytes. These electrolyte imbalances, which may be life threatening, may be the first

TABLE 3.3	Treatment of Sexually Transmitted Infections
Infection	**Treatment**
Gonorrhea, cervicitis, urethritis	Ceftriaxone 125 mg IM single dose *or* Cefixime 400 mg PO single dose *or* Ciprofloxacin 500 mg PO single dose *or* Ofloxacin 400 mg PO single dose
Chlamydia trachomatis, cervicitis, urethritis	Azithromycin 1 g PO single dose *or* Doxycycline 100 mg PO bid × 7 days *or* Erythromycin 500 mg qid × 7 days **(if pregnant)**
Trichomoniasis	Metronidazole 2 g PO single dose
Bacterial vaginosis	Metronidazole 500 mg PO × 7 days *or* Clindamycin cream 2%, 1 applicator intravaginally qhs × 7 days *or* Metronidazole gel 0.75%, 1 applicator intravaginally bid × 5 days
Vulvovaginal candidiasis	Topical clotrimazole, miconazole, terconazole, or nystatin at varying doses
Chancroid	Azithromycin 1 g PO single dose *or* Erythromycin 500 mg PO qid × 7 days *or* Ceftriaxone 250 mg IM single dose
Lymphogranuloma venereum	Doxycycline 100 mg PO bid × 21 days *or* Erythromycin base 500 mg PO qid × 21 days **(if pregnant)**
Syphilis	
Early (primary, secondary, < 1 year duration)	Penicillin G benzathine 2.4 million U IM single dose *or* Doxycycline 100 mg bid × 2 weeks
Late (> 1 year duration)	Penicillin G benzathine 2.4 million U IM weekly × 3 *or* Doxycycline 100 mg PO bid × 3 weeks
Neurosyphilis	Penicillin G 2.4 million U IV q4hr × 10–14 days
Epididymitis	Ceftriaxone 250 mg IM × single dose *plus* Azithromycin 1 g PO × single dose *or* Doxycycline 100 mg PO × 10 days

Pelvic inflammatory disease	As inpatient:
	    Cefoxitin 2 g IV q6hr *plus*
	    Doxycycline 100 mg PO bid × 14 days *or*
	    Erythromycin 500 mg PO qid × 14 days
	As outpatient:
	    Ofloxacin 400 mg bid × 14 days *plus*
	    Metronidazole 500 mg × 14 days *or*
	    Ceftriaxone 250 mg IM × 1 *plus*
	    Doxycycline 100 mg PO × 14 days

Herpes simplex	
First episode	Acyclovir 200 mg PO 5/day × 7–10 days *or* Acyclovir 400 mg PO tid × 7–10 days *or* Famciclovir 250 mg PO tid × 7–10 days
Prophylaxis	Acyclovir 400 mg bid *or* Famciclovir 250 mg bid *or* Valacyclovir 500 mg qd
Recurrent episode	Acyclovir 400 mg tid × 5 days *or* 200 mg 5/day × 5 days *or* 800 mg bid × 5 days Famciclovir 125 mg bid × 5 days *or* Valacyclovir 500 mg bid × 5 days

IM = intramuscularly; IV = intravenously; PO = orally; qd = every day; bid = two times per day; tid = three times per day; qid = four times per day; qhs = at night; q6hr = every 6 hours.

presentation of an eating disorder. Hyponatremia may be secondary to water intoxication in teenagers attempting to escape detection through rapid weight gain. Hypokalemia with a hypochloremic metabolic alkalosis occurs with vomiting. The hypokalemia develops with chloride and water depletion, leading to secondary hyperaldosteronism, and increases potassium excretion with sodium retention. Calcium, zinc, and magnesium deficiencies also occur. Starvation causes

TABLE 3.4 Effectiveness of Contraceptive Options for Adolescents

Method	Typical Failure Rate (%)
Condoms	12
Diaphragm	18
Cervical cap	18
Chance	85
Spermicide	21
Periodic abstinence	20
Withdrawal	18
Pill	
Combined	3
Progestogen only	0.5
Injectable progestogen	0.3
DMPA	
Implants: Norplant	0.04

DMPA = depot medroxyprogesterone acetate.

ketonuria and lower blood urea nitrogen (BUN) than expected, resulting from decreased muscle mass.

Cardiovascular symptoms are usually precipitated by electrolyte disorders. Prolonged QT interval on electrocardiography (ECG), which results from hypokalemia, can cause sudden death. Hypotension and bradycardia occur as a result of decreased blood volume. In addition, ipecac may cause a cardiomyopathy.

Amenorrhea may result from a disturbed hypothalamic pituitary axis, presumably secondary to malnutrition. Hypoestrogenism and hypercortisolism in anorexia nervosa decrease bone mineral density, leading to osteoporosis.

Iron deficiency may develop in anorexia nervosa as the result of malnutrition. Frequent vomiting may cause reflux esophagitis, Mallory-Weiss tears of the esophagus, parotid gland enlargement, and tooth decay from enamel erosion. Constipation resulting from decreased intestinal motility is a hallmark of anorexia nervosa. This may also cause abdominal cramps and lead to increased laxative use.

Clinical and Laboratory Evaluation

History
When interviewing all adolescents, the physician should inquire about daily diet and exercise routine. Teenagers should also describe their mood, because many individuals with eating disorders have depressive symptoms. Menstrual patterns should be a topic of inquiry in girls.

TABLE 3.5 Hormonal Contraception

Contraceptive Agent	How It Works	Possible Side Effects	Contraindications
Combined oral contraception (estrogen/progestin)	Inhibits ovulation Thickens cervical mucus Inhibits implantation	Spotting/breakthrough bleeding Amenorrhea Mood changes Weight change Headaches	Gallbladder disease Hepatic adenoma Active liver disease, including active mononucleosis Hypertension Pregnancy Breast cancer Estrogen-dependent neoplasia Liver tumor, cancer Previous thromboembolic event or cerebrovascular accident Ischemic heart disease Unexplained vaginal bleeding
Norplant (levonorgestrel) implant	Suppresses ovulation for 5 years	Visible implants Spotting Amenorrhea Headache	Pregnancy Allergic reaction to components Same as oral contraception
Depo-Provera (medroxyprogesterone acetate)	Injection suppresses ovulation for 12 weeks	Pain of injection every 3 months Irregular bleeding Amenorrhea Mood changes Headache Weight gain Osteoporosis	Pregnancy Allergic reaction to components Same as oral contraceptive pills

TABLE 3.6 Criteria for Diagnosis of Anorexia Nervosa and Bulimia Nervosa

ANOREXIA NERVOSA
- Refusal to maintain body weight at or above a minimally normal weight for age and height (weight loss leading to maintenance of body weight < 85% of expected or failure to make expected weight gain during period of growth, leading to body weight < 85% of expected)
- Intense fear of gaining weight or becoming fat, even though underweight
- Disturbance in body weight/shape experienced, denial of seriousness
- Current low body weight
- Three consecutive cycles of amenorrhea in postmenarchal girls

Restricting type: No regular binge-eating or purging behavior
Binge-eating type: Regular binge-eating or purging behavior

BULIMIA NERVOSA
- Recurrent episodes of binge eating
- Inappropriate compensatory behavior to prevent weight gain such as self-induced vomiting, misuse of laxatives, diuretics, enemas or other medications, fasting or excessive exercise
- Feelings of lack of control during binges
- Preoccupation with weight and body shape
- No occurrence during episodes of anorexia nervosa

Purging type: Self-induced vomiting or misuse of laxatives
Nonpurging type: Use of other inappropriate compensatory behaviors such as fasting or excessive exercise but not laxatives, self-induced vomiting, diuretics, or enemas

With any suspected eating disorder, careful inquiry into weight patterns over the past few months, exercise, and typical daily diet is essential. The clinician should ask girls if they feel happy with their bodies. Do they think that they are too thin or too fat? The weight of family members is also a topic for inquiry. It is also important to know whether boys and girls make themselves vomit or use ipecac or laxatives. Knowledge of family psychiatric history is appropriate, because many teenagers with eating disorders experience depression and affective or obsessive-compulsive disorders.

Physical Examination
Height and weight measurements are of paramount importance as part of the physical examination. A body-mass index [weight in kilograms/ height (meters) squared] less than the 5th percentile for age is a sign of anorexia nervosa. A patient with anorexia nervosa who has lost greater than 15% of ideal body weight appears sick, but a patient with bulimia may look well nourished. Malnutrition causes lanugo, brittle hair and nails, dry cold skin, loss of subcutaneous fat, and pedal or pretibial edema. Bradycardia, hypothermia, and hypotension may be evident.

Laboratory Evaluation
The purpose of laboratory tests is to determine whether a particular teenager with an eating disorder needs emergent medical attention. Usually, the history and physical examination allow the diagnosis of an eating disorder. Blood tests include serum electrolytes, hemoglobin, hematocrit, and white blood cell (WBC) count. Urinalysis is also necessary. The clinician should order an ECG to detect arrhythmias. Thyroid function tests are important if symptoms of hypothyroidism (e.g., bradycardia, thinning hair, cold intolerance) are present. Measurements of follicle-stimulating hormone (FSH) and luteinizing hormone (LH) are usually suppressed, causing amenorrhea.

Differential Diagnosis

Pediatric Pearl
Before making the diagnosis of an eating disorder, it is important to evaluate weight loss to exclude a systemic condition.

Weight loss or vomiting may not result from anorexia or bulimia. It may result from malignancy, malabsorption, inflammatory bowel disease, tuberculosis, cystic fibrosis, diabetes mellitus, and hyperthyroidism. Vomiting may be due to gastrointestinal (GI) obstruction, gastroenteritis, or increased intracranial pressure from a brain tumor, migraine headaches, or an aneurysm. Findings of weight loss or excessive vomiting together with an abnormal body image lead to the diagnosis of either anorexia nervosa or bulimia.

Management

The management of adolescents with eating disorders is most frequently accomplished on an outpatient basis unless there are severe metabolic or cardiac disturbances, dehydration, or the necessity for inpatient psychiatric care. Treatment for eating disorders is multidisciplinary, with a team consisting of a pediatrician, mental health professional, and nutritionist. The goals of hospitalization are correction of physiologic abnormalities, weight gain, and initiation of psychologic evaluation.

Weight gain may occur on an outpatient basis, by having the adolescent eat food or nutritional supplements. If weight gain through oral feeding is not possible, then trials of inpatient nasogastric or intravenous nutrition must proceed. Weight goals should be established within a certain time frame. Ongoing psychotherapy and, sometimes, family therapy are necessary.

SPORTS MEDICINE

Physical activity during adolescence benefits the musculoskeletal and cardiovascular systems, and participation in team sports fosters psychosocial development. Improvements in strength, flexibility, endurance, bone mineral density, perceptual motor skills such as eye–hand coordination, and cardiopulmonary function result from regular physical activity. In addition to fitness, organized sports encourage good health behaviors and social and team skills. Participation in sports may produce lifetime benefits in terms of disease prevention and quality of life.

EXTENT OF SPORTS PARTICIPATION AND SPORTS-RELATED INJURIES

In the United States, sports participation and sports-related injuries are common in adolescents, and their incidence is increasing. More than 30 million adolescents are enrolled in formal sports programs, and more than 30% of teenagers participate in competitive, organized high school sports—as many as 50% of boys and 25% of girls between 8 and 16 years of age (> 15 million teenagers participate in organized play each year).

More than 3 million sports-related injuries occur each year in adolescents, and 22%–39% of teenage athletes sustain injuries that temporarily restrict play.

Pediatric Pearl

Sports play is the most common cause of injury between 13 and 19 years of age.

Sport–related injuries are second to motor vehicle injuries as the cause of adolescent emergency department visits nationwide. Team-related sports account for the greatest number of, and the most serious injuries. Demographic statistics do not include injury rates due to participation in nonteam sports, but the medical literature cites in–line skating, trampoline use, weight lifting, surfing, martial arts, motor cross racing, and skiing as common causes of adolescent sports injury.

Injury rates are higher in some sports activities than others. For adolescent boys, the highest injury rates occur in football and wrestling, while for girls, the highest injury rates occur in soccer and gymnastics. In general, this reflects the demographics of sport participation. Some conditions are gender-related. For example, the triad of amenorrhea, eating disorder, and osteoporosis is well described in competitive female athletes. Postexertional breast tenderness, another gender-specific condition, affects about three-fourths of female athletes. Adolescent girls may also have higher injury rates. A 15-year longitudinal study of high school cross-country running injuries demonstrated the occurrence of significantly higher shin, hip, and foot injury rates and knee, calf, and foot reinjury rates in female runners than for males.

Other injuries are most common among teenagers. More than 75% of the 40,000 sports-related eye injuries that occur each year are in athletes under 25 years of age.

APPROACH TO ADOLESCENT ATHLETES WITH SPORTS-RELATED INJURIES

Sport–specific physical demands and technique and the adolescent sports "culture" all contribute to athletic performance and injury. Physiologic maturity is one of the intrinsic factors that determine an athlete's susceptibility to pathologic change. Other intrinsic factors include strength, flexibility, endurance, posture, and sport technique. Factors that relate to the environment and sport–specific demands are also important. These include the activity, position played (if applicable), and intensity of play or competition.

A sense of invulnerability and risk–taking behavior can encourage athletes in attempts to exceed their abilities or previous performances. Their identity and self–esteem may be connected to physical fitness or a specific sport or team. This can foster actions, including the use of steroids and related substances, which may lead to injury. The use of ergogenic aids, including dietary supplements and steroids, is common among high school and college athletes. An estimated 6%–10% of high school seniors (boys) use or have used anabolic or androgenic steroids beginning at 16 years of age or less. Use of creatine and anabolic or androgenic steroids is frequent in adolescence, despite the lack of proper guidelines.

Young athletes should avoid high–intensity training and sports specialization. This is contrary to the position taken by many serious athletes who exhibit a "win at all costs" mentality. It is typical for competitive athletes to improve their performance through year–round practice of one sport. Many people tend to view cross-training as an addition to, not a substitution for, the primary sport. Cross-training should be a strategy to vary physical activity and avoid injury or to maintain fitness while recovering from injury.

In September 2000, the Committee on Sports Medicine and Fitness of the American Academy of Pediatrics (AAP) summarized one of the most significant behaviors that contributes to sport–related pathology.

> "Young athletes who specialize in just one sport may be denied the benefits of varied activity while facing additional physical, physiologic, and psychologic demands from intense training and competition."

Pathophysiology

Several physiologic factors determine adolescents' vulnerability to injury. Growing athletes have less fat and connective tissue, and as a consequence a lower shock absorption capacity, than adults. As a result, the bone and viscera of adolescents receive a greater amount of force per unit area than in adults.

Pediatric Pearl

Most adolescent–specific injuries affect the epiphyseal plate.

The viscera of physically immature athletes are more closely packed, and the frequency of multiple organ injuries during sports play is inversely related to the athlete's age. While the youngest athletes are most susceptible to visceral and osseous injury, older athletes have a relatively greater vulnerability to soft tissue damage (see MUSCULOSKELETAL INJURIES).

Adolescent athletes also have a lower anaerobic capability than mature adults. To meet physical demands, teenagers have a relatively greater oxygen consumption, higher heart and respiratory rates, and decreased cardiac stroke volume. This increases the metabolic cost for endurance activities and reduces the injury threshold in teenagers.

Clinical and Laboratory Evaluation

Evaluation of adolescent athletes includes the screening preparticipation physical examination, a comprehensive medical and athletic history, and identification of the specific physical demands of intended play. Screening can identify disqualifying medical conditions, identify risk factors for injury, diagnose undetected disease, and suggest interventions that will allow successful sports participation. Screening for factors associated with a high rate of injury may help avoid serious morbidity. The value of the preparticipation physical examination varies. Reported statistics indicate that it is positive (disqualifies the athlete or requires modification of the sport) in 3.4% of junior high school athletes, 15.4% of high school, and 33.9% of college-age athletes, with an overall disqualification rate of about 1.7%.

History

Key elements of the medical history include details regarding prior injury and treatment, general medical status, and the athlete's past performance. Training schedules, frequency of competition, and the number of years of play are noteworthy. The history can help the physician obtain a sense of the athlete's level of competitiveness and identify external pressures (from peers, coaches, or family) to which the athlete is subjected. It is important to note any sports–related goals that the athlete may have such as a college athletic scholarship or playing in a professional league.

Questions about previous loss of consciousness or changes in memory, behavior, and personality are appropriate. Any prior surgery, allergies, exercise-induced asthma, medications, family history of sudden cardiac death, menstrual history, and lifestyle assessment (e.g., nutrition, substance abuse, performance anxiety) should be part of the athlete's medical record (Table 3.7).

The specific challenges of athletic play, equipment, or the playing field may also present a hazard to the athlete. For example, a cross-country runner may be at risk for ankle injury due to uneven terrain or improper footwear. The linebacker playing in August may be at risk for heat exhaustion, especially if obese.

TABLE 3.7 Contraindications to Sports Participation

Relative Contraindications

Exercise-induced angina, syncope, family history of sudden cardiac death, exercise-induced arrhythmia, mitral regurgitation, or prior embolic event

Atlantoaxial instability (especially juvenile rheumatoid arthritis or Down syndrome) [contact or partial contact sports]

Coagulopathy

Detached retina

Fever or acute illness

Repeated spine or brain trauma with residual deficits

Conditions Requiring Restricted Contact or Other Accommodation

Congenital absence of one kidney

Cystic fibrosis

Acutely enlarged spleen

Physical Examination

The physical examination should begin with an assessment of posture. Check symmetry at rest and during movement (static and dynamic symmetry). Abnormalities in posture, alignment, limb girth, or trunk contour help provide a focus for the examination, which should address strength, range of motion (ROM), and quality of motion. ROM should be full and smooth and proceed at a normal rate. Examine the neck, trunk, and joints of upper and lower extremities for ROM and strength. Look for swelling, tenderness, crepitus, or deformity. Use specific provocatory maneuvers when appropriate; for example, the Hawkins sign suggests supraspinatus tendinitis or subacromial bursitis as the cause of shoulder pain. Whenever practical, direct observation of the athlete performing specific sport tasks can be very illustrative.

In addition, obtain the adolescent's height and weight. Perform an abdominal examination and check for organomegaly; this may help identify the risk for heat exhaustion or visceral injury during contact sports. The blood pressure and pulse rate, along with cardiac auscultation for murmurs or arrhythmia, generally suffice for cardiac screening. Further cardiovascular screening such as exercise stress testing remains controversial.

Laboratory Evaluation

If anemia is suspected in the female athlete on the basis of history (e.g., menorrhagia) or examination (pale conjunctiva or mucosa, delayed capillary refill), determination of the hemoglobin or hematocrit may be useful. No other laboratory studies are generally necessary, although in special circumstances an athlete may be screened for doping (autologous transfusion to increase hemoglobin or hematocrit) steroid or other drug use.

Imaging, generally plain films or magnetic resonance imaging (MRI), is often helpful to assess bone and soft tissues. Radiographs have the added benefit of providing information regarding skeletal maturity. Most diagnoses can be made on a clinical basis. However, when tissue is disrupted (e.g., tear of the anterior cruciate ligament), MRI of the soft tissues provides information that cannot be elicited on examination because of edema or guarding.

Management

A knowledge of the demands of a particular sport allows the health care practitioner to work with athletes and coaches to develop strategies that minimize injury risk and, ideally, optimize performance. The generic management of adolescent sports injuries may be viewed as staged interventions. The earliest efforts seek to prevent injury. Education by the health care provider can help balance the emphasis placed on repetition and performance by trainers and coaches. Suggestions for maintaining strength and flexibility, warming up and cooling down, or managing minor aches and pains are valuable contributions that reduce injury and enhance athletic performance.

Treatment of acute injury follows the RICE protocol: **r**est, splint, or cast; **i**ce; compression or support; and **e**levation. The use of nonsteroidal anti-inflammatory agents (NSAIDs) or local corticosteroid injection should be considered. If tissue disruption is suspected (fracture, tear of tendon or ligament), imaging or orthopedic referral for surgical evaluation is appropriate. If strength or sensory deficits are apparent, referral for neurologic evaluation is important.

During the subacute stage of management (week 2–4 postinjury), bracing, taping, or splinting may provide stability or support to an injured body segment. Physical therapy can train the athlete in a balanced therapeutic exercise program of strengthening, stretching, and "work hardening." Repeated counseling about beneficial and harmful activities may be helpful. Involvement of athletes as well as coaches or trainers in setting goals and planning therapy is effective.

The chronic stage of care focuses on modification of equipment, training, or competition strategies. Individualization of specific care is necessary for each athlete and the injury.

SPECIFIC TYPES OF SPORTS-RELATED INJURIES

MUSCULOSKELETAL INJURIES

Musculoskeletal injuries are the leading cause of morbidity in adolescent athletes. Although the growing skeletal system of adolescents is highly vulnerable, the preponderance of injuries involve muscles, ligaments, tendons, and bursae. Both osseous and soft tissue injury occur more frequently during periods of rapid growth.

Sprains and strains remain the most common injuries affecting the adolescent athlete. Because these injuries correlate with the patterns of physical demand, they stratify according to sport. Low back pain occurs in competitive or recreational adolescents involved in rowing (crew, kayaking), with an estimated prevalence of 15%–25%. Knee and ankle sprains are common in adolescent soccer and basketball players, gymnasts, and boxers. Foot and ankle sprains, stress fractures, and compartment syndromes are common in runners and gymnasts. Shoulder trauma resulting in, for example, rotator cuff tendinitis, acromioclavicular sprain or scapular muscle strain has a high incidence in teenage swimmers, baseball pitchers, volleyball players, and participants in racket sports. Muscular neck or back pain in teenage golfers is common, although the exact prevalence is unknown (it approaches 90% in adults).

Pathophysiology

Sprain (tendon tear) and strain (a tear of muscle), as well as tendinitis, bursitis, and certain stress fractures result from three basic patterns of injury: (1) cumulative trauma due to repetitive motion, (2) cumulative trauma due to static strain, and (3) direct trauma. A tissue's inherent resistance to pathologic change determines its ability to recover from an applied force. Repetitive motion or static muscle tension (required for stabilization of a body segment) results in pathologic change when rest and recovery between activities is inadequate. In acute trauma, the delivery of a force that exceeds tissue resistance may result in a fracture or tear.

There are two patterns of tissue response to trauma: irritation or inflammation, or loss of tissue integrity (e.g., laceration or fracture). Lesions of muscle, tendon, joint capsule, and bursa characteristically manifest as pain, swelling, erythema, and guarding as a consequence of inflammation. Muscle, ligament, and tendon may tear, and bone may fracture. In these instances, the clinical presentation is usually more pronounced. When the injury is chronic or recurrent, long–term changes may become evident. These include shortening or incompetence of muscle, ligament and capsule with segmental changes in posture, instability, and degenerative joint disease.

Growing articular cartilage, as well as the physis and epiphysis of long bones, is especially vulnerable to both macrotrauma and microtrauma. During periods of accelerated growth (growth spurts), this vulnerability is greatest. Because skeletal maturity does not occur until late adolescence or early adulthood, the growth plates of young individuals are susceptible to injury. Until about 24 years of age, the strength of joint capsules and ligament exceeds that of bone, which explains the unique collection of epiphyseal fractures and osseous avulsion injuries seen in adolescent athletes. In addition to fractures of the epiphysis and physis (Table 3.8), stress fractures of the spine and metacarpal bones have been reported in adolescent athletes. Spondylolysis, usually at L4

TABLE 3.8	Salter-Harris Fracture Classification

Salter Classification	Description of Fracture
I	Epiphyseal separation from the metaphysis without bony fragment
II	Line of separation extending along physis and through portion of metaphysial bone; metaphyseal bone fragment is seen (Thurston Holland sign)
III	Intraarticular fracture of the epiphysis, with cleavage plane extending from joint surface to physis and parallel to growth plate
IV	Fracture line beginning at articular surface, extending through epiphysis and segment of metaphysis
V	Crush injury of epiphysis

or L5, affects 11%–15% of female gymnasts, compared with 2.0%–2.5% of the nonathletic female adolescent population.

Significant joint disease can occur as repetitive wear of articular cartilage exposes joint surfaces. Osteoarthritis of the knee has been demonstrated in 50% of soccer players after 5–15 years of competitive play and may potentially affect late adolescents. Injury and subsequent degenerative change is seen in the proximal interphalangeal joints of volleyball players.

Clinical and Laboratory Evaluation

History
Knowledge about an athlete's sport is important to both the prevention and understanding of the pathomechanics of injury. Sports may be classified as either full contact (or impact), limited contact or noncontact. The clinician should ask questions concerning the degree and type of effort involved in play: do the necessary muscle contractions require a large or small degree of force? Is this force sustained or explosive? How long is this force applied? It is important to identify the set of movements required for play, the joints involved and the required ROM, the demands for flexibility, and whether the activity involves repetitive movement or exposure to excessive external force. Upper extremity injuries such as shoulder tendinitis and impingement and elbow/forearm epicondylitis or myositis most commonly result from repetitive motion. Lower extremity injuries from running may result from repetitive motion, while basketball injuries are often related to intermittent, explosive lower extremity use. Sprains, strains, and stress fractures of the foot, ankle, and knee, along with other lower extremity injuries typically result from this type of trauma.

Physical Examination
Identify the joints involved and assess their ROM, strength of related musculature, and the athlete's overall endurance and flexibility. If possible, observe the specific activities of play and look for guarding, asymmetry and the quality of motion. Note any swelling, tenderness or ecchymosis (an indication of tissue disruption).

Laboratory Evaluation
Joint instability, locking or buckling of a joint, crepitus with movement, or persistent pain on weight-bearing may require imaging studies for precise diagnosis. Plain radiographs are appropriate initially.

Management

RICE, followed by rehabilitation, is appropriate for most injuries. If there is a fracture or tendon, ligament, or meniscal tear, referral to an orthopedist is important. The consultant pediatric orthopedist may believe that additional imaging studies, often including an MRI of the affected area, are appropriate.

NEUROLOGIC INJURIES

Central nervous system (CNS) trauma affects the brain or spinal cord. Serious neurologic injuries are more common in athletes older than 12 years of age compared with younger children. The incidence of spinal cord injury increases dramatically between 15 and 18 years of age, and 4%–14% of the reported spinal cord injuries occur as a result of participation in football, gymnastics, wrestling, or diving. Unfortunately, 30%–50% of these injuries involve the cervical spine and result in quadriplegia and severe disability. The literature regarding closed head or traumatic brain injury, concussion-related disorder, and postconcussion syndromes is extensive. Head trauma may affect performance, either physical or cognitive, or behavior (Table 3.9). One-fourth of all high school football players suffer a concussion each football season.

Fortunately, adolescent athletes more frequently sustain a less severe neurologic injury—the "burner" or "stinger." This injury is very common in high school and college athletes who play football, basketball, or hockey, or who engage in

TABLE 3.9 Long-Term Sequelae of Repeated Head Trauma		
Cognitive Sequelae	**Behavioral Sequelae**	**Motor Sequelae**
Memory loss	Emotional lability	Motor apraxia
Impaired learning	Disinhibition	Balance deficit
Dementia	Aggression or apathy	Other movement disorders

wrestling or weight lifting; in football players, it has a reported lifetime incidence of 18%–65%. The condition is usually self–limited, but recurrences are common. With multiple recurrences, a permanent neurologic deficit may result.

Pathophysiology

Neurologic lesions can result from traction or compression. Axial compression of the spine when force is applied to the head with the neck in flexion may lead to quadriplegia. In "burners" or "stingers," damage to the C5 or C6 nerve roots, the brachial plexus upper trunk, or a peripheral nerve occurs. Most of these lesions results in neurapraxia, and they resolve if they are not subjected to additional trauma.

Clinical and Laboratory Evaluation

History

Complaints of weakness, paresthesia (usually tingling in nature), decreased or altered sensation or burning pain may suggest neuropathology. A history of forced head flexion, traction on an abducted arm, or trauma to a peripheral nerve warrants further evaluation of the neurologic system (Table 3.10).

Physical Examination

Check muscle strength, light touch and position sense, tendon reflexes, motor control and coordination, and cognitive status. Between 15% and 20% of spinal cord injuries are spinal cord injury without radiographic abnormality (SCIWORA). The diagnosis of these injuries is made on the basis of clinical findings alone.

Athletes who have suffered a concussion warrant evaluation for antegrade and retrograde amnesia (Table 3.11). Evaluation should include assessing the athlete's ability to understand and respond appropriately to questions; orientation to person, place, and time; and the presence of headache or dizziness. With loss of consciousness due to head trauma, there may be an associated spinal injury.

Laboratory Evaluation

Any injury resulting in hypesthesia, paresthesia, weakness, or altered consciousness necessitates further evaluation. MRI is the imaging study of choice. However, if the suspected injury is close to bone, computed tomography (CT) provides the best assessment. Electrodiagnostic studies [e.g., electromyography (EMG), nerve conduction testing, evoked potentials] may provide insight into lesion location, severity, and prognosis when performed at least 10–14 days following injury.

Management

Management initially follows the RICE protocol, with splinting and bracing as needed. In most instances in which there is an apparent neurologic deficit, neurologic consultation is desirable (see Table 3.11).

CATASTROPHIC INJURY

Catastrophic (emergent or life-threatening) injuries may occur, although they are uncommon. Direct contact or projectile contact trauma results in a wide range of injuries, including ophthalmologic emergencies. Eye injuries result in

---

TABLE 3.10 Postconcussion Syndrome

History	Signs/Symptoms
Head trauma within 6 months Loss of consciousness at injury Posttraumatic amnesia	Attention deficits* Memory deficits* Rapid fatigue Disordered sleep Headache Dizziness Irritability Anxiety Depression Change in personality Apathy

*Required symptom.

TABLE 3.11 Concussion Severity and Activity Guidelines		
Concussion Severity	**Return to Play**	**Termination of Season**
Mild (grade I): no LOC	After being asymptomatic for 1 week; if second concussion, after 2 asymptomatic weeks	Third concussion
Moderate (grade II): LOC < 5 minutes or PTA > 30 minutes	After being asymptomatic for 1 week; if second concussion, after 1 month of rest (must remain asymptomatic during play)	Third concussion
Severe (grade III): LOC > 5 minutes or PTA > 24 hours	1 month rest (must remain asymptomatic during play)	Second concussion

LOC = loss of consciousness; PTA = posttraumatic amnesia.

about 40,000 emergency department visits per year.

Pediatric Pearl

Eye injuries are much more common in adolescent athletes than in adults.

The risk is greatest in baseball and basketball, followed by racket sports, hockey, combat sports, darts, archery, wrestling, the martial arts and boxing. There are reports of sudden death due to chest wall trauma in adolescents competing in baseball. Reports of similar injuries in hockey, lacrosse, and softball are less common. Pneumothorax has been associated with running, tennis, golf, bicycling, wrestling, weight lifting, and rowing.

Most sudden deaths affect male athletes. The highest rates occur in football, with nontraumatic deaths due to cardiac causes and thermal injury, and traumatic causes relating to head and neck trauma. Sudden cardiac death in athletes is usually the result of underlying cardiovascular disease; hypertrophic cardiomyopathy and congenital coronary artery anomalies are most common. Careful screening (i.e., preparticipation physical examination) should identify adolescents who are at risk prior to their sports participation (see Table 3.7).

ADOLESCENT SPORTS MEDICINE AND CHRONIC DISEASE

Although adolescents with chronic disease may require close medical supervision for participation in competitive or recreational sports, they potentially derive substantial health benefits and pleasure from the experience. Exercise may be an effective part of the treatment plan for teenagers with diabetes mellitus, asthma, hypertension, and obesity. For these athletes, strategies to minimize

risk and maximize performance are important. It is important to frequently monitor the serum glucose of adolescents with diabetes who participate in endurance activities until a baseline of glucose variation during play is established. The majority of athletes with asthma have exercise-induced disease, which may require premedication.

Exercise and sports play may not improve other conditions such as sickle cell disease, which requires careful attention to hydration and fatigue. However, with adequate medical supervision and care, affected adolescents can still participate and derive the cardiovascular, neuromuscular, respiratory, and psychosocial benefits associated with sports participation.

Disabled adolescents constitute a special category of athlete. Closely organized and supervised wheelchair sports or athletic programs associated with disability (e.g., Special Olympics programs) may prove beneficial.

SUGGESTED READINGS

Adkins SB, Figler RA: Hip pain in athletes. *Am Fam Physician* 61(7):2109–2118, 2000.

Alderman EM, Schonberg SK, Cohen MI: The pediatrician's role in the diagnosis and treatment of substance abuse. *Pediatr Rev* 1992;13(8):314–318.

American Academy of Pediatrics: Testing for drugs of abuse in children and adolescents. *Pediatrics* 98(2): 305–307, 1996.

American Academy of Pediatrics, Committee on Injury and Poison Prevention and Committee on Sports Medicine and Fitness: In-line skating injuries in children and adolescents. *Pediatrics* 101(4 Pt 1): 720–722, 1998.

American Academy of Pediatrics, Committee on Injury and Poison Prevention and Committee on Sports Medicine and Fitness: Trampolines at home, school, and recreational centers. *Pediatrics* 103(5 Pt 1):1053–1056, 1999.

American Academy of Pediatrics, Committee on Sports Medicine and Fitness: Athletic participation by children and adolescents who have systemic hypertension. *Pediatrics* 99(4):637–638, 1997.

American Academy of Pediatrics, Committee on Sports Medicine and Fitness: Climactic heat stress and the exercising child and adolescent. *Pediatrics* 103(1 Pt 1):158–159, 2000.

American Academy of Pediatrics, Committee on Sports Medicine and Fitness: Injuries in youth soccer: A subject review. *Pediatrics* 105(3 Pt 1):659–661, 2000.

American Academy of Pediatrics, Committee on Sports Medicine and Fitness: Intensive training and sports specialization in young athletes. *Pediatrics* 106(1 Pt 1):154–157, 2000.

American Academy of Pediatrics, Committee on Sports Medicine and Fitness: Medical concerns in the female athlete. *Pediatrics* 106(3):610–613, 2000.

American Academy of Pediatrics, Committee on Sports Medicine and Fitness. Mitral valve prolapse and athletic participation in children and adolescents. *Pediatrics* 95(5):789–790, 1995.

American Academy of Pediatrics, Committee on Sports Medicine and Fitness: Participation in boxing by children, adolescents and young adults. *Pediatrics* 99(1):134–135, 1997.

American Academy of Pediatrics Committee on Sports Medicine and Fitness: Safety in youth ice hockey: The effects of body checking. *Pediatrics* 105(3 Pt 1): 657–658, 2000.

American Academy of Pediatrics, Committee on Sports Medicine and Fitness; American Academy of Ophthalmology, Committee on Eye Safety and Sports Ophthalmology: Protective eyewear for young athletes. *Pediatrics* 98(2 Pt 1):311–313, 1996.

American Academy of Pediatrics, Committee on Substance Abuse: Indications for management and referral of patients involved in substance abuse. *Pediatrics* 106(101):143–148, 2000.

American Psychiatric Association: *Diagnostic and Statistical Manual of Mental Disorders,* 4th ed. Washington, DC: American Psychiatric Association, 1994.

Becker, AE, Grinspoon SK, Klibansk A, et al: Eating disorders. *New Engl J Med* 340(14):1092–1098, 1999.

Bernhardt DT, Landry GL: Sports injuries in young athletes. *Adv Pediatr* 42:465–500, 1995.

Briner WW Jr, Farr C: Athlete age and sports physical examination findings. *J Fam Pract* 40(40):370–375, 1995.

Centers for Disease Control and Prevention: CDC surveillance summaries. *MMWR* 49(SS-5), 2000.

Centers for Disease Control and Prevention: State-specific birth rates for teenagers—United States, 1990–1996. *MMWR* 46(36):1–24, 1997.

Deppen RJ, Landfried MJ: Efficacy of prophylactic knee bracing in high school football players. *J Orthop Sports Phys Ther* 20(5):243–246, 1994.

Dryfoos J: *Adolescents at Risk.* New York, Oxford University Press, 1990.

Hatcher RA, Trussell J, Stewart F, et al: Contraceptive Technology. New York, Ardent Media, Inc, 1998.

Herman-Giddens ME, Slora EJ, Wasserman RC, et al: Secondary sexual characteristics and menses in young girls seen in office practice: A study from the pediatric research in office settings network. *Pediatrics* 99:505–512, 1997.

Hickey GJ, Fricker PA, McDonald WA: Injuries of young elite female basketball players over a six-year period. *Clin J Sport Med* 7(4):252–256, 1997.

Hoffman A: Clinical assessment and management of health risk behaviors in adolescents. *Adolesc Med:* 1(1):15–29, 1990.

Jellinek MS, Snyder JB: Depression and suicide in children and adolescents. *Pediatr Rev* 19:255–264, 1998.

Jessor R, Jessor SL: *Problem Behavior and Psychosocial Development: A Longitudinal Study of Youth.* New York: Academic Press, 1977.

Kreipe RE, Dukarm CP: Eating disorders in adolescents and older children. *Pediatr Rev* 20:410–421, 1999.

Luckstead EF: Cardiovascular evaluation of the young athlete. *Adolesc Med* 9(3):441–455, 1998.

Malanga GA, Stuart MJ: In-line skating injuries. *Mayo Clin Proc* 70(8): 752–754, 1995.

McCoy RL, Dec KL, McKeag DB, et al: Common injuries in the child or adolescent athlete. *Prim Care* 22(1):117–144, 1995.

Metzl JD: Sports medicine in pediatric practice: Keeping pace with the changing times. *Pediatr Ann* 29(3): 146–148, 2000.

Metzl JD: Sports-specific concerns in the young athlete: Soccer. *Pediatr Emerg Care* 15(2):130–141, 1999.

Metzl JD: Strength training and nutritional supplement use in adolescents. *Curr Opin Pediatr* 11(4): 292–296, 1999.

Micheli LJ, Fehlandt AF: Overuse injuries to tendons and apophyses in children and adolescents. *Clin Sports Med* 11(4):713–726, 1992.

Neinstein L: *Adolescent Health Care—A Practical Guide,* 3rd ed. Baltimore, Williams & Wilkins, 1996.

Newacheck PW: Adolescents with special health needs: Prevalence severity and access to health services. *Pediatrics* 84(5):872–875, 1989.

Omey ML, Micheli LJ: Foot and ankle problems in the young athlete. *Med Sci Sports Exerc* 31(7 Suppl): S470–S486, 1999.

Ozer EM, Brindis CD, Millstein SG, et al: *America's Adolescents: Are They Healthy?* San Francisco: National Health Information Center, University of California, San Francisco, 1997.

Pelz JE, Haskell WL, Matheson GO: A comprehensive and cost-effective preparticipation exam implemented on the World Wide Web. *Med Sci Sports Exerc* 31(12):1727–1740, 1999.

Rauh MJ, Margherita AJ, Rice SG, et al: High school cross-country running injuries: A longitudinal study. *Clin J Sport Med* 10(2):110–116, 2000.

Saperstein AL, Nicholas SJ: Pediatric and adolescent sports medicine. *Pediatr Clin North Am* 43(5): 1013–1033, 1996.

Stanitski CL: Pediatric and adolescent sports injuries. *Clin Sports Med* 16(4):613–633, 1997.

Stevens-Simon C: Providing effective reproductive health care and prescribing contraceptives for adolescents. *Pediatr Rev* 19:409–417, 1998.

Stracciolini A, Metzl JD: Pediatric sports emergencies. *Phys Med Rehabil Clin North Am* 11(4):961–979, 2000.

Vaughn VC, Litt IL: *Child and Adolescent Development: Clinical Implications.* Philadelphia, WB Saunders, 1990.

Vinger PF: Sports medicine and the eye care professional. *J Am Optom Assoc* 69(6):395–413, 1998.

Weist MD, Ginsburg G, Shafer M: Progress in adolescent mental health. *Adolesc Med State Art Rev* 10(1): 165–173, 1999.

Wekesa M, Langhof H: The effect of a three-week sports training programme on the coordinative abilities of asthmatic children. *East Afr Med J* 70(11): 678–681, 1993.

West RV: The female athlete. The triad of disordered eating, amenorrhoea and osteoporosis. *Sports Med* 26(2):63–71, 1998.

Chapter 4

Principles of Pediatric Nutrition, Fluids, and Electrolytes

Steven P. Shelov, Patricia Castaneda,
Fatai Bamgbola, and Frederick J. Kaskel*

PRINCIPLES OF PEDIATRIC NUTRITION

This section of the chapter introduces medical students to the elements of nutrition and feeding of young infants and children that are useful beginning with the first interaction with parents. Often the discussion of optimum feeding practices begins at visits before an infant is born, with discussions about the advantages of breastfeeding versus bottle-feeding and what to expect in the first few days of the newborn's life. **These interactions are not only fruitful for establishing confidence and trust with parents; they are also a source of great satisfaction for pediatricians.**

In addition, this section also outlines the specifics of breastfeeding and formula-feeding in infancy, when and what to introduce as solid foods in the latter half of the first year, and elements of nutritional advice for toddlers and preschoolers. It also gives a brief overview of nutritional goals for school-age children. Several accessible, supportive references, listed at the end of this chapter, provide more complete information about any of these topics and can serve as resources for pediatricians and parents. **In addition, the American Academy of Pediatrics (AAP) maintains an active web site (www.AAP.org), which is a source of continually updated nutritional advice.**

Breastfeeding

After a number of years, it now appears that the message that breast milk is the optimum food for infants is more effectively reaching professionals and parents. As recently as 10 years ago, fewer

than 50% of new mothers stated that they were intending to breastfeed their new baby; most recent estimates now place this percentage at somewhere near 60% and apparently climbing. The AAP, longtime advocates for breastfeeding as the preferred method of infant nutrition, urges all of its 55,000 member pediatricians to reinforce this message at every possible encounter. It appears that the increasing percentage of women choosing this method of feeding their infant partially reflects a positive response to this strongly worded message.

Facts About Breast Milk

What are some of the advantages of breastfeeding? It is important to share several specific facts about breast milk and breastfeeding with new or expectant mothers:

- The nutritional components of breast milk, the carbohydrate (the sugar is lactose—a disaccharide of glucose and galactose), the protein (whey and casein in an 80:20 ratio), and the fat (cholesterol and a mixture of other triglycerides of varying lengths), are all of human origin and extremely well tolerated.
- The caloric content is 20 kcal/oz, ideal for the quantity ingested relative to weight.
- Breast milk is less allergenic, because the protein components (whey and casein) are human-based, not cow- or soy-based. This is significant, because cow's milk–protein intolerance has been associated with eczema, allergy-mediated diarrhea and vomiting, colic irritability syndrome, and microscopic blood loss in the gastrointestinal (GI) tract.
- The presence of protective bacteriophagic elements, including macrophages and antibodies, is an important factor. In addition to local antibody [immunoglobulin A (IgA)] contributing to GI immunity as well as additional antiviral immunity (against poliomyelitis, in-

*We would like to acknowledge Charles L. Stewart, MD, for his contributions to the first edition of this chapter.

"Principles of Pediatric Nutrition" was written by Steven P. Shelov.

fluenza), the normally present macrophages in breast milk can synthesize complement, lysozyme, and lactoferrin, with the latter acting as an inhibitor to *Escherichia coli* growth in the intestine.

- Through its lower pH, breast milk contributes to a greater degree of lactobacillus growth in the intestine, which also may be protective against certain pathogenic intestinal bacteria (*E. coli*).
- Breast milk contains sufficient iron stores for at least 6 months and sufficient vitamin D and fluoride for at least 4 months.
- Breast milk is readily available and an important part of close bonding and maximal contact between the mother and her infant. The psychologic benefits of being able to provide the caloric sustenance through physical contact cannot be overemphasized. Breastfeeding on demand not only fulfills the infant's nutritional needs but also the baby's and mother's nurturing and skin contact needs.

Pediatric Pearl

Contraindications to breastfeeding include truly inverted nipples, mastitis, severe fissuring or cracking of the nipples, and the need for pharmacotherapy (certain medications that enter breast milk and negatively affect the infant) [Table 4.1]. However, for the most part these contraindications occur very infrequently.

The Feeding Process

There is little need for special preparation of the breasts. Excessive nipple preparation or skin softening creams are only potentially injurious and sensitizing. In the first 2–3 days postpartum, the breasts secrete a thin, orange-tinted substance called colostrum, which is an electrolyte-, macrophage-, and nutrient-rich substance with a pre-milk composition. Colostrum is an extremely important component of the initial feeding experience of the newborn infant. With nursing taking place every 2–3 hours, the true milk supply usually comes in (milk "let down") at about the third day postdelivery. The mother knows when this is happening, because the breasts feel full, even engorged, quite quickly. It is most important that even with this initially slightly uncomfortable feeling, infants be encouraged to feed at 2–3-hour intervals to keep the milk flowing and provide the continued stimulus for ongoing milk production.

At first, the feeding process is often a bit awkward but very quickly becomes comfortable and relaxed. While the mother is either sitting or lying down, the infant is held and the face is brought directly facing the breast (Figure 4.1). Using the rooting reflex, the baby **latches onto the areola portion surrounding the nipple** and begins to suck (Figure 4.2). The sucking action is really a compression-milking action in which the milk is squeezed from the ductules into the ducts and then through the nipple into the baby's mouth. The infant may suckle in bursts and then take pauses in between. The first feedings usually last 5–10 minutes, usually with 5 minutes on each breast. **It is important that each feeding start on the breast on which the infant last nursed.**

In the course of the first month, the length of time for each feed, given a 2–3-hour interval between feedings, increases quickly to 20–30 minutes/feeding. Parents often want to be sure that the baby is getting enough milk. To reassure them that everything is going well, the clinician should ask the following questions: Is the infant wetting between four and six diapers each day? Is the infant gaining weight adequately? After each feeding, does the infant appear to be satisfied, or does the baby appear hungry by crying vigorously and sucking frantically on a fist? If there is any doubt about milk supply, it is often a good idea to see the baby at about 2 weeks of age to be sure that the child has at least regained her birth weight.

The 2-week visit is also a good opportunity to talk to the parents about any problems they might have been experiencing and to support their efforts during these expectantly stressful times. Reassurance and support go a long way during these fatiguing and, at times, seemingly endless feeling of the first weeks. Parents often need to hear several times how well you, the pediatrician, think things are going. **This period is often quite stressful for the new mother,** especially the first-time parent, because breastfeeding is not yet completely established and there is often a high degree of anxiety focused on the feeding process. It is crucial that pediatricians support the mother's positive attitude about her ability to breastfeed her baby successfully. Supportive literature or personnel (a doula or breastfeeding expert is a great resource) help the new mother through these often stressful first weeks. Often, previously successful breastfeeding mothers are great referrals for new mothers who may be struggling a bit with the process.

It is also important to remember that maternal fatigue is a major counterproductive force to establishing successful breastfeeding. The mother

TABLE 4.1	Effect of Maternal Drugs on Breastfed Infants	
Drug	**Effect**	**Comment**
Amoxicillin	None	Safe
Antimetabolites	Carcinogenic	Contraindicated
Aspirin	Rare complication of bleeding	Usually safe
Atenolol	None	Probably safe
Bromocriptine	Suppresses lactation	Avoid
Carbamazepine	Unknown	Probably safe
Cascara	Colic, diarrhea	Avoid
Chloramphenicol	Gray baby syndrome	Contraindicated
Codeine	Lethargy	Usually safe
Diazepam	Lethargy, apnea	High doses contraindicated
Digoxin	None	Safe
Ergot	Gangrene, vasospasm	Contraindicated
Furosemide	None	Safe
Gold salts	Hepatonephrotoxicity	Contraindicated
Meperidine	Lethargy	Avoid
Methimazole	Hypothyroidism	Contraindicated
Metoprolol	None	Probably safe
Metronidazole	Carcinogenic	Contraindicated
Phenindione	Hemorrhage	Contraindicated
Phenobarbital	Lethargy	Usually safe
Phenytoin	Usually none	May not be recommended
Prednisone	None	Probably safe
Propoxyphene	Lethargy	Usually safe
Propranolol	None	Probably safe
Propylthiouracil	Usually none; rare goiter	Probably safe
Radioactive material	Carcinogenic	Discontinue breastfeeding 1–2 wk
Tetracycline	Discolored teeth	Contraindicated

should get as much rest as possible and have help around the house with other chores. Minimizing fatigue allows her to relax more easily, and a relaxed mother can concentrate on the needs of both herself and her infant. It is essential to reduce such major disruptions as maternal fatigue, anxiety, and tension to ensure successful breastfeeding, and the pediatrician and the family can often creatively develop methods to accomplish these goals.

Breastfeeding is usually well established by the end of the first month. The routine is nursing every 3 hours or so with each feeding lasting around 30 minutes. It is reassuring to know that the majority (80%) of the milk at each feeding is probably consumed in the first 5 minutes of the feeding. This should help relieve some of the anxiety experienced when parents say that often their baby falls asleep after 10 or 15 minutes at the breast. Reassurance with continued good growth of the infant further helps reinforce the success of the breastfeeding, but the pediatrician must always remember that the need for such reassurance is often ongoing, especially in the first several months of the new baby's life.

Pediatric Pearl

In many instances, the breastfeeding process does not go well for many reasons, such as personal choice, difficulty with the process, and unrelenting anxiety about the baby's "not getting enough milk." When these signs appear, it is important to recognize them and know when to stop breastfeeding and switch to formula-feeding. A 2–4-week trial is usually sufficient to know whether breastfeeding is going to work for the mother and infant.

If breastfeeding continues to be "difficult" or anxiety-provoking, the optimum strategy is formula-feeding with equally unqualified support from family and pediatrician. It is most important that the mother, especially a first-time mother, not be made to feel guilty about the switch. Many mothers feel the need to do this. Once the baby is on formula, both the baby and mother find greater satisfaction, the desired goal of any feeding process.

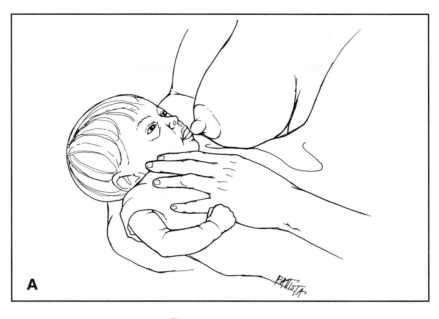

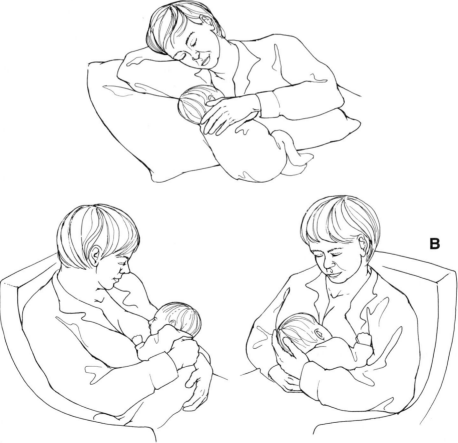

FIGURE 4.1. (*A*) The infant instinctively latches onto the nipple and begins to suck. (*B*) Different feeding positions. The infant's entire body, not just the head, should be facing the mother's body.

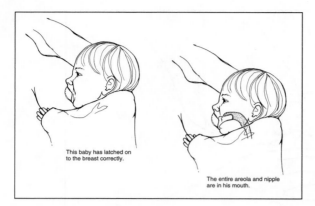

This baby has latched on to the breast correctly.

The entire areola and nipple are in his mouth.

FIGURE 4.2. Rooting reflex.

Formula-feeding

Formula is commercially prepared cow's milk–based infant feeding. For a variety of reasons, a large number of mothers (40% of new mothers by some estimates) choose not to breastfeed their new babies. There are some advantages to formula-feeding that some families find compelling and, as a result, would prefer to use for their infants.

Facts About Formula

The excellent alternatives available to breast milk have become increasingly more sophisticated and more "breast milk–like." Fortunately, these preparations have been designed to be similar enough to breast milk and yet available in a variety of safe and easy-to-use formulations that they may serve as perfectly acceptable alternatives to breast milk as the basic nutritional source for proper infant nutrition. The three basic components of milk in formulas—carbohydrate, protein, and fat—are similar to those found in breast milk, although not totally identical. Formulas vary in terms of their exact composition (Table 4.2).

What are some of the more general similarities and differences?

- Both provide the same caloric content, approximately 20 kcal/oz (0.67 kcal/ml).
- Both breast milk and regular formula [those marketed as Similac (Ross Laboratories), Enfamil (Mead Johnson), SMA (Wyeth), Good Start (Carnation), and Gerber's] contain the **disaccharide** carbohydrate lactose (glucose and galactose).
- Both contain whey and casein as the principal proteins. Different formulas have varying whey:casein ratios, although all are less than the 80:20 ratio seen in breast milk. In addition, the protein in formula is cow's milk–based protein and not human, and although it has been hydrolyzed and altered somewhat to make it more digestible and potentially less al-

lergenic (different brands do different things to the protein), the continued presence of cow's milk–based protein might trigger a sensitivity or allergy in those rare infants who might be allergic to cow's milk protein. For such situations, there are formulas available with a soy protein base that provide perfectly suitable nutrients for optimum growth.

- Both contain fats, but in formula, once the cow's milk is skimmed of all animal fat, which is quite poorly digestible, a variety of vegetable oils are added, including corn, coconut, and safflower oil, depending on the brand.
- In soy protein formulas, the protein is soy-based and not cow's milk–based, and the sugar is a corn syrup and sucrose, not lactose. Therefore, this type of formula is useful in lactose-intolerant situations and where milk protein intolerance may be suspected.
- The mineral contents are variably different from breast milk (see Table 4.2). However, each formula contains iron and vitamin supplements, eliminating the need for any additional supplementation in the first 6 months and in the latter half of infancy, as long as the infant is then given additional sources of iron-containing food.
- Fluoride supplementation remains controversial. The Committee on Nutrition of the AAP does not recommend fluoride supplementation for breastfed or formula-fed infants from birth to 6 months of age, regardless of the fluoride concentration in the community water. Currently, fluoride supplementation is recommended for children 6 months of age and older (Table 4.3).

The Feeding Process

Formula is available in three basic preparations. The most frequently used is a concentrate form, which requires an equal amount of water to be added to reconstitute it to full strength suitable

TABLE 4.2 Composition of Breast Milk and Infant Formulas

	Breast Milk (per dl)	Standard Formula (per dl)	Premature Formula (per dl)	Soy Formula (per dl)	Nutramigen (per dl)	Pregestimil (per dl)
Calories (kcal)	67–72	67	67–81	67	67	67
Protein (g)	1.2	1.5	2.0–2.4	2.0	1.9	1.9
(% calories)	(6%)	(9%)	(12%)	(12%)	(11%)	(11%)
Whey:casein protein ratio	80/20	60/40, 18/82	60/40	Soy protein	Casein hydrolysate, amino acid premix	Casein hydrolysate plus L-cystine, L-tyrosine, and L-tryptophan
Fat (g)	4.5	3.6	3.4–4.6	3.6	2.6	3.8
(% calories)	(56%)	(50%)	(45%)	(48%)	(35%)	(48%)
MCT (%)	0	0	40%–50%	0	0	20% Corn oil/60% MCT
Carbohydrate (g)	6.8	6.9–7.2	8.5–8.9	6.8	9.1	6.9
(% calories)	(38%)	(41%)	(42%)	(40%)	(54%)	(41%)
Source	Lactose	Lactose	Lactose/glucose polymers, corn syrup	Corn syrup, sucrose	Sucrose, tapioca starch	Corn syrup solids, corn starch, dextrose
Minerals (per L)						
Calcium (mg)	340	420–550	750–1440	700	635	640
Phosphorus (mg)	140	280–390	400–720	500	475	430
Sodium (mEq)	7.0	6.5–8.3	6.5–15	13	14	12
Vitamin D (IU)	Variable	400	510–1200	400	400	400
Osmolality (mOsm)	273	300	250–310	240–260	290	290
Renal solute load (mOsm)	75	100–126	122–150	126	175	125
Comments	Reference standard, deficient in vitamin K; may be deficient in Na⁺, Ca²⁺, protein, vitamin D for VLBW	Risk of milk protein intolerance, gastrointestinal bleeding, anemia, wheezing, eczema	Specifically fortified with additional protein, Ca²⁺, P, Na⁺, vitamin D, and MCT oil	Useful for lactose and milk protein intolerance; possible development of soy protein intolerance; development of rickets with VLBW	Useful for lactose and milk protein intolerance	Useful for malabsorption states as well as lactose and milk protein intolerance

MCT = medium-chain triglycerides; VLBW = very low birth weight.

TABLE 4.3 Fluoride Supplementation*			
Age	**< 0.3**	**Water Fluoride Content (ppm) 0.3–0.6**	**> 0.6**
Birth–6 months	0	0	0
6 months–3 years	0.25	0	0
3–6 years	0.50	0.25	0
6–16 years	1.00	0.50	0

*Fluoride daily doses are given in milligrams.

for feeding to infants. The "ready-to-feed" preparations in various sized bottles and cans are just that, ready to feed, but are more expensive; parents are basically paying for water. The availability of small (4–6-oz), ready-to-feed bottles that are very useful for travel or middle-of-the-night purposes are handy but are expensive as a regular, everyday procedure. Finally, many of the formula preparations come in a powder form that is also convenient for travel and comes with an easy-to-understand measuring spoon or scoop.

Formula preparation, whether it be from the ready-to-use cans or the concentrate, requires extreme care and cleanliness, especially in the first 3 months of an infant's life. The basic process most frequently used now is called the **terminal heating method.** In the first 3 months, there is usually rigid adherence to this process; after that, the single-bottle-at-a-time process is often the favored choice, although perhaps not quite as convenient in the middle of the night. Terminal heating does not require presterilization of any of the utensils. The terminal heating process involves the following steps:

1. Formula is poured into thoroughly washed and rinsed, wide-mouth glass (or plastic) bottles. If it is ready-to-feed formula, no additional water need be added; if it is the concentrate, an equal amount of water needs to be added. If the powder is used, it is important to follow manufacturer's directions.
2. With the desired amount of formula in bottles sufficient for a full day's feeding (Table 4.4), nipples are applied upside down and then

loosely secured with the bottle cap, often with a plastic piece on top underneath the screw cap. Different procedures are appropriate for other types of bottles with disposable, collapsible bags; manufacturer's instructions should be followed.
3. The bottles are then placed in a rack that is placed in a container large enough to allow the bottles not be touched by the lid.
4. Water is poured into the container up to the midpoint of the bottles. The container is then covered and placed over moderate heat. The water is allowed to boil gently for about 25 minutes.
5. Once the heating process is completed, the burner is turned off, and the bottles are taken out with tongs and allowed to cool, either in a pan of cold water for 10 minutes or in air. They are then placed in the refrigerator and are ready to be used during the next 24 hours.

There is some controversy about the need for this process at all, given the safe nature of the water supply throughout most communities in the United States. Certainly this method should be used in any household in which the risk of contamination of food is a reality.

In general, new infants are fed every 3–4 hours and take about 2–4 oz/feeding in the first several weeks. From the third week on, the feedings are increased in amounts (4–5 oz at a time) and generally follow a certain pattern (see Table 4.4). During the first 2–3 months, feeding usually continues every 4 hours or so through the night. Once infants are about 3 months of age, the evening feedings can many times be slightly increased in quantity to allow for a longer time between the late evening feeding and the early morning feeding, allowing the mother and infant (and father) to get a little longer stretch of continuous sleep. This first night that an infant "sleeps through the night" is usually heralded with much relief. The total amount of feeding per day usually approximates 150 ml/kg, which allows for approximately 120 kcal/kg, sufficient for good growth of the infant through these early months.

TABLE 4.4 Average Quantity of Feedings	
Age	**Average Quantity Taken in Individual Feedings**
1st and 2nd week	2–3 oz (60–90 ml)
3 weeks–2 months	4–5 oz (120–150 ml)
2–3 months	5–6 oz (150–180 ml)
3–4 months	6–7 oz (180–210 ml)
5–12 months	7–8 oz (210–240 ml)

Homemade Formula

A small number of families continue to make formula from whole cow's milk rather than use commercially prepared formula. If this is the case with your patient, the recommendation is to use *only* evaporated milk (*not* condensed milk). An easy way for parents to prepare milk-based formula is the following:

1. All utensils required for mixing and storing of formula should be sterilized by boiling in water for 5–10 minutes.
2. Rubber nipples and caps should be boiled for no more than 5 minutes.
3. Wide-mouth glass bottles and a thoroughly cleaned quart (32 oz) bottle are easiest to use.
4. After thorough cleaning of the quart bottle, pour in 1 can (13 oz) of evaporated milk. Fill the remainder of the jar with tap water. Then add 2 tablespoons of cane sugar or 4 tablespoons of Mead's Dextrimaltose. Stir well.
5. Pour the formula, once made, into bottles as in the steps above and terminally heat. This will make enough formula for 1 day of the infant's needs. Each supply must be made no more than 1 day at a time.

Second 6 Months of Life: Introduction of Solid Food

Breastfeeding or formula-feeding should continue throughout the second half of the first year of life. Numerous studies have indicated an intolerance to whole cow's milk when ingested by infants under 1 year of age. This intolerance has resulted in occasional episodes of vomiting, diarrhea, and, most significantly, occult blood loss through the GI tract, resulting in an iron deficiency state.

Beginning at about 5–6 months of age, additional foods usually supplement nutrition provided by breast- or formula-feeding. The first food usually recommended is iron-fortified, single-grain infant cereal. This cereal, especially prepared for infants, can be either rice, barley, or any other single grain. Initially, 3–4 level tablespoons can be diluted with 6 parts of breast milk or formula (about 108 kcal/dl) and fed to infants with a small baby spoon. Most often, this solid food supplementation is reserved for two feedings a day, but as additional solid foods are introduced, they can be spaced out into any of the feedings. The first feeding with the spoon is also a pretty sloppy affair, so parents should be warned to be prepared with lots of bibs and plastic on the floor. It takes a short while for infants to adjust.

After the introduction of cereals, additional specially prepared baby foods are introduced, one at a time, and again fed with a spoon. Although many parents have a tendency to put cereal and other foods into the bottle, this is not recommended; the potential for overfeeding of higher caloric dense solids is a common result. Strained fruits contain 45–70 kcal/100 g; strained vegetables, 25–65 kcal/g; and meat, 90–140 kcal/g. Some studies indicate that the addition of larger amounts of solid foods than calorically required can be one factor in the early predisposition to obesity later in childhood.

Toward the latter several months of the first year, the strained foods are generally less pureed and offered as "junior foods." However, as these commercially prepared baby foods are expensive and offer no advantage over homemade, freshly prepared and pureed foods, parents can certainly feel comfortable preparing their own foods for older infants, taking proper caution to keep all food preparation clean.

Feeding After the First Year: More Solid Food

With the beginning of the second year of life, infants become more mobile and active and motorically more facile. This means the feeding process is also a more active one. During this time, children show initiative with feeding, have food preferences, and have erratic food volume intakes, even from day to day. Unpredictable in their food choices as in their other activities, they may have a "favorite" meal one day and reject it totally the next day. They love to feed themselves; although self-feeding is often messy and disruptive, it should be encouraged.

They usually eat three meals and two snacks a day. In addition, their milk drinking (whole cow's milk is now acceptable, although 1%–2% can be used after the second year) has generally been shifted to a cup that they can hold (unless, of course, they are still breastfeeding). With the addition of table foods at all of the meals, milk no longer occupies such a central place in the diet.

Pediatric Pearl

One guideline for milk volume per day is never to allow more than 1 quart of milk. If a child is drinking more than this, a loss of interest in other types of foods may result, and a risk for nutritional deficiency could occur.

The diet should include foods from all the different food groups, and parents should match the degree of chewing required to children's ability to chew. It is most important *not* to allow foods that require too much chewing; the risk for choking is probably greatest at this age. The basic food groups are:

- Dairy products—milk, yogurt, cheese, and milk products
- Meat, fish, poultry, eggs, and legumes
- Vegetables
- Fruits
- Cereal grains, breads, pastas, and rice

It is not necessary that children have representatives of all the food groups every day, but they should be in the diet at least two to three times per week. Although food that are low in fat and cholesterol foods are recommended for adults, the AAP agrees that fat and cholesterol should not be limited until after 2 years of age.

The nutritional requirements of children in the preschool and school-age years are less specific and more reflective of the daily activities, personal and family likes and dislikes, and overall taste preferences. Regular meals, especially breakfast, are important not just as nutritional activities but also as social and family activities. In general, children's eating routines are integrally involved with the family. Continued attention to foods from the different food groups should guide nutritional food preparation, and now a greater watchfulness over the fat and cholesterol content of the diet should be a determining factor. There is no need for more than three cups of milk/day as a calcium source, and other milk and vegetable sources of calcium can consistently be ingested that are also sufficient.

It is also important to try and resist the natural temptation to replace some of the earlier, well-established sound eating principles with high-calorie snacks and fast foods. The eating of these foods is inevitable to some degree; ease, availability, and peer pressure are often hard to resist. It should occur as infrequently as possible. Even with the increased energy needs of children during the preschool and school-age years, the calories from a more balanced diet are sufficient, and variations on those early dietary principles can be limitless and still maintain the majority of the good aspects of those early nutritional behaviors and habits. Finally, it is important not to minimize the influence that family and adult dietary habits have on children's determination of their own dietary needs and fancies. Discussions about family feeding and food preparation as a "family health item," by definition, include the children and incorporate them into this most essential part of growing up in the family.

PARENTERAL FLUID AND ELECTROLYTE THERAPY

All infants and children require the adequate intake of fluid and electrolytes in order to thrive. For most children, this is accomplished without difficulty by oral ingestion of food and fluids. The goals of an organized approach to fluid and electrolyte therapy in children are twofold: (1) to supply fluids and electrolytes used or lost as a result of normal metabolism and (2) to replace or repair abnormalities in fluid and electrolyte balance incurred by a disease process or a behavior. Physicians and other health care professionals should promote, whenever possible, the enteral route of fluid and electrolyte administration; they should reserve parenteral (intravenous) fluid administration reserved for those children who cannot use enteral alimentation for medical or surgical reasons (Table 4.5). A major goal in the treatment plan for most of the children affected by the conditions listed in Table 4.5 is the resumption of enteral nutrition.

Fluid and electrolyte therapies (both enteral and parenteral) are frequently divided into several categories and subcategories, most commonly "maintenance" and "deficit replacement" phases. The following discussion of deficit fluid therapy focuses on diarrheal dehydration, although many of the concepts discussed apply to other causes of volume and electrolyte deficits.

Maintenance Fluid and Electrolyte Requirements

Children admitted to the hospital for any reason are usually on "maintenance" fluids, often unregulated and administered via the oral route. It is necessary to modify this, of course, if they are overhydrated, dehydrated, or have acute renal insufficiency. Before certain surgical procedures, children may need to receive their fluid and electrolyte requirements intravenously, as do children who are in the early stages of recovering from surgical procedures, especially thoracic, abdominal, and central nervous system (CNS)

"Parenteral Fluid and Electrolyte Therapy" was written by Patricia Castaneda, Fatai Bamgbola, Charles L. Stewart, and Frederick J. Kaskel.

TABLE 4.5 Conditions That May Require Parenteral Fluid and Electrolyte Therapy

Dehydration (see Table 4.10 for causes)*
Presurgical and postsurgical procedures
    Abdominal
    Neurosurgical
    Cardiovascular
Gastrointestinal diseases
    Bleeding
    Perforation of viscus
    Inflammatory bowel disease (uncommon)
Electrolyte abnormalities
    Hyponatremia (severe) [see Figure 4.3]
    Hypokalemia (severe)
    Hypernatremia
    Hyperkalemia
Acute hypovolemia, shock, or both
    Trauma
    Sepsis
    Gastroenteritis
    Hemorrhage (external or internal)
Metabolic abnormalities
    Diabetic ketoacidosis

*Enteral alimentation is preferred if feasible.

surgery. Children undergoing bowel surgery may require more than maintenance fluids secondary to bowel wall edema or inflammation, also known as "third spacing." CNS surgery occasionally warrants a decrease in the "normal" maintenance fluids in order to ameliorate possible cerebral edema. Many acute and chronic diseases impair the child's ability to ingest food and water or significantly depress appetite or mental status and may make oral consumption of food and fluids dangerous.

The goal of parenterally administered maintenance fluids is to keep total body water and electrolytes at "even" or "zero" balance. That is, the amount of fluid and electrolytes utilized and expended by the body (metabolism, growth, losses via skin, respiratory tract, GI tract, and urine output) should approximate the amount given to the child intravenously.

Method for Estimating Maintenance Fluid Needs

Numerous methods are being used to estimate maintenance fluid and electrolyte requirements in infants and children. The two most common techniques are based on either metabolic rate (the "caloric" method) or on body surface area ("per square meter" method). Each of these systems has many variations yielding similar but not the same results, and all methods must be considered estimates of actual requirements. Thus, each patient given intravenous fluid and electrolyte therapies requires frequent reassessment and monitoring and, sometimes, revision of the fluid prescription. This section of the chapter outlines the caloric method of fluid therapy.

The major components of maintenance fluid therapy are insensible fluid losses and urine output, with a small amount of fluid normally lost in feces (Table 4.6). Insensible water losses are related to energy expenditure by the body; under basal (resting) conditions, 45 ml of water are lost for every 100 kcal of energy metabolized per day. Two-thirds of these insensible losses occur through the skin (not sweat, which is an additional sensible loss of fluid), and one-third occurs via the respiratory tract.

Alterations in respiratory rate, ambient temperature, and inspired humidity may alter these values somewhat (Table 4.7). In general, few or no electrolytes are lost via the insensible route. The remainder of maintenance fluid requirements are water lost in stool and urine. Normal solid stools account for a very small amount of water loss—about 5 ml/100 kcal metabolized (see Table 4.6). Urine output typically varies according to daily oral fluid intake and solute load. The value used to estimate this component of maintenance requirements is a value that does not force the kidney to maximally concentrate or maximally dilute the urine; under basal conditions, this is estimated to be 50 ml/100 kcal of metabolic energy.

TABLE 4.6 Components of Maintenance Fluid Therapy

Water requirements (ml/100 calories metabolized/day)
    Insensible
        Skin = 30
        Lungs = 15
    Stool = 5
    Urine = 50
Electrolyte requirements (mEq/100 calories metabolized/day)
    Sodium = 2.5–3.0
    Potassium = 2.0–3.0
    Chloride = 4.5–5.5

TABLE 4.7 Conditions Altering Maintenance Fluid or Electrolyte Requirements and Ongoing Losses	
Condition or Problem	**Fluid Adjustment Needed**
Increased metabolic rate	
Fever	Increase caloric estimate by 12% per °C rise in body temperature
Hypermetabolic states (hyperthyroidism, salicylism)	Increase caloric estimate by 25%–50%
Decreased metabolic rate	
Hypothermia	Reduce caloric estimate by 12% per °C fall in fever
Hypometabolic states	Reduce caloric estimate by 5%–15%
Sweat	
Mild to moderate	Increase fluid requirement by 5–25 ml/100 calories metabolized; increase sodium requirement by 0.5–1.0 mEq/100 calories metabolized
Mild to moderate (cystic fibrosis)	Increase fluid as above; increase sodium by 1–2 mEq/100 calories metabolized
Urinary losses	
Oliguria	Adjust fluid allowance to replace insensible losses plus output
Polyuria	Increase water allowance to replace output (may need to decrease dextrose in replacement fluids)
Sodium- or potassium-wasting states	Adjust sodium or potassium to equal losses
Sodium- or potassium-retaining states	Reduce or eliminate sodium or potassium intake

Pediatric Pearl

The estimate of insensible water losses (45 ml/100 kcal metabolized), when added to stool and urine losses (55 ml/100 kcal metabolized), causes the emergence of a simplified, one-to-one relationship of fluid requirements and caloric expenditure: 100 ml of fluid lost (and therefore required) for each 100 kcal expended.

The estimate of caloric requirements is based on body weight in kilograms, which is reasonable for infants older than several weeks of age (Table 4.8). Children who weigh 10 kg or less expend 100 kcal/kg (and thus require 100 ml of

fluid/kg). Infants who weigh between 10 and 20 kg utilize an additional 50 kcal of energy/kg over 10 kg (thus, an additional 50 ml of fluid/kg are necessary). These children thus require 1000 kcal of energy (or 1000 ml of fluid) for the first 10 kg and 50 kcal (or 50 ml of fluid) for each kg between 10 and 20 kg. Children over 20 kg expend an additional 20 kcal in addition to the 1500 kcal (or 1500 ml) required for the first 20 kg (thus, they need an additional 20 ml of fluid).

The caloric method of estimating pediatric fluid requirements also allows estimation of sodium and potassium needs. Typically, children need 2.5 mEq of sodium and potassium (as chloride salts) per 100 kcal metabolized (see Table 4.6). If children are dehydrated, losses of electrolytes along with fluids have already occurred, and it is necessary to estimate these losses and replace them. In addition, it is essential to assess and replace fluid and electrolyte losses that occur via vomiting, diarrhea, nasogastric tube, and surgical drains (often called "ongoing losses"). Typically, parenteral maintenance fluids are given for a brief period of time only, and enteral feeding is begun as soon as appropriate. Although clinicians estimate caloric requirements to calculate fluid needs, the administered fluids rarely supply more than 20% of estimated caloric needs; if the GI route cannot be used for a prolonged pe-

TABLE 4.8 Caloric Requirements Based on Body Weight	
Body Weight (kg)	**Calories Expended (kcal/kg body weight/day)**
3–10	100
10–20	1000 calories + 50 per kg for each kg > 10
> 20	1500 calories + 20 per kg for each kg > 20

riod of time, consideration of parenteral hyperalimentation is warranted.

CASE 4.1

A 15-kg child requires intravenous fluid for several days following surgery. The child has normal hydration status, normal serum electrolytes, and normal kidney function. Assuming no unusual fluid losses, calculate maintenance parenteral fluid and electrolyte administration for 24 hours.

Maintenance fluids are 1000 ml (100 kcal or 100 ml/kg body weight for the first 10 kg) plus 250 ml (50 kcal or ml for each kg between 10 and 20 kg), which equals 1250 kcal or ml/24 hr. Maintenance electrolytes are 2.5 mEq of sodium and potassium per 100 calories metabolized, with 1250 kcal metabolized, which equals 2.5 times 12.5 or 31.25 mEq of sodium and 31.25 mEq of potassium to be given in the daily maintenance volume of 1250 ml.

The final 1-L infusion "bag" should then contain 5% dextrose with 25 mEq of sodium (as chloride) and 25 mEq of potassium, to infuse at a rate of 52.08 ml/hr. (Of course, the intravenous infusion rate should be reasonable; here, 52 ml/hr.)

CASE 4.2

Estimate maintenance fluid and electrolyte requirements for an infant weighing 6.8 kg.

Caloric expenditure is 100 kcal/kg/day for the first 10 kg of body weight; here, this would be 680 kcal. Thus, this child requires about 680 ml of fluid/24 hours. The sodium and potassium requirements are 2.5 mEq of each per 100 calories metabolized; here, this is 17 mEq of sodium and 17 mEq of potassium per day. The final solution would therefore be 1 L of 5% dextrose with 25 mEq of sodium/liter and 25 mEq of potassium/liter, to infuse at 28.3 ml/hr ("rounded off" to 28 ml/hr).

Many factors may alter maintenance requirements (e.g., sweat, fever, and increased respiratory rate, which increase fluid loss), and sick children may have or develop abnormal ongoing losses (e.g., new development of vomiting or diarrhea). In these cases, intravenous fluid requirements need to be adjusted (Table 4.9; see Table 4.7).

Dehydration

One of the most common reasons that parenteral fluid and electrolyte therapy is used in children is **dehydration,** which has many causes (Table 4.10). For most children with dehydration, fluid loss occurs via the GI tract with diarrheal stools, frequently accompanied by vomiting. **Viral (e.g., rotavirus) or bacterial (e.g., *Salmonella*, *Shigella*, or cholera) infections of the GI tract (gastroenteritis), which are frequent in children, are the most common cause of dehydration in most parts of the world.** Fluid loss via the GI tract is often accompanied by anorexia, with concomitant decreased intake of fluids. It should be emphasized that parenteral correction of dehydration is often not necessary, and oral rehydration has been successfully used in children with mild-to-moderate (and occasionally severe) dehydration.

Several important considerations in assessing and treating dehydration help formulate a reasonable therapeutic approach, such as:

- Is the child dehydrated, and if so, how much fluid has been lost?
- Does the child have an osmolar disturbance (usually, hyponatremia or hypernatremia) in addition to the fluid loss?
- Does the child have an acid–base abnormality, and should the child be given specific correction for this?
- Is the serum (or, sometimes better, plasma) level of potassium normal?
- Are the kidneys responding to the fluid and electrolyte abnormalities appropriately?

Determining the Extent of Dehydration

At present, no particular laboratory test can quantify or estimate the severity of dehydration. The more reliable physical signs of dehydration

TABLE 4.9 Gastrointestinal Losses of Fluid and Electrolytes				
Fluid	Na^+ (mEq/L)	K^+ (mEq/L)	Cl^- (mEq/L)	HCO_3^- (mEq/L)
Gastric juice	50	515	110	0
Pancreatic juice	140	5	75	110
Small bowel	140	5	110	30
Ileostomy	130	10	110	30
Diarrhea	50140	515	50110	1550

TABLE 4.10 Causes of Dehydration

Inadequate fluid intake
  Altered thirst (central nervous system lesion)
  Physical impairment (cannot access fluids)
  Altered mental status (lethargy, coma)
  Dysphagia
  Increased fluid needs
Increased gastrointestinal fluid losses
  Diarrhea
  Vomiting
  Ileostomy
  Nasogastric drainage
Increased insensible fluid losses
  Fever
  Thermal injury (burns)
  Sweating
  Cystic fibrosis
  Increased ambient temperature
  Increased respiratory rate
Increased renal fluid losses
  Osmotic diuresis (diabetes mellitus, mannitol)
  Diabetes insipidus (central or nephrogenic)
  Tubular concentrating defect (sickle cell disease, hypokalemia, hypercalcemia, congenital nephropathy)

are **reduced skin elasticity and prolonged capillary refill.**

Pediatric Pearl

Most commonly, the extent of dehydration (and thus the amount of fluid that needs to be replaced) is expressed as a percentage of body weight that has been lost acutely as a result of fluid loss (preillness weight minus admission or current weight, divided by preillness weight, multiplied by 100).

If a very recent preillness body weight is known, then the amount of weight lost when the child is seen for an acute diarrheal illness reflects the amount of body fluid lost. However, because the preillness weight is only rarely known, **the amount of fluid lost by the child is estimated based on physical examination and historical criteria** (Table 4.11); **it is usually expressed as a percentage.** Once the degree of dehydration has been estimated, an organized approach to the various components of intravenous (or oral) fluid therapy can be designed, with close attention paid to frequent reassessment of the patient after therapy is implemented.

Osmolar Considerations

An infant or child with dehydration **may have abnormalities in serum or plasma osmolality, usually resulting from hyponatremia or hypernatremia** that develop concomitantly with the dehydration. In the most common form of dehydration (iso-osmolar or isonatremic), the serum sodium concentration is normal or nearly normal (between 130 and 150 mmol/L). In these children, the amount of water and electrolytes lost from the body are proportional in concentration to electrolyte concentrations in the extracellular fluid space, or hypotonic fluid is lost from the body and is replaced orally with hypotonic fluid, so that serum sodium concentration remains stable. **Approximately 75%–85% of dehydration episodes are isonatremic.** Proportional losses of electrolytes in children vary depending on the degree of isonatremic dehydration (Table 4.12).

Infants with **hyponatremic dehydration (Na⁺ < 130 mEq/L) have had more electrolyte losses than proportional water losses; these infants have more compromised intravascular volume**

TABLE 4.11 Evidence of Dehydration Found on Physical Examination

Symptom/Sign	Mild	Moderate	Severe
Body weight loss			
Infants < 20 kg	5%	10%	15%
Older children	3%	6%	9%
Mucous membranes	Normal	Dry	Very dry, cracked
Tears	Normal	Absent	Absent
Urine output	Normal, concentrated	Decreased	Little or none
Capillary refill	Normal (< 2 sec)	Increased or normal	Increased
Skin elasticity	Normal retraction	Slow retraction	Delayed retraction, tenting
Blood pressure	Normal	Normal; may have orthostatic changes	Low
Heart rate	Normal or slightly increased	Orthostatic changes or increased	Increased; pulses thready

TABLE 4.12 **Estimated Fluid and Electrolyte Deficits in Iso-osmolar Dehydration**

% Dehydration	Water (ml/kg)	Sodium (mEq/kg)	Potassium (mEq/kg)
5	50	4	3
10	100	8	6
15	150	12	9

(more signs of shock) compared with infants with the same volume loss from isonatremia or hypernatremia. **Between 5% and 10% of diarrheal dehydration illnesses are hyponatremic,** and replenishing body stores of sodium is a major goal of therapy. It is possible to distinguish many other causes of hyponatremia on the basis of normal, reduced, or increased body fluid status (Figure 4.3). Significant hyponatremia results in certain clinical findings (Table 4.13).

Hypernatremic dehydration accounts for 5%–15% of diarrheal dehydration episodes; in such cases, intravascular volume is well maintained despite significant volume losses (caused by shifts of intracellular fluids into the extracellular and intravascular spaces because of the increased sodium concentration). **This results in fewer clinical signs typical of dehydration (i.e., less tachycardia and more preserved skin elasticity). Often, the skin texture in these infants**

has a "doughy" feeling. **Hypernatremia can have significant CNS and metabolic sequelae,** both acutely and with correction of the hypernatremia. When hypernatremia develops gradually or has been present for some time, **the cells within the brain begin to generate new osmolar substances (so-called "idiogenic" osmoles, mostly amino acids such as taurine);** these osmoles help to prevent brain cell shrinkage and possible hemorrhage.

Because of possible neurologic sequelae and the newly formed osmoles, **most authorities recommend slow rehydration of infants and children with diarrheal hypernatremic dehydration.** Some young infants (often with poor sucking reflexes or with inexperienced mothers) have developed hypernatremic dehydration with breastfeeding, and several mothers have been found to produce milk with abnormally high sodium concentrations; certainly, incorrect mixing of powdered formulas may also result in hypernatremia. Other conditions may cause hypernatremia (Table 4.14).

Acid–Base Considerations

In severe dehydration, which may be accompanied by peripheral circulatory failure, significant metabolic acidemia may ensue with a low blood pH (Table 4.15). Nevertheless, correction of the metabolic acidemia in this instance does not

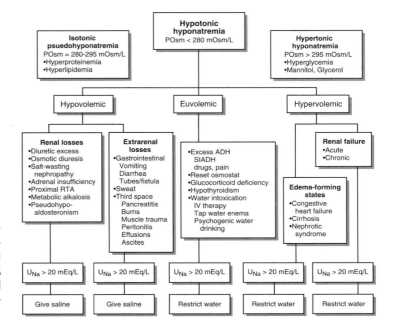

FIGURE 4.3. Classification, diagnosis, and treatment of hyponatremic states. ADH = antidiuretic hormone; IV = intravenous; RTA = renal tubular acidosis; SIADH = syndrome of inappropriate secretion of antidiuretic hormone.

TABLE 4.13 Osmolar Disturbance and Moderate Dehydration—Physical Findings

Symptom/Sign	Isonatremia	Hyponatremia	Hypernatremia
Mental status	Lethargic	Very lethargic	Irritable
Skin texture	Dry	Moist, clammy	Doughy
Heart rate	Increased	Markedly increased	Orthostatic or somewhat increased
Blood pressure	Normal or orthostatic	Low	Normal to orthostatic
Capillary refill (seconds)	1.5–3	> 3	2–3

warrant bolus alkali therapy, but rather, a slower correction of the bicarbonate deficit. The bicarbonate deficit may be estimated as follows:

$$[HCO_3^- \text{ deficit}] = (\text{desired serum } HCO_3^-) - (\text{current serum } HCO_3^-) \times \text{Weight (kg)} \times V_d$$

where V_d is the volume of distribution of HCO_3^- (0.7 in infants; 0.6 in children and adults). Only one-half to two-thirds of the estimated deficit should be replaced.

Children with significant vomiting (as in pyloric stenosis) may have hypochloremic metabolic alkalosis. There is an associated urinary loss of potassium from the distal tubules in an attempt to retain hydrogen ions for the correction of the alkalosis. Chloride-containing solutions (5% dextrose plus 0.45% isotonic saline with added potassium chloride) are used to repair the fluid and electrolyte defects in accordance with the degree of estimated dehydration. Chloride-responsive metabolic alkalosis (e.g., in excessive loss of hydrogen and chloride ions from vomiting, gastric suction, diuretic therapy, and excessive sweat loss from cystic fibrosis) is usually characterized by urinary chloride concentrations less than 10 mEq/L. Chloride-resistant metabolic alkalosis (in primary or secondary hyperaldosteronism such as in renal artery stenosis) is reflected by urinary chloride greater than 20 mEq/L. Aldosterone increases the amount of hydrogen and potassium ions secreted from the distal renal tubules in exchange for sodium reabsorption.

Potassium Considerations
Most patients with diarrheal dehydration require oral rehydration therapy for fluid and electrolyte correction. Virtually all oral rehydration preparations contain at least 20 mEq/L of potassium supplement. Furthermore, the advantage of early feeding in diarrheal manage-

TABLE 4.14 Causes of Hypernatremia

Sodium excess
   Ingestion of seawater
   Excessive parenteral sodium administration
   Improperly mixed infant formula
Water loss or deficit
   Diabetes insipidus
      Central
      Nephrogenic
   Sweating
   Lack of access to water
   Lack of thirst
   Excessive sweat
   Diabetes mellitus
Water loss in excess of sodium loss
   Diarrhea (all causes)
   Osmotic diuresis
   Obstructive uropathy
   Renal dysplasia

TABLE 4.15 Causes of Metabolic Acidosis

Normal anion gap
   Gastrointestinal loss of bicarbonate
      Diarrhea
   Renal loss of bicarbonate
      Renal tubular acidosis
      Renal dysfunction
   Ingestion of chloride acids
      Ammonium chloride
      Hyperalimentation
High anion gap
   Lactic acidosis
   Ketoacidosis
   Renal insufficiency
   Rhabdomyolysis
   Ingestions
      Salicylate
      Methanol
      Formaldehyde
      Ethylene glycol
      Paraldehyde

ment includes gradual restoration of potassium balance. Even when parenteral fluid therapy is needed, intravenous replacement of potassium is unnecessary if enteral feeding is tolerated and serum potassium is within normal limits. Patients with protracted poor feeding, persistent frequent vomiting, or high stool output (> 10 ml/kg/hr) require 20–40 mEq/L of potassium chloride (potassium acetate may be used if there is an associated metabolic acidosis; acetate is metabolized into lactate by the liver) added into the intravenous fluids, even if the serum potassium level is normal. The serum potassium level may not reflect the total body potassium (potassium is largely an intracellular cation); this is especially true for patients with failure to thrive or protein–energy malnutrition because of significant muscle wasting. Clinicians should add potassium to the intravenous fluids only after ensuring that urinary voiding has occurred.

It is essential to prevent iatrogenic hyperkalemia judiciously, because the danger of lethal cardiac arrhythmia is much greater with elevated serum potassium than with hypokalemia. Lethal arrhythmia is hardly ever seen in hypokalemic patients with normal hearts. Patients with rapid onset severe hypokalemia and those with hypokalemia associated with life-threatening symptoms [severe muscle weakness with or without hypoventilation, electrocardiographic (ECG) changes, and cardiac arrhythmia] may require bolus treatment with 0.5–1 mEq/kg/dose given as an infusion over 1–3 hours (intravenous rate $<$ 1 mEq/kg/hr). Intravenous bolus therapy of potassium should occur only in the intensive care unit (ICU) setting with a continuous cardiac monitor as well as frequent measurement of serum potassium (every 30–60 minutes).

Patients with chronic hypokalemia require slower correction of the deficit, and the daily requirement of potassium 1–2 mEq/kg is given as oral supplements. The dose is gradually increased according to the monitored serum level until normal potassium is achieved. Oral supplements can also be used to restore residual potassium deficit after intravenous correction in acute hypokalemia. Several useful oral preparations of potassium that contain sodium, potassium, and bicarbonate are available, including potassium chloride (40 mEq potassium = 3 g potassium chloride), potassium gluconate (40 mEq potassium = 9.4 g potassium gluconate), potassium phosphate, and Polycitra.

Renal Function Considerations

The most common cause of oliguria (urine output < 1 ml/kg/hr in infants; < 0.5 ml/kg/hr in children) is volume deficit, often secondary to dehydration. The resultant renal hypoperfusion may cause prerenal azotemia. Delay in treatment not only jeopardizes full recovery of renal function (with a progression to acute tubular necrosis) but may also cause damage to other major organs. Thus, aggressive fluid therapy is warranted in severe dehydration and peripheral circulatory failure. Furthermore, it may be difficult to differentiate between oliguria secondary to prerenal insufficiency and that due to intrinsic renal failure.

In the event of profound oliguria, it is safer to assume a prerenal insufficiency. It is necessary to give a fluid challenge with a crystalloid infusion using 20 ml/kg isotonic saline or lactated Ringer's solution (preferred in diarrheal dehydration because it provides a bicarbonate supplement) over 30–60 minutes. Clinical signs of improved tissue perfusion are capillary refill greater than 2 seconds; decreased brachial pulse rate; increased blood pressure; and most importantly, enhanced urinary output. In patients with altered mental status and those too young to allow accurate urinary output estimation, urethral catheterization may be necessary. If oligoanuria persists despite one or two doses of bolus crystalloid infusion, it is necessary to give intravenous furosemide 2–5 mg/kg with a repeated fluid challenge.

In most cases, oligoanuria that persists after three boluses of fluid therapy (with or without furosemide) may suggest intrinsic renal failure. It is important to ascertain that the poor urine output is not due to accumulation of urine in the bladder from lower urinary tract obstruction. It is possible to palpate or percuss a distended bladder in the suprapubic region or perform catheterization.

Several biochemical parameters may be useful in the differentiation between prerenal and intrinsic renal failure (Table 4.16). It is essential to interpret these indices in line with other previously obtained clinical information. Some parameters are less useful than others, depending on the clinical situation; for example, blood urea nitrogen (BUN) is affected in hypercatabolic or nutritional deficiency states. Fractional excretion of sodium (FE_{Na}) is the most sensitive parameter. Most of the indices are derived on the basis of intact renal tubular concentrating capacity in prerenal failure (in contrast to the intrinsic renal failure). Thus, urinary specific gravity and osmolality are both elevated in prerenal failure, while urine sodium and FE_{Na} are low.

TABLE 4.16 Biochemical Parameters Used to Differentiate Oliguria			
Laboratory Test	Prerenal Failure	Intrinsic Renal Failure	SIADH
Urine output	Oliguric	Oligoanuric/nonoliguric	Oliguric
Urine microscopy	Often normal	Granular/epithelial/RBC casts	Normal
Urine sodium (mEq/L)			
Children and adults	< 20	> 40	> 40
Neonates	< 40	> 40	> 40
Urine specific gravity			
Children and adults	≥ 1.020	< 1.010	> 1.020
Neonates	≥ 1.015	< 1.015	> 1.020
Urine osmolality (mOsm/L)			
Children and adults	> 500	< 350	> 500
Neonates	> 400	< 400	> 500
Urine:plasma osmolality ratio	> 1.5	< 1.5	> 2.0
BUN (mg/dl)	> 20	< 10	> 15
Creatinine (mg/dl)			
Children and adults	> 40	< 20	> 30
Neonates	> 20	< 15	> 20
BUN:creatinine ratio	> 20	10–20	—
RFI			
Children and adults	< 1.0	> 1.0	> 1.0
Neonates	< 3.0	> 3.0	> 1.0
FE_{Na}			
Children and adults	< 1.0	> 1.0	1.0
Neonates	< 2.5	> 3.0	1.0

BUN = blood urea nitrogen; FE_{Na} = fractional excretion of sodium $[(U_{Na} \times P_{Cr})/(U_{Cr} \times P_{Na}) \times 100]$; RBC = red blood cell; RFI = renal failure index $(U_{Na} \times 100/U_{Cr} \times P_{Cr})$; SIADH = syndrome of inappropriate antidiuretic hormone secretion.

✳ Pediatric Pearl

It should be noted that a primary glomerular disease (often distinguished by clinico-biochemical parameters) without significant tubular involvement may have a concentrated urine (low urinary sodium, high specific gravity, and urine: plasma osmolality ratio) and a low FE_{Na}, mimicking prerenal failure.

Transferred to the ICU is necessary for patients with persistent oligoanuria in spite of seemingly adequate fluid therapy for central line placement and monitoring of central venous pressure. Pressures less than 5 cm H_2O imply persistent hypovolemia; more fluid may be necessary. It is necessary to perform a careful search for the etiology of the circulatory failure, which may include septicemia (redistributive shock), hypoglycemia, and drug poisoning. Pressures more than 10 cm H_2O suggest inadequate cardiac output in spite of adequate preload (cardiogenic shock).

On establishing the diagnosis of acute (intrinsic) renal failure, oral and parenteral fluid replacement should be limited to insensible water loss and ongoing urinary output (as well as fluid output from other sources). In most pediatric patients, the daily fluid needed to maintain a zero balance can be calculated as:

$$M = UOP + ERL + IWL$$

where M is daily fluid requirement; UOP is urinary output, or the estimated urine output of the previous 24 hours (electrolyte content may be determined); ERL is extrarenal fluid loss, or fluid loss (estimated and analyzed for electrolyte composition) replaced accordingly; and IWL is insensible water loss of 400–500 ml/m^2/day.

A shorter period of urine collection and measurement (16, 8, or 4 hours) may be chosen for determination of a more physiologic fluid replacement. The smaller time interval should be used for younger patients (especially neonates) in view of the characteristically high fluid turnover rate.

Adequacy of fluid therapy is monitored by a strict input–output analysis, daily weight, physical assessment and serum sodium concentration. Most patients have a daily weight loss of 0.5%–1% due to a high catabolic activity or inadequate calorie intake. In patients with a stable sodium consumption, hyponatremia in the face of oliguria may reflect a positive fluid balance while hypernatremia signifies fluid deficit. Dilutional anemia may also indicate overhydration.

Approach to Parenteral Therapy in Dehydrated Infants or Children

Phases of fluid therapy in children are often described and provide a useful framework for organizing fluid therapy and (very importantly) following the results of the therapy.

Phase 1

The aim of the first phase of therapy is **restoration of the circulating intravascular volume in children with severe dehydration and shock.** If an infant or child has a history of volume deficit and is severely dehydrated or has signs of shock, **rapid intravenous infusion of a volume-expanding agent at 20 ml/kg body weight is appropriate.** (Usually this agent is isotonic saline, although lactated Ringer's or 5% albumin may be used.) Continuous monitoring during this therapy is necessary, and intensive nursing and medical support are required. After the infusion, repeat evaluation of vital signs and physical examination are essential, and it is necessary to repeat the "bolus" of isotonic saline until cardiovascular stability (improved capillary refill, lower heart rate, higher blood pressure, improved mental status) ensues. Typically, between one and three such infusions are necessary.

Children in hypovolemic shock should not receive inotropic agents unless restoration of the intravascular volume fails to improve cardiac output. Assessment of serum electrolytes, urea nitrogen, and creatinine should occur prior to fluid therapy, because these help guide the subsequent phases of fluid therapy. **Children with dehydration but no evidence of shock do not require "bolus" fluid therapy, and phase 1 can be eliminated.** Many physicians recommend subtracting the initial fluid boluses given to the infant from the maintenance and deficit fluids calculated for the initial 24 hours; this is optional and depends on the individual patient.

Phase 2

Phase 2 in fluid replacement therapy requires attention to several components of fluid therapy as discussed previously (see METHOD FOR ESTI-

MATING MAINTENANCE FLUID NEEDS). All children need maintenance fluid, and for children with isonatremic or hyponatremic dehydration, maintenance fluids should be calculated as described above. Maintenance therapy for children with hypertonic dehydration is described in the following section. **In addition to maintenance fluids, replacement of losses from ongoing diarrhea, vomitus, or nasogastric secretions is essential.** Accurate replacement involves measurement of the electrolyte content of these body fluids in the clinical laboratory, volume measurement at the bedside, and administration of appropriate replacement fluids. Table 4.9 gives typical values for these ongoing losses, which can be used as guidelines. If these ongoing losses are significant, frequent replacement (every 1–2 hours) is necessary; for less severe losses, less frequent replacement may be appropriate.

Deficit therapy (replacement of previously lost fluids) can be calculated in several ways for children with isonatremic or hyponatremic dehydration. If accurate and recent preillness body weight is known, then the amount of fluid needed to be replaced (as deficit) is simply the preillness weight minus the current weight (in kilograms). A body weight that decreases by 1 kg from diarrheal fluid loss requires 1 L of fluid replacement (1 L of water weighs 1 kg). **It is essential to give this and other deficit replacements in addition to "regular" maintenance fluids and replacement of ongoing losses.**

If preillness weights are not available, it is possible to estimate the percentage dehydration by using the physical examination criteria listed in Table 4.11. The preillness weight may be "back-calculated" according to the following formula:

$$\frac{x \text{ (preillness weight in kg)}}{\text{Current weight in kg}} = \frac{100}{100 - \% \text{ dehydration}}$$

The amount of fluid lost in the acute dehydration episode that should be replaced is then estimated as x (preillness weight) minus the current weight, which equals the volume of fluid to be replaced. **Alternatively, the amount of fluid deficit can be estimated in infants based on the percent dehydration, as outlined in Tables 4.11 and 4.12.** Table 4.12 also gives proportional electrolyte replacement needs for children with isotonic dehydration.

Fluid Calculations in Isonatremic Dehydration

 CASE 4.3

A male infant is seen in the emergency department because of diarrhea, decreased oral fluid intake, and irritability. The boy's weight at present is 8.1 kg; his mucous membranes are dry, and no tears are present when he cries. Parents report that the last urine output was about 12 hours prior to the emergency department visit. Blood pressure is 86/45 mm Hg, heart rate is 152 beats/min, capillary refill is 3 seconds, and skin elasticity is slow to retract. Based on these findings, you estimate the child to be 10% dehydrated and in need of urgent fluid resuscitation.

Question 4.3.1
What are the first steps in this child's rehydration therapy?

Answer 4.3.1
The first step involves obtaining vascular access and serum electrolytes. The second step involves giving 20 ml/kg body weight of isotonic saline and reassessing the child. The amount of isotonic saline is 20 ml/kg multiplied by 8.1 kg, or 162 ml; it should be given as quickly as possible (usually over 10–20 minutes).

The child responds to the fluid challenge with a decrease in heart rate to 115/min and improved capillary refill of 2 seconds, and urine output, although scant, is obtained and is concentrated, with a specific gravity of greater than 1.035. The child's serum sodium is 135 mEq/L.

Question 4.3.2
Now that the child is more stable, how would you proceed with the fluid therapy?

Answer 4.3.2
Because the child now weighs 8.1 kg and you have determined that he is 10% dehydrated, the preillness weight can be calculated accordingly:

$$\frac{x}{8.1 \text{ kg}} = \frac{100}{100} - 10$$

$$\times \text{ (preillness weight)} = 9 \text{ kg}$$

Therefore, the amount of fluid lost (deficit fluid) is 9 kg minus 8.1 kg, which equals 0.9 kg (or, in fluid, 0.9 L or 900 ml). The amount of sodium and potassium in the deficit fluids is outlined in Table 4.12; here, the amount of sodium that should be given in the 900 ml of deficit fluid is 72 mEq.

Maintenance fluids need to be given; 9 kg multiplied by 100 kcal (ml) equals 900 ml, with 22.5 mEq of sodium (see Table 4.6; 9 × 2.5 mEq sodium per 100 calories metabolized) for 24 hours.

The total 24-hour fluid estimation is then 900 ml (deficit) plus 900 ml (maintenance), which equals 1800 ml/24 hour (as mentioned, you may "subtract" the initial fluid bolus given, which reduces the 24-hour infusion volume to 1638 ml). The total sodium content is 72 mEq (deficit) plus 22.5 mEq (maintenance), which equals 94.5 mEq of sodium per day. A 1-liter container of 5% dextrose, with 54 mEq sodium chloride added, set to infuse at 75 ml/hr, gives 1800 ml of fluid over 24 hours, with the required sodium deficit and maintenance (or run at 68 ml/hr to give the total infusion minus the initial bolus therapy). This is approximately "5% dextrose with one-third normal saline," with potassium added to the intravenous solution after urinary voiding has been established.

Fluid Calculations in Hyponatremic Dehydration

As mentioned previously, children with hyponatremia often appear more ill than isonatremic children with similar volume deficits. The procedure for calculating the amount of fluid to be given is the same as described previously (see METHOD FOR ESTIMATING MAINTENANCE FLUID NEEDS); in fact, the only difference is that more sodium is given. It is necessary to approach children as if they have an isonatremic dehydration requiring replacement of the fluid deficit. Maintenance fluid and sodium requirements are outlined in Tables 4.6 and 4.12. The sodium deficit may be estimated using the following equation:

(Desired [Na] − observed [Na]) × weight (kg)
× 0.6 (volume of distribution of Na)

It is recommended not to raise the serum sodium concentration more than 10–15 mEq/day in order to avoid neurologic complications such as seizures and pontine demyelination. Hyponatremia presenting with neurologic manifestations requires rapid correction with 3% sodium chloride not to exceed 1–2 mEq/L/hr.

 CASE 4.4

A previously healthy female infant who weighed 10 kg on a well-child evaluation during the previous week has diarrhea with some vomiting for several days. On evaluation in the pediatric emergency department, she weighs 9 kg; in addition, she has sunken eyes, a capillary refill of 4 seconds, and dry mucous membranes. She is sleepy and lethargic. Blood pressure is 55/38 mm Hg with a heart rate of 160 beats/min. Laboratory studies indicate a sodium of 125 mEq/L, potassium of 3.8 mEq/L, chloride of 115 mEq/L, and bicarbonate of 9 mEq/L. Serum urea nitrogen is 32 mg/dl, and creatinine is 0.7 mg/dl.

Question 4.4.1

Should this child receive emergency fluid resuscitation?

Answer 4.4.1

The prolonged capillary refill and depressed mental status of this child, along with the clinical history, indicate significant hypovolemia and warrant emergency resuscitation. This child should receive 20 ml/kg body weight of isotonic saline (or lactated Ringer's solution) rapidly (over 10–20 minutes); this should be repeated if the response is not sufficient.

Question 4.4.2

If a single infusion of isotonic saline of 20 ml/kg reduces capillary refill to 2 seconds, increases blood pressure to 90/48 mm Hg, and decreases heart rate to 124 beats/min, what would the fluid and electrolyte requirements be?

Answer 4.4.2

The maintenance fluid requirement for a child weighing 10 kg is 1000 ml/day, and the maintenance sodium requirement is 25 mEq/day (2.5 mEq/ 100 kcal metabolized). Because 1 kg or 1000 ml of fluid have been lost (in a child who is 10% dehydrated), the fluid deficit is 1000 ml. Proportional sodium losses (as in isonatremic dehydration) are given in Table 4.12; there are 80 mEq of sodium (8 mEq of sodium/kg body weight in a child with 10% dehydration). Additional sodium losses are calculated based on the sodium deficit formula:

$$(\text{Desired Na} - \text{current Na}) \times \text{weight (kg)} \times 0.6 = \text{Na deficit}$$

Body weight (kg) multiplied by 0.6 is the commonly used formula for extracellular fluid volume of distribution for ions such as sodium. In this case, the sodium deficit is

$$(135 - 125) \times 10 \times 0.6 = 60 \text{ mEq Na}$$

The total 24-hour fluid requirement is then 1000 ml (maintenance) plus 1000 ml (deficit) or 2000 ml, and the total sodium requirement is 25 mEq (maintenance) plus 80 mEq (proportional losses) plus 60 mEq (sodium deficit) or 165 mEq sodium.

This child could receive 2000 ml of 5% dextrose over 24 hours in a solution that provides 165 mEq of sodium in that volume. The final 1-liter intravenous fluid container could include 5% dextrose with 82.5 mEq/L sodium, infused at a rate of 84 ml/hr.

An alternative is to give one-half of this deficit–maintenance solution in the first 8 hours (900 ml in 8 hours = 112 ml/hr) and the remainder over the ensuing 16 hours (900 ml in 16 hours = 56 ml/hr), assuming there are no significant ongoing losses. This solution is very close to the commercially available 5% dextrose with one-half "normal saline." Potassium should be added to the intravenous fluids after urinary voiding is observed, usually at 20–40 mEq/L.

When an infant or child requires parenteral fluid administration, every effort should be made to resume enteral feedings as soon as possible. Often, the fluid bolus or first few hours of parenteral fluids are all that is necessary. The important point to remember is that these fluid calculations are at best estimates of fluid and electrolyte requirements, and frequent reassessment of physical examination, vital signs, and blood chemistries is imperative.

Fluid Calculations in Hypernatremic Dehydration

Causes of hypernatremia are listed in Table 4.14. Children with diarrheal dehydration and hypernatremia have lost both water and sodium from the body, but the water loss is proportionally less than the sodium loss. Because many children have diarrheal stools with sodium contents of between 30 and 60 mEq/L, **loss of this hypotonic (relative to the extracellular fluid) diarrhea without adequate enteral replacement of hypotonic fluids can result in hypernatremic dehydration.** With hypernatremic dehydration, it remains reasonable to replace volume deficits slowly and to adjust maintenance fluid requirements, as described in Case 4.5.

 CASE 4.5

An infant boy with a recent weight of 10 kg has diarrhea and occasional vomiting and refuses all attempts at feeding. **He is becoming more irritable, and now has a somewhat high-pitched cry. His skin has a "doughy" feel,** the mucous membranes are dry, and muscle tone is somewhat increased. Capillary refill is slightly less than 2 seconds, blood pressure and heart rate are normal, and weight is now 9 kg. Blood pressure is 98/60 mm Hg, and heart rate is 122/min. The urine output for the last 24 hours has been minimal. **Serum electrolytes demonstrate a sodium level of 165 mEq/L.**

Question 4.5.1
Will this child require emergency fluids?

Answer 4.5.1
This child is certainly dehydrated, **with dry mucous membranes, altered mental status, and decreased urine output.** However, capillary refill is not significantly prolonged, and blood pressure and heart rate are normal. **Some physicians would opt for treatment with 10–20 ml/kg body weight of isotonic saline because of the low urine output.** Because of the high serum sodium (and con-comitantly high levels of antidiuretic hormone in response to the ensuing increase in osmolality), however, urine output is obligatorily low. The child may benefit from bolus infusion, but with this clinical scenario it is not mandatory.

Question 4.5.2
Assume that the attending physician did not want to give a bolus infusion but asks you to calculate maintenance and deficit replacement therapy for fluids and electrolytes. How would you do this for a child with hypernatremia?

Answer 4.5.2
Modifications in maintenance and deficit replacement fluids and electrolytes are required for children with hypernatremia. When the components of maintenance fluids were described earlier (see METHODS FOR ESTIMATING MAINTENANCE FLUID NEEDS), the major components were insensible body losses (respiratory and skin) and an allowance for urine output that is reasonable to excrete waste products but not force the kidney to maximally concentrate or maximally dilute the urine. In hypernatremic dehydration with hyperosmolality and a maximal secretion of antidiuretic hormone, urine output is obligatorily small. It is therefore reasonable to allow 65–70 ml (rather than 100 ml)/100 kcal metabolized as daily maintenance fluids and an additional 30–35 ml/100 calories metabolized as deficit replacement. The total amount of fluid to be given would then be 100 ml/100 calories metabolized per day (which in "normal" situations are maintenance require-ments). The sodium content of the intravenous fluids should be small (0.2%–0.3% isotonic saline).

It is essential that this volume be given at a uniform rate over a 48-hour period with no bolus or increased volume in the first 48 hours. The danger with too rapid expansion of the extracellular volume with too dilute a solution is that it may lead to a precipitous drop in the serum sodium and too rapid fluid shifts intracellularly. Seizures and cerebral edema could result.

A prospective study compared the use of hypotonic dextrose and saline (5% dextrose with 0.2% isotonic saline) at 100 ml/kg (estimated rehydrated) body weight per day with 5% dextrose and 0.2% isotonic saline given faster (150 ml/kg/-day) and 5% dextrose with 0.45 normal saline given faster (150 ml/kg /day). **Children given the fluids more rapidly and with more sodium had a significantly higher complication rate, with more seizure episodes during treatment and more edema.** Those given hypotonic saline more slowly had more controlled resolution of their hypernatremia with fewer adverse effects.

Children treated for hypernatremia require very close monitoring of their body weight, urine output, serum glucose, and calcium levels. **Hypocalcemia may require intravenous calcium replacement. In addition, hyperglycemia may require reducing the dextrose concentration to 2.5% rather than the usual 5%. Most physicians report that a sodium reduction of 0.5 mEq/L/hr or between 10 and 15 mEq/L/day are reasonable goals.** Serum electrolytes should be obtained frequently (every 2–8 hours, depending on the original sodium concentration, the severity of clinical illness, and the response to fluid therapy). It should also be remembered that urine output will be quite low until serum sodium levels are near the normal range, and urine output alone is not an adequate tool to monitor efficacy of therapy.

Approach to the Use of Oral Rehydration Solution

Oral rehydration solution (ORS) is necessary in all children with diarrhea or vomiting, except in conditions such as peripheral circulatory failure, frequent and persistent vomiting, and serious ill-ness with or without altered mental status (Table 4.17). Early initiation of ORS may prevent dehy-dration in most patients. On initial contact with the patients, it is necessary to perform a goal-oriented history and physical examination. As-sessment of dehydration status should be as-sessed based on suggested clinical parameters (see Table 4.11). The most sensitive of these pa-rameters include loss of skin turgor, dry oral mu-cosa, sunken eyeballs, and altered mental status. The degree of dehydration can be estimated more accurately if the premorbid weight is known.

It is necessary to administer ORS to correct the calculated fluid deficit plus the maintenance and the ongoing fluid loss over 4–6 hours. Esti-mates of ongoing fluid loss for every diarrheal

TABLE 4.17 Guidelines for Oral Rehydration Therapy

Patient eligibility

    All ages

    Any cause of dehydration

    Avoid with shock or near-shock, intractable vomiting, or altered mental status

Method

Estimate fluid deficit based on previous weight (if known) and percent dehydration (see Table 4.11).

Use rehydration solution with glucose content of 2.0–2.5 g/dl and sodium content of 60–75 mEq/L.

Give 6–8 hours of maintenance volume plus deficit fluid volume.

If stool losses continue, replace with rehydration formula.

After rehydration, reassess. If patient is still dehydrated, estimate deficit fluid, add maintenance fluids,
    and give over 6–8 hours.

Continue breastfeeding.

If rehydration is successful, change to maintenance formula.

Do not use rehydration solution for more than 4–12 hours.

If patient is hypernatremic, give replacement fluids over 24 hours.

For maintenance phase:

    Use solution with glucose of 2.0–2.5 g/dl and sodium of 40–60 mEq/L.

    Give as tolerated, making sure enough is taken to supply maintenance needs and ongoing losses.

    Offer half-strength formula within 24 hours after starting rehydration therapy; advance to full strength
        within 24 hours.

stool output are 50–100 ml and 100–200 ml for children younger than 2 years of age and older than 2 years of age, respectively. Alternatively, it is possible to weigh or quantify every stool output as 10 ml/kg body weight.

After 4–6 hours of rehydration, reassessment is appropriate. If the child is still dehydrated, it is necessary to administer a newly reestimated fluid requirement once again. Cycles continue until rehydration is adequate. Thereafter, ORS is

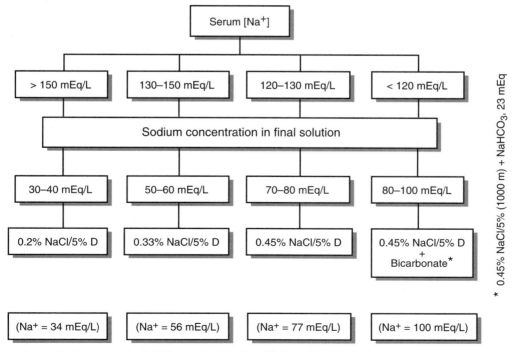

FIGURE 4.4. Decision tree for fluid therapy in dehydrated infants. D = dextrose.

given as the calculated maintenance requirement plus the ongoing fluid requirement.

For example: a 10-kg infant with a 10% weight loss following an acute onset of diarrhea that occurs every 3 hours would require a specific amount of ORS in the initial 6 hours based on the following calculations:

$$\text{Fluid deficit} = 1000 \text{ kg} \times 10\%$$
$$= 1000 \text{ ml ORS}$$

Maintenance
requirement $= 100 \text{ ml/kg/24 hr (first 10 kg)}$
$$= 25 \text{ ml/kg/6 hr} = 250 \text{ ml ORS}$$

Ongoing loss $= 2 \text{ stools in 6 hours (10 ml/kg/}$
$$\text{stool)}$$
$$= 200 \text{ ml ORS}$$

Therefore, the total amount of ORS required in the first 6 hours equals 1450 ml. On reassessment, the patient is well hydrated, and the diarrheal stool subsided after three bowel movements in the next 12 hours. Therefore, the "maintenance" and "ongoing" fluid replacement needed would approximate 500 ml and 300 ml, respectively. ORS can be given by spoon, cup, or bottle.

Maintenance ORS (next 12 hr) $= 25 \text{ ml/kg/12 hr}$
$$= 500 \text{ ml}$$

Estimate of ongoing loss $= 3 \text{ stools/12 hr}$
$$(10 \text{ ml/kg/stool})$$
$$= 300 \text{ ml}$$

Summary of Pediatric Fluid Therapy

The calculation of fluid requirements for dehydrated children can be complex, so a "decision tree" approach has been developed that works very well for children with moderate dehydration (Figure 4.4). Once the clinician has decided what fluids are necessary and implemented their administration, frequent physical examinations, vital signs (especially body weight), and certain "follow-up" laboratory parameters help ensure the achievement of the therapeutic goals of safe restoration of body fluid status and resumption of enteral alimentation.

SUGGESTED READINGS

Principles of Pediatric Nutrition
American Academy of Pediatrics: *Pediatric Nutrition Handbook.* Elk Grove Village, IL: American Academy of Pediatrics, 1993.

Lawrence RA: *Breast Feeding, a Guide for the Medical Profession,* 3rd ed. St. Louis: CV Mosby, 1989.

Martinez GA, et al: Nutrient intakes of American infants and children fed cow's milk or infant formula. *Am J Dis Child* 139:1010–1018, 1985.

Pittard WB III: Breast milk immunology: A frontier in infant nutrition. *Am J Dis Child* 133:83–87, 1987.

Shelov SP (ed): *Caring for Your Baby and Young Child, Birth to Age 5.* New York: Bantam Books, 1993.

Parenteral Fluid and Electrolyte Therapy
Adrogue H, Madias N: Hypernatremia. *N Engl J Med* 342(20):1493–1499, 2000.

Adrogue H, Madias N: Hyponatremia. *N Engl J Med* 342(21):1581–1589, 2000.

Jospe N, Forbes G: Fluids and electrolytes—Clinical aspects. *Pediatr Rev* 17(11):395–403, 1996.

Moritz ML, Ayus JC: The changing pattern of hypernatremia in hospitalized children. *Pediatrics* 104(32): 435–439, 1999.

Murphy MS: Guidelines for managing acute gastroenteritis based on a systematic review of published research. *Arch Dis Child* 79:279–284, 1998.

Sio JO, Alfiler CA: *Fluid and Electrolyte Management in Pediatrics.* Manila, Phillipines, Express Types and Prints, 2000.

Chapter 5

Behavioral Pediatrics and Child Abuse

Esther H. Wender

In the practice of pediatrics, the behavior of an infant, child, or adolescent is often the primary concern. Frequently, parents are seeking advice about managing that behavior. However, at times, they are concerned that the behavior might indicate a significant disorder and are anxious to know whether a problem exists and what should be done about it. Estimates indicate that as much as 50% of general pediatric practice is related to assessing and advising parents and others about children's behavior. This chapter is devoted to a review of the most common behavioral issues in children and their origins, assessment, and management. Child abuse is also reviewed as a separate, but related, issue.

Pathophysiology

Children's behavior is always a combination of neurobiologic and socioenvironmental influences. The degree to which any particular behavior or behavior pattern is subject to the influence of biologic or social and environmental factors varies and often fluctuates over time. The following discussion is a review of these neurobiologic and socioenvironmental factors and their interaction.

The most common sources of neurobiologic influence are listed in Table 5.1. Experts are only beginning to understand the precise manner in which neurobiology affects behavior. It is known that there is a significant genetic contribution to learning disabilities and attention deficit disorders. However, the precise nature of the genetic contribution is not known. Similarly, the exact mechanism involved in some prenatally acquired neurobiologic factors such as the effect of alcohol consumed in large quantities by pregnant women is unclear. Postnatally acquired disorders such as injuries or diseases affecting the central nervous system (CNS) are better understood, but their specific impact on behavior is still a mystery.

All behavior is simultaneously affected by socioenvironmental factors. Some of the most common sources of socioenvironmental influence are listed in Table 5.2. Complex interactions among the following three factors determine the degree to which any of these issues affects children's behavior.

1. Children and their vulnerability
2. Nature and timing of the environmental factors
3. Any counteracting influences that might be present

In addition, behavioral variations are due to development, which is itself a dynamic process resulting from neurophysiologic processes and environmental influences. Every behavior must be evaluated in its development context. For example, certain behaviors that may be quite normal at one developmental phase may represent a significant problem at another stage. Bed-wetting, which may be normal at 3 years of age, is usually perceived as a problem at 8 years of age. Some of the most commonly recognized "problems" of behavior are listed in Table 5.3, organized according to the most important reason for their appearance.

Developmental "crises" refer to normal developmental issues to which children may overreact or that frequently elicit caregiver stress, sometimes leading to inappropriate caregiver response. Although the behavior itself may be within normal limits, the potential for a maladaptive outcome leads to the need for preventive counseling.

"Developmental pattern" disorders are common and almost always associated with behavior problems. The general public (and physicians) often misunderstand the source of behaviors associated with developmental disorders. These behaviors are either intrinsic manifestations of the developmental problem or possibly reactions to the rejection and resulting poor self-esteem inherent in these conditions.

The sources of acute or chronic stress are extensive. Although the nature of the stress may be

TABLE 5.1 Neurobiologic Influences on Behavior in Children

Genetic conditions
Inherited temperament
Inherited cognitive potential
Genetically transmitted disorders

Prenatally or perinatally acquired conditions
Congenital infections of the CNS
Drug or alcohol effects
Birth injuries

Postnatally acquired conditions
Injuries to the CNS
Diseases affecting the CNS
Endocrine disorders
Exogenous toxins such as lead

CNS = central nervous system.

quite varied, the problematic behavioral reactions of infants, children, and adolescents are often quite similar. The source of the stress may be either in the family (e.g., abuse, personal loss such as death or divorce) or in the community (e.g., war or natural disaster). The stress may also be specific to the child (e.g., acute illness; loss of function as a result of injury; chronic illness, especially with uncertain outcome).

Clinical and Laboratory Evaluation

History

The evaluation of behavior is especially dependent on information gathered from the history. However, compared to the history of medical ill-

TABLE 5.2 Social or Environmental Influences on Behavior in Children

Rearing practices
Method of discipline
Type of emotional climate
Consistency and structure

Family environment
Clothing, shelter, food
Health care
Presence of abuse or neglect
Relationships with parents and siblings

Community environment
Culture
War, famine
Natural disaster

TABLE 5.3 Common Behavior Problems in Children

Problems associated with developmental "crises"
Sleep problems in infants and toddlers
Temper tantrums and defiant behaviors in toddlers and adolescents
Fears and anxieties in preschool and school-age children
Bed-wetting (enuresis) in early school-age children
Soiling (encopresis) in preschool and school-age children
Risky behaviors (sex, drugs, firearms, automobiles) in adolescents

Problems related to "developmental pattern" disorders
Aggressive behaviors in preschool children with specific language delays
Immature behaviors in children with developmental delay
Inattentive or hyperactive and impulsive behaviors in children with attention-deficit hyperactivity disorder
Inattentive or immature behaviors in children with specific learning disabilities

Problems associated with acute or chronic stress
Withdrawn and "regressed" behavior
Excessive anxiety or fear
"Acting out" or provocative behavior

ness, the history of behavior may be difficult to obtain. Some of the problem is language. If you ask a mother, "What was the child's temperature?" or "Where does it hurt?," the answer is usually straightforward. In contrast, if you ask, "What are the behaviors that worry you?," the answer may range from "I'm not worried" to "He's lazy" or "She's dumb." These words are loaded with psychologic issues and may mean something very different to the physician than to the parent(s) from whom the history is obtained. Obtaining a behavioral history is, therefore, an art that must be practiced. Certain questions are important (Table 5.4).

Pediatric Pearl

Obtaining an accurate history of behavior problems requires paying attention to the meaning of words parents use to describe a child's problem.

TABLE 5.4	**Important Questions in History-Taking**

How does your child compare with other children his age with regard to:
    Temper tantrums?
    Activity level?
    Aggressive behavior?
    Attention span?

What does your child *do* that makes you say he is:
    Aggressive?
    Lazy?
    Immature?

When did the behavior start?

What is the context of the behavior (e.g., what else is happening to the child when the behavior occurs)?

Do these behaviors affect your child's ability to:
    Get along with peers?
    Get along with adults?
    Achieve at school?
    Participate in age-appropriate activities such as sports and play?

The identification of many behavioral disorders requires obtaining the history of a pattern of behavior over time. For example, encopresis is a complicated disorder that often begins with constipation in infancy, then involves resistance to toilet training during the toddler period, and finally leads to retention of stool with resulting overflow soiling during the early school-age period [see BED-WETTING (ENURESIS) IN SCHOOL-AGE CHILDREN]. The pediatrician must learn to recognize behavior patterns that are associated with many of these disorders. In addition, the clinician must address parenting issues such as the following:

- The actions of the parents in response to the behavior
- The important events antecedent to the behavior
- The reaction of peers, siblings, and parents to the behavior

Each of the behavior problems associated with the developmental crises listed in Table 5.3 has common presenting history patterns, which are described in the following discussion.

SLEEP PROBLEMS IN INFANTS AND TODDLERS. Sleep problems in infants typically present as difficulty or slowness in being able to sleep through the night. Exceptionally brief episodes of sleep (i.e., 30 minutes rather than the expected 3–4 hours) and prolonged periods of fussing and crying (e.g., colic), which may be reported as children being "unable to sleep," are other presenting complaints. Older infants and toddlers most commonly present with resistance to going to sleep or waking up and then being unable to return to sleep. Rearing practices, especially the methods parents use to get their child to sleep and the steps parents take to keep their child from crying, significantly affect these behaviors. In turn, the parents' emotional reaction to their child's crying or resistance to sleep affects rearing practices.

TEMPER TANTRUMS AND DEFIANT BEHAVIORS IN TODDLERS AND ADOLESCENTS. All children occasionally have temper tantrums and defiant behaviors (e.g., saying "no," yelling, or striking out), which normally increase during the toddler period and in early adolescence. Both periods of development are associated with assertion of independence. The defiance is usually seen in response to parental requests or discipline. However, when this type of behavior is excessive for the child's age or is associated with frustration (e.g., the child cannot accomplish a task or is teased by peers), it may indicate more serious problems.

FEARS AND ANXIETIES IN PRESCHOOL AND SCHOOL-AGE CHILDREN. Beginning at approximately 3 years of age and extending into the middle school-age period, children normally experience a number of different fears and anxieties. Young preschool children typically see magical rather than rational reasons for everyday experience and, therefore, may be afraid, for example, of flushing toilets, air conditioning vents, and elevators. Clowns and people dressed up in costumes may be frightening. As children become older (5 or 6 years), they frequently become afraid of the dark, of monsters in closets or under the bed, and of animals and loud noises. School-age children typically fear death or dismemberment and go through periods of belief in superstition and frequent nightmares. Problems may occur when parents misunderstand and overreact to these common fears. Any of these normal fears or anxieties is a source of concern when it keeps the child from participating in age-appropriate activities.

BED-WETTING (ENURESIS) IN SCHOOL-AGE CHILDREN. The gradual acquisition of bladder control, first during the day and then at night, is part of the normal development of toddlers and preschool children, although there is considerable variation in speed of development and in parental approaches to training. By 5 years of age, about 20% of children still wet the bed at night, and 5% also wet during the day. These numbers gradually decrease as development proceeds. Enuresis is more frequent in boys and is clearly associated with developmental problems.

Pediatric Pearl

By the age of 18 years, approximately 1% of individuals still wet the bed in the absence of any significant medical problem.

Enuresis also has a significant genetic component. A very small but important percentage of children who are persistent bed-wetters have an underlying neurologic or anatomic problem. Stress clearly affects both the degree and the persistence of bed-wetting in those cases in which the condition has no biologic cause. In children with school problems, for example, enuresis may be better during summer vacation and worse during the school year. Secondary emotional problems may occur when parents are overly punitive in their response to bed-wetting or when the child feels shamed by the problem.

SOILING (ENCOPRESIS) IN PRESCHOOL AND SCHOOL-AGE CHILDREN. The development of soiling as a problem often follows a complex sequence of both biologic and child-rearing issues. The majority of children who develop encopresis are constipated in early childhood, even in infancy. During the toilet-training period, they frequently resist having bowel movements, and in many instances parent–child interaction problems develop around the coercion of toilet training. In the preschool period, children then have infrequent movements and gradually develop megacolon, which is a distention of the colon associated with a decrease in responsiveness to the neurologic signals that normally precede defecation. The presence of megacolon is often indicated by very-large-caliber stools passed infrequently (i.e., once every week or two). In the final stages, watery stool leaks from the proximal colon around the impacted stool in the distal colon, leading to soiling. This is the most common pattern, but encopresis may also result from rare neurologic abnormalities (Hirschsprung disease) or from inattention to the need to defecate but without stool impaction and megacolon in children with attention deficit problems. Finally, soiling may be a part of a serious psychopathology.

RISKY BEHAVIORS (SEX, DRUGS, FIREARMS, AUTOMOBILES) IN ADOLESCENTS. Part of the normal pattern of development in most adolescents is experimentation with "adult" (especially "forbidden adult") behavior preceding the establishment of a firm sense of identity (see Chapter 3, Adolescent Medicine). During this transition, adolescents commonly experiment with sexual expression, from kissing and petting in some to sexual intercourse in others. This sexual experimentation includes homosexual behavior in those destined to become homosexual as well as in many heterosexuals. Many adolescents experiment with smoking and alcohol. A lower but significant number try marijuana, and experimentation with other illicit drugs is less common but still fairly frequent. Adolescents are also very likely to explore the use of guns or other weapons and to participate in risky use of the automobile (e.g., joy riding, speeding).

For most adolescents, this period of experimentation is brief and quickly supplanted by a return to behaviors that are the cultural norm for their family or community. Unfortunately, accidental death or injury all too frequently results from this experimentation. Clearly, the greatest deterrents to a chronic pattern of substance abuse or risky behaviors are (1) a strong family attachment in which counteracting family cultural values have been clearly communicated, and (2) a good sense of self-esteem.

CHILD ABUSE. History may suggest the possibility of child abuse. Unfortunately, child abuse frequently first comes to the attention of the health care system when children present with an injury for which the explanation seems unlikely or suspicious. Another common presentation is physical findings or examination results that suggest previous episodes of intentional injury. Both of these presentations occur late in the cycle of chronic abuse, and the resulting injuries may be serious or even life threatening. Psychologic trauma from the abuse has already occurred by the time these discoveries are made. Nevertheless, the physician should be aware of the types of injuries, the typical physical findings, and the characteristic test results that suggest abuse (see PHYSICAL EXAMINATION).

The presenting behaviors of children involved in situations of child abuse are nonspecific, and corroboration by other evidence is essential. In general, children react to chronic or acute stress in three different ways. They may do one of the following:

- Become withdrawn or sad
- Develop new and excessive anxieties or fears
- Act out with anger and aggression

All of these behaviors deserve careful analysis, particularly if they represent a change from the previous state.

Various factors associated with a parent or the parent–child interaction often increase the risk of child abuse. Frequently, the parent was a victim of abuse as a child. Currently, the parent may be experiencing considerable stress and have few social supports; self-control may be compromised by the use of drugs or alcohol. Alternatively, certain types of behavior are more likely to provoke abuse such as patterns of difficult temperament or some of the immature or provocative behaviors that characterize children with developmental disorders.

☀ Pediatric Pearl

Child abuse often develops in situations in which a parent is highly stressed and the child is vulnerable because of immaturities or behavior problems associated with undetected developmental delays.

The interaction between the parent and child may be obviously hostile or volatile, and the parent's style of discipline is often excessively harsh, or there are unrealistic expectations of the child. These conditions are not necessarily associated with poverty, and child abuse is found in all racial groups and socioeconomic strata.

Physical Examination

The history is the most important tool of behavioral assessment, but physical findings can help in some conditions. For example, genetically transmitted disorders resulting in developmental delays often have characteristic physical findings. Fragile X disorder often produces a typical pattern of facial anomalies. Fetal alcohol syndrome also is associated with certain facial features. Developmental disorders also frequently produce neurologic findings referred to as "soft signs," which include poor coordination, difficulty executing patterned motor movements, and neurologic reflexes that are immature for age. Finally, physical findings characteristic of the acute or chronic disorder that is producing stress in the child may be evident. The presence of anemia, a common nutritional problem in early childhood that may result in lethargic, withdrawn behavior and an impaired attention span, is worthy of special mention.

Children may feel stressed in certain clinical settings, such as during a physical examination or a procedure conducted in the clinic or hospital when they have an injury or a significant medical problem. At stressful times, it is possible to observe behaviors that may suggest a problem. However, evaluating the significance of observed behavior requires considerable experience. Inexperienced physicians should report such observations to more senior staff before attempting to interpret their significance.

Physical findings suggestive of child abuse may lead to definitive identification of the problem. Table 5.5 lists some of these findings.

Laboratory Evaluation

In behavioral pediatrics, "laboratory" tests include examinations conducted by nonmedical professionals such as psychologists, speech and language pathologists, educational diagnosticians, and physical or occupational therapists. These assessments by professionals from related disciplines are often essential in establishing a diagnosis. Other relevant laboratory measures include (1) genetic tests such as chromosomal analyses and metabolic assessments needed to identify genetic disorders, and (2) the laboratory findings associated with chronic and acute medical conditions that may be responsible for a child's behavioral symptoms.

TABLE 5.5 Physical Findings Suggestive of Child Abuse

Skin
Round "cigarette burn" scars
Marks suggesting rope or strap burns
Suspicious scars at varying stages of healing
Burns in pattern suggesting immersion

Eyes
Retinal hemorrhages in otherwise normal
child, suggesting "shaken baby" syndrome

Radiographs
Multiple fractures at varying stages of healing
Hairline, tendon–avulsion fractures

Magnetic resonance images
Meningeal tears in absence of injury
Unexplained subdural hematoma

Management

Only a general approach to management of some common behavioral problems, which are discussed according to the groups presented in Table 5.3, is given here. Each of these behavioral problems has an extensive differential diagnosis, and several factors always influence the children's behavior (see PATHOPHYSIOLOGY). Management often involves a process of trying several therapeutic approaches and modifying those strategies based on children's response.

Behavior Problems Associated With Developmental Crises

Both prevention and direct counseling are the best approaches to these problems. These common developmental issues can and should be anticipated as part of well-child care. Pediatricians and their office staff should address these issues directly as well as provide literature and other forms of guidance aimed at preventing these problems.

An excellent example of a preventive approach would be the following response to sleep problems. *Before* the critical periods of development occur, the pediatrician should ask the parents how they prepare their child for naps or nighttime sleep and how they handle nighttime wakening. The clinician should encourage parents to let the child settle herself to sleep rather than rock her to sleep or have her sleep with them. However, if the problem has already developed, a fitting counseling approach would be to identify the factors that may contribute to the problem and make specific suggestions for change. Such counseling must include listening for emotional issues in the parents that may affect their ability to modify their own behavior.

Pediatric Pearl

When prevention and counseling are not effective, the possibility of referral to other, more specifically skilled professionals must be considered.

Behavior Problems Related to Developmental Pattern Disorders

For the purpose of good management strategy, a distinction must be made between behaviors that are direct expressions of the particular developmental disorder (e.g., short attention span, over-activity) and behaviors that are secondary to inappropriate expectations (e.g., excessively harsh discipline) or are direct expressions of poor self-esteem (e.g., sadness, self-loathing). Children might use self-critical comments when they do not complete tasks; this reflect low self-esteem.

Direct, rapid improvement of these latter behaviors may often result from changes in expectations or boosts in self-esteem. Behaviors that are more direct expressions of children's developmental problems (e.g., inattention, motor restlessness, immature social behavior) are much harder to change. Attention-deficit hyperactivity behaviors may be very responsive to stimulant medication, which should be considered in any child with this problem. Skilled behavioral management, including carefully applied programs of reward and consistent expectations, is also an effective management strategy. Both children and their parents may also need individual or group psychotherapy to deal with the stress of these conditions.

An additional and vital component of management is the provision of special educational experiences to deal with the cognitive or perceptual problems that frequently accompany these developmental disorders. This component of management requires collaboration with other disciplines and collaborative relationships with schools.

Behavior Problems Associated With Acute or Chronic Stress

The most important and obvious management strategy is relief from the stress. When the source of the stress is an acute or chronic illness, preventive measures and counseling strategies may be effective once appropriate medical therapy is instituted. For example, school-age children with significant injuries may improve with strategies aimed at putting them in control of their rehabilitation. Children with chronic but invisible illnesses such as asthma or diabetes can be taught to manage their own illness as much as possible, and strategies should be adopted that lead to inclusion in all possible age-appropriate academic and social activities. Primary prevention includes strategies such as good nutrition to prevent anemia and the elimination of environmental toxins such as lead.

In the case of suspected child abuse, relief from the stress often may involve removal from the home while the family issues are evaluated and any problems corrected. It is hoped that the removal is temporary. Most states require that physicians and other health care providers report suspected child abuse to the social service agency responsible for evaluating possible abuse. In some health care settings, if the parent refuses treatment, the physician may need to enlist the help of law enforcement to ensure that the child is kept in a safe environment. If the child is removed from the home, health care providers should recognize that such separation is itself a source of stress, although the child may now be in a safe situation. For a parent or child who is subject to chronic emotional stress (i.e., a history of abuse), psychotherapy is clearly indicated, although it is not always effective.

SUGGESTED READINGS

Blackman J (ed): Development and behavior: The very young child. *Pediatr Clin North Am* 38(2):1351–1560 (entire volume), 1991.

Christopherson E, Levine MD (eds): Development and behavior: Older children and adolescents. *Pediatr Clin North Am* 39(3):369–584 (entire volume), 1992.

Reece R (ed): Child abuse. *Pediatr Clin North Am* 37(4): 791–1013 (entire volume), 1990.

Schmitt BD: Your child's health: A pediatric guide for parents. New York, Bantam Books, 1987.

Schor E: *Children in the Middle Years—5–12 Years.* New York, Bantam, 1999.

Shelov SP, Hannemann RE (eds): *Caring for Your Baby and Young Child: Birth to Age 5.* New York, Bantam Books, 1998.

Chapter 6

Socioeconomic and Cultural Issues in Pediatrics

Fernando S. Mendoza

The role of pediatricians is to maintain children's health by preventing and curing disease. To achieve this goal, physicians have adopted the broad definition of health proposed by the World Health Organization (WHO): health is a state of complete physical, mental, and social well-being, not merely the absence of disease or infirmity. Pediatricians attempt to understand not only the science behind the disease process but also the illness itself, including the psychosocial effects of disease on children and families. These practitioners work as clinicians and child advocates to improve the environment in which children and their families live. To provide comprehensive health care, it is essential to understand the physical and social surroundings of the child and family, including the community in which they live. This means understanding the effects of social class, race, and ethnicity as well as the health care system on the health of children. The Academy of Pediatrics (AAP), through its policy statement on culturally effective pediatric care, and the Future of Pediatric Education II Task Force (AAP and other pediatric societies), with its focus on preparing pediatricians for the 21st century, acknowledge the importance of understanding a child's and family's cultural background and its influence on the child's health. These groups recommend that pediatricians take a child's socioeconomic class, race, and ethnicity into account.

This chapter will present a picture of diversity of children in the United States and how the characteristics that define that diversity relate to increased risk for poor health and reduced access to health care. The discussion will examine the health disparities associated with social class, race, and ethnicity. Moreover, it will focus on the practice of pediatrics in the 21st century by addressing the following questions:

- What should pediatricians do in assessing children from diverse backgrounds?

- What should pediatricians know about disease prevalence among different groups of children?
- How should pediatricians modify their management of a disease process when dealing with children from diverse backgrounds?

SOCIOECONOMIC DIVERSITY

In the United States, the primary measures of social class are the level of family income and parental education, which are highly correlated. Family income has been the most robust indicator of poor health in children. For example, is the family income above or below the poverty line? The **poverty threshold,** which is established by the federal government, is the income that can supposedly support a family of a certain size with food and shelter. (It should be noted that this does *not* include health insurance.) Children who live below the poverty threshold are more likely to have a higher probability of growth and development problems as well as a greater prevalence of disease. Consequently, the number of children who live below the poverty threshold is an approximate measure of those who are at risk for health problems.

One method for evaluating the effects of inequalities in family income involves classifying children based on their relationship to the poverty threshold. However, this method identifies only some of the at-risk children; it does not recognize those in families at or just above the poverty threshold (i.e., 100%–180% of the poverty income threshold), who are still considered to be at risk and frequently qualify for poverty assistance programs. Suppose that $10,000 is the poverty threshold. The range is $10,000–$18,000. Furthermore, in areas where the cost of living is high, even those significantly above the poverty threshold (i.e., > 200%) may find themselves homeless (and without health insurance).

Unprecedented economic growth has occurred in the 1990s. As a result of this economic upsurge, the percent of families living in poverty fell to 9.3% in 1999, the lowest level since 1979. The level of poverty in certain racial and ethnic groups is at its lowest point in a generation, but the rates are still two to four times higher than in non-Hispanic whites. For example, the 1999 poverty rate in non-Hispanic whites was 5.5%. In contrast, it was significantly higher in American Indians–Alaskan Natives (25.9%), African Americans (21.9%), Hispanics (20.2%), and Asian Americans–Pacific Islanders (10.3%). The percentage of all children living in poverty (16.9%) has also dropped to its lowest level since 1979. However, in terms of absolute numbers, non-Hispanic white children constitute the largest proportion of poor children.

In addition to race and ethnicity, **family structure** is also significantly associated with poverty. The economic impact of a two-parent versus one-parent household is apparent in all racial and ethnic groups; poverty rates are lower in two-parent families. Among all families with children, those headed by a woman are six times more likely to live in poverty than those headed by married couples (36% versus 6%). Again, African-American and Hispanic households with children and headed by a woman are significantly more likely to live in poverty than their non-Hispanic white counterparts (46% versus 25%). These data demonstrate that even in the best of economic times, a significant number of children and families live in poverty. Moreover, poverty has a disproportionate effect on children. Although children constitute only 26% of the U.S. population, they make up 40% of all individuals living in poverty.

RACIAL AND ETHNIC DIVERSITY

Currently, about one-third of all children in the United States are children of color: African American, Hispanic, Asian, or American Indian. The U.S. Census Bureau predicts that by the year 2020, approximately one-half of all U.S. children will be children of color. In certain states, such as California, this prediction has already become true. At present, 40% of all children in California are Hispanic, 15% are Asian, and 10% are African American. This demographic trend is also evident in many urban areas in other states for two reasons: (1) higher birth rates, and (2) immigration from Latin America and Asia. In the United States, non-Hispanic white women in the 15–45-year age group have the lowest fertility rate at 58

births/1000. Birth rates are higher in all other groups: Mexican American (112), Puerto Rican (76), African American (73), American Indian (71), and Asian–Pacific Islander (64). These higher fertility rates have a major implication for patient populations in obstetrics and pediatrics, particularly in those states and regions where these groups are concentrated. Furthermore, these higher fertility rates set the stage for continued diversification of the U.S. population independent of any changes in immigration policy.

Over the past 20 years, the number of children in the United States who are immigrants themselves or whose parents are immigrants has increased significantly. The recent report of the Institute of Medicine (National Academy of Sciences) on the health and well-being of children in immigrant families noted that one of every five children in the United States (14 million) is an immigrant or has immigrant parents. The great majority of these are from Latin American and Asia. However, every country in the world contributes to the immigrant population of the United States. (Each year, children in kindergarten classes in California speak more than 100 different dialects.)

This increase in the immigrant population poses a challenge to both educators and pediatricians. It is necessary to understand immigrant children and families not only with regard to their language and culture but also with respect to the issues they bring from their own country that may affect their health and well-being. These issues may include economic impoverishment; political persecution; or psychological trauma resulting from war, government-sponsored violence, or terrorism. As traditional borders become less well-defined, the practice of pediatrics develops a more international character.

HEALTH DISPARITIES IN CHILDREN

If all children throughout the world were equal and lived in similar environments, differences in disease and illness would be based on their genetic propensity for such disorders. This is not the case, and pediatricians must understand the various factors that contribute to poor health outcomes and how they lead to health disparities seen among children (i.e., the disproportionate distribution of illness).

Socioeconomic Disparities

Health disparities in children from all backgrounds are most often due to poverty. Children living in economically impoverished environments are more likely to suffer from growth abnormalities, impaired development, and increased exposure to infectious and environmental agents that either cause or contribute to disease processes. Using various national data sources, one researcher found that children from low-income families were two to three times more likely than those from the general population to suffer from a variety of illnesses and conditions (Table 6.1).

The effects of poverty on children begin before birth. Poor mothers have a higher risk of nutritional and health problems and limited access to quality prenatal care. These women are more likely to deliver low-birth-weight or premature infants, who are twice as likely to die in the first year of life.

Beyond infancy, the environment of poverty can significantly affect children's health. One of the most common medical problems among children that directly relates to the degree of economic impoverishment is impaired physical growth, which results from inadequate caloric and nutrient intake that leads to **malnutrition.** Worldwide, malnutrition affects one of every four children (150 million), with 70% of malnourished children living in Asia, 26% in Africa, and 4% in Latin America. Over the past decade, 37% of immigrants to the United States have come from Asia and 41% from Latin America.

Thus, it is not uncommon for a pediatrician in the United States to see a child with some form of malnutrition.

In 1998, the U.S. Census Bureau and the U.S. Department of Agriculture estimated that 12 million children in the United States suffer from **food insecurity** (i.e., hunger), meaning that they did not have access to enough food to meet their needs. Some of the children in the United States who suffer from hunger are not necessarily severely malnourished. However, many suffer from the condition known as "failure to thrive," the inability to maintain a normal growth velocity, which is estimated to occur in as many as 10% of U.S. children. Quite often children with failure to thrive also demonstrate significant developmental delays that relate to their relative malnutrition and impoverished environments. Still others who have no evidence of growth abnormalities have problems in concentrating and learning in school because of hunger.

Evaluating a child for malnutrition involves examining two parameters: (1) weight-for-height (a measure of **wasting,** or thinness for height), and (2) height-for-age (a measure of **stunting,** or shortness for age). Because poor children have fewer resources to maintain an adequate diet, they tend to have a greater probability of wasting (< 5th percentile in weight for height) and stunting (< 5th percentile in height

TABLE 6.1 Differences in Health Status Among Poor and Nonpoor Children	
Increased Frequency in Poor versus Nonpoor	
Low birth weight	Double
Teenage births	Triple
Delayed immunization	Triple
Asthma	Higher
Bacterial meningitis	Double
Rheumatic fever	Double–triple
Lead poisoning	Triple
Increased Severity of Health Problems in Poor versus Nonpoor	
Neonatal mortality	1.5 times
Postneonatal mortality	Double–triple
Child deaths	
Due to accidents	Double–triple
Disease related	Triple–quadruple
Complications of appendicitis	Double–triple
Diabetic ketoacidosis	Double
Complications of bacterial meningitis	Double–triple
Percent with conditions limiting school activity	Double–triple
Lost school days	40% more
Severely impaired vision	Double–triple
Severe iron deficiency anemia	Double

for age, or less than what would be expected genetically). Depending on the degree and duration of malnutrition, stunting may persist for years even after the establishment of adequate nutritional intake. In contrast, given adequate nutrition, wasting may resolve (i.e., weight may increase to a normal value) in a much shorter period. Because weight may catch up more quickly than height, previously malnourished children may have a greater weight-for-height (i.e., they may be overweight). Thus, although it may seem somewhat counterintuitive, some previously malnourished children may be overweight and present with a short, stocky physique.

It is well documented that persistent poverty from one generation to another can lead to malnutrition and stunting in parents and their children. The opposite is also true. If children grow up in a more favorable socioeconomic environment than their parents, they become taller than their parents. Evidence for this is apparent in children in the United States, who have grown taller each generation because of improved economic circumstances. For instance, comparisons of 1968 and 1980 surveys of height in Mexican-American children show a significant increase in stature, indicating improved economic status.

Comparing the growth patterns of children from developing countries, researchers have demonstrated that the height of children from upper socioeconomic classes is similar to U.S. norms, whereas the height of children living in poverty varies from the norm in proportion to the severity of poverty. For example, the heights of children in rural China are 1.5 standard deviations below U.S. norms. That is, 50% of rural Chinese children have a height below the 15th percentile of U.S. norms, and 35% of these children have a height below the 5th percentile of U.S. norms. In contrast, the height of children in urban China is only 0.6 standard deviations below U.S. norms. Thus, with less poverty, urban Chinese children grow taller.

These findings are important because they indicate that all children are capable of growing to U.S. norms and that U.S. norms should be used with all children independent of race, ethnicity, or country of origin. Indeed, the WHO has recommended that all studies of children's growth should use the U.S. growth curves developed by the National Center for Health Statistics and compare children to these curves by using Z scores (standard deviations).

Pediatricians have a unique opportunity to work with children who suffer from malnutrition and food insecurity (hunger). Usually, prolonged and multidisciplinary intervention is necessary. Management may involve the participation of nutritionists, social workers, public health nurses, and mental health workers, as well as nonprofessional support groups in the community. Health professionals should recognize that malnutrition is as much a social problem as a medical one and act accordingly.

Malnutrition is not the only health problem that may affect children from poor backgrounds. Children who live in poverty are also at greater risk of contacting pathogenic infectious and environmental agents. They are more likely to live in crowded, substandard housing, with increased exposure to individuals who may have untreated infectious diseases. In addition, if children are malnourished, they are at greater risk of contracting infectious diseases because the probability of their having an impaired immune system is greater. Limited access to health care and isolation from the health care system also contribute to the increased risk of transmission of contagious diseases among poor individuals. Outbreaks of tuberculosis, pertussis, and measles in poor and immigrant populations occur commonly.

Simple preventative measures such as immunization and screening can have a major impact on the spread of infectious diseases among poor children. Unfortunately, those children in the United States who are most often unimmunized are those who are poor or belong to minority or immigrant populations. The immunization of all children is good not only for the individual child but for the public at large as well.

Exposure to toxic environmental agents may occur as a result of living in substandard housing. In urban areas, lead is the most common environmental toxin. According to the latest national survey on lead levels in children, poor children are three to four times more likely than nonpoor children to have lead levels greater than 10 μg/dl, a level considered to be a risk for neurobehavioral and developmental delays. The risk is three times higher in inner cities than in rural areas. Lead levels are elevated in more than one-third of African-American children and one-fifth of Mexican-American children living in urban areas of greater than 1 million population. This compares to 6% of non-Hispanic white children in large metropolitan areas.

In rural areas, pesticides are a common environmental toxin. Many poor and immigrant families live and work in close proximity to the fields, so the risk of exposure is high. Children, particularly younger ones, usually accompany families to the fields. Unfortunately, it is difficult to determine whether pesticide exposure has occurred; the symptoms, which may involve the respiratory tract, the nervous system, and the skin, are nonspecific.

Recently, pesticide exposure has also become a concern for children living in the inner city because of efforts to control pests. Scientists do not yet completely understand the effects of these environmental agents on children, but clearly young children are the most vulnerable because of their rapid growth and greater hand-to-mouth contact. It thus becomes the pediatrician's responsibility to question families about environmental exposures or **pica** behavior (eating nonfood substances), particularly in children who are 3 years of age or younger.

With regard to chronic illness, the socioeconomic class of children has a variable effect. Most commonly, the occurrence of chronic illness in children is the result of genetic predisposition for a particular disease. For example, sickle cell anemia or cystic fibrosis affect children because of their genetic profile.

However, some chronic illnesses in childhood may be linked with socioeconomic background, specifically, those chronic illnesses that are the result of untreated infectious or acute illness. For example, the lack of treatment of pulmonary tuberculosis in a child may lead to an infection that subsequently spreads to the brain, resulting in meningitis and significant long-term consequences. Another example is chronic lead ingestion, which if untreated can cause learning and developmental problems that may be irreversible.

Yet poverty can also modify chronic illnesses that have a significant genetic component. Asthma, the most common chronic illness in childhood, has a genetic basis, but poverty can increase its prevalence and severity. This is particularly true for African-American and Hispanic children who live in urban areas. One study proposes a mechanism for this effect involving differences in access to health care, patterns of medical care, psychosocial stress, and environmental exposure. The National Cooperative Inner City Asthma Study (NCICAS), a study of poor inner city children with moderate to severe asthma, found that although most children had routine health care, 50% had difficulties obtaining follow-up care for their asthma, suggesting that their care was fragmented. Furthermore, only 50% received treatment according to the recommended national guidelines, indicating that the care may have been less than optimal. In addition, psychosocial stress in children and mothers in the NCICAS was high, with 50% of mothers and 35% of children meeting the criteria for referral to a mental health professional. Significantly, maternal and child psychosocial stress levels were correlated with each other and with the child's morbidity from asthma. Exposure to a higher level of environmental pollutants and allergens, a characteristic feature of poverty, may also have affected the prevalence and severity of asthma in children in the NCICAS. Of particular importance was exposure to cockroach antigen, which was found in 90% of homes. The study reported that 50% of the homes of these poor children had levels of exposure considered clinically detrimental.

Other external environmental factors beyond the children's own households may also have an impact on their health and development. Neighborhoods can be a positive influence on child development by providing a safe, nurturing environment for play and school. Unfortunately, poor neighborhoods suffer not only from substandard housing but frequently from crowded and neglected schools, lack of safe play areas, and high levels of crime.

In a study of children attending suburban and urban middle schools, investigators reported that children in poorer urban schools had higher rates of exposure to crime in that they knew or had witnessed someone being robbed, beaten, stabbed, shot, or murdered. Of children who attended a middle school in a poorer neighborhood, 96% knew someone who had witnessed one of the previously mentioned events, while 88% witnessed such an event. For middle class suburban school children, these same values were 89% and 57%, respectively. Sixty-seven percent of children attending the middle school in the poorer neighborhood reported being victimized themselves: 48% robbed, 21% stabbed, and 3% shot. Ninety-four percent of poor neighborhood children had heard gunfire in their neighborhood and 24% had been caught in gun crossfire. While the children from the poorer neighborhoods reported more violent events and experiences, the children from the middle class suburban neighborhoods also reported a greater-than-expected number of events.

Violence involving children has become a major public health issue in the United States and disproportionately affects poor children and adolescents. Children who witness a violent event experienced fear, sadness, anger, empathy with the victim, confusion, shock, and a desire to become involved in the altercation. Symptoms associated with somatization, depression, and posttraumatic stress syndrome, including stomach pains, headaches, trouble sleeping, trouble remembering, nightmares, nervousness, sadness, and a sense of a foreshortened future were common. Children rarely discuss these events with a health or mental health professional.

Some investigators recommend that health care and mental health professionals be more proactive in seeking a history of exposure to violence, particularly among poor children, and that they receive training about dealing with children and families who have been traumatized by violence. It is important to note that one of the leading causes of death of school-age children and adolescents, particularly in urban areas, is homicide.

Racial and Ethnic Disparities

Racial and ethnic factors, as well as socioeconomic characteristics, may also influence pediatric care. Racism, whether overt or covert, may affect the health of children in one or more of the following ways:

- By forcing them to live in neighborhoods in which health risks are greater
- By causing stressful experiences involving discrimination
- By forcing them to develop under an imposed stigma of inferiority
- By causing bias (unintentional) on the part of health care providers (i.e., when a particular provider deals with patients of a different racial or ethnic group)

Racial discrimination and housing practices designed to limit integration of racial and ethnic groups have led to the segregation of neighborhoods on the basis of race and ethnicity, as well as socioeconomic factors (i.e., income). Such separation can reinforce children's feelings of isolation from the rest of society, which may have a negative health effect on the people who live in the neighborhood by producing a stigma of inferiority and visible signs of discrimination. Several laws have been adopted to limit segregation, but the results of this practice are still apparent in some communities. Bias among physicians, although unintentional, should not be unexpected; physicians are raised in the same society that has created these biases and stereotypes. A recent review of the literature by the Institute of Medicine (National Academy of Sciences) affirms that one of the reasons for health disparities among minorities is physician bias and prejudice, usually unintentional. Nevertheless, physicians are called on to rise above these prejudices, but to do so they must understand their own biases.

Although the segregation of neighborhoods has definite negative health effects, the existence of concentrations of people of similar cultural and ethnic backgrounds may have some positive health effects. The maintenance of the culture of the country of origin appears to have a greater positive health effect than the negative effect caused by the isolation from the mainstream culture. For example, in Mexican-Americans, newly immigrant children appear to do better, as measured by a variety of parameters, than later generation children, even though newly immigrant children and their families have higher rates of poverty, lower levels of parental education, and less access to health care than later generations. Two findings in newly immigrant Mexican-American mothers are interesting: (1) similar prevalence of low birth weight infants compared with middle class non-Hispanic white women, and (2) similar or better infant mortality rates than their middle class counterparts. Apparently, this results from maintenance of cultural health habits with respect to pregnancy and child care. However, it is important to note that as these Mexican-American women become acculturated to American society, the health parameters of low birth weight and infant mortality appear to worsen and approach the norms of later generations. The cultural buffer to the detrimental effects of poverty that exists for these mothers and children appears to lessen as American cultural practices replace those of the country of origin.

Poverty is a strong predictor of poor health, but some families can buffer some of its negative health effects by creating their own cultural milieu. Researchers have noted that this phenomenon, termed the "immigrant paradox," occurs in many other immigrant groups (e.g., immigrants from Asia and Africa). Reportedly, it affects low birth weight, infant mortality, and health behaviors of immigrant children. The "immigrant paradox" is believed to result from positive, culturally based family health practices, which receive support from the community; these measures may help buffer the negative effects of poverty. A community that is supportive of the family culture and provides children and their families with a positive self-image and identity can be a significant health resource and create a positive psychosocial environment. Social organizations (e.g., religious groups, clubs, sport groups, school–parent associations, local businesses) may act as such resources.

Disparities in Access to Health Care

The principal determinant of children's access to health care is the ability to obtain health insurance, which in turn depends on their parents' ability to obtain health coverage. This assumes that if parents work, their jobs offer health insurance, or that if the parents are unable to work, then their children qualify for a social welfare program that provides access to health care.

Unfortunately, neither of these two assumptions is necessarily true. In a recent analysis using national data, investigators found that ethnic minorities were much more likely than non-Hispanic whites to be uninsured. Hispanics were the most likely to be uninsured (37%), followed by African Americans (23%), Asian Americans–Pacific Islanders (21%), American Indians–Alaskan Natives (17%), and non-Hispanic whites (14%). Although 87% of uninsured Hispanics work, they are much less likely to receive employment-based health insurance, regardless of how much they work or the size of their firm or industry. Hispanic non-U.S. citizens are very likely to be uninsured (58%), but even Hispanic U.S. citizens have a high rate (27%). Similarly, African Americans have lower rates of job-based health insurance compared to non-Hispanic whites, 53% versus 73%. Among children alone, the relative numbers of uninsured were similar to those for all individuals in their group: Hispanic (29%), African American (19%), Asian Americans–Pacific Islanders (15%), American Indians–Alaska Natives (13%), and non-Hispanic whites (11%). This translates into less acute care and preventive care for children. In addition, uninsured patients are less likely to follow minimum care recommendations.

If children are not able to obtain health insurance through their parents, they may receive financial assistance for medical care depending on family income and on immigration status (i.e., whether a child is a U.S. citizen or a legal resident). States usually determine income eligibility; in many states an income of up to 250% of the poverty threshold qualifies a family for health care insurance through a state or federal program. A family of four can make as much as $42,625 per year and qualify for a government health insurance program. (This may seem high, but a family of four living in the San Francisco Bay area needs $46,000 just to meet basic housing and living needs.) The requirement for citizenship or legal residence also has been a major deterrent, particularly for children of immigrant families. In the mid-1990s, welfare reform excluded immigrant children from participation in federal and many state programs. For example, in California, undocumented immigrant children were ineligible for the state's Medicaid program except in emergencies. However, they do have access to a preventive health screening program (Children's Health and Disability Prevention program) and to a program to aid families with chronically ill children (California Childrens Services).

It is hoped that increased awareness of the need to provide decent health care for all children will result in adequate health care for all immigrant children. It is of interest that three-fourths of all children in immigrant families are U.S. citizens, but frequently families are fearful of obtaining government-sponsored health insurance because of the implication it has for the efforts of noncitizens to obtain citizenship. Thus, it is important that pediatricians become familiar with various state and federal programs so that they can better serve as advocates for this diverse population of children.

ASSESSING AND TREATING CHILDREN FROM DIVERSE BACKGROUNDS

The information presented in the first part of this chapter indicates that pediatricians should learn how to adapt their clinical care to better meet the diverse needs of children and families, both for their patients' benefit and their own professional satisfaction. Diversity occurs in the form of socioeconomic class, race, ethnicity, and immigration status. Each of these affects the physician–patient interaction through the process of verbal and nonverbal communication and differences in the health beliefs. Ultimately, they affect the overall outcome: patient satisfaction, compliance with medical recommendations, and improved patient health.

Communication: Verbal and Nonverbal

Obtaining an accurate and comprehensive history from patients is the cornerstone of clinical care. The history not only provides the data necessary to understand a patient's complaint and disease process, but it also allows physicians to assess the patient's understanding and response. In pediatrics, this also includes understanding a family's knowledge of and response to a child's disease. Obtaining a pediatric history involves an interaction between several individuals: the physician, the patient, and the parents or other caregivers. As with any human interaction, each party has its own set of communication skills, expectations, unspoken understandings, and personal biases. Effective pediatricians attempt to identify the patient's or caregiver's background and determine how it interacts with their own.

Initially, it is necessary to determine whether patients, parents, and providers are fluent in the same language. Frequently, they are not. In such situations, it is essential to obtain the services of an accurate and culturally sensitive interpreter. This seems obvious, but often no interpreter is available, resulting in the use of either family members or ad hoc interpreters (i.e., nonmedical personnel working in the area). In a review of the literature, one researcher found that the lack of a professional interpreter has a significant negative impact on patients' understanding of their disease and satisfaction with care. Furthermore, the inability to communicate with a patient effectively resulted in errors in diagnosis and in increased morbidity.

However, even when interpreters are available, using them in a clinically effective manner requires conscious understanding that an interpreter is a tool to establish a relationship with the patient, and should not be used just to gather information from the patient. The personal rela-

tionship of the pediatrician with the patient or parent is the basis of all clinical interactions (Table 6.2).

Language is just one part of a social interaction. In a review of cultural interactions, investigators encourage physicians to see the office visit as an interaction between two cultures, that of the patient and that of the provider. They state that clinicians must be cognizant of the historical, political, and economic factors of patients' families. Patients and providers each have unspoken understandings about their particular roles, and if both are from similar sociocultural backgrounds, these understandings about roles and expectations usually coincide. However, if they are not, socioeconomic, racial or ethnic biases, or stereotypic views may influence patient and provider perceptions. Most frequently, these barriers to effective communication are transmitted through nonverbal communication. For example, parents or patients who are silent after being asked whether they have any questions, never smile, or have only negative interactions with a provider may be trying to communicate their displeasure about how a physician has interacted with them. Having a socioculturally sensitive interpreter who can interpret these nonverbal signs or directly asking parents or pa-

---

TABLE 6.2 **Guidelines for the Effective Choice and Use of Interpreters in Clinical Settings**

INTERPRETER CHOICE

Always use trained interpreter unless thoroughly fluent in patient's language.

Avoid using strangers from waiting room or untrained staff as interpreters because of potential problems with accuracy, confidentiality, and medical terminology.

If trained interpreters are not available, use adult relatives or friends brought specifically to translate as acceptable alternatives, but problems with accuracy, confidentiality, medical terms, and disrupted social roles may occur.

Use children as interpreters of last resort because of problems with disruption of social roles, sensitive issues, and accuracy.

Always ask patient whether designated interpreter is acceptable.

INTERPRETER USE

Position clinician, interpreter, and patient/parent in equilateral triangle so important nonverbal cues can be appreciated.

Speak to and maintain eye contact with patient/parent, not interpreter.

Ask interpreter to translate as literally as possible.

If mistranslation or misunderstanding is suspected, return to issue later using different wording.

Emphasize key instructions and explanations by repetition.

Use visual aids (charts and diagrams) whenever possible to verify quality and comprehension of translation, and have patient/parent repeat information through "back translation."

AT END OF MEDICAL VISIT

Have interpreter write lists of instructions for patient/parent, particularly for prescriptions and other therapeutic interventions.

Indicate to pharmacists that prescription instructions should be printed in patient/parent's language.

Always have interpreter accompany patient/parent to schedule follow-up appointments with receptionist.

tients about their satisfaction with care helps the pediatrician acknowledge and lower any barriers to effective health care.

Health Beliefs

Everyone has a notion of what it means to be healthy, and in some ways an understanding of what keeps us healthy or makes us sick. Depending on their exposure to Western medicine, many people share some of the same views about medical treatment. However, based on their individual health beliefs, people not uncommonly use alternative therapies [complementary and alternative medical care (CAM)]. One researcher found that 33%–50% of adults in the United States report using CAM therapy. Among some ethnic groups, folk remedies or CAM therapies may be more common. This is particularly true for new immigrants, who bring their health beliefs and therapies from their country of origin with them. Although at times, these CAM therapies may seem exotic and contrary to Western medicine, practitioners should acknowledge these attempts on the part of parents to help their children. If these measures are not harmful, clinicians should try to integrate them into the medical management of the patient. Clearly, parental education is necessary to prevent the use of folk remedies that have any harmful effects (i.e., lead-containing folk remedies; greta, azarcon, or albayalde treatment for empacho in Mexican Americans).

Unfortunately, parents or patients often never tell pediatricians about the use of alternative treatments, because they feel uncomfortable relaying such information to physicians. Therefore, pediatricians need to open discussions by asking patients or parents what they believe is wrong with the child's health, what do they think is causing it, and what have they done to make it better. It is also useful to normalize the use of folk or alternative medicines by saying "Many people use. . . . for your child's condition. Have you heard of it? Have you used it?" In these ways, physicians can make themselves aware of patients' or parents' health beliefs, thus enabling them to integrate them into the therapeutic plan.

SUGGESTED READINGS

American Academy of Pediatrics: Culturally effective pediatric care: Education and training issues. *Pediatrics* 103(1):167–170, 1999.

Brody D, et al: Blood lead levels in the US populations. Phase I NHANES III. *JAMA* 272(4):277–283, 1994.

Brown E, Ojeda V, Wyn R, et al: *Racial and Ethnic Disparities in access to Health Insurance and Health Care*. Los Angeles, UCLA Center for Health Policy Research, 2000.

Campbell C, Schwarz D: Prevalence and impact of exposure to interpersonal violence among suburban and urban middle school students. *Pediatrics* 98(3):396–402, 1996.

Eggleston P: Urban children and asthma. *Immunol Allergy Clin North Am* 18(1):75–84, 1998.

Flores G: Culture and patient–physician relationship: Achieving cultural competency in health care. *J Pediatr* 136(1):14–23, 2000.

Food Research and Action Center: Hunger in the United States. http://www.frac.org/index.html

The Future of Pediatric Education II: Organizing pediatric education to meet the needs of infants, children, adolescents and young adults in the 21st century. *Pediatrics* 105(1):163–210, 2000.

Gahagan S, Holmes R: A stepwise approach to evaluation of undernutrition and failure to thrive. *Pediatr Clin North Am* 45(1):169–187, 1998.

Hernandez DJ, Charney E (editors), with Committee of the Health and Adjustment of Immigrant Children and Families of the Board of Children, Youth, and Families (Institute of Medicine, National Research Council): *From Generation to Generation: The Health and Well-Being of Children in Immigrant Families*. Washington, DC, National Academy Press, 1998.

Kemper K, Cassileth B, Ferris T: Holistic pediatrics: A research agenda. *Pediatrics* 103(4):S902–909, 1999.

Kinsman S, Mitchell S, Fox K: Multicultural issues in pediatric practice. *Pediatr Rev* 17(10):349–355, 1996.

Lewit E, Baker L: Race and ethnicity—Changes for children. *The Future of Children. Critical Health Issues for Children and Youth* 4(3):134–144, 1994.

Martorell R, Mendoza FS, Castillo RO: Genetic and environmental determinants of growth in Mexican-Americans. *Pediatrics* 84(5):864–871, 1989.

Martorell R, Mendoza FS, Castillo RO: Poverty and stature in children. In *Linear Growth Retardation in Less Developed Countries*, Nestle Nutrition Workshop Series, vol 14. Edited by Waterlow JC. New York: Vavey/Raven Press, 1988, pp 57–73.

Mendoza FS, Fuentes-Afflick E: Latino children's health and the family–community health promotion model. *West J Med* 170(2):85–92, 1999.

Pachter L: Culture and clinical care: Folk illness, beliefs, and behaviors and their implications for health care delivery. *JAMA* 271:690–694, 1994.

Schulman K, Berlin J, Harless W, et al: The effects of race and sex on physician recommendations for cardiac catheterization. *N Engl J Med* 340:618–626, 1999.

Starfield B: Childhood morbidity: Comparisons, clusters, and trends. *Pediatrics* 88(3):519–526, 1991.

U.S. Census Bureau: Poverty in the United States 1999. Current Population Reports P60–210. Washington, DC, U.S. Department of Commerce, 2000.

Williams D: Race, socioeconomic status, and health: The added effects of racism and discrimination. *Ann N Y Acad Sci* 896:173–188, 1999.

World Health Organization (WHO)/Department of Nutrition for Health and Development: WHO Global Database on Child Growth and Malnutrition. http//www.who.int/nut/pem.htm

Chapter 7

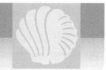

Ethical Issues in Pediatric Practice*

Alan R. Fleischman

Children are a precious resource and in a real sense represent the future of our society. Pediatricians play a special role in society because they are both caregivers of and advocates for children. The practice of pediatrics involves concern for the physiologic health of children as well as the emotional and psychosocial development of children within families. This role is quite different from the responsibilities faced by physicians caring for adults and creates significant challenges for the practice of pediatrics.

In the past 20 years, the role of the physician in American society has changed from that of the highly respected and rarely questioned paternalistic decision maker, to that of a collaborator who is expected to provide recommendations for health care decisions made by patients and families. Patients have become consumers of physicians' services, expecting to be fully informed and increasingly responsible for decisions about their own health care. This respect for a person's fundamental right of self-determination or autonomy has resulted in the practice of allowing adults to make health care decisions for themselves, even if the physician disagrees and, more importantly, even if the physician perceives that the decision is not in the patients' best interest. This principle, known as "respect for persons," incorporates two ethical convictions: that individuals should be treated as autonomous agents and that persons with diminished autonomy are entitled to protection. This fundamental idea maintains that all persons capable of participating in decision making have the right to determine what happens to their own bodies. Furthermore, individuals with diminished autonomy who are incapable of participating in decision making for themselves are entitled to additional protection

from harm. In general, society believes that children have diminished autonomy and require protection.

The doctrine of informed consent, an expression of this respect for a person's right of self-determination, assumes that patients can understand the risks and benefits of alternative treatments and can make informed choices. When the process of informed consent relates to children or to any individuals who lack the capacity to decide for themselves, it involves the use of a proxy or surrogate. Any proxy consent is based on another person's perception of the appropriate choice, not on an individual's choice. Many people have argued that the respect for a person's fundamental right of self-determination should extend to the family, who could be viewed as an autonomous unit. In this view of self-determination, the judgments of family members could substitute for those of members who cannot participate in decision making.

When applied to children, this extension of the principle of respect for persons may occasionally be problematic. The principle of informed consent for autonomous adults is extremely powerful; it allows capable adults to refuse treatments despite negative consequences. However, parental refusals of treatments that are deemed beneficial for their children do not carry the same weight as refusals by competent adults for treatments for themselves. Parental refusal of necessary therapy does not relieve physicians or other health care providers from an ethical duty to children, particularly if the refusal of such treatment puts them at significant risk.

This ethical duty derives from the principle of "beneficence," which states that ethical treatment involves not only respecting the decisions of patients and protecting them from harm but also making efforts to secure their best interests or well-being. Beneficent actions attempt to maximize possible benefits and to minimize possible harms. To fulfill beneficence obligations to chil-

*Parts of this chapter were adapted from Fleischman AR, Nolan K, Dubler NN, et al: Caring for gravely ill children. Pediatrics 94:433–439, 1994.

dren and to preserve their future right to autonomous decision making, another concept, known as the principle of the "best interests of the child," has evolved. This principle promotes decision making for the benefit of children, even if, in rare occurrences, it conflicts with parental beliefs. The "best interests" standard presupposes that decision makers are able to consider the interests of children as primary, regardless of their own interests and those of other family members.

Although the "best interests of the child" is the appropriate standard for treatment decisions, it is important to realize that what is in the best interests of any individual is often uncertain. When faced with lack of clarity about what is effective or beneficial, it can be argued that those who bear the burden of the decision (e.g., in the case of children, the families) should play the major role in making the choice. Families play an important, if not vital, role in deciding the future outcome of children. Their input and support is crucial in optimizing the environment in which children live. Thus, it seems that the "best interests" standard for children must incorporate recognition of the interests of families and a commitment on the part of society to provide the resources that allow families to support children's interests without creating an undue burden.

ETHICAL ISSUES IN NEWBORNS

 CASE 1

The pediatric team is called to the delivery room to resuscitate a 675-g (1½-pound), 25-week-gestation, premature male infant who has just been born. This infant, just past the threshold of viability, has a reasonable (50%) chance to survive with aggressive intervention and greater than a 50% chance of being normal if he survives. He may suffer all the complications of prematurity, including cerebral palsy, mental retardation, impaired vision and hearing, and chronic lung disease. Should the pediatricians resuscitate the infant? Should the medical team allow the family to choose whether treatment is initiated? If treatment begins, under what circumstances may the clinicians withdraw it? Who should make these decisions and by what process?

Dramatic changes in the technologic care available to newborn infants have resulted in the ca-

pability of saving the lives of the majority of even the sickest, smallest neonates. In most neonatal centers, the survival rate of newborns as young as 24 weeks gestational age and weighing 500 g is greater than 20%. Infants born at 1000 g and 28 weeks gestation, thought to be at the threshold of viability in the 1960s and 1970s, now have a greater than 90% survival rate. In addition, the development of new surgical techniques in the past two decades has allowed for the correction or amelioration of congenital anomalies of the heart, kidneys, intestine, liver, and brain. With intravenous parenteral nutrition, infants can grow and gain weight with normal development for weeks, months, or years without oral intake. These advances in neonatal medicine have enhanced the lives of countless children, yet at the same time they have also resulted in saving the lives of some children who are left with severely disabling and handicapping conditions. (See Chapter 10, Neonatology.)

It is frequently difficult to predict which infants will survive and thrive with a good future quality of life and which infants will suffer irreversible damage, resulting in devastating chronic illness. American author, Jeff Lyon, in his book *Playing God in the Nursery*, graphically portrays the dilemma of this uncertainty:

> If it is hard to justify creating blind paraplegics to obtain a number of healthy survivors, it is equally hard to explain to the ghosts of the potentially healthy that they had to die in order to avoid creating blind paraplegics.

In general, American neonatologists have evolved a decision-making strategy that deals with this uncertainty by ranking the death of an infant who could have lived a reasonable life as worse than the saving of an infant who becomes devastatingly disabled. Both outcomes may be viewed as equally tragic. In general, pediatricians believe that neonates with any chance of survival deserve resuscitation in the delivery room, followed by stabilization in the neonatal intensive care unit (NICU) until data concerning the certainty about future outcome become available. When death or drastically impaired future quality of life seems likely, physicians may recommend withdrawing treatment or withholding future treatment. This approach to the uncertainty of neonatal outcome contrasts with the vitalist approach, which advocates aggressive intervention for all infants, or a statistical approach, which seeks to minimize the number of infants who die slow deaths or live with profound handicaps by treating only those infants who satisfy minimum weight or gestational age criteria.

At the core of all discussions concerning appropriate treatments for critically ill neonates is the question of how much people value members of society who have disabling and handicapping conditions. All infants have an inherent worth that deserves respect, regardless of the extent of their physical defect or future cognitive impairment. Physicians should discuss all treatments that may potentially enhance the interests and well-being of infants with family members. However, this respect for infants does not mean that because a treatment is available, a physician must provide it.

Assessment of what is in the best interests of a particular infant includes analysis of the potential benefits and burdens of the treatment plan, the future expected quality of life of the child, and the views and values of the family. If the potential for ultimate survival is small, the burdens of a proposed treatment great, or the future quality of life likely to be poor, a recommendation not to provide a particular treatment may be appropriate. The parents of neonates should be the ultimate decision makers, unless they are choosing a course of action that is clearly against the best interests of the child. The birth of an abnormal newborn may be tremendously stressful for parents, but it is possible to educate almost all parents about their infant's condition so that they can make decisions that put the child's interests first.

Most hospitals now have bioethics committees that review complex, value-laden decisions in order to assist parents and professionals in the determination of what is in the best interests of infants. These multidisciplinary committees include physicians, nurses, social workers, ethicists, clergy, and other professionals who are interested in protecting and promoting the interests of particular children. Some physicians have opposed bioethics committees; they contend that the best person to make such complex decisions is the treating physician at the bedside, who is most knowledgeable of the medical facts as well as the infant's interests and the family's wishes. However, clinicians who have used infant bioethics committees believe that the committees enhance the decision-making process by reviewing the medical facts and protecting infants' interests while invoking ethical principles, and not merely intuition, in decision making. Infant bioethics committees may also enhance the role of parents in decision making by supporting parental choices in ambiguous cases in which it

is uncertain as to what is in the best interest of a particular child. In addition, such committees can provide ethical comfort to both families and health care professionals who are ultimately responsible for both making and implementing difficult decisions.

When parents refuse what the health care providers and the ethics committee believe to be clearly in a child's interests, procedural mechanisms involving the courts have been developed to override parental choice. These legal approaches are the embodiment of the physician's beneficence obligations to a child, protecting an infant from inappropriate cessation of treatment. An example of this type of intervention is the court-ordered administration of blood products to save the life of a child whose parents' religion prohibits transfusions.

Increasingly, a new type of ethical dilemma is occurring in NICUs. Physicians who have become comfortable with families having the discretion to choose to withhold or withdraw life-sustaining treatments from critically ill newborns are concerned about families who insist that their infants receive life-sustaining treatments that are deemed by the professionals to have minimal, if any, benefit. What should happen when physicians disagree with a parental request for treatment that will be life-prolonging but possibly not life-enhancing? When a treatment has no potential benefit and will only inflict pain and prolong suffering, physicians are not obligated to provide or even offer such interventions even if requested by parents. However, when parents request a treatment that offers a low likelihood of benefit, even in the face of significant burden, health care professionals should not make this decision themselves.

In general, when caring, concerned parents request continued attempts to save or prolong the life of their child, physicians should not impose their views over the values of the family. Clinicians should give broad latitude to parental discretion regarding choices for children when there is honest uncertainty concerning the ratio of benefits to burdens of continued therapy. However, parental discretion in demanding treatment should not be unlimited. Physicians and other health care providers, based on their own strongly held personal beliefs, have the right to opt out of the care of children for whom they believe the benefits of treatment do not outweigh the burdens. In addition, society has the right through its laws, regulations, and institutions to limit individual resource allocation for patients unlikely or unable to benefit from continued treatment.

ETHICAL ISSUES IN YOUNG CHILDREN

 CASE 2

A 6-year-old girl with diabetes no longer wishes to cooperate in testing her blood sugar and taking insulin injections. Lack of insulin will cause the child to lose weight and eventually become seriously ill. Her parents seek advice from the pediatrician on what to do. Should the pediatrician respect the child's refusal? Should the parents punish the child for noncompliance?

Although most young children lack the capacity to make binding choices, their individual needs, interests, and perspectives must still be the central focus of health care decisions. Certain aspects of treatment and decision making permit, and sometimes even require, the participation of young patients. The proper role of children in planning care depends less on chronologic age than on developmental and personal capacity. For example, although 10-year-old children are usually less able to understand abstract concepts than adults, some may act or think quite maturely. Children even younger than 10 years of age often have a keen appreciation of their own clinical situations and options. Although very young children may be unable to envision the future benefits of a treatment that may justify its associated burdens (e.g., pain, discomfort, hospitalization), adults should not ignore children's perceptions of those burdens. Physicians should encourage children to verbalize their feelings and to choose methods to enhance their comfort or acceptance of painful or unpleasant procedures.

As children become older and more perceptive, they should be involved more fully in decision making concerning their care. Children may have religious or other values that shape their responses to illness, and they often are able to articulate personal goals and even views of death that warrant respect. There is no simple formula for determining whether and to what extent children are capable of participating in planning their own care. Parents and pediatricians should jointly decide how much weight to give children's treatment preferences, taking into account not only the child's level of understanding and ability to anticipate future consequences of present actions but also the gravity of the decision in question, the likelihood of benefit, and the probability and severity of the burdens of treatment. Adults should respect children's right to disagree. However, on occasion, parental wishes must prevail for the best interests of the child.

For example, take the case of the 6-year-old girl with diabetes who is refusing to cooperate with the treatment regimen. The girl's inability to fully assess the consequences of her actions is a sign of immaturity, and she is at significant risk of serious harm if her pediatrician and family accept her choices. The clinician, in concert with the family, must provide treatment while working with the child to help her understand why this particular regimen is being followed.

At the very least, physicians or parents should inform children, in terms appropriate to their developmental level, about the nature of their condition, the proposed treatment course, and the expected outcome. By asking children about their hopes and fears, health care professionals and families may gain understanding about what the illness means to an individual child, and it may also provide valuable insights into how well children process information and form opinions. Such efforts foster children's cooperation and involvement and increase children's feelings of self-esteem and respect.

Because of parents' desire to protect, they may object to informing their children about a disease, proposed treatment plan, or prognosis. Health care professionals have an obligation based on an independent relationship with children to ensure that they receive adequate information. At the same time, these professionals should help parents understand that a conspiracy of silence rarely succeeds, often leaves children with unanswered questions and fears, and may be harmful to children's development of trust.

Regardless of children's level of participation in planning care, physicians should give young patients as much control over actual treatment decisions as possible. Even 2- and 3-year-old children may be able to help manage their treatments or at least determine the order in which various procedures are performed. Physicians and parents should not mislead or deceive children about their degree of authority. If a negative answer is unacceptable, then health care professionals and caregivers should avoid asking for children's approval. If a procedure is necessary, honesty demands that physicians offer children a more limited but feasible range of options (e.g., choosing in what order to receive a series of tests or whether or not to have a parent present).

Many childhood illnesses are chronic in nature with acute exacerbations and times of quiescence of disease. Young children faced with such chronic illnesses may develop and articulate clear sets of values and desires concerning future treatments and future quality of life. Children's perspective should be an integral part of planning care. The goal for health care of chronically ill children should be to prolong and normalize their lives, optimize their functioning, and enhance their future potential productivity. These goals are not always attainable, and some physicians and parents may wish to provide all available therapeutic interventions, even those that offer only the slimmest possibility of achieving short- or long-term survival. Aggressive treatments that hold out little hope of success may be excessive and cause children to suffer pain, fear, and isolation for little potential benefit. Physicians and parents must deal with the difficult issue of knowing when to decrease technologic intervention and to increase palliative and comfort care. Continued unsuccessful attempts at treatment may divert children and families from integrating the inevitability of impending death.

An increasing number of chronically ill children are dependent on technology such as respirators, intravenous feeding, and dialysis machines. These infants and children are often "graduates" of neonatal and pediatric intensive care units and beneficiaries of new life-saving technologies. Because they will require technologic assistance for many years, perhaps for the duration of their lives, many people contend that these children are better off living at home. Thus, programs that allow for the home care of technology-dependent children have developed throughout the United States.

Many families have accepted the responsibility of caring for technology-dependent children in the nurturing environment of the home. Such families are motivated by a clear desire to have their children at home as part of the family, and for the most part, the family provides the majority of the child's care. It has become increasingly clear that it costs less to care for technology-dependent children at home than at an acute care hospital or chronic care facility. This realization has created an important ethical dilemma. In order for society to spend fewer dollars for the care of children, it has become common to ask families to assume the burden of care, with consequent family cost and disruption.

Society must address and define the limits of parental obligation to chronically ill, technology-dependent children. Those families who make great sacrifices deserve praise, but at the same time, do those who do not wish to or cannot provide this extraordinary level of commitment to their child warrant condemnation? Should society take custody of a child away from parents because they cannot provide adequate home care for a technology-dependent child? Even if a family has the ability to provide such care, does this imply that they are obligated to keep their children at home when this will dramatically affect the lives of others in the family? If home care for children is a good that society wishes to foster, families should receive adequate social support and financial incentive to make caring for children within the family an experience that enhances the interests of all concerned. Families who object should not be forced to care for children at home; society should provide creative alternatives to care for such technology-dependent children while allowing parents to maintain their legal and emotional ties to their children.

SPECIAL PROBLEMS OF ADOLESCENTS

 CASE 3

Samantha is a 15-year-old girl newly diagnosed with leukemia. She and her family want her doctors to do everything to cure her of this serious disease. However, she and her parents are Jehovah's Witnesses and will not accept blood or platelet transfusions if they should become necessary secondary to complications of the aggressive chemotherapy required to eradicate the leukemic cells. Should the pediatrician respect the adolescent's and family's wishes concerning transfusion? Should the pediatrician allow the family and the child's wishes to result in her death?

Adolescence is a period of intense physical growth and maturation, accompanied by rapid changes in cognitive capacity, abstract thinking, and moral development. As children move into adolescence, they interpret the values inculcated by their family and develop opinions of their own. They shape their opinions first through comparisons to their peer group and later by a firmer sense of self and the ability to assess options and understand the consequences of actions. Increasingly, they base moral choices on abstract values, but peer influences sometimes override internal concepts of right and wrong. Adolescents are well known for an increased propensity for risk-taking behavior, which results from their curiosity, sense of omnipotence, and a drive to establish independence from parents and other authority figures. Illness itself may be a major influence on adolescent development and the capacity to make health-related decisions. Although certain diseases or therapies may impair cognitive function and limit the ability to participate in decision making, experience with an illness over time may empower adolescents with clear understanding of both the choices and consequences of a given health care decision.

Age alone is not a sufficient determinant of intelligence, experience, maturity, or perception, and physicians and parents should not use age as the sole criterion when deciding whether teens are capable of participating in health care decisions. Even cognitive ability alone is not sufficient. The combination of maturity and the ability to weigh the risks and benefits of alternative courses of action with an understanding of future consequences is the key to assessing the ability of adolescents to make independent decisions. Decisions of adolescents about their own health care deserve great consideration if the teenagers are able to:

- Make virtually all decisions about their daily affairs
- Come and go reasonably independently
- Make and keep medical appointments
- Articulate needs and follow recommendations
- Appear to understand the benefits and risks of proposed treatments

Physicians should respect the wishes of this 15-year-old girl, unlike those of the 6-year-old girl in Case 2, if the teenager has a fully developed view of her religious beliefs and the ability to understand the consequences of her choices. Careful assessment of the adolescent's ability to make decisions and an assessment of her independence from parental coercion must be performed before deciding to allow her view to prevail. Adults are given the right to refuse any treatment based on respect for their autonomy, including the right to refuse treatment even with grave consequences. It may be difficult for pediatricians to accept that adolescents have reached the level of maturity required to make such choices, but many teenagers do have the capac-

ity to make hard decisions, and their views warrant respect. This is particularly true when adolescents and their parents are in agreement, as in this case, and their views and values conflict with physicians' recommendations.

Ideally, decisions concerning adolescents should be collaborative and include patients, parents, and health care professionals. If adolescents disagree with their parents about the best course of treatment, and health care professionals believe that this choice is reasonable, physicians should respect the young persons' position after a careful assessment of the adolescent's capacity and mental health. At the same time, clinicians should attempt to work with the families to develop a reasonable plan of management. Pediatricians should not accept parents' surrogate decision making for patients whom they believe to be functionally autonomous.

If adolescents request confidentiality in an attempt to prevent their parents from learning of impending death or to hide certain behaviors that have resulted in an illness or injury, health care professionals are faced with another ethical dilemma. Physicians should explain the full scope of the problem to their patients, emphasizing that it may be more difficult to maintain confidentiality as the condition progresses, and there will be an increasing need for continuous support from a caring adult, preferably a parent. Most often, adolescents will benefit from the emotional support of parents and other family members, and health care professionals can help young persons by explaining this and creating a plan that ensures family involvement. Many professionals who work with adolescents believe that if teenagers insist on maintaining confidentiality, physicians should comply with their patients' request not to share information with parents. Physicians who are unwilling to maintain confidentiality should explain this to adolescents. Clinicians should not violate adolescents' trust by informing their parents and asking them not to tell a child of their knowledge of the matter.

Some adolescents are, by law, considered emancipated minors capable of making legal and binding decisions concerning their own health care. In general, these emancipated minors live independently, are in the military, or are parents of their own children. In addition, in most jurisdictions, even adolescents who are not emancipated may legally consent to medical treatment for sexually transmitted diseases, pregnancy and its prevention, and abortion services. It is clear that many older adolescents possess sufficient maturity and should be allowed to consent to or refuse care without parental involvement. The appropriate role of health care professionals who are caring for adolescents is to respect their patients' evolving autonomy and foster the young persons' role in decision making whenever possible.

END-OF-LIFE CARE

Sadly, there may come a time in the care of critically or chronically ill children when parents and health care professionals may need to question the appropriateness of continued treatment or the initiation of new treatment. Concerned adults may value children's intrinsic worth and want to support their interests, but they must also face the reality of the impending death of a child.

When considering allowing children to die, many physicians believe that withdrawing a treatment is legally and morally less justified than withholding one, but this distinction is erroneous. In the real world, bad deeds seem to occur more often because of someone's action rather than from lack of action. However, in the physician–patient relationship, with its implied contract to help and to provide appropriate treatment, there is no moral difference between withholding and withdrawing a treatment if the expected result of either action is the death of the patient. If there is a good reason to withhold a particular treatment from a particular patient, then it is equally defensible to withdraw that treatment if it is ineffective after it has been begun. Conversely, if a treatment is morally indicated, it is just as wrong to withhold that therapy as it would be to withdraw it. There is no question that it is psychologically more difficult to withdraw a treatment than to withhold one, but this psychologic difference does not create an ethical distinction. In addition, although many physicians believe that there is a legal difference between withholding and withdrawing treatments, in the opinion of most legal scholars, nothing in the law makes stopping treatment a more serious legal issue than not starting it in the first place.

In recent years, some medical professionals have contended that withdrawing a treatment that proves ineffective is morally superior to withholding a treatment because of its uncertain efficacy. Physicians often make decisions to withhold therapy in emergent situations in which uncertainty of outcome is quite great and contemplative discussion is impossible. On the other hand, they may base decisions to withdraw a treatment after a trial of therapy on additional information and perhaps more thoughtful discussion with patients or parents.

Some parents regard survival of severely ill or debilitated children as undesirable, and they sometimes resist proposed therapies that are unlikely to restore fully their children's health and function. Other parents believe that life has value under any circumstances, regardless of suffering, disability, or handicap, leading to requests for any and all treatments that can conceivably prolong children's biologic survival. Ascertaining what constitutes the best interests of children in these uncertain circumstances can be extremely difficult.

Perhaps the clearest example of such a case is that of children who have been diagnosed as brain dead and whose organ function can be maintained only by technologic support. In virtually all jurisdictions in the United States, determinations of death are possible after the irreversible cessation of circulatory and respiratory functions or the irreversible cessation of all functions of the entire brain, including the brainstem. There are specific brain death criteria for children; a degree of caution is necessary when applying them in very young infants. After a competent determination of brain death, children are deemed to be dead and, therefore, to have no interest in continued treatment. In such circumstances, most experts believe that no treatment should be provided even if requested by parents. Technologic intervention may continue for a short period of time for psychosocial support of the family or for maintaining organs for transplant donation but not in the interests of the deceased child.

Children who have no cortical function and no conscious ability to respond to the external environment but who do not fulfill the criteria for brain death (e.g., a child in a persistent vegetative state) present a more complex case. The only possible benefit of continued treatment is the prolongation of physical survival or the hope of an error in the diagnosis of irreversibility. Careful neurologic examination with reference to the cause and circumstances of the illness or injury can make misdiagnosis extremely unlikely. Because such children presumably cannot experience either suffering or joy or interact with the environment, they have few interests, if any, to which a "best interests" standard might apply, except the interest in being maintained in a comfortable and dignified manner. In these cases, in which there is no interaction with the environment and yet no pain and suffering, the "best interests" standard requires a supplementary standard that considers the presence or absence of basic human capacities. The ethical principle that justifies this additional standard is the proposition that biologic human life is only a relative good in the absence of certain distinctly human capacities such as self-consciousness and the ability to relate to others. Professionals may counsel parents faced with such tragic circumstances to withhold or withdraw all life-sustaining medical treatments from their children on the basis of a perception of the child's interests and possible future quality of life, as well as the potential minimal benefits of continued treatment. However, it remains the parents' choice whether treatment should be withdrawn or continued.

Decision making is more complicated when the prospect of successful outcome is less certain or the degree of burden is high. Parents, physicians, and others may quite reasonably become distressed by the pain and suffering caused by treatments expected to be of marginal usefulness. A small statistical chance of survival may not seem worth the agony of such treatment, especially if the course of therapy is prolonged. At some point, acceptance of likely death by physicians and parents as well as children may be preferable to exerting all efforts to avoid it. There is no easy way to determine when the burdens of treatment become sufficiently great to warrant a change in management away from attempts at cure solely toward the promotion of comfort. However, sound decision making requires that parents and their children, in consultation with health care professionals, make a judgment about the proportion of benefits to burdens. When they recognize that attempts at cure or restoration of function are no longer reasonable, the promotion of comfort becomes the primary goal of medical management; the health care team must devote its efforts to helping children and their families cope with the process of dying. Providing adequate pain relief is crucial in this endeavor, because both pain and the fear of pain create tremendous suffering for everyone involved. In the care of terminally ill children, when promotion of comfort is the primary goal, most health care professionals do not hesitate to utilize full and effective doses of pain medication, even if a possible secondary effect is sedation, depression of respiration, and the possible hastening of death. Careful titration of pain medication is intended to promote comfort and should not be mistaken for an act of killing.

In addition, it is important to determine where children should spend their last days. Many children experience a less traumatic and more com-fortable death at home than in the hospital. If families receive adequate support and are prepared to deal with pain relief and the signs and symptoms associated with impending death, home care may be appropriate. Many hospices offer support services to aid families who wish to support dying children at home. Alternatively, the hospital or inpatient hospice may be the appropriate setting for children whose families do not wish to cope with a terminally ill child at home. Death in the midst of loved ones and without the burdens of technologic intervention is possible in a hospital, either in an inpatient hospice unit or through special arrangements on pediatric units. It is important to develop an environment that facilitates continuing emotional and spiritual support for children and families before the child's death; this should continue through the grieving process to assist families in coping with the profound impact of a child's death.

ETHICAL ISSUES AND MANAGED CARE

In addition to all of the ethical dilemmas raised by the interaction of pediatricians with patients and their families, there are serious ethical issues in the actual practice of pediatrics. Ask any patient, physician, or health care administrator what he thinks about the present system of financing and organizing health care delivery, and you will hear an avalanche of complaints. Many of the complaints inevitably stem from managed care, the nation's most far-reaching attempt to restrain the costs of medical care. Managed care, which was conceived to integrate the financing and delivery of health care, promised to enhance the quality of care while containing or even lowering costs. There is much dispute about whether current managed care organizations have put these two laudable goals on equal footing.

Several factors account for this feeling of dissatisfaction, including:

- Loss of choice
- Fear of undertreatment
- Concern about being unable to provide optimal care for children
- Out-of-pocket costs for uncovered services
- Greater physician work for lower income
- Complex contracting arrangements

The public is distrustful of the health care system, physicians are depressed and angry, and administrators are fearful about the future of their institutions.

Physicians face unprecedented challenges to their professional identities as healers in trusting relationships with their patients and families. Rising health care costs and unexplained variations in medical practice patterns across the country have often forced physicians to be dual agents, with responsibilities to both patients and payers. The health care system places individual practicing physicians in the difficult position of serving as advocates for the interests of their patients while facing significant financial and bureaucratic impediments. Patient advocacy now includes educating families about coverage limits and appeals processes, disclosing financial incentives to families, assessing the evidence of efficacy of recommended services for insurers, and aggressively contesting denials of medically recommended treatments.

Of course, there are limits to the duty of physicians to work as advocates for their patients. No one can be expected to spend an inordinate amount of time obtaining marginally beneficial diagnostic and treatment services for patients. Similarly, patients should not expect physicians to lie for them (or to them). Misrepresentation or even outright lying to insurers or patients may harm patients and certainly affect the trust that is critical to the physician–patient relationship. Although good intentions may be the motive behind such actions, and they may benefit individual patients, ultimately, lying does not solve the problems of the health system and demeans the medical profession.

SUGGESTED READINGS

Arras JD: Toward an ethic of ambiguity. *Hastings Center Report* 14:25–33, 1984.

Committee on Bioethics, American Academy of Pediatrics: Ethics and the care of critically ill infants and children (RE9624). *Pediatrics* 98:149–152, 1996.

Committee on Fetus and Newborn, American Academy of Pediatrics: The initiation or withdrawal of treatment for high-risk newborns (RE9532). *Pediatrics* 96:362–363, 1995.

Duff RS, Campbell AGM: Moral and ethical dilemmas in the special care nursery. *N Engl J Med* 289:889–894, 1973.

Emanuel EJ, Dubler NN: Preserving the physician–patient relationship in the era of managed care. *JAMA* 273(4):323–329, 1995.

Fleischman AR: An infant bioethical review committee in an urban medical center. *Hastings Center Report* 16:16–18, 1986.

Fleischman AR, Nolan K, Dubler NN, et al: Caring for gravely ill children. *Pediatrics* 94:433–439, 1994.

Hastings Center: Guidelines on the termination of life sustaining treatment and the care of the dying. Briarcliff Manor, NY, Hastings Center, 1987.

Kleigman RM, Mahowald MB, Youngner SJ: In our best interests: Experience and workings of an ethics review committee. *J Pediatr* 108:178–187, 1986.

Lorber J: Results of treatment of myelomeningocele. *Dev Med Child Neurol* 13:279–303, 1971.

Lyon J: *Playing God in the Nursery.* New York, WW Norton, 1985.

Mechanic D: Managed care and the imperative for a new professional ethic. *Health Affairs* 19(5):100–111, 2000.

Morreim EH: Gaming the system: Dodging the rules, ruling the dodgers. *Arch Intern Med* 151:443–447, 1991.

National Commission for the Protection of Human Subjects: The Belmont report. Washington, DC, U.S. Government Printing Office, 1979.

President's Commission for the Study of Ethical Problems in Medicine and Biomedical and Behavioral Research: Deciding to forego life sustaining treatment. Washington, DC, U.S. Government Printing Office, 1983.

President's Commission for the Study of Ethical Problems in Medicine and Biomedical and Behavioral Research: Defining death. Washington, DC, U.S. Government Printing Office, 1981.

Report of Special Task Force: Guidelines for the determination of brain death in children. *Pediatrics* 80:298–299, 1987.

Rhoden NK: Treating Baby Doe: The ethics of uncertainty. *Hastings Center Report* 4:34–42, 1986.

Shaw A, Randolph SG, Manard B: Ethical issues in pediatric surgery: A nationwide survey of pediatricians and pediatric surgeons. *Pediatrics* 59:588–599, 1977.

Chapter 8

Health Care Economics and Managed Care

Steven P. Shelov and Elizabeth K. Kachur

Health care economics is rarely discussed in traditional textbooks for medical students because it does not seem to be relevant to clinical medicine. However, the current times clearly dictate a broader orientation for the successful practice of medicine. This must include at least some understanding of the economics of health care in our current world.

It is important for medical students to become familiar with the language of health economics (Appendix 8.1). Additional glossaries appear in many reference books (e.g., Kongstvedt, Wenner, Nelson and Minon) and on the Internet (see SUGGESTED READINGS). As the health care system changes, some terms fall into disuse, and new concepts emerge. Yet, all health care providers must keep up with this terminology to effectively negotiate the system for patients and themselves. Without a firm understanding of who pays for health care, how insurance companies determine what they can provide, how the health care market works, and what life is like in a managed care setting, future pediatricians will find themselves at a distinct disadvantage.

This chapter provides some of this necessary information. It begins with a description of how the health care market differs from others and what purchasers of health care would be likely to get for the money they spend.

HEALTH CARE: AN ATYPICAL MARKET

The health care market is intrinsically different from the traditional supply-and-demand market. Typical market purchases result in direct satisfaction to the consumer with few externalities (secondary gains or spillover effects). Usually buyers are knowledgeable about the items they purchase, make rational choices, and are fairly certain about the outcome. For example, buying a lawn mower usually involves doing research and purchasing the most suitable machine available. The lawn mower will cut grass, and the consumers know what they are "getting for their money." Although variations in price may influence the type of machine people buy, no one would buy more lawn mowers just because they are becoming less expensive.

Purchasing health care involves an entirely different series of decisions and rationales.

Pediatric Pearl

It is health that gives satisfaction, not the purchase of health care.

Buying more health care may be an attempt to achieve good health, but it certainly does not guarantee it. The purchase of health care may have many spillover effects. For example, not only are families who receive immunizations healthier, but they do not infect others who might be susceptible. (Buying a particular lawn mower has little effect on anyone but the consumer.)

There is no perfect guide to the purchase of health care, and consumers may be poorly informed. Although health care–related information is certainly better than it used to be, there are still few guarantees and many differences of opinion. In the past, people depended on providers and believed this was sufficient. Now, they seek information from insurance companies, advertisements, the Internet, the media, and other patients. Yet their education is rarely comprehensive, which may contribute to the excessive or needless purchasing of health care services.

The purchase of a computer may simulate the atypical health care market most closely. In many cases, people still derive a sense of satisfaction when they buy a fancy computer with extensive capabilities well beyond their skills level. Often there is excessive buying or upgrading with marginal improvement in computer literacy.

Health does not permit a series of rational choices. When it comes to their health, many people say, "there is no limit to what I would spend." However, the purchase of more health care services does not always result in better health or an improved quality of life.

APPENDIX 8.1

Selected Terms Used in Health Care Economics*

Benchmark—measurable variable used as baseline or reference in evaluating the performance of an organization or program.

Capitation—fixed amount paid per enrollee per month to cover a defined set of services over a specific period of time, which may be more or less than the cost of the actual services provided.

Carveout—set of medical services that are contracted for separately or left out of the basic arrangement (e.g., mental health or substance abuse services).

Case management—coordination of patient care to ensure appropriateness, efficiency, speediness, and prevention of complications.

Continuous quality improvement (CQI)—form of *quality management* that uses a systems approach and targets internal operating procedures to improve efficiency and effectiveness.

Coordination of benefits (COB)—procedure that prevents double payment for services when a subscriber has coverage from two or more sources (e.g., additional insurance from spouse).

Copayment—cost-sharing arrangement in which the patient pays a flat charge for a specific service.

Current Procedural Terminology (CPT)—five-digit codes for all types of physician services and procedures used for reporting and billing.

Deductible—amount a patient has to forfeit directly to a provider before an insurance plan begins to pay benefits.

Demand curve—graphical representation of the relationship between price and quantity requested. The higher the price, the lower the consumption.

Demand management—decision and behavior support system (e.g., self-care intervention, health promotion, educational tools, telephone help lines) for encouraging patients to use medical services appropriately.

Diagnosis related groups (DRGs)—classification system instituted by the *Health Care Financing Administration* (*HCFA*) to establish *Medicare* hospital reimbursement rates. Patients are categorized by principal diagnosis, type of surgical procedure, presence or absence of significant comorbidities or complications, or other relevant criteria to determine the amount that *Medicare* will pay for their treatment.

Direct Medical Education (DME) Reimbursement—part of the *Graduate Medical Education* (*GME*) payment that hospitals receive for training residents. DME consists of salaries and fringe benefits for trainees.

Disease management—a systematic approach to provide care to a group of patients with a certain condition (usually chronic) for the purpose of managing their health problem over time, improving outcomes, and lowering costs. Such management programs may involve patient and provider education, guidelines for applying alternative therapies, patient monitoring, and outcome assessments.

Enrollment—recruitment of *members* to an insurance plan.

Externalities (spillover effects, secondary gains)—costs or benefits that impact society but are not included in the market price of a good or service. Negative externalities have negative consequences (e.g., pollution), and positive externalities have positive consequences (e.g., the cost of immunizing one child does not include the extra benefits of preventing the spread of disease in the community).

Fee-for-service (FFS) plan—insurance system in which providers and hospitals receive direct payment for their billed charges, either from the patient or the insurance company (see Table 8.6).

Formulary—list of selected pharmaceutical agents believed to be most useful and cost-effective for patient care. Closed formularies limit clinicians to prescribing the drugs on the list, whereas open formularies serve more as a recommendation.

For-profit entity—company or organization that aims to benefit financially from the services it provides; opposite of non-profit or *not-for-profit*.

Gatekeeper—first contact provider (usually primary care practitioner), who determines the appropriate level and delivery of care for each patient by making the initial diagnosis; administering treatment; and authorizing referrals, tests, and hospitalization.

Graduate Medical Education (GME) Reimbursement—*Medicare* and *Medicaid* funds that are given to hospitals that train residents. The reimbursement consists of two portions: *Direct Medical Education* (*DME*) and *Indirect Medical Education* (*IME*) payments.

Gross domestic product (GDP)—current terminology for the total market value of all goods and services produced within a country during a given period of time, usually 1 year. The GDP equals the *gross national product* (*GNP*) plus income from other countries. In the United States, this figure is tabulated and reported by the Department of Commerce.

Gross national product (GNP)—total market value of all goods and services produced by the

(continued)

Selected Terms Used in Health Care Economics* *(Continued)*

citizens of a country during a given period of time, usually 1 year. The GNP was once the official measure of how much output the U.S. economy produced. In the early 1990s, the term was replaced by *gross domestic product* (*GDP*), which excludes or does not include foreign income.

Health Care Finance Administration (HCFA)— branch of U.S. Department of Health and Human Services that administers *Medicare* and oversees the state-run *Medicaid.* This agency, which introduced the *diagnosis related groups* (*DRGs*), also provides *GME* reimbursements.

Health maintenance organization (HMO)— managed care organization that provides comprehensive health care to a certain population of patients for a prepaid, fixed sum (see Table 8.6).

Health Plan Employer Data and Information Set (HEDIS)—standard measures of health plan performance (e.g., access, patient satisfaction, membership, utilization).

ICD-9-CM (International Classification of Diseases, 9th edition, Clinical Modification)— list of diagnoses and identification codes used by physicians to report patient diagnoses to health plans.

Indemnity plan—insurance plan in which the insured person or provider is reimbursed for all or part of the covered expenses after a service is provided; the opposite of a *prepaid plan.*

Independent practice association (IPA)—type of *health management organization* (*HMO*) that contracts with physicians who see its *members* in their own offices, together with their other patients (see Table 8.6).

Indirect Medical Education (IME) Reimbursement—part of the *Graduate Medical Education* (*GME*) payment that hospitals receive for training residents. It covers expenses incurred from excessive test ordering and other inefficiencies. IME also supplements the salaries of attending physicians for their teaching activities.

Intermediate care facility (ICF)—facility that provides less comprehensive care than hospitals or skilled nursing facilities but more comprehensive care than can be given at home.

Management services organization (MSO)— company that provides administrative, managerial, financial, and managed care contracting services to providers, especially those in group practices. MSOs are used by hospitals to assist their affiliated physicians.

Medicaid—state-sponsored health insurance for poor individuals. Medicaid is administered by state health departments but is overseen by the

Health Care Financing Administration (*HCFA*), a federal agency.

Medical necessity—judgment by a clinical expert that specific care is required to preserve the life or health of a patient.

Medicare—governmental health insurance for individuals older than 65 years of age and those with a permanent disability. It is centrally administered by the *Health Care Finance Administration* (*HCFA*), a federal agency.

Member—person enrolled in a managed care plan.

Not-for-profit entity—organization or company that reinvests the majority of its profits in itself. It does not focus on enriching its owners or shareholders. Such institutions are subject to special regulations, but they also receive special tax benefits.

Patient panel—*members* assigned to a single provider or a group of health care providers.

Per member per month (PMPM)—measurement unit for operating statistics: one *member* enrolled in a *health maintenance organization* (*HMO*) for 1 month (whether or not the *member* receives services). (Two member months may be one *member* who enrolls for 2 months or two members who sign up for 1 month each.)

Personal Health Care Expenditure—average amount of money spent on health care by an individual in a given year.

Physician hospital organization (PHO)— collaboration of physicians and a local hospital or group of hospitals to contract with managed care organizations.

Point of service (POS) plan—managed care plan in which *members* can choose from a *health maintenance organization* (*HMO*), *preferred provider organization* (*PPO*), or *indemnity plan* at the time health care is needed. Thus they do not have to make a decision at the time of enrollment (see Table 8.6).

Practice guidelines—systematically developed statements on medical practices that assist with clinical decision making for specific medical conditions.

Precertification—prospective review for the purpose of granting or withholding permission for diagnosis or treatment coverage.

Preferred provider organization (PPO)— managed care plan that contracts with independent providers who render services to *members* at discounted rates (see Table 8.6).

Premium—amount paid to an insurer or health care plan for providing coverage for a certain level of services during a specific time period. It may be paid by either an individual or

Selected Terms Used in Health Care Economics* *(Continued)*

an employer or it may be shared by both parties.

Prepaid health plan—entity that contracts to provide certain medical services to enrollees in exchange for *capitation* payment.

Profiling—systematic method for collecting and analyzing patient data to develop provider-specific practice information.

Provider—health care professional or organization that offers health care services.

Quality management—formal set of activities (e.g., quality assessment, corrective actions) to ensure the quality of services provided.

Report card—tool for policy makers and health care purchasers to understand and compare the performance of health plans or providers (e.g., quality and utilization, consumer satisfaction, administrative efficiency, financial stability, cost control).

Risk sharing—apportionment of chance of incurring financial loss by insurers, managed care organizations, health care providers, and patients.

Third party payor—insurance plan (e.g., *Health Maintenance Organization* (*HMO*), *Medicaid*, *Medicare,* traditional insurance company) that pays *providers* for care. It acts as intermediary between the employer (who pays for health coverage) and the individual/*member* (who uses health care services).

Utilization review—a process that measures the use of resources (e.g., professional staff, facilities, services) to determine cost effectiveness and conformity to criteria of optimal use.

Welfare loss—loss to society that is incurred by the purchase of unnecessary services.

*Italicized terms are also defined in the glossary.

For all of these reasons, the **health care market is atypical** (Table 8.1). Individuals who can afford to overpurchase care often do, with no true guarantee that this will result in better health. As a matter of fact, in 1996 the top 1% of the U.S. population who spent money on health care accounted for 27% of all expenditures, while the bottom 50% of those who spent money on health care accounted for only 3% of all expenditures (Figure 8.1). In 1996 dollars, the annual expenditure of the bottom 50% of the U.S. population was $122 per person, and it was $56,459 per person in the top 1%. This pattern has been fairly stable over the past few decades. Because the managed care environment prides itself on investing in preventive care, one might have ex-

pected a greater balance between the top and bottom spenders.

THE INFLUENCE OF INSURANCE ON THE DEMAND FOR HEALTH CARE

Insurance has permitted health care consumers to utilize increasing amounts of services, often with little regard for actual cost. Only deductibles and copayments force consumers to assume some real costs for their health care, which may reduce excessive utilization. Figure 8.2 reflects some of these effects. If the cost of health care is completely assumed by the consumer (P_1), then the quantity demanded is (Q_1). If health care is completely covered (i.e., no cost to the consumer)

TABLE 8.1   **Characteristics of Typical Markets and Atypical Health Care Markets**

Typical Market	Atypical Health Care Market
Direct satisfaction to customer	Satisfaction from health, not medical care per se
No externalities or spillover effects	Externalities or spillover effects
Well-informed consumer (certainty concerning outcome of purchase)	Poorly informed consumer (little knowledge about competence of provider; significant degree of uncertainty about outcome)
Rational consumer	Health is not a rational series of choices

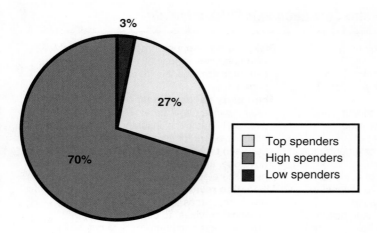

FIGURE 8.1. Distribution of health care expenditures, which has remained surprisingly stable over the past 50 years regardless of changes in the health care system. Looking at the total amount of health care dollars spent (represented by the pie), it is evident that the top and high spenders (50% of the population) are responsible for 97% of the United States health care expenses. The top spenders (only 1% of the population) account for 27% of health care payments; many of these patients are old or very ill. The low spenders (50% of the population) account for only 3% of the health care expenditures.

[P_0], demand for health care is at a maximum (Q_4). Imposing a deductible forces consumers to pay up to P_2 before their insurance takes effect.

If insurance picks up a significant portion of the costs, and consumers are responsible only for the copayment (e.g., as little as $5), they will most likely want more health care (Q_3), than if they had to pay full price. Suffice it to say that price (cost) is a powerful influence on the purchase of health care.

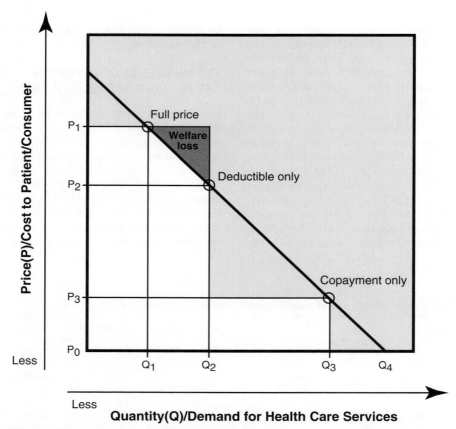

FIGURE 8.2. The effect of insurance on the demand for health care services. See text for explanation.

Pediatric Pearl

Factors such as deductibles and copayments influence how people purchase health care and are one way that insurance companies have attempted to influence the excessive utilization of health care—to limit the number of dollars spent.

Copayments and deductibles make people feel as if they are paying less. The lower the price, the more health care people demand (see Figure 8.2). Because there is no real way to determine whether health itself is actually being purchased, there is a tendency to simply buy more, which creates a situation known as welfare loss (*shaded triangle*). This extra amount of health care purchased probably does not result in better health but only generates waste or loss to the greater society.

With some economic understanding of the atypical nature of the health care market and how people could achieve optimum health by purchasing health care wisely, this chapter now explores how the macroeconomic trends over the past 60 years have led to the current health care environment and what the economic future may be.

WHO PAYS FOR HEALTH CARE?

Health care expenditures have changed greatly since the beginning of the 20th century. In 1929, $3.6 billion were spent on health care, a mere 3.5% of the U.S. gross national product (GNP), as it was then called. The per capita (per person) health care expenditure was only $29. The percent of the U.S. gross domestic product (GDP), as it is now called, and per capita spending has increased dramatically since then. In 1998, health expenditures exceeded one trillion dollars, or 13% of the GDP. The average per capita expenditure, also known as the Personal Health Care Expenditure, rose dramatically, too (Figure 8.3).

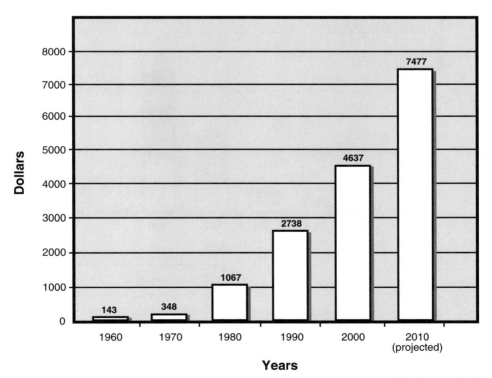

FIGURE 8.3. Personal Health Care Expenditures—what is the per capita cost for health care in the United States? In 1960, each person spent an average of $143 on health care. By 2000, that amount had risen to an average of $4637, and it is expected to almost double by 2010. The sharpest rise occurred between 1970 and 1980, when the individual amount paid for health care tripled.

Pediatric Pearl

Each year, health care costs have increased by 5%–11%. This has created an environment in which consumers and providers need to seriously examine the source of these increases and develop methods for limiting them.

Physician services account for a significant percent of health care expenses, but by no means the majority. Over the past 40 years, expenses for physicians have amounted to an average annual increase of 10%–11%, which has remained steady compared to other health care costs (Figure 8.4).

The most significant source of health care spending is hospital care. In 2000, while physician and clinical services accounted for $286 billion, hospitals costs accounted for $412 billion. Both categories together accounted for 54% of all health care dollars spent. As many different interest groups, especially the payors, have become concerned about the inflationary spiral of

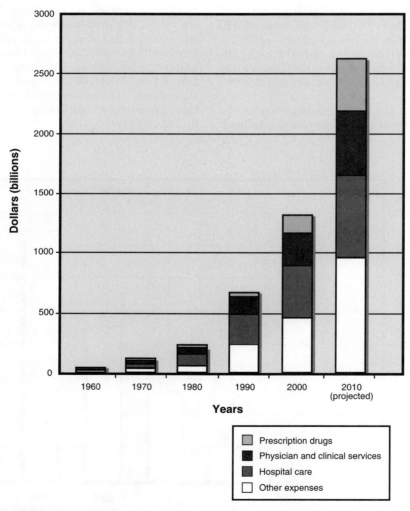

FIGURE 8.4. National health expenditures—how much money does the United States spend on health care? This graph illustrates the sharp rise in national health care expenditures over the past 40 years. The breakdown into different types of expenses illustrates that some are rising more quickly than others. Most expense categories double each decade, but the monies spent for prescription drugs seem to triple during these periods and are of special concern. "Other expenses" include dental services, nursing homes, durable medical equipment, and government public health activities.

health care costs, these expenditures have become obvious targets as sources of savings.

Just as important as the increase in costs are the shifts in who pays for health care (Figure 8.5). In 1929, individuals and families paid for health care almost entirely out of their own pockets. The government accounted for only 4% of the payments, mostly for those veterans who had fought in previous military conflicts. In 1960, the sources of payment for the growing health care costs shifted markedly to include a rising private insurance business (21%) and government support (21%). However, individuals continued to carry the majority of the burden. The Medicare legislation of 1965 changed those ratios once again, setting the stage for the marked shift in who pays for health care.

Before 1965, the poorest population in the United States was the elderly. This group, which was far smaller than it is today, was often forgotten in their needs. They and their children viewed health care costs as an onerous burden at best, cruel at worst. Both the Kennedy and Johnson administrations recognized the need for reform. The resulting Medicare legislation of 1965 changed the health care landscape forever for the elderly, the nation, and health care providers at all levels. By 1970, federal, state, and local governments (in combination) paid for 35% of all health care costs; the individual contribution dropped to 40% (see Figure 8.5).

Finally, the government began health care coverage for the very poor, known as Medicaid, which further transformed the relative amounts that governments and individuals pay for health care. Currently, the share of the health care dollar paid for by the government accounts for almost 50%. Individuals assume about 20%,

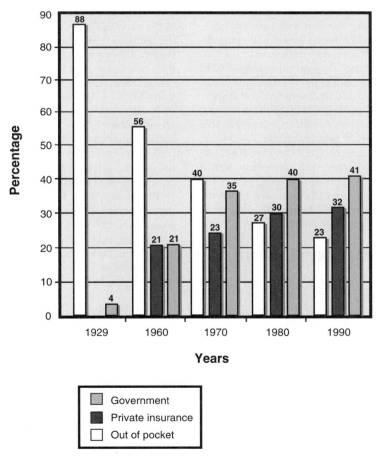

FIGURE 8.5. Bar graph that shows the shift in the source of health care payments since 1929, when individuals paid for most of their health care themselves. By 1990, health care was financed primarily by private insurance and the government (state and federal combined).

and private health insurance pays for the remainder.

The Medicare legislation also instituted additional support for Graduate Medical Education (GME). Many people still do not realize that the Medicare legislation of 1965 was so broad in scope. The creators of that landmark ruling envisioned that physicians-in-training at academic health centers would provide much of the health care for individuals older than 65 years of age or those who were very poor. These trainees (residents) would receive supervision from senior physicians, who would be spending their time educating and not providing patient care. If they were not subsidized, trainees would be extremely costly since they are inherently less efficient, utilize more tests, and burden the system in other indirect ways.

The government assumed the financial responsibility of many of these GME costs by allocating money through Medicare and Medicaid. Training hospitals and medical schools receive a special amount per resident that varies by geographic region and poverty level of the population served. GME dollars are divided into two basic bundles: Direct Medical Education (DME) reimbursement, which is the salaries and fringe benefits for the residents themselves, and Indirect Medical Education (IME) reimbursement, which covers the costs resulting from excessive test ordering, partial salaries of teaching physicians, and other inherent inefficiencies of a training program. DME and IME payments, which have become an integral and growing part of the government's support of health care expenses, now account for over $7 billion of reimbursement to training programs annually.

THE HEALTH CARE ENVIRONMENT SINCE 1970

This marked change in who pays for health care in the United States has had a profound impact on every element of the health care industry: consumers, health care providers, insurance companies, businesses, and all levels of government. Until the late 1980s, when concerns about raising health care costs came into national consciousness, the various groups who had a stake in health care engaged in behaviors that in many ways aided and abetted the inexorable increase in annual expenditures (Table 8.2). All participants in the health care setting played some role in the rising costs. By passing along these charges to other groups with little insight into the true implications of this practice, every par-

ticipant contributed to the sense that the growing expenses for increased utilization and technology could be ignored. People realized that this situation, which involved excessive health care use with little regard for quality of outcomes and true marginal gain, was no longer affordable.

Some of the key factors of health care inflation are amenable to intervention, and others are unavoidable (Table 8.3). By the 1970s, and certainly into the 1980s, the rapidly increasing health care inflation spiral could no longer be overlooked, especially in the midst of the economic downturn of that time. Each of the parties in Table 8.2 had to modify its behavior to make spending practices conform to a more rational and disciplined model of care. Some of the corrections have been excessive and some have been insufficient; the situation is still evolving.

COST REDUCTION STRATEGIES

In the early 1970s, as people began to appreciate the consequences of the rampant health care inflation, the system of care and affordability of that care began to erode. Several different cost containment approaches emerged during these years (Table 8.4). Hospitals, the greatest source of health care expenses, began to impose increasing restrictions on spending, personnel, and equipment. Capital purchases and building projects came under greater scrutiny, and personnel inefficiency and excessive technology purchases were sharply curtailed or altered.

Physicians were forced to begin to look at their practices with a greater degree of financial accountability. They began to form different types of group practices, partially in response to payor shift and partially out of desire to maintain quality and income. Multispecialty groups, hospital-purchased practices, and preferred provider organizations (PPOs) became part of the moving force. Finally, performance measured against definable outcomes, either good or bad, increasingly became part of physicians' everyday worlds.

The federal government imposed changes in reimbursement strategies and began to move away from straight-cost reimbursement to other methods such as using diagnosis related groups (DRGs); scrutinizing lengths of stay; and questioning procedures, tests, and other heretofore unchallenged elements of medical practice. As a result, health care costs as a political agenda began to gather momentum and culminated in the early 1990s in Bill Clinton's

TABLE 8.2 **Attitudes and Behaviors in Health Care Stakeholders That Led to Increased Health Expenditures**

EMPLOYERS/BUSINESSES
Used health care coverage as important benefit for employees
Could deduct health care premiums paid for employees from taxes
Raised prices for goods and services to cover premium increases
Used health care benefits as substitute for wage increases (given tax-deductible nature of paid premiums, government implicitly subsidized such increases)
Rarely held employees accountable for their health services utilization
Rarely held physicians or hospitals accountable for health services provided
Exercised little control over escalating health care costs
INSURERS
Covered health care liberally; increased costs were passed on to employer/individual through premiums
Had little concern for outcomes
Did not require health care providers to account for costs
Had little concern for evidence-basis of health care practices
Were eager to insure low-risk patients and reluctant to insure those with potential health care needs ("cherry picking")
Were willing to pay:
    Physicians and hospitals for a percent of charges
    Physicians on a fee-for-service basis, offering incentives for providing more services
    Hospitals on a cost- (sometimes cost-plus) basis defined by hospitals
    For new technology indiscriminately
PHYSICIANS
Lived in a world where few questioned their authority
Had several different, often conflicting incentives
Kept patients free from illness
Maintained and grew personal income
Used the most modern techniques, technologies, medicines
Maintained a competitive advantage over other physicians
Grew market shares by expanding practices
Tried to see more patients and provide more services to receive more payment from third party payors

Were minimally accountable for their income
Had few requirements for timely, clear and comprehensive documentation
Maintained quality standards that were individually determined and not scrutinized
Subscribed to a strong personal ethic to do well by individual patients, and to do no harm
Had little need to worry about competition from nonphysician providers
Were conscious of malpractice potentials but did not live in fear of it
Practiced in solo or group practices, controlled by physicians who dictated costs, cost structure, and practice
Held a prominent stature in communities and society
Lived under the basic assumption that physicians were untouchable
HOSPITALS
Attempted to provide quality care, costs were secondary
Allowed wide disparity of physician practices without accountability for outcomes
Could usually pass on increased costs to payors, either government or private insurance
Purchased new technology with little regard for redundancy within geographic settings
Exercised little oversight of quality of care
Assumed M.D. or D.O. degrees provided sufficient credential for quality
Depended on physician self-monitoring over practices and outcome
Often received reimbursement on a cost or cost-plus basis from payors
Expanded capital improvement through low-cost loans and by passing on costs to payors (especially not-for-profit hospitals)
Operated with few cost restrictions (especially for-profit hospitals)
CONSUMERS (formerly called patients)
Used precious health care resources in nondiscriminating fashion
Tended to overuse resources, since there was little impact on personal finances
Were protected by insurance from understanding the true value (cost) of health care
Remained naive and uneducated about details of health care (quality, comparable options, actual outcomes)
Were less interested in true prevention
Depended on health care providers for making health decisions

TABLE 8.3	Causes of Health Care Inflation

UNAVOIDABLE FACTORS
Aging of population
Technology and its success in prolonging life
Service cost inflation
DISCRETIONARY FACTORS
Medically uneducated, insufficiently price-sensitive consumers
Highly fragmented insurance industry with little expertise in medical management
Massive excess hospital capacity, exacerbated by the proliferation of outpatient care
Wildly varying standards of medical practice
Resource focus on acute rather than preventive care
Insufficient medical outcome data
Oversupply and overuse of physician specialists
Heroic attempts to save virtually hopeless cases
Malpractice fears and pressures
Few effective pharmaceutical formularies

successful run for the presidency. Health care became a legitimate target for change; all participants, patients, providers, hospitals, employers, and payors (including federal, state, and local governments) had a stake in seeing these costs come under control, without sacrificing quality. The United States has spent billions of dollars on health care, but the country does not fare well in terms of public health indicators such as longevity, child survival, and immunization rates.

The old health care system was inaccessible to millions of people, rewarded costly intervention as opposed to prevention and fiscal prudence, and allowed individual providers to work regardless of practice conventions and scientific evidence. The Clinton administration attempted to pass legislation to create a universal health care system that would permit risk sharing among the entire population and would bring in those people who increasingly slip through the health care safety net. The purpose of universal coverage is to allow all individuals to have health insurance, including those at highest risk for developing a medical condition.

☀ Pediatric Pearl

By having everyone in the same pool, the premiums from low-risk individuals (those less likely to get sick in any given year) could cross-subsidize those of high risk.

Spreading out the risk pool through universal coverage could achieve a lower per capita cost that would be financially bearable for all individuals except the poor. Government funding would underwrite the costs for the truly indigent population.

Although the legislation failed for a variety of reasons, the focus on health care expenditures became a national imperative. The aim to institute a unified health care system for all remains a priority for many people, and it will probably reemerge in some politically satisfactory way within the next decade. In the interim, the health care financing world continues to be one with very mixed signals that is still unable to properly care for a significant portion of the population. This uninsured and underinsured group includes many needy children and families who are above the Medicaid level but cannot afford an insurance system that covers even minimum benefits.

After the health care initiatives of 1993 failed, managed care, which began decades earlier, grew substantially and became a major force. Not only did the managed care system make payors and providers scrutinize costs more carefully, it also created entirely new reimbursement strategies. At first, many hospitals and physician providers found these methods onerous, and they tried to hold on to the status quo that had proved profitable for the health professions for so long. These care providers are now being blamed for having squandered valuable opportunities for the medical profession to take an active stance in improving the health care system.

On the other hand, corporate entities demonstrated more responsibility for the cost of care and a better appreciation of service outcomes. As a result, much of the control over spending on health care is out of the hands of physicians and physician groups and in the hands of corporations, some of which are for-profit and some are not-for-profit.

The following section outlines the managed care system and describes how this novel approach to health care has simultaneously driven the industry to new levels of certainty and uncertainty.

WHAT IS MANAGED CARE?

The term "managed care" refers to the new era in health care, but it does not have a simple definition. As the U.S. health care system is undergoing rapid transformations (see COST REDUCTION STRATEGIES), managed care is also changing

TABLE 8.4 Cost-cutting Measures Initiated by Different Health Care Stakeholders

BUSINESSES

Raised copayments and deductibles on traditional insurance plans

Encouraged employees to join HMOs

Jawboned down HMO price increases to 0%–3%

Monitored the quality of HMO services (e.g., with HEDIS)

Replaced traditional insurance companies with HMO-based point-of-service plans

Integrated group health and workers compensation

Cut back Medicare supplement benefits for retirees, encouraging them to join HMOs

Joined business coalitions to coordinate cost-containment and purchasing strategies

Encouraged preventive care and wellness programs

Carved out psychiatric and pharmaceutical benefits (would not pay for undercovered benefits)

GOVERNMENT PROGRAMS (MEDICARE/MEDICAID)

Arbitrarily and capriciously reimbursed providers at 50%–75% of fee-for-service rates

Held down Medicare price increases to 0%–2%

Provided reimbursement of pharmaceuticals for Medicaid recipients and received 15%–20% discounts

Conducted quality or outcome audits

Excluded low quality hospitals or physicians

Provided extra incentives to join HMOs

Forced Medicaid HMOs to market on an individual basis, rather than mandating that all beneficiaries join HMOs

Arbitrarily changed annual Medicare HMO price increases within an excessively wide range of 2%–10%

Explored the closing of Veterans Administration hospitals

Mandated HMO/insurance carriers (but not self-insured plans) to provide extra benefits and pay premium taxes

HEALTH MAINTENANCE ORGANIZATIONS (HMOs)

Moved physician contracting from discounted fee-for-service to capitated arrangements

Increasingly insisted that contracted physicians are board certified

Contracted with narrow provider networks to lower costs and improve quality

Required approval before covering costly procedures (precertification)

Paid hospitals on a per-diem or capitated basis

Focused on disease management to reduce costs and increase quality of care for patients with asthma, diabetes or other chronic diseases

Selectively integrated vertically into primary care physician offices

Employed a dedicated sales force for marketing to Medicare, Medicaid, and small employer group populations

Published report cards on service performance, preventive programs, and patient outcomes

Better-coordinated healthcare to avoid waste

HOSPITALS

Reengineered patient care by encouraging physicians to establish and follow protocols

Instituted continuous quality improvement (CQI)

Reduced the number of registered nurses, while increasing the number of lower-cost licensed practical nurses and aides, cross-trained support staff

Consolidated department overhead structures

Committed volume guarantees to medical suppliers in return for price concessions or utilization controls

Integrated horizontally by acquiring local hospital competitors, managing services regionally, rationalizing cost structures, eliminating redundant services

Integrated vertically into subacute care, rehabilitation, home care, and psychiatric care

Established PHOs or MSOs or purchased medical groups to contract with managed care insurers in collaboration with physicians

Gained market shares with HMOs by cutting prices in return for incremental patient volume

PHYSICIANS

Rapidly formed single-specialty and multi-specialty group practices to share overhead, standardize care, negotiate with HMOs and manage risks

Expanded regionally to better serve managed care payors

Improved physician productivity through more effective patient scheduling and increased use of physician assistants and nurse practitioners

Began to design standard patient protocols, particularly for high-cost chronic care cases

Began to publish their own patient report cards

Established hospital risk pools in collaboration with HMOs to hold down hospital utilization

Individual physicians cut prices to HMOs (but without improving their own productivity their income and market share declined)

CONSUMERS (formerly called patients)

Became better informed about health care matters

Requested generic drugs

Became more selective about health care purchases

Discriminated more concerning quality of provider chosen

Asked about outcomes

Scrutinized quality of care

Challenged previously not discussed medical opinions

HEDIS = Health Plan Employer Data and Information Set; HMO = health maintenance organization; MSO = management services organization; PHO = physician–hospital organization.

continuously. This new approach to health care delivery and financing has several building blocks. Some of the key elements are presented in Figure 8.6. As mentioned earlier, the system is still under construction and will take a while before it stabilizes.

In *Principles of Managed Care,* the American Medical Association (AMA) defines managed care as

> . . . processes or techniques used by any entity that delivers, administers, or assumes risk for health services in order to control or influence the quality, accessibility, utilization, cost and prices, or outcomes of such services provided to defined populations.

The general concept arose from the desire to "manage" care, to make it more organized, coordinated, and efficient than what it had become during a fee-for-service reimbursement system.

At present, "managed care" is the established name, but different names (e.g., care management) are under consideration to eliminate the negative emotional baggage associated with this

term. With the help of a new name, some people hope it will be possible to capitalize on the many positive innovations of the past few decades and make the still much-needed health care reforms.

Managed care began over 70 years ago (Table 8.5). In 1929, a physician established the first prepaid group practice plan in rural Oklahoma. Farmers who joined a corporation as shareholders received medical care at a discounted rate. In the next three decades, a variety of other plans replicated this model, but overall managed care growth was slow. Paul Ellwood, a physician from Minneapolis who lobbied for passage of the 1973 Health Maintenance Organization Act, first coined the familiar term health maintenance organization (HMO).

In the past 15 years, enrollment in managed care plans has grown tremendously (Figure 8.7). Initially, many physicians tried to resist the movement toward managed care and HMOs but were forced into participating because of growing competition. If they did not join a plan or collaborate to create one of their own, they were at risk for losing many of their patients.

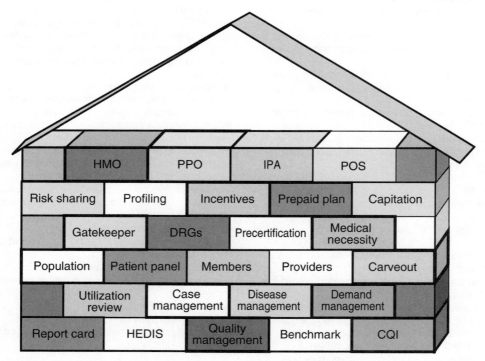

FIGURE 8.6. The building blocks of managed care, which are some of the key concepts and strategies that developed through managed care. CQI = continuous quality improvement; DRG = diagnosis related group; HEDIS = Health Plan Employer Data and Information Set; HMO = health maintenance organization; IPA = independent practice association; POS = point of service; PPO = preferred provider organization.

TABLE 8.5 **Some Key Developments in the History of Managed Care**

1929	Michael Shadid, MD, developed the first prepaid group practice insurance plan for a rural farmer's cooperative in Elk City, OK.
1929	Donald Ross, MD, and H. Clifford Loos, MD, started a prepaid plan for the Los Angeles Department of Water and Power.
1933	Sidney Garfield, MD, and associates started a prepaid plan for a California aqueduct construction project, a forerunner of Kaiser Permanente.
1937	The Group Health Association (GHA) was developed for employees of the Federal Home Loan Bank in Washington, DC.
1943	GHA won a lawsuit against medical societies that were convicted of criminal conspiracy in restraint of trade.
1945	The Kaiser plan opened for community enrollment.
1947	The Group Health Cooperative of Puget Sound, opened up for the Grange, the Aeromechanics Union, and local supply and food cooperatives in Seattle, WA.
1947	The Health Insurance Plan of Greater New York (HIP) was developed for city employees with much support of Mayor Fiorello LaGuardia.
1947	The American Medical Association (AMA) lost an antitrust lawsuit because of their aggressive opposition to the development of prepaid health plans.
1954	The San Joaquin County Medical Society in Stockton, CA, created the prototype individual practice association (IPA) to counter competition from Kaiser Permanente.
1957	The Group Health Plan of Minneapolis was initiated.
1965	The Medicare and Medicaid Acts were passed by the U.S. government.
1971	The Nixon administration initiated a new grants and loan program to foster the development of health maintenance organizations (HMOs).
1973	The HMO Act was passed by Congress to allocate funds for HMO development. It preempted state laws that banned prepaid groups, and required companies with at least 25 employees to offer a federally qualified HMO.
1980	The Reagan administration discontinued the Office of Health Maintenance Organizations, which oversaw 118 federally qualified HMOs.
1993	The Clinton administration tried to revamp the health care system, but concerns about excessive government involvement pushed toward a resolution of the health care crisis in the market place, bringing managed care to the forefront.
1998	Medicaid and Medicare managed care bills were passed, initiating a movement toward managed care in these two governmental programs.

Over the past decade, with the overall tightening of the economy, came a major push to managed care plans from employers, who eagerly embraced newly emerging organizations that promised health care delivery for a lower cost. Indeed, in the mid- to late 1990s, there was a sharp drop in their premiums for employees. However, that cost is increasing again, and now, the corporate world is contemplating its general ability to offer health care benefits.

Several types of health care plans are currently operating in the United States (Table 8.6). They range from minimal cost and quality control in fee-for-service plans to a maximum of structure and control in HMOs.

The seemingly simple change in the payment system from fee-for-service to prepayment resulted in a redistribution of risks and a revamping of emphasis from paying providers to deliver diagnosis and treatment to paying them for keeping patients well. Each provider receives a preset amount of money (capitated payment) to care for a predetermined number of patients (a population) in a given period of time. A provider who does less work (e.g., because patients are healthy or services become more efficient) can keep the extra money. In contrast, another provider, whose patients are ill more frequently, may have to work more, exceeding the fees received.

With HMOs, the financial risk of having to expend health care resources shifts to providers and hospitals rather than remaining with insurance companies. Because physicians are a key element in the distribution of health care, the overutilization of health care resources that had been a problem in the past quickly became a concern about underutilization. Health care providers were encouraged to order fewer rather than more tests and to prescribe less expensive rather than more expensive medications—not always on the basis of scientific evidence.

National HMO Enrollment

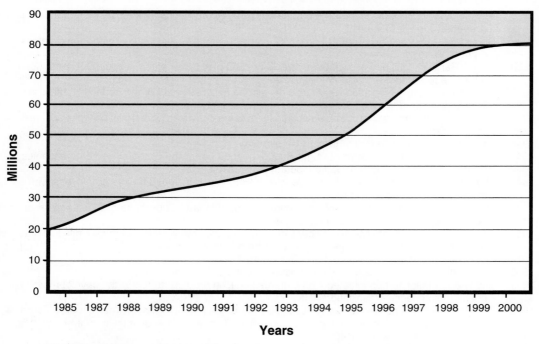

FIGURE 8.7. Enrollment in managed care plans. This graph illustrates the dramatic increase in individuals who are enrolled in managed care plans. In 1985, such plans had 20 million participants, and by 2000, this numbered had quadrupled.

Initially, it was assumed that because health care plans had an incentive to keep their members healthy, they would heavily invest in prevention. However, the combination of requiring care by a selected number of providers and having health care insurance linked to employment created a problem. Members, the contracted patients, were not long-term participants; they were disenrolled when they lost their jobs or changed employment or when they got older or sicker. This reduced the incentive to invest in prevention, which requires a long-term perspective.

Because data are essential for "managing," information technology and evidence-based medicine (EBM) have become a major backbone of managed care. The former focuses on the availability and processing of performance data (e.g., number of patients seen, types of treatments provided), and the latter addresses the management of knowledge that can be derived from the fast growing literature of medicine. In its classic definition by Sackett et al, EBM is the " . . . conscientious, explicit and judicious use of current best evidence in making decisions about the care of individual patients." Many websites promote the use of EBM in daily practice, and some even focus on pediatrics (see SUGGESTED READINGS).

Until recently, pediatrics has been relatively unaffected by the national health care changes. In part, this can be attributed to the fact that proportionally less money is needed for the care of children, because they are less likely to require costly interventions. In addition, some experts argue that there has been a lack of outcome data. One, fewer drug trials assess whether one medication is better and more cost effective than another. Two, Medicaid, the primary governmental insurer of children, is administered by the individual states, unlike Medicare, which is a federal agency; this makes the accumulation and sharing of information more difficult and less useful.

The case of a child with asthma helps illustrate how some of the benefits of managed care translate to an individual patient (Table 8.7). If the system works well, the child should receive more coordinated care. Furthermore, there would be a multitude of resources aimed at making the child and the family more knowledgeable and self-sufficient and thus less reliant on costly physician and hospital care.

TABLE 8.6 Types of Health Care Organizations			
Increasing Control of Cost and Quality →			
Indemnity, Fee-for-Service (FFS) Plan	**Preferred Provider Organization (PPO)**	**Point of Service (POS) Plan**	**Health Maintenance Organization (HMO)**
Provider is reimbursed for number and type of services performed	Selected panel of providers who agree to discounted fee schedule	Combines HMO and indemnity options	Prepaid, comprehensive health coverage for hospital and physician services
Provider's income is directly related to volume and intensity of units of service rendered	Provider reimbursement is fee-for-service	Selection is made when need arises	Members are required to use participating providers
	Patients are not required to have primary care provider or seek prior authorization for services	Additional costs to patient if non-HMO providers are used	Primary care providers act as gatekeepers
Insurer may pay percentage of charges or utilize predetermined fee schedule		All provider reimbursement is fee-for-service	In staff model HMOs, physicians are employees (e.g., Lovelace Health Systems of New Mexico)
	Patients can obtain care from providers outside of plan but have higher copayments		In group model HMOs, physicians work in a group practice and contract with HMO (e.g., Kaiser Permanente)
			In an Independent Practice Association (IPA) model HMO, physicians maintain their independent offices while contracting with HMO
Example: Blue Cross Blue Shield	Examples: CIGNA Health Care, CAN Managed Care PPO	Example: Tufts Total Health Plan	Example: Aetna US Healthcare

Many of the HMOs that started in the 1940s to 1960s were not-for-profit. On the other hand, some of the newer companies were for-profit, and thus their central focus became stockholder shares, rather than investing in patient care. Methods of cost control entailed the exclusion of sicker patients, micromanagement of clinical decisions, denial of beneficial but expensive care to some patients, perverse incentives for providers, and pitting specialists and primary care physicians against each other. Quickly new ethical concerns arose about "squeezing care to expand profits." It is unethical to waste resources, but it is just as unacceptable to withhold them unnec-

essarily. Managed care, one single health care innovation, led down two opposite paths; a comparison was made between "Dr. Jekyll and Mr. Hyde" care.

HEALTH CARE IN THE FUTURE

Gradually the health care system will stabilize. Not all corporate entities are drawn to managed care just because of the potential of making money; many see this as an opportunity to increase access and advance health care delivery. Laws and regulations are being enacted to ensure that the rights of patients and health care

TABLE 8.7 A Child With Asthma: Example of How a Patient May Receive Effective and Efficient Medical Care*,†

A 5-year-old boy with no significant past medical history is brought to the emergency department by ambulance. The mother says that her son is usually in good health. However, 3 days ago, he developed a mild cough that progressively worsened. He was playing outdoors when he suddenly came inside the house and told his mother that he found it difficult to breathe. The patient's mother noted that he was coughing and short of breath. She became scared and called for an ambulance. The boy received one treatment of albuterol nebulizer from the emergency medical technicians on the way to the hospital.

In the emergency department:
1. Vital signs are temperature, 98.8°F; heart rate, 140 bpm; and respiratory rate, 32/min.
2. Oxygen saturation is 90% on room air.
3. Physical examination shows that the patient is alert but in moderate respiratory distress. HEENT, within normal limits; chest, symmetric with intercostal and supraclavicular retractions; lungs, diffuse wheezing bilaterally; cardiovascular system, normal S_1 and S_2, with no murmurs; abdomen, benign.
4. The patient receives the following medications: albuterol nebulizer × 3, ipratropium bromide × 2, and prednisolone × 1.
5. The chest radiograph shows hyperinflation bilaterally with increased peribronchial markings.
6. The diagnosis is reactive airway disease. The boy is admitted for further management, and he stays in the hospital for 24 hours. Both parents are educated about asthma management prior to discharge.

Under a new and improved health care system that may be referred to as "managed care," the following services are also routinely available for patients with asthma:
1. Asthma education for parent and patient prior to hospital discharge.
2. Regular visits to the primary care physician for check-ups. The frequency of visits varies with the severity of asthma.
3. Provision of an individualized, written Asthma Action Plan.
4. Telephone services to provide support from medical staff.
5. Enrollment in a disease management program that includes parent and patient support groups and a visiting nurse to inspect the home for environmental triggers.
6. Peak flow scores for children 5 years of age or older, according to the ability of the child.
7. Referral to a specialist if the asthma is poorly controlled despite the primary care physician's and parents' efforts.
8. Reviews of the patient's medications, emergency department visits, and hospitalizations by the National Committee on Quality Assurance or a similar organization. There is some increased accountability for quality of care provided and adherence to standards for preventive strategies. Ideally, the Primary Care Physician is contacted and instructed to make adjustments if the quality of care is viewed as less than ideal. These organizations also monitor the number of patients who:
   - Receive a written Asthma Action Plan
   - Use medications with a spacer
   - Use a home peak flow meter
   - Receive instructions on the correct use of inhalers
   - Receive counseling on the role of environmental irritants
   - Receive annual pulmonary function tests

---

*This case was created by Valerie A. London, MD, when she was completing a managed care rotation during the third year of her pediatrics residency at Maimonides Medical Center in Brooklyn, New York.
†Sources: Charles JH: Asthma disease management. *New Engl J Med* 337:1461–1463, 1997.
Bodenheimer T: Disease management—promises and pit falls. *New Engl J Med* 340:1202–1205, 1999.
Wagner EH: The role of patient care teams in chronic disease management. *BMJ* 320:569–572, 2000.

providers are not compromised. For example, the "gag rule," which forbids providers to take any actions or make any communications that could undermine the confidence of enrollees or the public in a health care plan (e.g., reveal incidences where cost-cutting measures would inhibit proper care) was quickly abandoned. Consumers also seem to be able to exert some influence. The initial efforts to control the resources through gatekeepers was met with much resistance and resulted in a gradual relaxation of such rules.

Movement from the focus on individual patients to the welfare of populations does create

TABLE 8.8 Managed Care Learning Needs Survey			

Please indicate where you stand in each of these competency domains.*

Competency Domains Important for Succeeding in the New Health Care Environment	Know little/ must get acquainted with the topic	Know something but should learn more	Know a lot/no need to include in my current learning agenda
1. Health Care System (e.g., organization, reimbursement systems, allocation of resources)			
2. Population-based Care (e.g., definition and description of populations, organization of databases, responsibility toward enrolled members or community)			
3. Quality Measurement and Improvement (e.g., definitions of quality and outcomes, methods for measuring performance, measurement of patient satisfaction)			
4. Medical Management (e.g., infrastructure for the delivery of care, guidelines, evidence-based medicine, utilization management, disease management)			
5. Preventive Care (e.g., delivery of preventive and health maintenance services, healthy lifestyles–prevention–health care cost link, employment of non–office-based approaches)			
6. Physician–Patient Communication (e.g., management of patient and family expectations regarding referrals and procedures, communication with groups of patients, behavioral change strategies)			
7. Teamwork and Collaboration (e.g., individual roles and processes required to work collaboratively, team leadership skills, group dynamics, delegation)			
8. Information Management and Technology (e.g., access and management of medical information, profiles of patient populations and practice patterns)			
9. Practice Management (e.g., business aspects of managing medical practice, managed care contracts, time management and patient flow)			

*These competencies were derived from Halpern R, Lee MY, Boulter PR, et al (see Suggested Readings).

some tension. Physicians find themselves in a new role that includes advocacy for social justice. Population-based medicine does not come naturally to a profession that prescribes to an oath that puts the single patient "front and center." However, it is necessary to be able to make such shifts to control health care inflation and move medicine to the next level.

Because of the changes in health care delivery, the training of physicians requires adjustments. A new set of competencies has become essential. The self-assessment tool in Table 8.8 provides an opportunity to set a learning agenda. The numbered categories represent the key competencies based on several national reports.

Health care economics continues to evolve as a science. Children still are not the economic priority when it comes to health care.

Pediatric Pearl

Over 6 million children remain uninsured or poorly insured, and certain subpopulations (e.g., minorities) are even more at risk for poor health coverage and health outcomes.

The health care of children in the United States is not satisfactory. An ultimate solution must provide universal coverage for the entire population, spreading the risk to those who do not need as much care and can afford to pay from those who do need the care and cannot afford it. Children and families must become a national priority, just as the elderly became through the landmark Medicare legislation. Pediatricians remain the primary advocates for children's health; their outspoken voices on behalf of children are a crucial building block for the overall health of children in the United States and throughout the rest of the world. It is hoped that the next decade will see a truly universal health care system evolve to benefit children, providers, and society.

SUGGESTED READINGS

American Medical Association (Council on Medical Service): *Principles of Managed Care*, 4th ed. 1999. www.ama-assn.org/ama/upload/mm/363/principles.pdf

Berk ML, Monheit AC: The concentration of health care expenditures, revisited. *Health Aff* (*Millwood*) Mar–Apr, 4420(2):9–18, 2001.

Centres for Health Evidence. www.cche.net

Clancy CM, Brody H: Managed Care. Jekyll or Hyde. *JAMA* 273(4):338–339, 1995.

Halpern R, Lee MY, Boulter PR, et al: A synthesis of nine major reports on physicians' competencies for the emerging practice environment. *Acad Med* 76(6):606–615, 2001.

Health Care Financing Administration (HCFA): National Health Care Expenditure. www.hcfa.gov/stats.nhe-oact

Heffler S, Smith S, Won G, et al: Trends: Health Spending Projections for 2001–2011: The Latest Outlook. *Health Aff* (*Millwood*) 21(2):207–218, 2002.

Integrated Health Care Association: *Managed Health Care—A Brief Glossary*. www.iha.org/gloss.htm

Kongstvedt PR: *Essentials of Managed Care*, 4th ed. Gaithersburg, Aspen Publishers, 2001.

Letsch SW, Lazenby HC, Levit KR, et al: National health expenditures, 1991. *Health Care Finance Rev* 14(2):1–30, 1992.

Levit K, Smith C, Cowan C, et al: Inflation spurs health spending in 2000. *Health Aff* (*Millwood*) 21(1):172–181, 2002.

Managed Care Online: *Managed Care Fact Sheets*. www.mcareol.com/factshts/factnati.htm

Nelson RP, Minon ME (eds): *A Pediatrician's Guide to Managed Care*. Elk Grove Village, American Academy of Pediatrics, 2001.

PedsCCM/org: www.Pediatric Critical Care Medicine.com. pedsccm.wustl.edu

Sackett DL, Richardson WS, Rosenberg WM, et al: *Evidence-Based Medicine: How to Practice and Teach EBM*. London: Churchill-Livingstone, 1997.

Texas Medical Association: *Glossary of Managed Care Terminology*. www.texmed.org/ata/ste/mcg.asp

Tufts Managed Care Institute: *Managed Care Glossary*. www.tmci.org/other_resources/glossary.htm

Wenner WJ: *The Pediatrician's Managed Care Manual*. Boston, Total Learning Concepts, 1999.

Pediatric Subspecialties

Chapter 9

Infectious Diseases

Kathleen Gutierrez

APPROACH TO EVALUATION OF THE FEBRILE CHILD

Physicians routinely encounter children with febrile illnesses. Fever is not harmful in itself; it is a symptom of underlying disease. Most fever in children results from underlying infection. Auto-immune disease, drugs, and neoplastic processes are less common causes. Rare causes of fever include central nervous system (CNS) abnormalities, thyrotoxicosis, and overheating (heat stroke).

Fever is an elevation in body temperature that occurs when the thermoregulatory center in the anterior hypothalamus is reset to a higher level. Cytokines produced in response to infection or inflammation induce production of prostaglandin E_2 and mediate fever. Normal body temperatures are subject to diurnal variation, with slightly higher (0.5°C–0.9°C) [0.9°F–1.6°F] core temperatures in the afternoon compared to early morning. Temperatures taken by a rectal thermometer reflect true core temperature, whereas oral and axillary temperatures are approximately 0.5°C and 1.0°C (0.9°F and 1.8°F) lower, respectively. The upper limit of normal body temperature in children is 37.9°C (100.2°F); a rectal temperature greater than 38.0 (100.4°F) represents fever. Temperature elevation rarely exceeds 41.1°C (105.9°F) even in the absence of antipyretic therapy. Very young infants, unlike older children, are often unable to mount a febrile response to infection and may instead become hypothermic.

Viral infections cause most febrile illnesses. However, **serious bacterial infections (SBIs)** affect a small proportion of children. By definition, SBIs include meningitis, pneumonia, bone and joint infection, urinary tract infection, bacterial gastroenteritis, and sepsis and occult bacteremia. Children with **occult bacteremia** usually have only high fever but no other localizing findings on the basis of careful history and physical examination. Some cases of occult bacteremia resolve spontaneously without antibiotic therapy, others lead to development of SBIs, most commonly urinary tract infections.

Pathophysiology

Infants less than 3 months of age are prone to infection with pathogens acquired around the time of delivery, when colonization by organisms present in the mother's rectal or vaginal area occurs. *Escherichia coli, Klebsiella pneumoniae, Enterococcus* species, and *Streptococcus agalactiae* (group B streptococci) are the usual pathogens. In addition, *Listeria monocytogenes* may cause bacteremia and meningitis.

Older infants and children between 3 and 36 months of age are prone to infection with encapsulated bacteria such as *Streptococcus pneumoniae, Neisseria meningitidis,* and, in incompletely immunized children, *Haemophilus influenzae* type b. Frequency of infection with *Streptococcus pyogenes* [group A beta-hemolytic streptococcus (GABHS)] increases as children reach school age.

Pediatric Pearl

Widespread use of *Haemophilus influenzae* type b conjugate vaccine and recent recommendations for use of pneumococcal conjugate vaccine makes bacteremia caused by these organisms less common in the completely immunized child.

In older children and adolescents, bacteremia is infrequent, and *N. meningitidis* is the most common cause of serious infections. *Staphylococcus aureus* is the most common cause of bone and joint infections in children of all ages.

The likelihood of SBI varies depending on age. The usual cause of fever is viral rather than bacterial (58% versus 8%, as reported in one study). In febrile infants less than 3 months of age, the incidence of bacterial infection is 0.7%–18.5%. In febrile children between 3 and 36 months of age, the risk of occult bacteremia ranges from 3% to 11%. The organism most commonly isolated from blood culture is *S. pneumoniae* (> 90%), with *N. meningitidis, Salmonella* spp., and other species isolated in fewer than 10% of cases.

Clinical and Laboratory Evaluation

Information used to determine risk of SBI or occult bacteremia includes the clinical appearance of the child and the results of laboratory tests. The chance of obtaining a positive blood culture increases with high fever (> 39.0°C [102.2°F]), ill appearance, and abnormal laboratory findings. Other factors associated with increased risk of SBI include underlying chronic illness and immunodeficiency.

However, neither laboratory studies nor careful observation are totally sensitive for detection of serious illness in febrile children. Therefore, each child warrants careful, thoughtful evaluation. It is necessary to make every attempt to avoid unnecessary laboratory testing and overuse of antibiotics while providing appropriate care and antibiotic therapy for patients identified as high risk.

History

Identifying febrile children at risk for occult bacteremia or SBI requires conscientious attention to parental concerns. It is necessary to question parents regarding duration and height of fever, method of measurement, and use of antipyretics. Inquiries about the child's behavior, appetite, and activity level are also appropriate. Previously healthy children who interact well, are playful and consolable, and have the ability to drink or eat and are interested in doing so are less likely to be seriously ill. Signs of serious illness include irritability, poor eye contact, failure to recognize parents, and poor interaction with people or the environment.

Physical Examination

Abnormalities in vital signs include fever or hypothermia, tachypnea, irregular respirations, apnea, tachycardia or bradycardia, and hypotension. It is important to examine the skin and mucous membranes for cyanosis, poor perfusion, and petechial or purpuric rash. The clinician should also examine the child for signs of meningeal irritation (Kernig and Brudzinski signs), pneumonia, heart murmur, abdominal infection, and musculoskeletal infection.

Careful documentation in the medical record of specific findings on physical examination is important. It is better to note, for example, that instead of being "responsive," a child smiles, plays with the stethoscope, or takes a bottle from his mother. Similarly, use of the word "toxic" is less informative than saying the child is difficult to awaken and has cyanosis and poor capillary refill.

Laboratory Evaluation

Febrile infants less than 1 month of age should have a **sepsis evaluation,** which includes a complete blood count (CBC), blood culture, urinalysis and urine culture, as well as examination of spinal fluid with culture. If diarrhea is present, a stool sample for polymorphonuclear (PMN) cells and bacterial culture is appropriate.

Recommendations for laboratory evaluation of febrile children between 1 and 3 months of age vary. A complete sepsis evaluation is necessary in ill-appearing children. The extent of testing necessary in non–ill-appearing children depends on the risk of SBI. Children with low risk of SBI include those with a white blood cell (WBC) count of 5000–15,000 cells/mm^3, a normal urinalysis, and no PMN cells on stool examination (if diarrhea is present). Laboratory findings associated with occult bacteremia or SBI include an elevated or depressed WBC count [> 15,000 cells/mm^3 or < 5000 cells/mm^3], an elevated sedimentation rate (ESR) or C-reactive protein, and an abnormal urinalysis or stool examination. Children with a high risk of disease should have a full sepsis evaluation.

Suggested guidelines for laboratory evaluation and management of nontoxic-appearing febrile children between 3 and 36 months depend on whether their temperature is above or below 39.0°C (102.2°F). In general, non–ill-appearing children with a temperature less than 39.0°C (102.2°F) and no focal findings on physical examination can be observed without laboratory evaluation. The laboratory evaluation of children with a temperature greater than 39.0°C (102.2°F) depends on the child's clinical appearance. Some clinicians defer initial laboratory tests and observe the child carefully; others choose to obtain a screening CBC. If the WBC is greater than 15,000 cells/mm^3, a blood culture, urine culture, stool culture, and chest radiograph may be appropriate. Any child who is very ill appearing should have a full sepsis evaluation, including lumbar puncture.

Differential Diagnosis

Often, a careful history and physical examination reveals the presence of a readily identifiable viral illness (e.g., croup, chickenpox). A well-appearing child between the ages of 6 months and 2 years with high fever with no source may have roseola caused by infection with human herpes virus-6 (HHV-6) [see ROSEOLA]. Typically, the rash usually appears just as the fever resolves. Meningitis carries a high risk of morbidity and mortality and requires early antibiotic therapy, so it is often considered in the differential diagnosis of children with fever or signs of sepsis.

Management

Important management considerations include age, clinical appearance, reliability of the family, and results of screening laboratory tests. **Antibiotics should never be initiated until appropriate cultures are obtained and should not be used in well-appearing older children whose laboratory results are unremarkable.** Hospitalization for intravenous antibiotics or careful observation pending culture results is appropriate for infants less than 1 month of age. Hospitalization and empiric parenteral antibiotic therapy is also recommended for high-risk children between 1 and 3 months of age (see LABORATORY EVALUATION). Antibiotic therapy is a consideration in nontoxic-appearing children over 3 months of age with high fever and elevated WBC pending blood culture results; however, studies have not demonstrated that antibiotic therapy is effective in preventing meningitis. Hospitalization and empiric intravenous antibiotics are warranted for ill-appearing children over 3 months of age.

Antipyretics are indicated for children who are uncomfortable. However, infants should not receive antipyretics until they have undergone a complete medical evaluation for the source of fever. Several different preparations of antipyretics are available. It is crucial that parents and physicians appreciate the differences between formulations made specifically for infants and children, including "junior strength" preparations. They should use only the dosing instructions that accompany the product. Many over-the-counter cold and cough preparations may contain acetaminophen or ibuprofen, and parents should take this into account before giving additional antipyretic therapy. Acetaminophen inhibits centrally mediated prostaglandin formation and release; the recommended dose is 10–15 mg/kg/dose every 4–6 hours, not to exceed five doses in 24 hours. Ibuprofen exerts its antiprostaglandin effect peripherally; the recommended dose is 5–10 mg/kg/dose every 6–8 hours. Aspirin is not recommended as an antipyretic in children because of the associated risk of Reye syndrome.

It may be possible to identify a focus of infection on the basis of history and physical examination. If so, management proceeds according to recommended guidelines for the specific infection.

ACUTE OTITIS MEDIA

Acute otitis media (AOM), the most common disease diagnosed in children, accounts for approximately 30,000,000 provider visits/year. In AOM, infection of the middle ear occurs when bacterial pathogens that colonize the nasopharynx multiply in the enclosed space. Studies show that more than 75% of children experience at least one episode of AOM. The primary reason for dispensing antibiotics is treatment of AOM. Several factors place children at risk for the development of AOM (Table 9.1). Additional risk factors for frequent AOM include underlying palatal or craniofacial abnormalities.

Pathophysiology

Young children are more prone to AOM because they have shorter eustachian tubes, which lie in a more horizontal position. The eustachian tube protects the middle ear from nasopharyngeal secretions, provides drainage of middle ear secretions into the nasopharynx, and equilibrates air pressure in the middle ear with atmospheric pressure. In AOM, viral upper respiratory tract infection causes swelling of eustachian tube mucosa and prevents normal drainage of fluid from the middle ear to the nasopharynx. Other factors that impede normal eustachian tube drainage include enlarged adenoids or functional obstruction associated with decreased cartilage support of the tube in infants.

The most common bacterial cause of AOM is *S. pneumoniae*. The number of episodes of AOM secondary to drug-resistant *S. pneumoniae* parallels the nationwide increase in isolates with intermediate [minimum inhibitory concentration (MIC) = 0.12–1.0 μg/ml] and high level (MIC $\geq$ 2.0 μg/ml)

TABLE 9.1 **Risk Factors Associated with the Development of Acute Otitis Media**

Age 6–18 months
Older sibling
Family history
Bottle fed
Pacifier use
Upper respiratory infection
Day care
Birth in the fall
Cigarette smoke
Allergies
Immunodeficiency
Native American race
Lower socioeconomic class

resistance to penicillin. Risk factors for infection with drug-resistant *S. pneumoniae* include residence in a community with high resistance rates, day-care attendance, antibiotic use within the past 3 months, and age less than 2 years. It is possible to isolate nontypeable *H. influenzae* and *Moraxella catarrhalis* from infected middle ear fluid. Gram-negative enteric bacteria may also cause middle ear infection in neonates.

Recent evidence proves a specific viral etiology in many cases of AOM; respiratory syncytial virus (RSV) is isolated most frequently. Other viruses isolated from middle ear fluid include parainfluenza and influenza viruses.

Clinical and Laboratory Evaluation

The basis of diagnosis of AOM involves assessment of specific clinical findings and eardrum appearance.

History

Affected children often have a history of preceding or concurrent upper respiratory tract symptoms, fever, and irritability. Older children complain of ear pain, whereas younger children may manifest only irritability.

Physical Examination

Physical examination of a child's ears requires practice and patience. If the patient is unable to remain still, it may be necessary to ask the parent for assistance in restraining the child. Complete visualization of the tympanic membrane involves gentle removal of cerumen with an ear curette or irrigation of the ear canal with warm saline or 3% hydrogen peroxide.

The correct diagnosis of AOM involves the use of a pneumatic otoscope. Physical findings seen on examination include erythema and thickening of the tympanic membrane, engorgement of blood vessels around or crossing the tympanic membrane, loss of a normal light reflex and bony landmarks, and decreased mobility of the tympanic membrane.

☀ Pediatric Pearl

Fever and crying cause the tympanic membrane to appear hyperemic. However, a diagnosis of AOM should not be made unless other features, particularly decreased mobility, are present.

The American Academy of Pediatrics (AAP) has constructed a virtual classroom to assist clinicians in the correct diagnosis of AOM. The Inter-

net address is *http://www.aap.org* (section on professional education).

Laboratory Evaluation

The diagnosis of AOM is made by clinical examination. Tympanocentesis to identify a specific bacterial pathogen is considered in immunocompromised children, in neonates, in the presence of a concomitant CNS infection, or in an infection that is refractory to multiple courses of antibiotics.

Differential Diagnosis

Conditions that warrant consideration in the diagnosis of AOM and ear pain are otitis media with effusion (OME), otitis externa, mastoiditis, furuncle, foreign body, and referred pain (Table 9.2). It is essential to make the distinction between AOM and OME, which does not necessitate the use of antibiotics (Table 9.3).

Management

The current standard of care for AOM is antibiotic therapy, which is indicated **only in children with evidence of AOM.** (See Chapter 26 for discussion of management of OME.) Several antibiotics are currently approved for treatment of AOM (Table 9.4). Amoxicillin, the drug of choice, is effective for treating infections with penicillin-susceptible *S. pneumoniae* and beta-lactamase–negative nontypeable *H. influenzae*. It has a narrow spectrum of activity. Higher-dose amoxicillin (80 mg/kg/day) is effective for treatment of *S. pneumoniae* with intermediate resistance to penicillin.

None of the oral cephalosporins is reliable against resistant pneumococci. Cephalosporins are active against beta-lactamase–producing *H. influenzae* and *M. catarrhalis*. Treatment of AOM with one to three doses of intramuscular ceftriaxone is as effective as several days of oral antibiotic therapy. Children less than 2 years of age are at increased risk of treatment failure, and 10–14 days of treatment is recommended. Children older than 2 years of age may warrant shorter courses of treatment (5–7 days).

In untreated AOM, the tympanic membrane becomes erythematous. After 24–36 hours exudate behind the tympanic membrane appears. Perforation occurs in 5% of cases. Consequences of lack of treatment include delay in resolution of pain as well as potential reemergence of complications formerly commonly associated with AOM, including mastoiditis, meningitis, extradural abscess, subdural empyema, brain abscess, and lat-

TABLE 9.2	Differential Diagnosis of Ear Pain	
Diagnosis	**Physical Examination Findings**	**Management**
Otitis externa	Swelling of external canal, discharge in canal	Keeping canal dry and clean
	Pain with movement of tragus, normal TM	Antibiotic and steroid drops
Mastoiditis	Erythema and pain over mastoid	CT scan of mastoid
	Usually signs of acute otitis media ± otorrhea	Surgical evaluation
	Anterior displacement of pinna	IV antibiotics
Furuncle	Visible in external canal, normal TM	Oral antistaphylococcal antibiotics
Foreign body	Visible in external canal, normal TM	Removal of foreign body
Referred pain	Normal examination of external canal and TM	Treating source of pain
	Other source (e.g., dental abscess) found	

CT = computed tomography; IV = intravenous; TM = tympanic membrane.

eral sinus thrombosis. Because spontaneous resolution occurs in 60% of cases of AOM, withholding treatment is a consideration in selected cases. Spontaneous resolution rates for *M. catarrhalis, H. influenzae,* and *S. pneumoniae* are 75%, 50%, and 15%, respectively. AOM caused by *S. pneumoniae* is least likely to resolve spontaneously, so it is most likely to be associated with suppurative sequelae.

Antibiotic prophylaxis for AOM is considered only in children with three or more episodes in 6 months or four or more episodes in 1 year. Duration of prophylaxis should not exceed 6 months. Antibiotics used include sulfisoxazole (50 mg/kg/day) or amoxicillin (20 mg/kg/day).

PHARYNGITIS

Sore throat occurs as a result of inflammation or infection of the tonsils, uvula, soft palate, and posterior oropharynx. Pharyngitis is more likely in older children; it is uncommon in infants and children younger than 2 years of age.

Pathophysiology

Several microorganisms are associated with pharyngitis (Table 9.5). Viral infection causes most cases, which occur during the winter, when many respiratory viruses are circulating. *S. pyogenes* (GABHS) is the most common bacterial cause. Pharyngitis in children 2–5 years of age is most of-

ten the result of infection with respiratory viruses. Older children and adolescents are more likely to have GABHS or Epstein-Barr virus (infectious mononucleosis).

Clinical and Laboratory Evaluation

History

Viral pharyngitis occurs in association with other symptoms of respiratory tract infection. Children with a viral syndrome typically have fever, rhinorrhea, cough, and mild pharyngitis. Fatigue, anorexia, and abdominal pain may be present. Family members or playmates may be ill with similar symptoms.

GABHS pharyngitis frequently manifests as acute onset of fever, headache, sore throat, and abdominal pain. Rhinorrhea or cough is uncommon. There may be a history of classroom exposure.

Physical Examination

Several clinical characteristics are associated with some of the organisms that cause pharyngitis (Table 9.6). Careful examination of the oral mucosa, tongue, and pharynx is important. The presence of an enanthem (lesions in the mouth), appearance of the tongue, tonsillar size, color, symmetry, and presence of an exudate are noteworthy.

Infection with enterovirus (**herpangina**) is associated with small ulcers on an erythematous

TABLE 9.3	Clinical Findings in Acute Otitis Media and Otitis Media with Effusion
Acute Otitis Media	**Otitis Media With Effusion**
Fever	Nonspecific signs of viral infection
Pain	Rhinitis, cough, diarrhea
Bulging yellow or red tympanic membrane	Middle ear effusion*
Middle ear effusion*	

*Always use pneumatic otoscopy or tympanometry to confirm middle ear effusion.

TABLE 9.4 Antibiotics Used for Treatment of Acute Otitis Media

Drug	Daily Dose	Taste*
Amoxicillin		
(Usual dose)	40–45 mg/kg/day tid	++
(High dose)	80 mg/kg/day bid	
Trimethoprim–sulfamethoxazole	8–12 mg/kg/day trimethoprim bid	++
Erythromycin–sulfisoxazole	50 mg/kg/day erythromycin tid or qid	++
Amoxicillin–clavulanic acid[†‡]	40 mg/kg/day amoxicillin component bid	++
	6.4 mg/kg/day clavulanate bid	
Second-generation cephalosporins		
Cefaclor	40 mg/kg/day tid or bid	++
Cefuroxime axetil suspension[†]	30 mg/kg/day bid	+
Cefprozil	30 mg/kg/day bid	++
Loracarbef	30 mg/kg/day bid	+++
Third-generation cephalosporins		
Cefpodoxime[†]	10 mg/kg/day bid	+
Cefixime	8 mg/kg/day q day	+++
Ceftibuten	9 mg/kg/day q day	+++
Cefdinir	14 mg/kg/day q day	+++
Ceftriaxone (IM)[†]	50 mg/kg/day q day for 1–3 days	N/A
Macrolides		
Azithromycin	10 mg/kg/day on day 1	+++
	5 mg/kg/day q day on days 2–5	
Clarithromycin	15 mg/kg/day bid	++

*Most palatable (+++).
[†]Best activity against both *Streptococcus pneumoniae* and beta-lactamase–producing bacteria.
[‡]Dose of amoxicillin–clavulanic acid varies depending on formulation used.

base found on the tonsillar pillars, soft palate, and uvula. Vesicles in the anterior portion of the mouth and on the lips are associated with herpes simplex type 1 (HSV-1) infection. Lesions in some cases of primary HSV-1 infection extend to the posterior oropharynx. Large tonsils with exudate are common with Epstein-Barr virus infection. In GABHS, the tonsils initially appear beefy

TABLE 9.5 Infectious and Noninfectious Causes of Acute Pharyngitis

Viral	Bacterial	Other
Rhinovirus	*Streptococcus pyogenes* (group A)	Allergies
Adenovirus	Beta-hemolytic streptococci (groups C and G)	Chronic sinusitis
Coronavirus	*Mycoplasma pneumoniae*	Kawasaki disease
Parainfluenza	*Arcanobacterium haemolyticum*	Foreign body
Influenza	*Chlamydia pneumoniae*	Environmental irritant
Respiratory syncytial virus	*Neisseria gonorrhoeae*	Neoplasm
HSV 1 or 2	*Neisseria meningitidis*	Stevens-Johnson syndrome
Epstein-Barr Virus	*Corynebacterium diphtheriae*	Behçet disease
Cytomegalovirus	*Francisella tularensis*	PFAPA
HIV	*Borrelia burgdorferi* (Lyme disease)	
Measles	*Streptobacillus moniliformis* (rat-bite fever)	
Rubella	*Salmonella typhi*	
	Treponema pallidum	
	Coxiella burnetii (Q fever)	
	Yersinia enterocolitica	
	Yersinia pestis (bubonic plague)	

HIV = human immunodeficiency virus; HSV = herpes simplex virus; PFAPA = **p**eriodic **f**ever, **a**phthous stomatitis, **p**haryngitis, cervical **a**denitis (syndrome).

TABLE 9.6 | **Clinical Characteristics of Selected Infections Associated with Pharyngitis**

Organism	Clinical Findings
Rhinovirus	Scratchy sore throat, rhinitis, cough
Coronavirus	Scratchy sore throat, rhinitis, cough
Adenovirus	Pharyngitis, often with significant pain, erythema and exudate, conjunctivitis
Coxsackie A	Summer/fall, prominent fever, coryza, vesicular lesions posterior pharynx, rash (including hands and feet)
Influenza A, B	Winter season, abrupt onset of high fever, myalgia, then pharyngitis, dry cough
EBV	Infectious mononucleosis, with fatigue, anorexia, fever, headache, severe pharyngitis, lymphadenopathy, hepatosplenomegaly, palatal petechiae, tonsillar exudate, periorbital edema, rash with ampicillin/amoxicillin. (Younger children may be asymptomatic.)
Cytomegalovirus	Similar to EBV except pharyngitis and lymphadenopathy less prominent, may have higher fever, more fatigue
HIV	Primary infection presents as mononucleosis–like illness with fever, pharyngitis, lymphadenopathy, rash, fatigue, arthralgia. Tonsils are red but no exudate is seen.
Streptococcus pyogenes	Peak incidence late winter or spring, sudden onset sore throat, fever, headache, abdominal pain, tonsillar exudate, palatal petechiae, strawberry tongue, sometimes rash or urticaria
Neisseria gonorrhoeae	Sexually active adolescents or adults, rash, arthralgia
Corynebacterium diphtheriae	Nonimmunized patients, low-grade fever, mild sore throat, gray-white adherent membrane seen on tonsils and posterior pharynx, weakness, lymphadenopathy, "bull neck," respiratory distress, cardiac and neurologic abnormalities
Arcanobacterium haemolyticum	Seen in adolescents and young adults, exudative pharyngitis, scarlatiniform rash, no palatal petechiae or strawberry tongue, desquamation rare
Mycoplasma pneumoniae	Headache, fever, sore throat, cough, coryza, sometimes tracheobronchitis or pneumonia
Chlamydia pneumoniae	Fever, cough, sore throat

EBV = Epstein-Barr virus; HIV = human immunodeficiency virus.

red. As disease progresses, a yellow-white exudate within the anterior tonsillar crypts is apparent. The tongue may become coated with a white membrane with protrusion of prominent red papillae ("strawberry tongue"). Anterior cervical lymph nodes are often enlarged and tender. In infectious mononucleosis, diffuse lymphadenopathy and splenomegaly are present.

Skin findings may be associated with different infectious causes of pharyngitis. In GABHS, a characteristic scarlatiniform rash may be evident (see BACTERIAL EXANTHEMS). With infection caused by certain types of enteroviruses, a diffuse erythematous maculopapular skin eruption and vesicular or pustular lesions on the hands and feet may be present.

Laboratory Evaluation

The clinical distinction between viral and GABHS pharyngitis is sometimes difficult; cough, rhinorrhea, or diarrhea are more likely to be symptoms of viral infection. Throat culture is the diagnostic test of choice. The clinician should vigorously swab the patient's posterior pharynx and tonsils. If GABHS is present, beta-hemolytic colonies of bacteria appear after 18–48 hours of incubation onto sheep blood agar. Definitive identification of GABHS is made by the presence of a zone of inhibition around a Bacitracin disk. The sensitivity of the throat culture is greater than 90%; fewer than 10% of cultures are falsely negative. However, the number of colonies of GABHS cannot distinguish between true infection and a carrier state.

A number of rapid tests for detection of group A streptococcal antigen are available. These tests generally use immunoassay or latex agglutination techniques to detect the presence of group A polysaccharide antigen from the bacterial cell wall. The specificity of most rapid tests is excellent (>95%), but the sensitivity is variable (70%–85%). Accuracy of the test depends on the kit used, the skill of the person performing the test, and the quality of the throat swab. Newer tests utilizing optical immunoassay techniques or chemiluminescent DNA probes may prove to have greater sensitivity. A confirmatory culture is usually performed when a child with suspected GABHS disease has a negative rapid streptococcal test.

Serologic testing is sometimes used to confirm infection with GABHS. Rising antibody titers against streptolysin O or DNAse B are seen during the first month after infection and decline to normal 6–12 months after infection. Antibody to DNAse B remains elevated longer than the antistreptolysin O titer.

Other infectious causes of pharyngitis may be diagnosed by use of special culture techniques. *Arcanobacterium haemolyticum,* a gram-positive or gram-variable nonsporulating bacillus, is best isolated using human or rabbit blood agar incubated for 72 hours. *Corynebacterium diphtheriae* is isolated from nose, throat, and membrane swabs inoculated onto select media. *Neisseria gonorrhoeae* is isolated using selective agar (chocolate agar with antibiotics).

Most cases of viral pharyngitis are self-limited, and viral culture is not necessary. Specific circumstances in which viral culture may be useful include cases of suspected HSV-1 or HSV-2 gingivostomatitis or in possible enteroviral disease with other manifestations (meningitis).

Diagnosis of Epstein-Barr virus infection **(infectious mononucleosis)** is made by Monospot and specific Epstein-Barr virus serology. Infection with Epstein-Barr virus stimulates an immunoglobulin (Ig) M heterophile antibody response. Serum from patients with infectious mononucleosis agglutinates sheep red blood cells (RBCs) after absorption with guinea pig kidney antigens. Production of heterophile antibodies is induced by Epstein-Barr virus, but the antibodies are not directed toward any known Epstein-Barr virus antigen. Several specific serologic antibody tests for Epstein-Barr virus are available. The Monospot test may be negative in children less than 4 years of age with infectious mononucleosis, who are less likely to generate a heterophile antibody response.

Differential Diagnosis

The differential diagnosis of sore throat is broad. Serious infections to consider include **peritonsillar abscess, retropharyngeal abscess,** and **epiglottitis**. Noninfectious causes of pharyngitis include allergy, trauma to the pharynx, burns, inhaled or swallowed toxins, smoke, psychosomatic illness, and referred pain.

A history of pharyngitis often precedes signs and symptoms of a **peritonsillar abscess,** which typically involves the superior pole of one tonsil. Children exhibit high fever, difficulty swallowing, and changes in speech. Physical examination reveals an acutely ill child with unilateral peritonsillar and tonsillar swelling. The uvula is displaced away from the affected tonsil, and the neck is often held in a rigid position with marked ipsilateral cervical adenitis. Bilateral abscess formation rarely occurs. Timely diagnosis is important to prevent rupture and possible aspiration of purulent fluid. Organisms within the abscess include GABHS, *S. aureus,* and aerobic and anaerobic mouth flora. Treatment is intravenous antibiotics and surgical drainage.

A **retropharyngeal abscess** occurs when lymph nodes located in potential space between the prevertebral fascia and posterior pharyngeal wall become infected and suppurate. Symptoms of retropharyngeal abscess are similar to those of peritonsillar abscess. Children appear ill with high fever, difficulty swallowing, and dyspnea. Careful examination of the mouth and pharynx reveals swelling of the posterior pharynx. Lateral neck films reveal retropharyngeal swelling. Treatment is similar to that of a retropharyngeal abscess.

Acute epiglottitis, a rapidly progressive disease, is now uncommon because of universal immunization with *H. influenzae* type b vaccine. The disease occurs in unimmunized patients. *S. pneumoniae; S. aureus;* nontypeable *H. influenzae; H. parainfluenzae;* and groups A, B, and C betahemolytic streptococci are rare causal organisms. Affected children have acute onset of high fever and sore throat, and within several hours they have difficulty swallowing and exhibit drooling and respiratory distress. Diagnosis is made by noting the appearance of a swollen, cherry-red epiglottis with laryngoscopy.

☀ Pediatric Pearl

If epiglottitis is suspected, it is imperative that a skilled physician perform the examination in a setting where emergent intubation or tracheostomy can be carried out.

Ideally, a pediatric anesthesiologist and surgeon are alerted to the situation and available at the time of the examination. After epiglottitis is diagnosed, intubation and observation in an intensive care unit with administration of intravenous antibiotics are necessary until swelling resolves.

The syndrome of periodic fever, aphthous stomatitis, pharyngitis, cervical adenitis **(PFAPA)** is characterized by periodic high fever occurring at regular intervals of about 3–4 weeks. Fever [temperature ≥ 39.0°C (102.2°F)] continues for 3–6 days, during which time, the child appears remarkably well. Aphthous stomatitis occurs in two-thirds of patients. Ulcers are typically smaller and more shallow than lesions seen in Behçet disease. Tonsils are moderately enlarged, erythematous, and without exudate. Cervical adenitis is often present. It is not known whether PFAPA is an infectious or immunologic disorder.

Management

Treatment of viral pharyngitis is symptomatic, with antipyretics (if the patient is uncomfortable), fluids, and rest. Treatment of GABHS pharyngitis involves antibiotics to decrease duration of symptoms, reduce spread of infection, and prevent **acute rheumatic fever** and **poststreptococcal glomerulonephritis**. Penicillin remains the drug of choice. It is safe, inexpensive, and has a narrow spectrum of coverage. In addition, it is proven to prevent both suppurative and nonsuppurative complications of infection with GABHS. When given within 9 days of onset of symptoms, penicillin prevents development of acute rheumatic fever. Therefore, a short delay while awaiting rapid antigen or culture results does not increase the risk of acute rheumatic fever. If compliance is a concern, intramuscular benzathine penicillin G is appropriate.

Amoxicillin is an effective substitute for penicillin. No isolates of GABHS are yet resistant to β-lactam antibiotics. Macrolide antibiotics including erythromycin, clarithromycin, and azithromycin are used in β-lactam antibiotic–allergic patients, although strains of GABHS resistant to macrolides have been identified. Tetracyclines and sulfonamides are not effective.

Routine throat culture after treatment is not necessary. Some children continue to have small numbers of GABHS present in their oropharynx; they are carriers. Generally, they do not have symptomatic disease, rarely spread disease to others, and are not retreated with antibiotics. Rare circumstances in which eradication of the carrier state is considered include: community outbreaks of acute rheumatic fever or poststreptococcal glomerulonephritis, family history of acute rheumatic fever, multiple or recurrent episodes of GABHS pharyngitis in families or closed communities, or a case of GABHS-caused toxic shock syndrome or necrotizing fasciitis in a family. Antibi-otics used with variable success to eradicate the carrier state include clindamycin, amoxicillin–clavulanic acid, or penicillin plus rifampin.

UPPER RESPIRATORY TRACT INFECTIONS

Most children have as many as 3–8 colds each year. Several viral species cause the common cold (Table 9.7). Rhinovirus is the most common viral agent associated with colds; at least 100 different serotypes have been identified. Symptoms are due to primary infection or reinfection with the same antigenic type.

Pathophysiology

Infection is spread by either airborne, droplet, or contact transmission. **Airborne transmission** is dissemination of evaporated microorganism-containing droplets, which are suspended in air for long periods of time. Organisms transmitted by airborne transmission include rubeola (measles), varicella-zoster virus, and *Mycobacterium tuberculosis*. **Droplet transmission** is propelling of relatively large microorganism-containing drops from infected children into the host's conjunctivae or nasal mucosa by sneezing, coughing, or talking. Viruses usually spread by droplet transmission include adenoviruses, coronaviruses and influenza viruses. **Contact transmission** is touching of infected secretions by noninfected individual, who autoinoculates the eyes, nose, or mouth. Viruses spread by contact transmission include RSV, parainfluenza virus, enterovirus, and rhinovirus.

After a virus is inoculated onto respiratory epithelium, local viral replication begins. This period, called the incubation period, typically ranges from 2 to 5 days. Symptoms of the common cold are due in part to production of inflammatory mediators such as histamine, kinins, and interleukins. Submucosal edema, vasodilation, and impaired mucociliary transport result in symptoms of nasal stuffiness, throat irritation, and sneezing. Subsequent sloughing of the respiratory epithelium results in nasal discharge. Local gamma-interferon production limits spread of infection to respiratory mucosa of the upper and lower respiratory tract, sinuses, and eustachian tubes. Viremia does not occur. Secretory IgA and serum IgG produced in response to infection prevent future infection with viruses of the same antigenic type. Viral shedding is greatest during the first few days of illness, with the highest concentration of virus present in nasal secretions.

TABLE 9.7 Viruses That Cause Upper and Lower Respiratory Tract Infections

Organism	Serotypes	Season	Clinical Manifestations
Rhinovirus	> 100	Year round, with autumn/spring peak	Rhinorrhea, malaise, headache, low-grade fever (common cold) Mild pharyngitis, occasionally otitis media, wheezing
Coronavirus	2	First type (winter) Second type (winter)	Rhinorrhea, malaise, headache, low-grade fever (common cold) Mild pharyngitis, occasionally otitis media, wheezing
Respiratory syncytial virus	Subtypes A and B	November–April	Bronchiolitis/pneumonia in infants and young children Upper respiratory tract illness in older children and adults
Parainfluenza	Types 1–4	Type 1 (autumn) Type 2 (autumn) Type 3 (spring/summer) Types 4A/4B (sporadic)	Croup, upper respiratory tract symptoms, bronchiolitis Bronchiolitis, croup Bronchiolitis, croup Mild upper respiratory tract infection
Adenovirus	51	Year round (increased in late winter/spring/early summer)	Common cold, pharyngitis, pharyngoconjunctival fever, otitis media, keratoconjunctivitis, croup, pertussis-like illness
Influenza	Three antigenic types (A, B, C)	Winter	Sudden onset of fever, headache, myalgia, nonproductive cough, then pharyngitis, rhinorrhea Abdominal pain, nausea and vomiting occasionally seen

Clinical and Laboratory Evaluation

History

Most respiratory viruses cause similar signs and symptoms. Children typically have low-grade fever and mild irritability. Other symptoms include nasal discharge, which progresses from clear to cloudy in a few days. An initially dry cough eventually becomes productive.

Physical Examination

Patients do not appear seriously ill. The presence of a mucopurulent nasal discharge, which is part of the normal progression of respiratory infection, does not necessarily imply an underlying bacterial sinus infection. The pharynx may be erythematous with mildly enlarged tonsils. Otitis media resulting from secondary bacterial infection or viral infection is occasionally evident. The chest is usually clear but wheezes may be heard. A viral exanthem is seen in association with enterovirus or adenovirus. Adenovirus infection is sometimes associated with high fever, prominent pharyngitis, and conjunctivitis.

Laboratory Evaluation

Because of considerable overlap in symptoms caused by respiratory viruses, it is difficult to make a specific diagnosis. Viral culture is usually not performed. Results are typically not available for days to weeks after the child is evaluated and the illness has resolved. Rapid diagnostic tests are available for diagnosis of RSV, parainfluenza, influenza, and adenovirus. These tests are not used routinely in outpatient settings. However, they are useful in evaluation of severely ill or immunocompromised children.

Differential Diagnosis

Sinusitis is a possibility when symptoms persist beyond 10–14 days, particularly when the condition is associated with cough, low-grade fever, facial pain, headache, or bad breath. In children who have not received the diphtheria and tetanus toxoids and pertussis (DTP) vaccine, **pertussis** begins as a mild upper respiratory tract illness (catarrhal stage) and progresses to severe paroxysms of cough (paroxysmal stage) associated with vomiting.

Management

Management of viral respiratory infections is supportive, with fluids and rest. Over-the-counter medications that contain antihistamines, decongestants, cough suppressants, and expectorants are available for treatment of colds. None of these preparations appears to have clear benefit in alleviating symptoms. Vitamin C may not prevent colds but may have modest benefit in reducing symptoms. Zinc gluconate inhibits viral replication in vitro but studies of clinical benefit have shown mixed results. Antibiotics are not indicated for treatment of viral respiratory illness but are used if secondary bacterial infection such as AOM or sinusitis is present.

☀ Pediatric Pearl

Good attention to handwashing, avoidance of touching mucous membranes, and decontamination of fomites decrease spread of infection.

BRONCHIOLITIS

Bronchiolitis is an obstructive pulmonary disease of infants and young children, caused most often by infection with RSV. Approximately 100,000 infants are hospitalized with RSV infection annually; mortality rates range from 0.5%–1.5%. The severity of illness caused by RSV ranges from mild upper respiratory symptoms to bronchiolitis or pneumonia. Bronchiolitis is most common in children younger than 1 year of age, with a peak incidence at 2–6 months.

Pathophysiology

RSV is the primary cause of bronchiolitis. Parainfluenza viruses and adenoviruses are less commonly associated with the disease. RSV, an RNA virus in the genus Pneumovirus of the family Paramyxoviridae, receives its name from the characteristic cytopathic effect (syncytial appearance) noted several days after inoculation of infected material into cell culture. The RSV genome codes for at least 10 polypeptides, including the envelope proteins F and G. Fusion protein (F) facilitates cell penetration and cell-to-cell spread in the respiratory tract, and the G protein helps with attachment to sialic acid residues on respiratory epithelial cells. RSV, which is divided into types A and B based on differences in the G protein, attaches to and infects respiratory epithelial cells.

Viral proliferation in the respiratory epithelium leads to edema and necrosis of the epithelial lining of the airway, sloughing of ciliated cells, and formation of mucous plugs. Intense peribronchial lymphocytic proliferation occurs. Possible distal air-way obstruction may lead to ventilation–perfusion mismatch, hyperinflation, atelectasis, hypoxemia, respiratory failure, and in some cases, death.

High levels of functional neutralizing serum antibody to RSV F and G proteins correlate with protection against disease. Lower levels of maternal neutralizing antibody are associated with more severe disease in young infants. Appearance of RSV-specific secretory IgA coincides with termination of RSV shedding. By the age of 3 years, virtually all children have formed antibody to RSV, although this antibody is not totally protective, and reinfection may occur. Severity of illness decreases as children become older, and infection involves primarily the upper respiratory tract in later life.

In the United States, RSV infection occurs during November through April. Types A and B strains may circulate together during a single respiratory season, although A strains are more virulent and tend to predominate. Recurrent infection with the same strain is possible. Children at highest risk for severe disease include premature infants, patients with complicated congenital heart disease, bronchopulmonary dysplasia, cystic fibrosis, and immunodeficiency; those who have received bone marrow and solid-organ transplants; and those receiving chemotherapy.

Clinical and Laboratory Evaluation

History

Clinical manifestations depend on the age of the child and underlying medical conditions. Infants may present with bronchiolitis or pneumonia. Lethargy, irritability, and apnea are major symptoms. Poor feeding results from increased work of breathing. Older children and adults have symptoms of the common cold (prolonged), wheezing, croup, tracheobronchitis, or pneumonia (uncommon). Alternatively, they may be relatively asymptomatic.

Physical Examination

The focus of the physical examination is to determine whether a child requires symptomatic treatment at home or closer observation in the hospital. Some children appear to be relatively well, with nasal congestion and mild cough. Those with more severe illness present with lethargy or respiratory distress. Vital signs reveal low-grade fever, increased respiratory rate, and increased heart rate. Children with significant respiratory distress feed poorly and have signs of weight loss or dehydration. AOM may be present, either from bacterial superinfection or RSV infection. Mucous membranes may be dry or cyanotic. It is necessary to observe the chest for supraclavicular, intercostal, and subcostal retractions. Rales, wheezes, rhonchi, or decreased breath sounds may be audible on auscultation.

Laboratory Evaluation

Diagnostic tests are generally not performed if children appear well. If testing is necessary, rapid diagnostic methods, including immunofluorescent and enzyme immunoassay techniques, are available. The sensitivity of most of these tests ranges from 80% to 90%. These rapid diagnostic tests are useful for appropriate "cohorting" of children admitted to the hospital.

It is possible to grow RSV by conventional viral culture techniques, although results are not available for 3–5 days. Some laboratories offer RSV culture by shell vial (centrifugation) with results available in 48 hours.

Pulse oximetry or arterial blood gases are used to determine if hypoxia is present in children with respiratory distress. Abnormal findings on chest radiograph include hyperinflation and atelectasis (usually right upper lobe and right middle lobe). An alveolar infiltrate is often present in immunocompromised children. An enlarged cardiac silhouette suggests a primary cardiac problem, although a concomitant acute infection with RSV may be present.

Differential Diagnosis

The differential diagnosis of RSV bronchiolitis includes infection with other viruses and some bacteria. Parainfluenza, adenovirus, and rhinovirus cause similar symptoms. *Chlamydia trachomatis* infection may produce similar symptoms in infants between 1 and 4 months of age, although fever is uncommon. Bacterial superinfection is rare, but occasionally clinical and chest radiographic findings of RSV bronchiolitis or RSV pneumonia are similar to those of bacterial pneumonia. Congestive heart failure leads to respiratory distress that may be indistinguishable from bronchiolitis; children wheeze on physical examination. Aspirated foreign body may mani-

fest as respiratory distress, wheezes, and atelectasis on chest radiograph.

Management

In most cases, treatment of healthy infants and children with symptoms of upper respiratory tract disease is supportive.

Medical Treatment

Hospitalization may be appropriate for children who appear ill, dehydrated, in respiratory distress, or in whom it is not possible to rule out SBI. Inpatient treatment may also be necessary for children with congenital cardiac or pulmonary disease when RSV is suspected because of the potential for rapid deterioration. Supplemental oxygen and bronchodilators are useful in reversing hypoxemia. Mechanical ventilation is sometimes necessary, particularly in premature infants or those with underlying cardiac or pulmonary disease.

Use of drugs is generally reserved for severely ill or immunocompromised children. Ribavirin, a synthetic nucleoside analog, has in vitro activity against RSV. Administration is by the aerosolized route. Corticosteroids are not effective and are not indicated.

Prophylaxis

Clinicians should consider prophylaxis against RSV disease in two groups of patients: (1) infants and children less than 2 years of age with chronic lung disease requiring medical therapy within 6 months of the start of the anticipated RSV season and (2) children born at less than 32 weeks' gestation. Children with severe immunodeficiency may benefit from prophylaxis; however, this has not been studied. Currently, no vaccines for prevention of RSV disease are available.

Two products that reduce hospitalization in RSV are available: (1) RSV intravenous immune globulin (RSV-IGIV) and (2) RSV monoclonal antibody [palivizumab (Synagis)]. RSV-IGIV, which is obtained from donors with high neutralizing antibody titer to RSV, is administered intravenously on a monthly basis during RSV season. It reduces hospitalization in high-risk infants with RSV by 41%. Palivizumab, a humanized mouse monoclonal antibody that binds to the F protein of RSV, is given intramuscularly on a monthly basis. Studies have found that it reduces hospitalization of high-risk infants with RSV by 55%. Compared to RSV-IVIG, palivizumab is more cost-effective and easier to administer. Neither RSV-IVIG nor palivizumab is licensed for use in children with cyanotic congenital heart disease.

CROUP

Croup, or laryngotracheobronchitis, is a common childhood illness. Hospitalization occurs in fewer than 2% of children, and only 0.5%–1.5% of these children require intubation. The majority of cases occur in boys in their first 3 years of life during late fall or early winter.

Pathophysiology

Croup is an acute respiratory illness resulting from inflammation and narrowing of the subglottic region of the larynx. In most cases, parainfluenza viruses 1, 2, or 3 are the causal agents. Less common causes are influenza, RSV, adenoviruses, measles, and *Mycoplasma pneumoniae*. Viral infection of the upper respiratory tract spreads to involve the respiratory epithelium of the larynx and trachea. Swelling and edema contribute to narrowing of the subglottic space. Inflammatory debris, mucus, and exudate contribute further to vocal cord dysfunction and subglottic obstruction.

Clinical and Laboratory Evaluation

History
The history should focus on understanding the tempo of the illness, prodromal symptoms, and likelihood of possible foreign body aspiration. Preceding symptoms include several days of mild upper respiratory tract illness. Children have a barking (or "croupy") cough, hoarseness, and inspiratory stridor. Fever is almost always present. Illness gradually subsides within 3–7 days. Disease progression occurs in some children, with respiratory distress, hypoxia, and ultimately respiratory failure.

Physical Examination
The child should be comfortable and sitting during the examination. It is important to pay special attention to evaluation of the severity of airway obstruction to rule out potentially life-threatening causes of stridor and airway obstruction. Children may appear relatively well with only rhinorrhea, hoarseness, and a barking cough. However, they may be cyanotic with intercostal retractions and respiratory distress. Restlessness and agitation are signs of hypoxia. Fever, increased respiratory rate, and increased heart rate may be present.

Some clinicians use croup scores to assess severity of illness and response to therapy. Scoring systems assign points for abnormal findings on physical examination. Parameters evaluated include stridor, retractions, decreased air entry, cyanosis, level of consciousness, presence of cough or dyspnea, and increased heart and respiratory rates.

Laboratory Evaluation
The diagnosis of croup is mostly based on clinical signs and symptoms. When obtained, the CBC is usually normal. Neck radiographs and chest radiographs are useful for eliminating other causes of stridor such as retropharyngeal abscess or foreign body aspiration. It is possible to isolate virus from nasopharyngeal secretions using conventional virus cultures. Rapid antigen detection assays are available for diagnosis of parainfluenza virus infection; however, the sensitivity of tests varies.

Differential Diagnosis

Viral croup is one of several causes of airway obstruction and stridor. Other diagnostic considerations include *H. influenzae* type b epiglottitis (see PHARYNGITIS, DIFFERENTIAL DIAGNOSIS), bacterial tracheitis, retropharyngeal abscess, and laryngeal foreign body (Table 9.8).

Management

Treatment of viral croup is supportive. Cool, humidified air is helpful in alleviating stridor. Nebulized racemic epinephrine reduces airway obstruction in hospitalized patients. Steroid therapy (parenteral dexamethasone, oral dexamethasone, inhaled corticosteroids) decreases the severity and duration of symptoms and the rate of hospitalization. Specific antiviral therapy is not available.

INFLUENZA

Infections with influenza virus are common in children. A short incubation period of 1–3 days and a long duration of viral shedding (1–2 weeks) facilitate spread of influenza virus. School-age children have the highest attack rates. However, 90% of deaths occur in persons over 65 years of age. Hospitalization for conditions related to influenza (~ 110,000/year) is more common in older persons (> 65 years) or in very young children (< 1 year).

Pathophysiology

The causal agent is the influenza virus, a single-stranded RNA virus in the family Orthomyxoviridae. Influenza viruses are classified by type (A, B, C), host of origin (if nonhuman), geo-

TABLE 9.8	Differential Diagnosis of Stridor/Upper Airway Obstruction				
	Viral Croup	Epiglottitis	Bacterial Tracheitis	Retropharyngeal Abscess	Laryngeal Foreign Body
Age	0.5–3 years	3–6 years	Any (usual 2–4 years)	<4 years	Any
Etiology	Parainfluenza Respiratory syncytial virus Influenza	*Haemophilus influenzae* type b	*Staphylococcus aureus* *S. pyogenes* *S. pneumoniae*	*S. aureus* *S. pyogenes* *S. pneumoniae* Anaerobic oral flora	Foreign object
History of onset	Viral prodrome	Abrupt	Viral prodrome, then sudden worsening of symptoms	Abrupt	Abrupt
Temperature	< 39°C	> 39°C	> 39°C	>39°C	Afebrile
Respiratory distress	Mild	Moderate to severe	Moderate to severe	Moderate to severe	Mild to severe
Cough	Present	Absent	Present	Absent	Present
Voice	Hoarse	Muffled	Hoarse	Muffled	Occasionally aphonia
CBC	Normal	↑WBC	↑WBC	↑WBC	Normal

CBC = complete blood count; WBC = white blood cell count.

graphic source, strain number, and year of appearance. The viruses have important surface glycoproteins such as hemagglutinin (H) to facilitate attachment and neuraminidase (N) to facilitate release of viral progeny from infected cells. The M2 proteins that occur in influenza A strains maintain acidity of the Golgi apparatus in infected cells and allow the virus to be uncoated.

Influenza A viruses are classified into subtypes on the basis of the surface antigens H and N. Immunity to the surface antigens of influenza reduces the likelihood and severity of infection. Antibody against one influenza type or subtype gives little or no protection against another type or subtype.

Both influenza A and B are associated with significant clinical illness and yearly epidemics. Influenza A is found in a wide range of animals, including humans, birds, ducks, pigs, horses, and marine mammals. Influenza B is predominantly a human pathogen. Influenza C infection is asymptomatic or causes mild respiratory illness in humans. Influenza viruses circulate during the winter in temperate and subarctic regions and year round in warmer tropical and subtropical climates.

Influenza viruses undergo frequent antigenic changes. **Antigenic shift,** an abrupt change, occurs after a circulating influenza A subtype disappears and is replaced by a subtype with one or both surface proteins (H or N) new to humans.

Antigenic drift, a gradual change, occurs in both influenza A and B and results from a series of genetic mutations. Both antigenic shift and antigenic drift allow influenza virus to escape host immune responses. As a result, humans are susceptible to influenza virus infection throughout their lives. Continual antigenic drift, which occurs more often than antigenic shift, causes seasonal epidemics of influenza. However, when antigenic shift does occur, large numbers of the population have no immunity to the virus. Pandemics result from the appearance of a novel influenza virus capable of rapid transmission in humans; in 1918, influenza type A subtype H1N1 led to more than 20 million deaths worldwide. New viruses with limited transmissibility are associated with relatively few cases of disease.

Infection of the respiratory epithelium by the influenza virus causes significant cellular necrosis, edema, and inflammation. The infection spreads rapidly to involve both the upper respiratory tract and the smaller airways of the lower respiratory tract. Systemic symptoms of malaise and myalgia relate to the production of interferon. Bacterial superinfections are more often seen with influenza infection than with other respiratory viruses. Otitis media occurs in 10%–50% of cases. *S. pneumoniae* and *S. aureus* may cause pneumonia or bacterial tracheitis.

Complications, including viral pneumonia,

myocarditis, meningoencephalitis, and Guillain-Barré syndrome, are more likely in individuals with underlying respiratory, cardiac, renal, metabolic, or immune disorders or in the elderly. Muscle pain (especially involving the calves), rhabdomyolysis, and rarely renal failure occur in association with influenza B infection. **Reye syndrome,** a hepatoencephalopathy, is associated with both influenza and varicella virus. This condition is more common in children who receive aspirin during the acute phase of influenza illness.

Clinical and Laboratory Evaluation

History
Young children have symptoms of influenza that are similar to those seen with infection with other respiratory viruses (see UPPER RESPIRATORY TRACT INFECTIONS). Older children and adults typically have abrupt onset of fever, headache, myalgia, sore throat, and nonproductive cough. Gastrointestinal (GI) symptoms are more frequent in children. Fever is present for 3–5 days. Myalgia and cough persist up to 2 weeks.

Physical Examination
The patient with influenza appears ill with high fever. Special care is given to examination of ears, lungs, heart, abdomen, CNS, and musculoskeletal systems to identify complications of disease and to identify presence of bacterial superinfection.

Laboratory Evaluation
The diagnosis is based on history and physical examination. Viral cultures of nasopharyngeal secretions are positive after 2–6 days. Cultured isolates provide specific information on circulating strains of influenza virus. Several rapid diagnostic tests are available for detection of influenza A and B viruses. The sensitivity of these tests is 62%–73%, and the specificity is 80%–99%. If bacterial superinfection is suspected, a CBC, blood culture, and chest radiograph warrant consideration.

Management

Supportive treatment is generally recommended for children with uncomplicated illness and normal immune function.

Antiviral Agents
Antiviral therapy decreases the severity of influenza and the duration of symptoms. Several antiviral drugs are available.

Amantadine and rimantadine, which prevent viral uncoating by blocking ion-channel activity of the viral M2 protein, are effective against influenza A but not B. Antiviral prophylaxis may be appropriate in high-risk patients who were immunized after influenza A began circulating, in immunodeficient patients with poor antibody response to vaccines, and in persons in whom the influenza vaccine is contraindicated (e.g., individuals with anaphylactic hypersensitivity to egg protein).

Zanamivir and oseltamivir, analogs of sialic acid, inhibit the neuraminidase activity of both influenza A and B viruses. Both drugs are effective for treatment of influenza A and B infections; oseltamivir is approved for prophylaxis. Zanamivir, which is available as a dry powder for inhalation, is generally not recommended for use in patients with underlying respiratory disease because of reports of wheezing and decreased pulmonary function.

Vaccination
Influenza virus vaccine is used to protect individuals from infection with circulating strains of influenza virus. An inactivated vaccine that consists of three viral strains (usually two type A and one type B), which are produced in embryonated eggs, is currently available. Experts select viral strains based on worldwide surveillance of circulating strains. Vaccine efficacy ranges between 50% and 95%, depending on how closely it matches circulating strains of virus. The optimal time for administration of vaccine is October through mid-November.

Adverse effects of vaccine administration include local pain, swelling, and redness in 10%–64% of recipients. Low-grade fever and myalgia may begin 6–12 hours after vaccination and persist for 1–2 days. In general, it is not appropriate to immunize children with a severe anaphylactic reaction to egg protein.

Adolescents and adults should receive whole virus vaccine, which is prepared from intact purified virus particles. Children under 13 years of age should receive the subvirion and purified surface antigen vaccines ("split-virus"), which have fewer side effects. Children over 9 years of age and children who have been previously immunized should receive one dose of vaccine, and children less than 9 years of age (no previous immunization) should receive two doses of vaccine 1 month apart. Influenza vaccine is not immunogenic in infants less than 6 months of age.

Studies have found that use of a cold-adapted trivalent intranasal influenza vaccine in children is effective in the prevention of influenza. Preliminary studies show that vaccine efficacy against certain strains of influenza is greater than 90%. In addition, this vaccine reduces the incidence of AOM by 30% and the incidence of febrile illness with concomitant use of antibiotics by 29%. The vaccine is under consideration for licensure by the US Food and Drug Administration (FDA).

PNEUMONIA

Pneumonia is infection or inflammation of the lung parenchyma. Most episodes of acute pneumonia in young children result from viral infection; a smaller percentage results from bacterial infection.

Pathophysiology

The organisms that cause viral pneumonia are also common causes of viral upper respiratory tract infections. The bacterial causes of pneumonia vary depending on age of the child (Table 9.9) and are similar to causes of other SBIs (see AP-PROACH TO EVALUATION OF THE FEBRILE CHILD). Intracellular organisms such as *Chlamydia trachomatis*, *C. pneumoniae*, and *M. pneumoniae* cause lower respiratory tract disease.

The lower airways are typically sterile. Infection occurs as a result of defects in host defenses protecting the lung, inhalation of a large inoculum of virus or bacteria, or infection of the lung by hematogenous dissemination. Infection of the bronchial epithelium is associated with cell death, sloughing, local inflammation, and edema with airway narrowing. Alveoli become filled with fluid, and infection spreads to involve adjacent lung parenchyma.

Recurrent bacterial pneumonia suggests underlying disease. Examples include immunodeficiency, anatomic abnormalities (e.g., cleft palate, tracheoesophageal fistula), foreign body aspiration, ciliary dysfunction, cystic fibrosis, and chronic aspiration.

Clinical and Laboratory Evaluation

History

The presentation of **viral pneumonia** involves prodromal symptoms of rhinorrhea, cough, low-grade fever, and pharyngitis. Affected children may be lethargic, refuse to play, or have difficulty feeding because of tachypnea or cough. Very young children may become apneic. Pneumonia is suspected when symptoms progress to signs of increasing respiratory distress.

The typical presentation of **bacterial pneumonia** is more abrupt. Older children and adults present with acute onset of high fever, cough, chest pain, and shaking chills. Younger children and infants may have a several-day history of upper respiratory tract symptoms followed by an acute increase in fever and respiratory distress. Cough is initially nonproductive. As infection progresses, hypoxia and delirium may develop.

Pediatric Pearl

In some cases of bacterial pneumonia, particularly of the right lower lobe, significant intra-abdominal pathology such as acute appendicitis is often the initial suspicion.

Neck pain and stiffness are seen with upper lobe pneumonia. Systemic findings of sepsis, including shock and multisystem organ involvement, may occur in some cases.

TABLE 9.9	Age-Related Differences in Etiology of Infectious Pneumonia

Age	Pathogens
0–1 months	*Streptococcus agalactiae*, gram-negative enteric bacteria, *Staphylococcus aureus*, *Listeria monocytogenes*
1–3 months	Viral,* *S. agalactiae*, Enterobacteriaciae, *S. aureus*, *Streptococcus pneumoniae*, *Chlamydia trachomatis*
3 months–5 years	Viral,* *S. pneumoniae*, *S. aureus*, *Streptococcus pyogenes* (rare), *Mycoplasma pneumoniae*
>5 years	Viral,* *M. pneumoniae*, *Chlamydia pneumoniae*, *S. pneumoniae*, *S. aureus*, *S. pyogenes* (rare)

*Viruses most often associated with pneumonia include respiratory syncytial virus, influenza, adenovirus, and parainfluenza viruses. Cytomegalovirus and herpes simplex virus may cause severe pneumonia in infants or immunocompromised children.

Physical Examination

Children with **viral pneumonia** may often be irritable, with nasal flaring, subcostal or intercostal retractions, and mucous membranes that appear cyanotic. Vital signs reveal fever (temperature usually < 39.0°C [102.2°F]), tachypnea, and sometimes tachycardia. In young children in whom auscultation of the lungs is difficult, tachypnea may be the only sign of underlying pneumonia. Findings on auscultation include rales and wheezes. Mild hepatosplenomegaly may be evident in infants if the lungs are hyperinflated.

Children with **bacterial pneumonia** may be toxically ill or anxious, with high fever (temperature > 39.0°C [102.2°F]), tachycardia, tachypnea, and occasionally hypotension. Nasal flaring and cyanosis of mucous membranes or skin may be present. The signs and symptoms of *M. pneumoniae* pneumonia include fever, headache, and cough. Typically, children do not appear to be very ill. Diffuse rales are evident on physical examination, and a rash is present in 10% of cases.

Careful examination of the lungs focuses on **appearance** of the chest, **palpation, percussion,** and **auscultation**. The clinician should note the rate and rhythm of breathing and presence of retractions.

Palpation of the chest produces tenderness. **Tactile fremitus,** which refers to palpable vibrations transmitted through the chest when a patient speaks, is decreased when a pleural effusion is present and increased over consolidated lung.

Dullness to percussion is present over consolidated lung or with a pleural effusion.

Bronchophony describes an increase in the clarity of spoken words as heard through the stethoscope. **Egophony** describes the change in transmission of patient's "eee" sounds to "aay." **Bronchial breath sounds** are best heard over the trachea. Expiration is greater than inspiration and is unusually high-pitched and loud. **Rales** are crackling noises heard over the area of infection. As infection resolves, cough becomes more productive, and rales and rhonchi are more prominent.

Signs of dehydration such as tachycardia, decreased perfusion, decreased skin turgor, and history of poor urine output may be present. Fever, poor fluid intake, and increased respiratory rate often cause dehydration.

Laboratory Evaluation

The diagnostic laboratory workup for children with suspected pneumonia is extensive (Table 9.10). WBC counts are typically greater than 15,000 cells/mm³, with a predominance of PMNs in bacterial pneumonia. Values of up to 40,000

TABLE 9.10 Diagnostic Workup of Pneumonia

1. Complete blood count with differential
2. Blood culture (if bacterial pneumonia suspected)
3. Chest radiograph
4. Sputum (only useful in children > 12 years of age) for Gram stain, bacterial culture, acid fast bacilli (AFB) smear, and AFB culture
5. Direct viral examination of nasopharyngeal specimens (if viral pathogen suspected)
6. *Mycoplasma pneumoniae* IgM and IgG
7. Pulse oximetry/arterial blood gas if children are ill-appearing, cyanotic, or in respiratory distress

Ig = immunoglobulin.

---

cells/ mm³ are not uncommon with pneumococcal and staphylococcal pneumonia. Blood cultures are positive in 10%–30% of cases of bacterial pneumonia. Typical chest radiographic findings for viral, mycoplasma, and bacterial pneumonia are distinctive (Table 9.11).

Infants less than 2–3 months of age are at risk for infection with *S. agalactiae,* gram-negative enteric bacteria, *L. monocytogenes,* and *S. aureus.* If bacterial pneumonia is a possibility, diagnostic workup includes blood culture and urine culture, and lumbar puncture is considered.

A positive rapid diagnostic test for RSV, parainfluenza, influenza or adenovirus may suggest a viral etiology for pneumonia but does not definitively rule out a bacterial superinfection. Diagnosis of *M. pneumoniae* involves serology for specific IgM and IgG. *C. trachomatis* involves isolating the organism from epithelial cells in tissue culture or noting the blue-stained intracytoplasmic inclusions in epithelial cells from conjunctival scrapings stained with Giemsa stain. Nucleic acid amplification is useful for evaluating urethral and cervical specimens but has not been evaluated adequately for detection of *C. trachomatis* in nasopharyngeal specimens. No reliable diagnostic test for *C. pneumoniae* is commercially available.

Pulse oximetry is useful for determining presence of hypoxia. If pulse oximetry is abnormal, arterial blood gas sampling is required. Bronchial alveolar lavage or lung biopsy may be necessary for diagnosis of complicated pneumonia not responding to empiric antimicrobial therapy.

Differential Diagnosis

Signs and symptoms of viral and bacterial pneumonia overlap considerably. Some features of the history and physical examination help distinguish between these two conditions (see Table 9.11).

TABLE 9.11	Distinguishing Features in Pneumonia: Bacterial verus Viral				
Organism	Prodrome	Onset	Signs and Symptoms	Laboratory Studies	Chest Radiograph
Streptococcus pneumoniae	None or URI Influenza	Abrupt	Temp > 39°C Mild-to-severe illness	WBC↑ Blood culture positive (10%–30%↑)	Lobar consolidation ± empyema Less common: bronchopneumonia, interstitial infiltrate, pneumatocele
Staphylococcus aureus	None or URI Influenza	Abrupt	Temp > 39°C Moderate-to-severe illness	WBC↑ Blood culture positive (rare)	Lobar consolidation Empyema Pneumatocele/abscess
Mycoplasma pneumoniae	Malaise Headache	Subacute	Fever Cough Pharyngitis Lymphadenitis Mild-to-moderate illness	WBC normal	Patchy consolidation Interstitial infiltrates Hilar adenopathy Effusion
Chlamydia pneumoniae	Malaise Headache	Subacute	Fever Pharyngitis Hoarse voice Mild illness	WBC normal	Unilateral patchy infiltrate
Chlamydia trachomatis	Conjunctivitis	Gradual	Afebrile Staccato cough Rales/wheezes	WBC normal	Diffuse infiltrates Peribronchial thickening Lobar consolidation
Mycobacterium tuberculosis	None or fever	Gradual	Fever Weight loss Cough Mild illness	WBC normal + PPD	Primary complex Hilar adenopathy Atelectasis/consolidation
Respiratory viruses	Rhinorrhea Cough	Gradual	Temp < 39°C Mild-to-moderate illness	Normal WBC	Perihilar infiltrates Hyperinflation Patchy consolidation

WBC = white blood count; URI = upper respiratory infection.

Management

Antimicrobial treatment of bacterial pneumonia is appropriate (Table 9.12). Outpatient management may be sufficient. Close observation is necessary until children improve. Decisions regarding hospitalization are based on the severity of symptoms. It is usually appropriate to admit the following patients: (1) infants less than 2–3 months of age for observation or empiric antibiotic therapy pending culture results, and (2) children with underlying immunodeficiency, metabolic disease, or cardiopulmonary disease, who are at risk for complications of pneumonia, for parenteral antibiotics. Other criteria for admission include respiratory distress, hypoxia or hypercarbia, sepsis, dehydration, and poor compliance.

LYMPH NODE ENLARGEMENT

Infections causing enlargement of single or multiple lymph nodes are common in children.

TABLE 9.12	Antimicrobial Treatment of Pneumonia
Etiology	**Treatment**
Respiratory syncytial virus	Supportive
	Consider ribavirin in severely ill children
Parainfluenza	Supportive
Adenovirus	Supportive
CMV	Ganciclovir IV plus CMV hyperimmune globulin in immunocompromised children
HSV	Acyclovir IV
Chlamydia trachomatis	Erythromycin
Chlamydia pneumoniae	Erythromycin
	Doxycycline in children > 8 years
	Azithromycin
Mycoplasma pneumoniae	Erythromycin
	Doxycycline in children > 8 years
	Azithromycin
Streptococcus pneumoniae	Penicillin/amoxicillin
	Second- or third-generation cephalosporin
Staphylococcus aureus	Nafcillin/dicloxacillin
	First-generation cephalosporin
	Clindamycin
	Vancomycin (only if methicillin-resistant *S. aureus* suspected)

CMV = cytomegalovirus; HSV-1 = herpes simplex virus type 1; IV = intravenous.

Pathophysiology

Reactive adenopathy, defined as diffuse mild inflammation of lymph nodes, occurs in response to systemic or local infection. The rubbery, mobile nodes have a diameter of less than 2 cm. Several conditions, both infectious and noninfectious, may cause reactive adenopathy (Table 9.13).

Lymphadenitis, defined as infection of the lymph node itself, occurs primarily as the result of bacterial infection; *S. pyogenes* and *S. aureus* cause 80% of cases. Affected nodes are poorly mobile, with associated soft tissue edema and erythema, have a diameter typically larger than 2 cm. Illness is characterized by painful rapid enlargement of the lymph nodes. Tonsillar and anterior cervical nodes are primarily involved. When dental disease is the initial source of infection, anaerobic bacteria may be found in infected submental and submandibular nodes.

Lymphadenitis is a common presentation of **catscratch disease.** Most patients have a history of a scratch by flea-infested cats or kittens, which are infected with the causal pathogen *Bartonella henselae*; young cats (< 1 year) are more often infected with the bacterium. The incidence of disease is greatest in fall and winter. A characteristic red papule is present at the site of the scratch, with regional adenitis noted proximal to the in-

jury. Children are often highly and persistently febrile. Infection can disseminate to cause retinal lesions, liver and spleen abscesses, bone lesions, and rarely encephalitis.

Lymphadenitis may also occur as the result of atypical mycobacteria in children less than 4 years of age. Submandibular, preauricular, anterior cervical, inguinal, or epitrochlear lymph nodes may be involved. Bilateral adenitis is not present. Affected children appear well with no fever or systemic symptoms. The lymph nodes are mildly tender with little warmth or inflammation, and after several weeks they become fixed and discolored. Spontaneous suppuration with formation of a sinus tract may occur.

Other bacteria associated with lymphadenitis include *Francisella tularensis* (the ulceroglandular form of tularemia), *Yersinia pestis* (bubonic plague), and *Pasteurella multocida*. *M. tuberculosis*, a cause of lymphadenitis in patients of any age, is always a consideration (see TUBERCULOSIS).

Clinical and Laboratory Evaluation

History
Important historical information includes rate of enlargement of lymph nodes, associated systemic illness, travel, illness in family members (rule out tuberculosis), and animal contact (cat-

TABLE 9.13 **Infectious and Noninfectious Causes of Lymphadenopathy***

Viruses
Epstein-Barr virus
Cytomegalovirus
Measles
Rubella
Varicella-zoster virus
Herpes simplex virus
HIV
Adenoviruses

Malignancy
Lymphoma
Leukemia
Neuroblastoma
Histiocytosis

Bacteria
Streptococcus pyogenes (pharyngitis)
Brucella spp.
Leptospira spp.
Ehrlichia spp.

Parasites
Toxoplasma gondii
Trypanosoma cruzi

Other
Medications
Juvenile rheumatoid arthritis
Systemic lupus erythematosus
Chronic granulomatous disease
Infection-associated hemophagocytic syndrome
Sarcoidosis

---

*Diffuse or regional nodes < 2 cm in size.
HIV = human immunodeficiency virus.

scratch disease, tularemia, bubonic plague). The clinician should question sexually active adolescents about risk factors for human immunodeficiency virus (HIV) infection.

Physical Examination

Detailed examination of lymph nodes is necessary, along with a careful written description of the nodes involved, and their appearance, consistency, and mobility. Measurement of the size of the nodes is also essential. An understanding of the anatomy and regional drainage of lymph nodes helps discern possible sources of infection (Table 9.14). An enlarged spleen or liver suggests systemic infection with Epstein-Barr virus or cytomegalovirus. A skin rash occurs in viral causes of reactive adenopathy such as rubella.

Laboratory Evaluation

The WBC count may be increased with bacterial lymphadenitis. The ESR is also elevated with bacterial lymphadenitis and adenitis caused by *M. tuberculosis*. The chest radiograph is often abnormal with *M. tuberculosis* infection but normal in infection with atypical mycobacteria. If tuberculosis is suspected, a purified protein derivative (PPD) test is appropriate. Additional studies based on history and physical examination include serology for *B. henselae*, toxoplasmosis, and Epstein-Barr virus. Culture of urine, nasopharynx, or peripheral blood mononuclear cells for cytomegalovirus may be appropriate if the illness is similar to **infectious mononucleosis** (fever, pharyngitis, reactive lymphadenopathy, splenomegaly) but Epstein-Barr virus serology is negative.

If the diagnosis is unclear and the patient does not respond to empiric therapy, biopsy or needle aspiration of the lymph node is appropriate, with material sent for pathology and culture. Incision and drainage of lymph nodes infected with *Mycobacterium* species may lead to chronic drainage and sinus tract formation. If these organisms are suspected, lymph node excision or fine needle aspiration is recommended.

Differential Diagnosis

The differential diagnosis of lymphadenitis includes the enlarged lymph nodes seen with **Kawasaki disease,** branchial cleft cyst, thyroglossal duct cyst, thyroid goiter, lymphoma or Hodgkin disease, and rhabdomyosarcoma.

Management

Management of reactive lymphadenopathy depends on the underlying illness. Specific management of lymphadenitis depends on the infectious cause (Table 9.15).

CENTRAL NERVOUS SYSTEM INFECTIONS

BACTERIAL MENINGITIS

Acute bacterial meningitis is a potentially life-threatening illness. Despite antibiotic therapy and supportive care, mortality is 5%–10%. Almost 50% of survivors of bacterial meningitis have long-term sequelae that range from mild to severe. Mortality and neurologic sequelae are highest with *S. pneumoniae* meningitis.

TABLE 9.14 Regional Drainage of Lymph Nodes

Site of Infection	Site of Drainage
Nasal and oropharyngeal infections	Tonsillar and anterior cervical nodes
Superficial facial infection or cellulitis	Anterior cervical nodes, preauricular nodes, submental nodes
Scalp infection	Occipital, posterior cervical, preauricular and postauricular nodes
Conjunctival infection	Preauricular nodes
Teeth, gingivae, tongue	Submental and submandibular nodes
Neck	Anterior or posterior cervical nodes
Breast and chest wall	Anterior axillary nodes
Hand and arm	Midaxillary nodes
Back	Posterior axillary nodes
Fingers, hand, forearm	Epitrochlear nodes
External genitalia, anus, umbilicus, lower abdomen, lower back, buttocks, upper thigh	Inguinal nodes
Foot and lower leg	Femoral nodes

The epidemiology of bacterial meningitis has changed significantly over the past 15 years. Historically, most cases of bacterial meningitis occurred in children under 5 years of age, and *H. influenzae* type b was the predominant pathogen, followed by *S. pneumoniae* and *N. meningitidis*. Immunization with *H. influenzae* vaccine has virtually eliminated *H. influenzae* type b as a cause of meningitis. As a result, in the United States, bacterial meningitis is now seen more often in adults than in young children.

Pathophysiology

The bacteria that cause meningitis include enteric pathogens in infants and encapsulated bacteria in older infants and children (Table 9.16). To infect the CNS, bacteria must evade several layers of defense provided by the host immune response. Organisms initially colonize and invade respiratory mucosal epithelium. To attach to the respiratory epithelium, encapsulated bacteria make IgA proteases that render secretory

TABLE 9.15 Management of Lymphadenitis*

Suspected Etiology	Antibiotics		Surgical Management
	Oral	Intravenous	
Bacterial adenitis	Dicloxacillin	Nafcillin	Incision and drainage if no response to antibiotic therapy. Send material for culture and pathology.
Staphylococcus aureus or	Cephalexin	Cefazolin	
Streptococcus pyogenes	Amoxicillin–clavulanate	Ceftriaxone	
	Clindamycin	Clindamycin	
Atypical mycobacteria	None	None	Surgical excision of affected nodes. (Incision and drainage may lead to chronic suppuration.)
Mycobacterium tuberculosis	Antituberculous medications		None
Bartonella henselae	Not necessary for mild cases		Usually excision is not necessary.
For more severe illness:	Azithromycin or rifampin or TMP/SMZ or ciprofloxacin or doxycycline (> 8 years of age) or intravenous gentamicin		Needle aspiration is performed in some cases.

*Nodes > 2 cm in size.
TMP/SMZ = trimethoprim–sulfamethoxazole.

TABLE 9.16 Infectious Causes of Meningitis

Organism	Microscopic	Typical Cerebrospinal Fluid Findings		
		Cell count (/mm³)	Glucose (mg/dl)	Protein (mg/dl)
Bacteria				
Age 0–3 months				
Streptococcus agalactiae	Gram-positive cocci in chains	> 100 to several thousand, with > 80% PMNs	< 40	100–500
Escherichia coli	Gram-negative rods	> 100 to several thousand, with > 80% PMNs	< 40	100–500
Enterococcus spp.	Gram-positive cocci	> 100 to several thousand, with > 80% PMNs	< 40	100–500
Listeria monocytogenes	Gram-positive rods (negative in 60%)	5 to > 1000, with usually > 60% PMNs	<40 in 40%	> 45
Age 3 months–5 years				
Streptococcus pneumoniae	Gram-positive diplococci	> 100 to several thousand, with > 80% PMNs	< 40	100–500
*Neisseria meningitidis**	Gram-negative diplococci	> 100 to several thousand, with > 80% PMNs	< 40	100–500
Haemophilus influenzae type b*	Gram-negative cocco-bacillary organisms	> 100 to several thousand, with > 80% PMNs	< 40	100–500
Age > 5 years				
S. pneumoniae	Gram-positive diplococci	> 100 to several thousand, with > 80% PMNs	< 40	100–500
N. meningitidis	Gram-negative diplococci	> 100 to several thousand, with > 80% PMNs	< 40	100–500
Any Age				
Mycobacterium tuberculosis	Negative Gram stain	10–500; PMNs early, lymphocytes later	< 40	100–500
Viruses				
Enterovirus spp.	Negative Gram stain	Usually < 1000 with early PMNs, then mononuclear cells	Normal	20–100
Fungi				
Coccidioides immitis	KOH usually negative	50–1000, lymphocytes, eosinophils	10–39	50–1000
Candida albicans	Gram-positive yeast			
Cryptococcus neoformans	Positive India Ink stain	> 20 lymphocytes	< 40	> 40

*Small gram-negative coccobacillary organisms such as *N. meningitidis* or *H. influenzae* type b may be difficult to see.

KOH = potassium hydroxide; PMN = polymorphonuclear neutrophil.

IgA nonfunctional. After attachment, bacteria invade mucosal barriers by endocytosis or through separations in tight junctions of columnar epithelial cells.

Once bacteria enter the intravascular space, capsular polysaccharide enables them to evade the alternative complement pathway. The bacteria then replicate in the blood and eventually penetrate the blood–brain barrier and infect the cerebrospinal fluid (CSF). Small blood vessels that enter the brain carry the infection to the cerebral cortex. Thrombosis of intracerebral vessels leads to hypoxia and infarction. Intracranial pressure rises as a result of increased permeability of the blood–brain barrier, toxins released by bacteria or neutrophils, and decreased CSF outflow. Replicating bacteria induce local release of interleukin-1 and tumor necrosis factor. Stimulation of neutrophils migrating into the CSF results in their degranulation, releasing toxic oxygen metabolites. Some studies suggest the host inflammatory response to infection is responsible for the long-term sequelae of meningitis.

Meningitis is also the result of direct bacterial invasion of the CNS after penetrating trauma or through a congenital malformation. Congenital malformations that lead to increased risk of meningitis include **dermoid sinus tract** or **meningomyelocele,** which are associated with recurrent or polymicrobial meningitis. A fracture through a sinus or a skull fracture may lead to CNS infection with respiratory pathogens.

Clinical and Laboratory Evaluation

Even after a careful history and physical examination, the diagnosis of meningitis sometimes remains in question. Careful and frequent evaluation is then indicated.

History

A history of recent symptoms of viral upper respiratory tract illness, head trauma, recurrent bacterial infections, documented immunodeficiency, or contact with other ill individuals may be present. N. meningitidis and H. influenzae type b infection occur in clusters among family members or close contacts.

Symptoms in infants and young children include irritability, anorexia, vomiting, and inconsolable crying. As illness progresses, lethargy, seizures, or focal neurologic signs develop. Older children complain of headache, back pain, stiff neck, and photophobia and may become increasingly confused and disoriented.

Physical Examination

Careful examination, focusing on the child's general appearance, vital signs, and neurologic status, is crucial. Observation of patients from across the room is helpful; children who happily play with toys in the waiting room but are fussy when examined by a physician are less likely to have meningitis. Fever is present in most children with meningitis, but hypothermia may occur in infants. With increased intracranial pressure, bradycardia and hypertension develop.

Signs of meningeal irritation, including pain and limitation of range of motion of the neck, may not be evident in children less than 18 months of age. Positive Kernig and Brudzinski signs are indicative of meningeal inflammation. A **Kernig sign** is elicited by having a child lie on her back with the knee flexed and the hip flexed so that the thigh is perpendicular to the trunk. If meningeal irritation is present, extension of the knees causes pain. A **Brudzinski sign** occurs when the hips and knees spontaneously flex after passive flexion of the neck.

It is necessary to perform a detailed neurologic examination with assessment of mental status, examination of cranial nerves, reflexes, muscle strength, and gait (if applicable). A bulging anterior fontanelle is sometimes apparent in young infants. Pulmonary, cardiac, abdominal, and bone and joint examination may reveal the presence of other sites of infection. Petechiae or purpura may be evident on skin examination. A careful retinal examination may detect presence of papilledema.

Laboratory Evaluation

Ninety-nine percent of children with bacterial meningitis have CSF abnormalities, and the initial diagnosis of acute bacterial meningitis is based on analysis of CSF findings (see Table 9.16). The normal range of cells, glucose, and protein in the CSF varies by age and is shown in Table 9.17. In bacterial meningitis, the CSF is typically cloudy. The cell count is more than 1000 cells/mm^3, with a differential revealing a predominance of PMNs (usually > 80%). (Some authorities consider the presence of at least one neutrophil/mm^3 as possibly indicative of bacterial meningitis.) Protein is elevated as a consequence of disruption of the blood–brain barrier. Glucose is low because the transport mechanisms responsible for carrying glucose from the peripheral circulation to the choroid plexus and into the CSF are impaired. Gram stain shows organisms if more than 10^3 bacteria/ml are present. Culture of CSF is positive in virtually all

TABLE 9.17	Normal Cerebrospinal Fluid Indices			
Age	WBC count (/mm³)	PMNs	Glucose (mg/dl)	Protein (mg/dl)
Preterm infant	0–25	0%–57%	24–63	65–150
Term infant	0–22	0%–61%	34–119	20–170
Older infant/child	0–5	0	40–80	5–40

WBC = white blood cell; PMN = polymorphonyclear neutrophil.

cases of bacterial meningitis, provided the child did not receive antibiotic therapy prior to the lumbar puncture. If possible, an extra tube of CSF is obtained for additional diagnostic tests if routine tests do not confirm bacterial meningitis.

A CBC with differential shows a predominance of PMN cells and an increase in band forms. Blood cultures are positive in the majority of cases; however, because time to positivity ranges from 24–72 hours, they do not aid initial diagnosis. Serum electrolytes may show decreased sodium secondary to the **syndrome of inappropriate (secretion of) antidiuretic hormone (SIADH).** Electrolyte abnormalities may also be a consequence of diarrhea, vomiting, or poor fluid intake. Bacterial latex agglutination may be useful in cases of partially treated meningitis. Polymerase chain reaction (PCR) for enterovirus or herpes simplex virus (HSV) may be helpful in cases of suspected viral meningitis.

Computed tomography (CT) or magnetic resonance imaging (MRI) scans detect complications of meningitis such as subdural empyema, venous thrombosis, infarction, and hydrocephalus. Routine CT scan before lumbar puncture is not necessary unless children are comatose or have papilledema or focal neurologic findings. If these findings are present, blood culture is obtained and empiric antibiotic therapy is started prior to the imaging procedure. If there is no evidence of cerebral edema or mass lesion on CT scan, lumbar puncture can be performed. Imaging studies are useful for identifying a contiguous focus of infection such as chronic otitis media or chronic sinusitis. MRI is useful in the diagnosis of some forms of fungal (*Coccidioides immitis*) and bacterial meningitis (*M. tuberculosis*) that show predominance of basilar and brainstem inflammation.

Differential Diagnosis

Other causes of fever, headache, and abnormal neurologic signs include aseptic meningitis, fungal meningitis, encephalitis, brain abscess, or brain tumor. Viruses as well as bacteria and fungi may cause aseptic meningitis (Table 9.18). Enteroviruses are the leading recognizable cause of aseptic meningitis. In temperate climates, enteroviruses circulate during summer and fall and are transmitted by fecal–oral spread. Mild respiratory or GI symptoms or a rash precede development of meningeal signs.

In children with aseptic meningitis, CSF usually shows a predominance of mononuclear cells, and routine bacterial cultures are negative. Recent data indicate that many patients with enteroviral meningitis have a predominance of PMNs. With viral meningitis, the total number of WBCs in the CSF is typically less than 500 cells/mm³. CSF glucose and protein are likely normal.

Management

All children with suspected bacterial meningitis should have a lumbar puncture and be admitted to the hospital. Treatment of acute disease includes antimicrobial therapy and management of sequelae of CNS infection and inflammation. Research efforts are directed toward therapeutic approaches that decrease the inflammatory response in addition to treatment with antibiotics.

The initial empiric choice of antibiotic therapy depends on the age of the child (Table 9.19). Parenteral therapy is given for the entire duration of treatment to achieve adequate CSF concentration of drug. Duration of therapy depends on the organism and the child's response (see Table 9.19). CSF concentrations of antibiotics commonly used to treat bacterial meningitis are approximately 5%–15% of serum levels.

Dexamethasone given before the first dose of antibiotic therapy may reduce the inflammatory response and prevent sensorineural hearing loss in *H. influenzae* type b meningitis. Studies have not clearly demonstrated the benefit of this agent in other types of bacterial meningitis. Children generally remain in the hospital until antibiotic therapy is complete. Seizures, SIADH, stroke, and subdural empyema may develop during treatment.

The most common sequela of meningitis is

TABLE 9.18 Infectious and Noninfectious Causes of Aseptic Meningitis

Infectious		Noninfectious
Viruses	**Bacteria**	**Immunologically Mediated Diseases**
Enteroviruses*	*Rickettsia* spp. (RMSF and typhus)	Sarcoidosis
Arboviruses	*Borrelia burgdorferi*	Systemic lupus erythematosus
Epstein-Barr virus	*Brucella*	Rheumatoid arthritis
HIV	*Treponema pallidum*	
LCM	*Leptospira* spp.	**Neoplasms**
Cytomegalovirus	*Bartonella* spp.	Leukemia
Adenovirus	*Mycoplasma pneumoniae*	Lymphoma
Influenza virus		Brain tumor
Measles virus	**Parameningeal focus**	
Parainfluenza virus	Brain abscess	**Drugs**
Varicella-zoster virus	Epidural abscess	Intravenous immunoglobulin
	Mastoiditis	OKT3
Fungi	Sinusitis	Isoniazid
Cryptococcus neoformans		Ibuprofen
Coccidioides immitis		

*Serotypes most likely to cause CNS infection include: coxsackie serotypes B2, B4, B5 and echovirus 4, 6, 7, 11

HIV = human immunodeficiency virus; LCM = lymphocytic choriomeningitis virus; RMSF = Rocky Mountain spotted fever.

sensorineural hearing loss. Other sequelae of bacterial meningitis include seizures, hemiparesis, hydrocephalus, ataxia, behavior disorders, and cognitive abnormalities.

ENCEPHALITIS

Encephalitis is an acute inflammatory process of brain tissue. Children and elderly adults are most often affected.

More than 100 different viruses are reported to cause encephalitis. HSVs are the leading cause of severe encephalitis. Encephalitis caused by either HSV-1 or HSV-2 is seen in infants less than 6 weeks of age, who acquire infection around the time of birth or in utero (rare) if the mother has genital lesions. Risk of infection is 33%–50% after primary maternal infection as opposed to less than 5% if the mother has a history of recurrent HSV infection. Infants can acquire infection after contact with a caregiver with cold sores or herpetic whitlow. Older infants and children develop HSV-1 encephalitis after reactivation of latent HSV-1 in the trigeminal ganglion or after primary infection.

Arboviruses are RNA viruses that cause either aseptic meningitis or encephalitis. Transmission occurs during summer or fall via mosquito or tick bites. The number of cases of encephalitis reported each year ranges from 150 to 3000. In the United

TABLE 9.19 Empiric Antibiotic Therapy for Bacterial Meningitis

Age	Pathogen	Empiric Antibiotic Therapy	Duration of Therapy
0–12 weeks	*Streptococcus agalactiae, Escherichia coli, Klebsiella pneumoniae, Enterococcus* spp., *Listeria monocytogenes*	Ampicillin plus cefotaxime or Ampicillin plus an aminoglycoside	*E. coli, K. pneumoniae,* and *Enterococcus* spp. 21 days (minimum) *L. monocytogenes* and *S. agalactiae* 14–21 days
3 months–18 years	*Neisseria meningitidis, Streptococcus pneumoniae (Haemophilus influenzae* type b)	Cefotaxime or ceftriaxone plus vancomycin**	*N. meningitidis* 7 days *H. influenzae* type b 7–10 days *S. pneumoniae* 10–14 days

**Vancomycin is discontinued if culture is positive for *N. meningitidis, H. influenzae* type b, or *S. pneumoniae* susceptible to penicillin or third-generation cephalosporin.

States, the most common types of arboviral encephalitis are St. Louis encephalitis; western equine encephalitis; eastern equine encephalitis; California encephalitis (LaCrosse strain); and recently, West Nile Virus. Neurologic sequelae are most common after infection with eastern equine encephalitis and St. Louis encephalitis. Mortality is highest with eastern equine encephalitis infection.

Enteroviruses typically cause aseptic meningitis but occasionally cause infection with focal neurologic signs and obtundation more typical of encephalitis. The nonpolio enteroviruses most likely to cause CNS infection include enterovirus 71;, coxsackievirus B5; and echoviruses 7, 9, 11, and 30. Infection is most common during summer or fall.

Pathophysiology

Initial viral infection occurs at a site distant from the CNS such as the respiratory tract or GI tract; arboviral infection involves direct inoculation into skin. The virus replicates locally and spreads to regional lymphoid tissue. Distribution throughout the body occurs during the primary viremic phase, with subsequent high-level viral replication. Symptoms of fever, malaise, and headache are associated with a secondary viremia. Some viruses reach the CNS by bypassing the blood–brain barrier during the secondary viremia. Other viruses such as HSV and rabies reach the CNS by retrograde axonal transport from peripheral sites. Direct viral infection of neural cells and associated perivascular inflammation leads to destruction of gray matter. Meningeal inflammation and CSF pleocytosis often accompany encephalitis.

A syndrome of **postinfectious encephalomyelitis** (acute disseminated encephalomyelitis) may follow infection with certain viruses or bacteria. It is possible to distinguish this autoimmune process from acute encephalitis by the primary pathologic finding of demyelination of white matter.

Clinical and Laboratory Evaluation

History

Important historical considerations include history of travel, recent insect bites, other illnesses in the family, and possible drug or toxin ingestion. Initial signs and symptoms of encephalitis are nonspecific and include fever, irritability, lethargy, and anorexia. Rhinorrhea, pharyngitis, cough, diarrhea, vomiting, or rash may be present. Several hours to days after the occurrence of these initial symptoms, abnormal neurologic conditions that range from mild to severe develop. These include headache, behavioral disturbances, cranial nerve deficits, hemiparesis, dysphagia, seizures, obtundation, and coma.

Physical Examination

A careful neurologic examination is performed to assess level of consciousness, presence of cranial nerve abnormalities, hemiparesis, movement disorders, and ataxia. It is necessary to examine skin and mucous membranes for signs of enterovirus infection or vesicular lesions consistent with HSV infection.

Laboratory Evaluation

In viral encephalitis, the CSF typically shows a lymphocytic pleocytosis, elevated protein, and normal or mildly decreased glucose. In some cases, the CSF is normal. MRI may detect focal abnormalities consistent with HSV encephalitis, including temporal lobe edema or hemorrhage. MRI findings suggestive of white matter demyelination on T2-weighted images assist in differentiation of acute encephalitis from postinfectious encephalomyelitis. Tests used for identification of a specific virus include culture, PCR, serologic studies, and immunocytochemical studies of brain tissue.

Differential Diagnosis

Noninfectious causes to consider in children with abnormal neurologic findings include intracranial hemorrhage, collagen vascular disease, metabolic disease, or exposure to drugs or toxins.

Management

Treatment of HSV encephalitis requires intravenous acyclovir for at least 3 weeks. Treatment of arboviral or enteroviral encephalitis is supportive; no antiviral drugs are licensed for therapeutic use in these conditions. In cases of suspected postinfectious encephalomyelitis in which acute viral, bacterial, and fungal infections have been reasonably excluded, some experts advocate a trial of steroid or immunoglobulin therapy, although these methods have no proven benefit.

BONE AND JOINT INFECTIONS

INFECTIOUS ARTHRITIS

Infection and inflammation of the joint is caused by bacteria, fungi, or viruses. **Pyogenic, or septic, arthritis** is the result of bacterial infection of the joint space (Table 9.20). **Reactive arthritis** is an inflammatory response in the joint space that occurs as the result of infection elsewhere in the body (Table 9.21).

Pyogenic arthritis occurs in all age groups but is most common in children younger than 3 years of age. Joints of the lower extremities, including knees, hips, and ankles, account for more than 75% of cases. Usually a single joint is affected. If multiple joints are infected, *N. meningitidis*, *Salmonella* spp., or *S. aureus* is suspected. Infection with *H. influenzae* type b, and *Kingella kingae* often follows an upper respiratory tract illness.

Pathophysiology

Joint infection in pyogenic arthritis occurs as a result of hematogenous spread of bacteria to the vascular synovium. An inflammatory response to bacterial endotoxin occurs within the joint space. The release of cytokines, including tumor necrosis factor and interleukin-1, stimulates production of proteinases by synovial cells. Leukocytes produce neutrophil elastases, which cause destruction of cartilage.

Pyogenic arthritis is less often the result of contiguous spread from adjacent osteomyelitis. The joint capsules of the hip and shoulder, which overlie the metaphysis of the femur and the humerus, respectively, allow extension of infection from the bone into the joint space. Contiguous spread of infection is more likely in infants or young children because of the presence

TABLE 9.21	Infectious Causes of Reactive Arthritis

Organisms that cause both pyogenic arthritis and reactive arthritis
  Streptococcus pyogenes
  Neisseria meningitidis
  Neisseria gonorrhoeae
  Salmonella spp.

Organisms that typically cause primary infection elsewhere with associated reactive arthritis
  Shigella spp.
  Yersinia enterocolitica
  Campylobacter spp.
  Chlamydia trachomatis

of transphyseal blood vessels. Direct inoculation of organisms into the joint space after puncture wound, trauma, or surgical intervention less often leads to pyogenic arthritis.

Clinical and Laboratory Evaluation

History

It is important to focus the history on information that helps distinguish between acute pyogenic arthritis, reactive arthritis, and **juvenile rheumatoid arthritis.** It is necessary to question caregivers regarding underlying illness (e.g., sickle cell disease, immunodeficiency); recent travel or exposure history (e.g., tick exposure, pet rats or reptiles); recent illness (e.g., pharyngitis, scarlet

TABLE 9.20	Bacterial Causes and Treatment of Pyogenic Arthritis and Osteomyelitis	
Age	**Organism**	**Empiric Antibiotic Therapy**
0–3 months	*Streptococcus agalactiae*, gram-negative bacteria, *Staphylococcus aureus*	Nafcillin plus cefotaxime
3 months–5 years	*S. aureus, Streptococcus pneumoniae, Streptococcus pyogenes, Kingella kingae*	Nafcillin plus cefotaxime or Cefuroxime
> 5 years	*S. aureus, S. pyogenes, Neisseria gonorrhoeae*	Nafcillin, cefazolin, clindamycin; ceftriaxone if *N. gonorrhoeae* suspected
Special circumstances		
Child with sickle cell disease	*Salmonella* spp., *S. aureus*	Nafcillin plus cefotaxime
Puncture wound through sneaker	*Pseudomonas aeruginosa*	Ticarcillin–clavulanate ± aminoglycoside
Bite wound	*Eikenella corrodens* (human bite) *Pasteurella multocida* (cat, dog) *S. aureus* and oral flora including anaerobes	Ampicillin–sulbactam

fever–like rash, upper respiratory tract infection, diarrhea, weight loss, or previous joint pain); and history of trauma. Adolescents should be interviewed regarding their sexual history.

Children with pyogenic arthritis typically present with acute pain in the affected joint. Initial symptoms in very young children or infants include crying with diaper changes, refusal to move the affected limb, or refusal to bear weight or walk. Fever is usually present.

Physical Examination

A careful musculoskeletal examination reveals the source of infection. The affected joint is swollen, warm, and tender. Range of motion is decreased. It may be difficult to diagnose pyogenic arthritis of the hip, because no redness or swelling of the joint is often apparent. Pain may be referred to the knee. The child may prefer to hold the hip in a flexed, externally rotated, abducted position. Differentiation of pyogenic arthritis of the hip from other causes of hip pain (e.g., transient synovitis) is crucial, because treatment of pyogenic arthritis of the hip requires immediate joint space drainage and intravenous antibiotic therapy.

Additional important physical examination findings include weight loss (inflammatory bowel disease), presence of skin lesions or rash, heart murmurs (endocarditis), abdominal pain (inflammatory bowel disease), or abnormal eye findings (juvenile rheumatoid arthritis or Behçet disease). It is necessary to perform a genital examination in adolescents to rule out sexually transmitted disease.

Laboratory Evaluation

The ESR, WBC, and C-reactive protein are elevated. Blood cultures are positive in 40% of cases. Analysis of joint fluid cell count, Gram stain, and culture is helpful in differentiating pyogenic from other causes of joint inflammation (Table 9.22). Gram stain and culture of joint fluid are diagnostic in 60%–70% of cases of pyogenic arthri-

tis. Isolation of *K. kingae* is enhanced by direct inoculation of joint fluid into a blood culture bottle.

Plain radiographs of the affected joint reveal soft tissue swelling and widening of the joint space. Ultrasound is sometimes used to detect fluid within the hip joint. MRI is a sensitive method for detecting fluid within the joint space and identifying associated bone or soft tissue involvement; however, it does not differentiate between infectious and noninfectious causes of joint space inflammation. Technetium phosphate radionuclide scans are not recommended except in cases where physical examination and plain radiographs cannot localize the site of infection (as in infection of the sacroiliac joint).

Differential Diagnosis

Illnesses that present with limb pain or refusal to walk include pelvic osteomyelitis, disk space infection (diskitis), vertebral osteomyelitis, primary or metastatic malignancies, trauma, and reactive or autoimmune arthritis.

Management

Hospitalization is appropriate for children with pyogenic arthritis. Management should occur in conjunction with an orthopedic surgeon. Goals of therapy include decompression and sterilization of the joint space. Immediate drainage of an infected hip joint is crucial to prevent vascular compromise and subsequent avascular necrosis of the femoral head. Aspiration of other joint spaces is recommended to obtain synovial fluid for cell count and culture and to facilitate decompression.

Pediatric Pearl

Immediate drainage of an infected hip joint is crucial to prevent vascular compromise and subsequent avascular necrosis of the femoral head.

TABLE 9.22 **Typical Synovial Fluid White Blood Cell (WBC) Counts Seen with Infectious Arthritis**

	WBC (cells/mm³) [usual range]	Polymorphonuclear Cells
Normal	< 150	< 25%
Pyogenic arthritis	10,000–300,000 (> 50,000)	> 90%
Lyme arthritis	180–100,000 (40,000)	> 75%
Viral arthritis	3000–50,000 (15,000)	< 50%

Empiric intravenous antibiotic therapy is based on age (see Table 9.20). Once culture results are available, antibiotic coverage is narrowed to treat the identified organism. Intravenous therapy is continued until fever resolves and joint swelling and tenderness improve. Because antibiotics penetrate into the joint space in high concentration, oral antibiotic therapy may be used to complete a course of therapy, providing the parents appear to be compliant and children take the medicine. Typical duration of antibiotic therapy (intravenous plus oral), which depends on the causal pathogen, ranges from 3 to 4 weeks. On appropriate therapy, serum C-reactive protein normalizes after about 7 days, and children display steady clinical improvement.

OSTEOMYELITIS

Inflammation of bone is usually the result of bacterial infection, although fungal organisms are occasionally responsible.

Pathophysiology

In children, osteomyelitis is usually the result of hematogenous dissemination of bacteria to bones, which are growing rapidly and have a rich vascular supply. Organisms deposited in metaphyseal capillaries replicate and spread to cortical bone. In some cases, a subperiosteal abscess forms and extension of infection into adjacent soft tissue may occur. Osteomyelitis may also occur as a result of contiguous spread of infection after trauma or from bite wounds. Anaerobic osteomyelitis of the skull or face is seen with extension of infection from sinuses, chronic otitis media, or dental abscess.

Approximately 50% of cases of hematogenous osteomyelitis occur in children less than 5 years of age. Males are twice as often affected as females. As with pyogenic arthritis, the long bones of the lower extremities are more likely affected. *S. aureus* is the most common cause of hematogenous osteomyelitis in all age groups. Other bacterial causes along with predisposing conditions are listed in Table 9.20.

Clinical and Laboratory Evaluation

History

Systemic symptoms of fever and malaise are usually present. Children may refuse to bear weight, walk, or move the affected extremity (**pseudoparalysis**). A past medical history of such underlying conditions as sickle cell disease or immunodeficiency is relevant. A history of travel may suggest infection with fungal organisms endemic in certain geographic regions (*C. immitis, Histoplasma capsulatum, Blastomyces dermatitides*). History of animal exposure leads to consideration of infection with *B. henselae* (cats) or *Salmonella* (reptiles). A history of congenital heart disease suggests bacterial endocarditis as a possible source of infection. A recent history of pharyngitis or chickenpox leads to consideration of infection with *S. pyogenes*.

Physical Examination

Some children with hematogenous osteomyelitis are afebrile and relatively well-appearing, whereas others have high fever and are moderately to severely ill. A careful bone and joint examination is required to localize the infection. Often swelling, redness, and warmth is evident over the affected portion of bone. Palpation of the bone reveals the site of maximum tenderness.

In osteomyelitis of the pelvis or lower back, which is difficult to diagnose, gait abnormalities or referred pain to the hip or abdomen is present. Rocking the pelvic girdle or direct palpation of the affected vertebral body elicits pain. Range of motion of the hip is normal.

Laboratory Evaluation

The WBC is either normal or elevated, with a predominance of PMN cells. The ESR and C-reactive protein are increased in more than 90% of cases, and blood cultures are positive in more than 50% of cases. Culture of infected bone increases the chance of making the appropriate bacteriologic diagnosis.

Plain radiographs reveal soft tissue swelling around affected bone within the first few days of illness. Bone destruction is not noted until approximately 50% of bone is demineralized. Therefore osteolytic changes are not seen until 10–20 days after onset of symptoms. Sclerosis of the bone is evident 1 month or more after onset of infection.

Radionuclide scans using technetium-labeled methylene-diphosphonate isotope are useful in the early diagnosis of osteomyelitis. Osteoblastic activity in infected bone enhances uptake of the isotope. The sensitivity of the bone scan is 80%–100%. A positive bone scan is not specific for infection, because malignancy, infarction, trauma, or soft tissue cellulitis overlying the bone may cause increased uptake of the isotope. The bone scan may be falsely normal in neonates and very early in the course of infection.

MRI detects changes in bone marrow caused by infection. The sensitivity for detection of osteomyelitis is greater than 90% but as with radionuclide scans, similar marrow abnormalities are present with malignancy, fracture, or infarction.

Differential Diagnosis

Causes of bone pain other than osteomyelitis include trauma, bone infarction, bone tumors, leukemia, and lymphoma.

Management

Hospitalization for intravenous antibiotics and evaluation by an orthopedic surgeon is usually necessary. Empiric antibiotic therapy pending a bacteriologic diagnosis is outlined in Table 9.20. β-lactam antibiotics, clindamycin, and vancomycin achieve levels in bone that are adequate for treatment of the usual pathogens. Theoretically, aminoglycosides are not used because of poor activity in an environment of tissue hypoxia and acidosis. Intravenous antibiotics are continued until fever resolves, local findings of pain, warmth, and erythema improve, and C-reactive protein and ESR are returning to normal.

Eventually, it is possible to consider a change to oral antibiotic therapy. Factors to consider before initiating this change include the ability of children and families to be compliant with medication regimens and to attend follow-up appointments. The choice of oral antibiotic depends on the organism isolated, and it should have approximately the same spectrum of coverage as the intravenous antibiotic to which the child responded. The dose of oral β-lactam antibiotics used is approximately two to three times the usual recommended dose. However, because of the excellent bioavailability of clindamycin, it is not necessary to alter the recommended dose of the drug. Duration of therapy ranges from 4 to 8 weeks.

Surgical intervention is recommended in the setting of persistent fever, erythema, swelling and pain. It is also recommended with a periosteal or soft tissue abscess, a draining sinus tract, or suspected necrotic bone.

VIRAL EXANTHEMS

Pediatric exanthems (rashes) may be viral or bacterial in origin. The classic viral exanthems result from infection with measles virus, rubella virus, HHV-6 and HHV-7, parvovirus B19, and varicella-zoster virus. Viral illnesses associated with exanthems have distinctive microbiologic and clinical characteristics (Tables 9.23 and 9.24). The pathogenesis of the rash varies depending on the inciting organism. Skin eruptions are caused by direct infection of the epidermis (measles), dermis (rubella), or vascular endothelium (rickettsial disease), circulating bacterial toxin (*S. pyogenes, S. aureus*), host immunologic response (parvovirus B19), or a combination of factors.

When assessing children with rashes, it is important to take a complete history regarding the rash. To establish the diagnosis, information regarding prodromal symptoms; the onset, spread, and evolution of the rash; and associated systemic symptoms is necessary. The clinician must obtain a history of travel, ill contacts, immunizations, allergies, medications, and insect or tick bites. It is essential to document the following characteristics of the rash: color and texture, location, and pattern (e.g., is it symmetrical?); involvement of the hands and feet; and manner and extent of spread. In addition, the clinician should also note whether the rash is painful, painless, or itchy; whether it blanches; and whether any mucous membranes are involved. Observation of abnormalities such as fever, respiratory symptoms, pharyngitis, lymphadenopathy, heart murmur, and joint abnormalities aid in the diagnosis.

MEASLES (SEE TABLE 9.24)

Measles (also known as "hard" measles, rubeola, red measles, and nine-day measles) is highly contagious, with most cases occurring in winter or spring. In the United States, the incidence of measles has dropped dramatically since the vaccine was licensed in 1963.

Pathophysiology

Skin eruptions result from direct viral infection of the epidermis. Bacterial superinfection may develop, and complications may occur. Death due to either respiratory or neurologic complications occurs in 1–3 of every 1000 cases in the United States. Mortality rates are higher in other countries. **Subacute sclerosing panencephalitis,** a progressive fatal degenerative CNS disease, occurs after wild-type measles. It is associated with a prolonged incubation period (10.8 years on average). Symptoms include progressive changes in behavior, cognitive deterioration, and seizures.

Clinical and Laboratory Evaluation

History
The history should focus on immunization status, travel, or contact with other individuals with rash-associated illnesses. Children are moder-

TABLE 9.23 **Viral Exanthems: Microbiologic Characteristics**

Virus	Disease	Transmission	Pathogenesis of Infection	Incubation Period
Measles Paramyxovirus family	Measles	Droplet/airborne	Replication in respiratory tract → lymphatics → viremia → RES → secondary viremia → dissemination to multiple organs, including skin	7–18 days
Rubivirus Togaviridae family	Rubella	Droplet/contact	Same as measles	12–23 days
Varicella-zoster virus Herpesviridae family	Chickenpox Varicella zoster (shingles)	Airborne/contact	Inoculation of respiratory tract → replication in lymph nodes → viremia → RES → secondary viremia → mononuclear cells transport virus to skin, replication in epidermal cells Latency established	10–21 days
Human herpes virus 6 Herpesviridae family	Roseola	Contact	Infects mature T lymphocytes Establishes latency	9–10 days
Parvovirus B19 Parvoviridae family	Fifth disease	Contact/droplet	Replicates in respiratory tract → viremia → infects RBC precursors	4–21 days
Enteroviruses*	Hand, foot and mouth disease	Contact (respiratory or stool)	Replicates in respiratory and GI tract → transient viremia → RES → secondary viremia to target organs (CNS, heart, skin)	3–6 days
Herpes simplex virus Herpesviridae family	Neonatal herpes simplex virus	Perinatal/contact	Skin or mucous membrane penetration → neuronal spread → viremia → organ involvement → latency	2–14 days (neonatal herpes simplex virus presents from day of life 0 to 6 weeks)

*Usually coxsackie virus A16, sometimes enterovirus 71 or other strains.
GI = gastrointestinal; RBC = red blood cell; RES = reticuloendothelial system.

ately to seriously ill, with symptoms of high fever, dry cough, coryza, and conjunctivitis with clear discharge. A distinctive rash develops following the prodromal symptoms.

Physical Examination

Measles is distinguished by a pathognomonic enanthem (**Koplik spots**) characterized by tiny white dots on a red base, which appears on the buccal mucosa 1 or 2 days prior to onset of rash. Mucous membranes and pharynx are red. Skin rash appears 3 to 4 days after onset of prodromal symptoms. The dark red raised morbilliform (measles-like) rash begins at the hairline and spreads to involve the trunk, arms, legs, and eventually hands and feet. Individual lesions become confluent as illness progresses. Lesions initially blanch but progress to darker nonblanching lesions as a result of capillary leak. The rash fades over 7–9 days with subsequent fine desquamation. Children appear ill and may complain of photophobia.

TABLE 9.24 Viral Exanthems: Clinical Characteristics

Disease	Prodrome	Enanthem	Exanthem	Complications
Measles	Cough, coryza, conjunctivitis, high fever	Koplik spots	Red, raised morbilliform rash	Otitis media, pneumonia, croup diarrhea, acute encephalitis, death, subacute sclerosing panencephalitis
Rubella	Malaise, posterior auricular nodes, low-grade fever	Red macules, soft palate	Red, raised rash, less intense than measles	Congenital rubella syndrome, polyarthralgia, arthritis, encephalitis, thrombocytopenia
Varicella	Malaise, anorexia, Headache (mild)	Vesicles may involve mucous membranes	Papules → vesicles → crusted lesions appear on scalp/face/neck Spread to trunk, extremities	Disseminated disease, pneumonia, hepatitis, coagulopathy, pneumonia, encephalitis, bacterial superinfection with *Streptococcus pyogenes*, *Staphylococcus aureus*
Roseola (HHV-6, 7)	High fever	Red macules soft palate	Red maculopapular rash on trunk Rash appears after resolution of fever	Seizures, (disseminated disease in immunosuppressed hosts)
Parvovirus (Fifth Disease)	Low fever, malaise	None	Slapped cheeks, lacy reticular rash trunk and extremities	Arthritis/arthralgia, transient aplastic anemia in patients with hemolytic anemia, fetal infection, chronic infection in immunosuppressed
Enteroviruses	Mild upper respiratory or gastrointestinal symptoms	Small vesicles or ulcers in posterior pharynx	Pustular or vesicular lesions on hands and feet, maculopapular rash	Aseptic meningitis, myocarditis
Neonatal HSV	Poor feeding, lethargy	Vesicular lesions	Grouped vesicles on an erythematous base	Disseminated infection causing hepatitis, pneumonia, disseminated intravascular coagulation, death, encephalitis

Laboratory Evaluation

Diagnosis is based on clinical findings, exposure, and immunization history, as well as positive serology. IgM antibody against measles is present for approximately 1 month after the onset of symptoms. Paired acute and convalescent sera demonstrating a significant rise in measles IgG are diagnostic. It is possible to culture measles virus from nasopharyngeal specimens, urine, and blood. It is important to notify the local health department immediately about suspected cases of measles to expedite processing of specimens and to identify possible sources and contacts.

Differential Diagnosis

The differential diagnosis of measles includes other viral and bacterial exanthems, Kawasaki disease, and drug allergy.

Management

Treatment

Supportive treatment is appropriate for most cases of measles. If bacterial superinfection is suspected, antibiotic therapy is necessary. Generally, specific antiviral therapy is not recommended. Ribavirin, which has in vitro activity against measles virus, has been used in intravenous or aerosolized form in some cases of severe disease.

Severe measles may occur in children with decreased serum levels of vitamin A. Although vitamin A deficiency is not a major problem in the United States, supplementation is considered in young children ($\geq$ 6 months of age) who either have complications of measles, malnutrition, immunodeficiency, and impaired intestinal absorption or who are recent immigrants from countries with high mortality rates due to measles.

Prevention

Effective prevention of measles involves vaccination. The AAP recommends that children receive two doses of live attenuated measles vaccine, one at 12–15 months of age and one at 4–6 years of age (see Figure 2.10). The trivalent measles, mumps, and rubella vaccine (MMR) is most commonly used in the United States. The measles vaccine is a live attenuated vaccine, which means that it is not appropriate for immunosuppressed children and pregnant women, except in the case of HIV-positive children who are not severely immunologically impaired. Transmission of measles virus by vaccine does not occur, so there is no contraindication to immunization of household con-

tacts. Adverse effects of vaccine include fever, rash, and thrombocytopenia.

The "Red Book" published by the Committee of Infectious Diseases of the AAP contains details about the measles vaccine, including guidelines for its use in epidemic circumstances or in susceptible adolescents and adults. Immunoglobulin products interfere with serologic response to measles vaccine. Clinicians should consult the AAP recommendations if they have a patient who has received an immunoglobulin product or blood transfusion to determine the appropriate interval before vaccine may be administered.

To prevent the development or decrease the severity of symptoms of measles in exposed nonvaccinated individuals, intramuscular immune globulin is useful. To be effective, the agent must be given within 6 days of exposure.

RUBELLA (SEE TABLE 9.24)

Rubella (German measles, **third disease**) is a moderately contagious disease, with most cases seen in late winter or early spring. The disease is now uncommon in the United States. During 1964, an epidemic of rubella resulted in over 12 million cases of rubella and 20,000 cases of **congenital rubella syndrome**. After rubella vaccine was licensed in 1969, the number of cases of the disease declined by 99%. Most rubella infections are seen in unimmunized Hispanic young adults, and all recent cases of congenital rubella syndrome have occurred in children of unvaccinated women born in Latin America.

Pediatric Pearl

It is important to recognize and diagnose rubella infection, because transmission of rubella virus to pregnant nonimmune women often results in severe congenital infection.

Pathophysiology

Skin eruptions in rubella result from direct infection of the dermis. The most common complications of rubella are arthritis and arthralgia. Joint abnormalities are rare in children but occur often in adult women. Fingers, wrists, and knees are most frequently affected.

Rubella infection during the early part of pregnancy is disastrous, leading to fetal death, premature delivery, or multiple congenital anomalies. All fetal organs may be affected. Abnormalities seen in congenital rubella syndrome include sensorineural hearing loss, cataracts, heart defects [usually patent ductus arteriosus (PDA), pulmonic artery stenosis, pulmonic valve stenosis], microcephaly and mental retardation, splenomegaly, hepatitis, and thrombocytopenia. Diabetes mellitus and progressive panencephalitis are late complications of congenital rubella syndrome.

Clinical and Laboratory Evaluation

History
It is important to obtain an immunization and contact history about any child who presents with a nonspecific viral exanthem. The prodrome, which does not occur in all cases, consists of low-grade fever, malaise, lymphadenopathy, and upper respiratory tract infection.

Physical Examination
Children appear well or mildly ill. Lymphadenopathy involving posterior auricular, suboccipital, and posterior cervical nodes may be present; the nodes remain enlarged for several weeks. An often pruritic rash, which occurs 1–5 days after prodromal symptoms, begins on the face and progresses caudally. It is fainter than the rash seen with measles and does not coalesce.

Laboratory Evaluation
Diagnosis is difficult, because many patients appear to have a nonspecific viral illness. Serology is the usual method for confirming a case of rubella. Reliable evidence of acute infection includes the presence of rubella IgM or a significant rise in rubella IgG demonstrated on paired acute and convalescent sera. Rubella virus is cultured from nasal specimens, throat swabs, blood, urine, and CSF. It is important to alert the laboratory about suspected rubella to facilitate appropriate testing. As with measles, it is necessary to notify local health departments about suspected cases of rubella.

Differential Diagnosis

The rash of rubella is difficult to distinguish from other viral rashes such as those seen with enterovirus, parvovirus B19, HHV-6, and Epstein-Barr virus infection.

Management

Supportive treatment is appropriate for rubella. Prevention involves vaccination. Rubella vaccine is a live attenuated viral vaccine administered as MMR at 12–15 months of age and 4–6 years of age (see Figure 2.10). All pregnant women have rubella serology as part of routine prenatal screening, and any woman found to be rubella nonimmune receives vaccine during the postpartum period. Vaccine is not appropriate for pregnant women. Recent administration of immune globulin preparations or blood products interferes with antibody response to vaccine. Children with altered immunity should not receive live virus vaccine during the time they are immunosuppressed. Adverse effects of vaccine include fever, lymphadenopathy, joint pain, and thrombocytopenia.

ROSEOLA (SEE TABLE 9.24)

Roseola (exanthem subitum, sixth disease), which results from infection with HHV-6 and occasionally HHV-7 virus, is an acute febrile illness followed by a rash. Infection with HHV-6 is common, and seroprevalence in most countries approaches 100% in children over 2 years of age. HHV-6 has two variants (A or B) based on genetic and phenotypic variations; variant B (HHV-6B) causes roseola.

Complications are uncommon. Seizures occur in 10%–15% of children during the febrile period (see Table 9.24). Occasionally, roseola infection in healthy children results in a mononucleosis-like syndrome characterized by lymphadenopathy and hepatitis.

Pathophysiology

Acute primary infection with HHV-6 occurs in infants who are 4–6 months of age or older. Virus is acquired from close contact with infected saliva from parents or siblings. After primary infection, the virus remains latent in mononuclear cells and likely persists in other tissue. Replication of virus in salivary glands accounts for the salivary route of transmission. Reactivation of virus is rarely associated with symptoms unless children are immunosuppressed. Symptoms associated with reactivation include fever, bone marrow suppression, hepatitis, pneumonia, and encephalitis.

Clinical and Laboratory Evaluation

History
Parents report a history of few prodromal symptoms and abrupt onset of high fever. The fever lasts for 3–7 days. Disease is typically mild. Occasionally respiratory or GI symptoms are present.

Physical Examination

Children have a high fever and are mildly ill or irritable. Except for the high temperature, vital signs are normal. Cervical lymphadenopathy or AOM may be present. Skin perfusion is normal. It is necessary to perform a careful examination to exclude SBI. Resolution of fever is followed by development of an erythematous maculopapular rash that resolves spontaneously. The rash may not appear until 1–2 days after fever breaks.

Laboratory Evaluation

Diagnosis of roseola is based on clinical findings. The CBC, if obtained, shows lymphocytosis and neutropenia. Serology is difficult to interpret, because a significant increase in HHV-6 IgG is seen after both primary infection and reactivation of disease. Techniques for culture of virus from peripheral blood mononuclear cells or detection of virus by PCR are available in some research laboratories. So far no technique has proved useful in differentiating primary infection from reactivation.

Differential Diagnosis

Conditions to be ruled out include occult bacteremia or another hidden source of bacterial infection such as a urinary tract infection.

Management

Supportive treatment, with antipyretic therapy, is appropriate.

PARVOVIRUS B19 (SEE TABLE 9.24)

Infection with parvovirus B19, which is known by a variety of different names, including **erythema infectiosum, fifth disease,** and **slapped cheek disease,** causes mild illness. Approximately 20% of infected persons are asymptomatic.

By the time they are 15 years of age, about 50% of children have antibody to parvovirus B19, with increasing rates of seroprevalence through adulthood. The usual mode of transmission is by contact with respiratory secretions. In addition, transmission by percutaneous exposure to blood or by mother-to-fetus also occur. Mother-to-fetus transmission causes fetal hydrops and death; however, risk is low (~ 5%).

Pathophysiology

The rash associated with parvovirus B19 is the result of an immune-mediated response. Children are most contagious during the prodromal period before the rash appears. After initial infection of the respiratory tract, viremia occurs with subsequent viral attachment to the P antigen on RBC precursors. Appearance of parvovirus-specific IgG correlates with protection from disease.

Arthralgia and arthritis may develop in adult women as the result of infection with parvovirus B19. Commonly affected joints include those of the hands, wrists, and knees. Joint pain and swelling usually resolve after 1–2 weeks, although symptoms may persist for months.

Because parvovirus B19 infects RBC precursors, most infected children experience mild and transient anemia. Children with disorders characterized by increased RBC turnover (e.g., sickle cell disease, glucose-6-phosphate dehydrogenase deficiency, autoimmune hemolytic anemia) develop transient aplastic crisis. Patients with immunodeficiency are at risk for chronic parvovirus infection and bone marrow failure. Parvovirus B19 infection is also reported to cause neutropenia and thrombocytopenia.

Clinical and Laboratory Evaluation

History

Children come to medical attention only after the rash appears. Illness is usually mild. Most children have a prodrome of low-grade fever, upper respiratory tract symptoms, and mild malaise.

Physical Examination

Children are well-appearing, with a low-grade fever or sometimes none at all. A red, flat rash on the cheeks and a lacy, reticular, often pruritic, rash on the trunk and extremities is notable. The rash becomes more intense if children are exposed to warm temperatures (e.g., a bath). The duration of the rash is approximately 7–10 days.

Examination of the joints for presence of arthralgia or arthritis is warranted. Complications of erythema infectiosum are uncommon in healthy children.

Laboratory Evaluation

Diagnosis in healthy children is made by clinical signs and symptoms. Laboratory work reveals mild anemia and a low reticulocyte count. Severe anemia is present in aplastic crisis. Serum IgM is more than 90% sensitive in identifying recently infected individuals, and serum IgG indicates previous infection and immunity. Serum DNA PCR is the preferred method of detection of parvovirus B19 infection in immunocompromised hosts.

Differential Diagnosis

The differential diagnosis of parvovirus B19 infection includes rubella, enterovirus infection, and drug reaction. If arthritis is present, juvenile rheumatoid arthritis or other collagen vascular diseases must be considered.

Management

Treatment is not necessary in most children.

Pediatric Pearl

In patients with parvovirus, when the rash appears, children are not contagious, and it is not necessary to keep them home from school or day-care facilities.

Isolation for 7 days is necessary for children with transient aplastic crisis, who often have no rash. Hospitalized, immunosuppressed children require isolation for the duration of hospitalization because of risk of prolonged viral shedding. Intravenous immune globulin may be effective in children with immunodeficiency or transient aplastic crisis. Intrauterine blood transfusion has been useful in the treatment of hydrops fetalis resulting from parvovirus B19.

CHICKENPOX (VARICELLA) [SEE TABLE 9.24]

Chickenpox results from primary infection with varicella-zoster virus.

Pathophysiology

Infection is characterized by a generalized pruritic vesicular rash. Children are contagious from 1–2 days prior to the onset of the rash until the lesions have crusted. During primary infection, varicella-zoster virus establishes latency in dorsal root ganglia. Reactivation of virus results in **herpes zoster (shingles)**.

The most common complication of chickenpox is bacterial superinfection with *S. pyogenes* or *S. aureus*. Parents of children who suffer from this complication often report that children were improving and afebrile with crusting lesions when they developed a new fever late in the course of illness. SBIs include pyogenic arthritis, osteomyelitis, pneumonia, bacteremia, and necrotizing fasciitis. Nonbacterial complications of chickenpox include pneumonia, cerebellar ataxia, encephalitis, hepatitis, hemorrhagic varicella, and arthritis. Disseminated varicella-zoster virus infection may cause death in immunocompromised patients as well as in healthy patients with a history of recent steroid therapy.

Clinical and Laboratory Evaluation

History

Children with chickenpox have a history of contact with another infected person within the previous 10–21 days. Although mild cases of varicella may occur in children who have been vaccinated against the disease, children usually have no history of varicella immunization. Prodromal symptoms include fever and malaise.

Physical Examination

Fever is often present. The child appears mildly to moderately ill. In cases of disseminated chickenpox or bacterial superinfection, the child may appear very ill. The rash begins on the neck, face, or upper trunk and spreads outward over the next 3–5 days. Mucous membranes may be involved. Lesions initially appear as small papules on an erythematous base. The papules evolve into vesicles that eventually form crusts. The rash is often intensely pruritic. It is important to inspect the rash for signs of hemorrhage or infection.

Lung examination may reveal signs of pneumonia caused by varicella-zoster virus or bacteria. Careful examination of the bones and joints may indicate infection caused by *S. aureus* or *S. pyogenes*. Neurologic examination may reveal cerebellar ataxia.

Laboratory Evaluation

Diagnosis of varicella is based on clinical findings. If the diagnosis is uncertain, it may be necessary to send scrapings of the bases of vesicular lesions for direct fluorescent antibody testing specific for varicella-zoster virus. A Tzanck smear reveals multinucleated giant cells; however, it is not specific for varicella-zoster virus and is less sensitive and accurate than direct fluorescent antibody. It is also possible to culture virus from lesions, but results are not immediately available.

Blood culture is warranted if bacterial superinfection is suspected. Chest radiograph, CBC, coagulation screen, and liver enzymes may be appropriate in ill-appearing children.

Management

Supportive treatment is appropriate for uncomplicated chickenpox in normal hosts. Acyclovir is useful in immunocompromised patients or patients with complications of disease. Antibiotics with activity against *S. pyogenes* and *S. aureus* may be effective in cases of suspected bacterial infection.

Prevention involves varicella vaccine, which is a live attenuated viral vaccine approved for children 12 months of age or older. The vaccine is not recommended for use in immunocompromised individuals or pregnant women; its use is under consideration in immunologically normal HIV-infected children. Varicella-zoster immune globulin is used for passive immunoprophylaxis in patients exposed to varicella who are at risk for severe disease. Administration should occur within 96 hours of exposure. Candidates include susceptible pregnant women, newborns whose mothers develop chickenpox shortly before or after delivery, premature infants, and immunocompromised children.

BACTERIAL EXANTHEMS

STREPTOCOCCUS PYOGENES INFECTION

The rash of **scarlet fever** results from the vascular effects of streptococcal pyrogenic exotoxins A, B, and C produced by *S. pyogenes*. This organism also directly infects skin and soft tissue, causing **impetigo, cellulitis, erysipelas,** and **necrotizing fasciitis**. Various clinical findings are associated with these conditions (Table 9.25).

TABLE 9.25 **Skin and Soft Tissue Manifestations of *Streptococcus pyogenes* and *Staphylococcus aureus***

Organism	Disease	Clinical Findings
Streptococcus pyogenes (GABHS)	Scarlet fever	See text
	Impetigo	Afebrile, honey-crusted pustular skin lesions
	Erysipelas	Fever, well-demarcated erythematous advancing superficial skin infection
	Cellulitis	Fever, pain, deeper infection of subcutaneous tissue
	Necrotizing fasciitis	Fever, pain out of proportion to skin findings, bullous lesions or erythema, tissue necrosis
	STSS*	Fever, erythematous macular rash, hypotension, renal impairment, coagulopathy, liver dysfunction, respiratory distress, soft tissue necrosis
Staphylococcus aureus	Staphylococcal scarlet fever	Same as *S. pyogenes* scarlet fever except no pharyngitis or enanthem
	Impetigo	Afebrile, honey-crusted pustular skin lesions
	Folliculitis	Infection of hair follicle
	Staphylococcal scalded skin syndrome	Fever, tender erythematous skin, bullous lesions, positive Nikolsky sign
	Toxic shock syndrome	Fever, erythroderma (sunburn-like rash), hypotension, mucous membrane hyperemia, vomiting and diarrhea, myalgia, renal and hepatic dysfunction, thrombocytopenia, altered level of consciousness

GABHS = group A beta-hemolytic streptococcus; STSS = streptococcal toxic shock syndrome.

Clinical and Laboratory Evaluation

History

Prodromal symptoms of scarlet fever include fever, pharyngitis, chills, and abdominal pain. The rash appears 1–2 days after initial symptoms.

Physical Examination

Most children with scarlet fever are only mildly ill. The rash of scarlet fever is erythematous and blanching, with fine, sandpaper-like papules on palpation. It is most prominent in warm, moist areas such as the neck, axillae, and groin and spares the area around the mouth (circumoral pallor). Other skin findings include petechiae and areas of hyperpigmentation in skin creases (Pastia lines). Approximately 1 week after the rash appears, fine desquamation begins on the face and spreads to the trunk and extremities.

Laboratory Evaluation (see PHARYNGITIS)

Differential Diagnosis

Other causes of a rash resembling scarlet fever may occur after infection with *S. aureus* or *A. haemolyticum*. A scarlet fever–like rash may also occur in association with streptococcal disease other than pharyngitis (e.g., bone or joint infection, pneumonia, streptococcal toxic shock syndrome).

Management (see PHARYNGITIS)

Parenteral antibiotics administered in the hospital are necessary for treatment of serious infections associated with scarlatiniform rash.

STAPHYLOCOCCUS AUREUS INFECTION

Infection with *S. aureus* causes a variety of skin manifestations (see Table 9.25). Strains of this bacterium produce an exfoliative toxin that cause **bullous impetigo, staphylococcal scalded skin syndrome,** or a **scarlatiniform eruption** similar to the rash seen with streptococcal scarlet fever. **Cellulitis,** which occurs after direct infection of skin and subcutaneous tissues with *S. aureus,* is usually the result of trauma to the skin but occasionally occurs with hematogenous dissemination of bacteria. A diffuse sunburn-like rash (**erythroderma**) is seen with staphylococcal **toxic shock syndrome** (TSS) caused by TSS toxin-1–producing strains of *S. aureus.*

Pathophysiology

Pathogenesis of infection is either by direct invasion of tissue or by effects of toxin-producing organisms distant from the site of the skin lesion.

Clinical and Laboratory Evaluation (see Table 9.25)

S. aureus is easily cultured from skin lesions or other sources of infection. If *S. aureus* is isolated from blood, tissue, or CSF, susceptibility testing to identify possible methicillin resistance is necessary.

Management

Treatment for **impetigo** is either a topical antistaphylococcal ointment such as mupirocin or an oral antistaphylococcal antibiotic such as dicloxacillin or a first-generation cephalosporin. Treatment for **cellulitis** or other serious staphylococcal infection is intravenous antibiotics. Drugs used include nafcillin, cefazolin, and clindamycin. Vancomycin is useful for suspected methicillin resistance. Treatment for suspected **TSS** involves admission for supportive care and intravenous antibiotics, with identification and removal of the source of infection (e.g., tampon, staphylococcal abscess).

ROCKY MOUNTAIN SPOTTED FEVER (*RICKETTSIA RICKETTSII*)

Rocky Mountain spotted fever is a rickettsial infection associated with skin rash. Despite its name, this disease is reported throughout the United States, although it is most commonly seen in Oklahoma, Kansas, Missouri, Arkansas, North Carolina, and Tennessee, particularly from late spring through fall.

Pathophysiology

Inoculation of *R. rickettsii* into the dermis, with subsequent infection of endothelial cells, occurs via a tick bite. The incubation period is 2–14 days. After replication and dissemination of bacteria, vascular inflammation is associated with a petechial or maculopapular rash. Unrecognized and untreated infection results in multisystem organ involvement, vascular obstruction, disseminated intravascular coagulation (DIC), and occasionally death.

Clinical and Laboratory Evaluation

History

Children may have a history of tick exposure in an endemic area. Prodromal symptoms are nonspecific and include headache, fever, and malaise. Nausea, vomiting, abdominal pain, and diarrhea may be present.

Physical Examination

Children are febrile and ill appearing. **The rash, which appears after the third day of illness, is unique in that it begins peripherally on the wrists, ankles, and lower legs and spreads centrally.** The soles and palms may be involved. Initial lesions are erythematous blanching macules or papules that evolve over several days into petechiae or purpura. A small percentage of patients with Rocky Mountain spotted fever do not have rash.

Laboratory Evaluation

A rickettsial group-specific serologic test confirms the diagnosis. A skin biopsy of petechial lesions detects *R. rickettsii* antigen. A CBC may reveal thrombocytopenia and leukopenia.

Management

Children with suspected Rocky Mountain spotted fever warrant admission to the hospital for administration of antibiotics, ideally, before day 5 of the illness. Antibiotics used to treat other childhood bacterial infections (e.g., penicillins, cephalosporins, macrolides) have no activity against *R. rickettsii*. Use of tetracyclines, including doxycycline, is generally not recommended in children 8 years of age or younger because of risk of discoloration of tooth enamel. However, with suspected Rocky Mountain spotted fever, the benefit of using doxycycline outweighs the small risk of tooth discoloration.

NEISSERIA MENINGITIDIS INFECTION

N. meningitidis, a small gram-negative diplococcus, causes a spectrum of diseases, including chronic bacteremia, acute bacteremia with sepsis, meningitis, and localized infection (pneumonia, arthritis). Chronic meningococcal infection is characterized by recurrent episodes of fever, rash, and arthralgia.

Pathophysiology

N. meningitidis causes disease when bacteria disseminate through the upper respiratory tract into the bloodstream.

Clinical and Laboratory Evaluation

History

Children with acute bacteremia often have a prodrome of fever, pharyngitis, and headache. They may have a history of contact with a family member or friend with *N. meningitidis* infection.

Physical Examination

Children are febrile and appear mildly to severely ill. Hypotension, poor perfusion, and cyanosis may be present. Petechial or purpuric skin lesions occur in approximately 70% of children; clinicians have reported finding other types of skin rash, including maculopapular and pustular lesions. Signs of meningitis, pneumonia, or joint infection may be evident.

Laboratory Evaluation

Diagnosis of meningococcal disease is made by isolation of the organism from blood or CSF.

Differential Diagnosis

Differential diagnosis of petechial rash includes enteroviral infection, idiopathic thrombocytopenic purpura, and leukemia.

Management

Hospital admission for antibiotics and supportive care is necessary. Penicillin remains the drug of choice for treatment. In the United States, some isolates with decreased susceptibility to penicillin have been reported and resistance is widely reported in other parts of the world. Third-generation cephalosporins are acceptable alternatives for therapy.

It is necessary to notify the local health department immediately about suspected or proven cases of meningococcal disease. Close contacts of index cases are at high risk for colonization with *N. meningitidis* and are candidates for prophylaxis. Antibiotics used for prophylaxis include rifampin, ceftriaxone, and ciprofloxacin.

OTHER INFECTIOUS DISEASES

PEDIATRIC HUMAN IMMUNODEFICIENCY VIRUS INFECTION

Since the beginning of the **human immunodeficiency virus (HIV)** epidemic, over 16,000 children in the United States have been infected with HIV. **Acquired immunodeficiency syndrome (AIDS)** is the severe end of the clinical spectrum of disease caused by HIV. Over 90% of pediatric cases of AIDS result from perinatal transmission. A small percentage of children acquire HIV through contaminated blood transfusion or blood products. An increasing number of adolescents acquire the virus through intravenous drug use or heterosexual and homosexual contact.

The number of children with perinatally acquired HIV infection has decreased steadily since 1992. The decline in the transmission of HIV that has occurred over the past 10 years is attributed to the use of zidovudine and other antiretroviral agents in pregnant women. Approximately 25%–30% infants born to untreated HIV-positive mothers are infected with the virus. Zidovudine treatment of mothers during pregnancy and delivery with prophylaxis of newborns decreases the rate of transmission to approximately 8%. The rate of transmission is likely even lower if the mother is receiving highly active antiretroviral therapy and has a low or undetectable HIV viral load.

Pathophysiology

HIV is a member of the Retroviridae family in the genus lentivirus. The initial cellular targets of HIV are Langerhans cells in the genital mucosa; viral glycoprotein 120 attaches to the CD4+ molecule on the cells, and coreceptors (either CCR5 or CXCR4) facilitate entry of the virus into the cell. Infected cells fuse with CD4 lymphocytes and spread to deeper tissues. After virus is internalized in the host cell and uncoated, viral reverse transcriptase facilitates transcription of viral RNA into DNA. The DNA is transported into the nucleus of the host cell and subsequent synthesis of new viral polyprotein occurs. HIV protease must cleave the large polyprotein into several smaller proteins for newly synthesized virions to mature and become infectious. Mature HIV virions are released from the host cell and reinitiate the life cycle by infecting other CD4+ target cells.

Virus is detectable in regional lymph nodes within 2 days of infection and in plasma 4–11 days after infection. An initial rapid rise in plasma viremia occurs with a subsequent marked reduction in plasma viral RNA to a "viral set point." The amount of viral RNA (or viral load) is usually higher in infected infants than in older children and adults.

Clinical and Laboratory Evaluation

History

It is necessary to obtain a careful social history from the child's parents to elicit risk factors for disease. However, the absence of apparent risk factors does not rule out HIV disease. It is important to discuss previous HIV test results and exposure history (intravenous drug use, sexual behavior, transfusions) in a sensitive and confidential manner. Partners and extended family members are often unaware of an individual's risk factors. A negative HIV antibody test during pregnancy is reassuring but does not rule out infection after testing was performed.

Pediatric Pearl

It is important to offer HIV testing to all pregnant women, because appropriate antiretroviral therapy during pregnancy and delivery and antiretroviral prophylaxis for the infant is proven to prevent perinatally acquired HIV infection.

Signs of primary HIV infection are rare in infants. Adolescents and adults often have symptoms of an acute illness similar to infectious mononucleosis (Table 9.26). Children with perinatally acquired HIV infection are often asymptomatic at birth but develop signs and symptoms of disease as they grow older; most have historical and clinical findings of HIV infection by 18–24 months of age. A small number of infected children come to medical attention within the first 2 or 3 months of life when they develop *Pneumocystis carinii* pneumonia (PCP) or disseminated cytomegalovirus infection. Medical history of the child may reveal poor growth, recurrent otitis media or respiratory infections, mild developmental delay, diarrhea, chronic thrush or diaper rash.

Physical Examination

Several abnormalities are apparent on physical examination (Table 9.27).

TABLE 9.26 **Signs and Symptoms of Acute Human Immunodeficiency Virus Infection in Adolescents and Adults**

Clinical features
Fever
Fatigue
Rash
Headache
Lymphadenopathy
Pharyngitis
Myalgia or arthralgia
Nausea/vomiting/diarrhea

Laboratory findings
Thrombocytopenia
Leukopenia
Elevated hepatic enzymes

TABLE 9.27 Abnormalities on Physical Examination Seen in Children with Perinatal HIV Infection

General
Failure to thrive

HEENT Examination
Acute or chronic otitis media
Eye abnormalities (cytomegalovirus retinitis)
Thrush, aphthous stomatitis
Chronic parotid gland enlargement
Diffuse cervical lymphadenopathy

Lungs
Chronic cough
Adventitial sounds on auscultation including wheezes, rhonchi

Heart
Tachycardia
Irregular rhythm

Abdomen
Hepatomegaly
Splenomegaly

Neurologic examination
Spasticity
Developmental delay

Skin
Diaper rash
Seborrhea
Eczema
Papillomavirus (warts)
Molluscum contagiosum

HEENT = head, eye, ear, nose, and throat; HIV = human immunodeficiency virus.

Laboratory Evaluation

Before testing children for HIV, it is necessary to obtain informed consent from a parent or legal guardian. For **exposed infants,** testing involves the use of the PCR for HIV viral DNA. Testing is performed within 48 hours of birth and repeated at 1 month and at 3 months of age. Some experts recommend repeat testing at 2 weeks of age. Serologic testing of perinatally exposed infants confirms exposure but not infection, because a positive test may reflect transplacentally acquired antibody. It is necessary to repeat a positive HIV test to confirm the diagnosis.

For **children over 18 months of age,** standard serologic testing is sufficient. Serologic tests are negative until 3–4 weeks after acute infection. A positive enzyme-linked immunoassay (ELISA) test is confirmed by Western blot. For **adoles-**cents and adults, diagnosis of acute HIV syndrome involves detection of HIV viral RNA in plasma. Viral RNA is detectable in plasma 1–3 weeks before the antibody test is positive.

After establishing the diagnosis of HIV infection, it is appropriate to determine a child's immunologic status based on the percent of CD4+ lymphocytes and clinical symptoms (Table 9.28). Children infected with HIV typically have a decrease in the number of CD4+ lymphocytes and an increase in the number of CD8+ lymphocytes, which results in an inverted CD4+:CD8+ ratio (usually < 1.0). The normal number of CD4+ and CD8+ lymphocytes varies with age, with higher numbers in infants.

Routine laboratory tests are appropriate. A CBC may reveal mild leukopenia, anemia, or thrombocytopenia. Transaminases may be mildly elevated.

Management

Although there is no cure for HIV infection, the use of highly active antiretroviral therapy is successful in suppressing viral load and preventing destruction of CD4+ lymphocytes. Three classes of antiretroviral drugs are currently licensed (Table 9.29).

The **nucleoside analog reverse transcriptase inhibitors** (NRTIs) prevent transcription of viral RNA into DNA. They compete with cellular deoxynucleoside triphosphates, and after being incorporated into the growing DNA strand, they cause premature termination of the HIV DNA intermediate. The thymidine analogs stavudine (d4T) and zidovudine (AZT) target activated CD4+ cells, and the nonthymidine analogs didanosine (ddI) and lamivudine (3TC) target resting CD4+ cells. A general principle regarding therapy with NRTIs involves pairing a thymidine analog with a nonthymidine analog (e.g., AZT plus 3TC). The **nonnucleoside analog reverse transcriptase inhibitors** (NNRTIs) prevent transcription of viral RNA into DNA by noncompetitive binding of viral reverse transcriptase. The **protease inhibitors,** which bind to specific cleavage sites on the HIV polyprotein, prevent viral protease from cleaving the larger polypeptide into smaller mature virions.

Recommendations for initial therapy should take into account the child's immunologic status, viral load, and ability and willingness to comply with medication regimen. Poor compliance contributes to development of resistant virus. Compliance is better with twice-daily dosing.

In HIV-infected children, initial antiretroviral

TABLE 9.28 Clinical and Immunologic Categories of Pediatric Human Immunodeficiency Virus Infection

CLINICAL CLASSIFICATION

N   No signs of symptoms of illness
A   Mild signs and symptoms
B   Moderate signs and symptoms
C   Severe signs and symptoms

IMMUNOLOGIC CATEGORY

	CD4+ Count (μl) By Age (%)		
	< 12 months	**1–5 years**	**6–12 years**
No evidence of suppression	≥ 1500 (≥ 25)	≥ 1000 (≥ 25)	≥ 500 (≥ 25)
Moderate suppression	750–1499 (15–24)	500–999 (15–24)	200–499 (15–24)
Severe suppression	< 750 (< 15)	< 500 (< 15)	< 200 (< 15)

HIV = human immunodeficiency virus.

treatment typically includes two NRTIs plus either a protease inhibitor or an NNRTI. For example, zidovudine/lamivudine plus either nelfinavir or efavirenz might be appropriate. In infants born to HIV-positive women, prophylaxis with AZT is essential, and babies should receive oral AZT 2 mg/kg/dose four times a day for 6 weeks. HIV virus is present in breast milk; therefore, breastfeeding is not recommended. A specialist in pediatric HIV infection should follow all infants exposed to HIV.

After the initiation of therapy, it is necessary to monitor children monthly for immunologic and virologic response and for adverse drug effects. During the first 3–6 months of treatment, the clinician may expect to see an increase in CD4+ lymphocyte count and significant decrease in viral load (often to undetectable levels). Adverse effects of antiretroviral therapy include anemia, elevated transaminases, pancreatitis, and hyperlipidemia. The most common complication of AZT prophylaxis in infants is anemia.

Children with HIV infection are at risk for opportunistic infections such as PCP, infection caused by *Mycobacterium avium-intracellulare*, *Cryptococcus neoformans*, cytomegalovirus, and toxoplasmosis. Infants exposed to HIV at birth receive prophylaxis for PCP beginning at 4–6 weeks of age until the diagnosis of HIV is excluded. If the child is infected, prophylaxis is continued until 12 months of age. After 12 months of age, the decision to give PCP prophylaxis is based on the CD4+ lymphocyte count. (For specific recommendations concerning prophylaxis, see SUGGESTED READINGS.)

TABLE 9.29 Antiretroviral Drugs Most Commonly Used in Children

Nucleoside analog reverse transcriptase inhibitors

Zidovudine (ZDV, AZT/Retrovir)
Stavudine (d4T, Zerit)
Didanosine (ddI, Videx)
Lamivudine (3TC, Epivir)
Abacavir (ABC, Ziagen)

Nonnucleoside analog reverse transcriptase inhibitors

Nevirapine (Virammune)
Efavirenz (Sustiva)

Protease inhibitors

Nelfinavir (Viracept)
Ritonavir (Norvir)
Saquinavir (Fortovase)
Indinavir (Crixivan)
Lopinavir/ritonavir (Kaletra)

TUBERCULOSIS

Worldwide, infection with *M. tuberculosis* causes an estimated 1.3 million cases of disease and 450,000 deaths annually among children younger than 15 years of age. In the United States, the incidence of tuberculosis is highest in nonwhite racial and ethnic groups, particularly in low socioeconomic populations or urban areas. Tuberculosis in young children differs from that in adolescents and adults. Children are at increased risk of extrapulmonary disease due to lymphohematogenous spread of bacteria. The risk of disseminated disease (miliary and CNS) is greatest in children younger than 4 years of age.

> ### Pediatric Pearl
>
> **The diagnosis of tuberculosis infection or disease in a child is a sentinel event signaling the presence of other cases in the household or community.**

The source of infection in children is usually a household contact. Casual contact such as in school or a day-care center is less frequently the source of transmission. Children younger than 12 years of age are unlikely to transmit infection, because they rarely have cavitary lesions with large numbers of organisms, and they usually do not cough or produce sputum. It is worth noting that an individual whose sputum smear is positive for acid-fast bacilli is more contagious than one who has a positive culture but a negative sputum smear.

By definition, children who have recently been in contact with a person who has contagious pulmonary tuberculosis have been exposed to the disease. In asymptomatic individuals, latent tuberculosis infection is defined as a positive tuberculin skin test (PPD). The chest radiograph is either normal or shows granulomas or calcification in the lung and regional lymph nodes. Individuals with tuberculosis disease have a positive PPD, symptoms, abnormal findings on physical examination, and an abnormal chest radiograph or evidence of extrapulmonary disease. Many clinical forms of tuberculosis exist (Table 9.30).

Pathophysiology

Tuberculosis is transmitted when a contagious person coughs and releases infected droplets of mucus into the air. Infection begins when the infected droplet nucleus reaches a pulmonary alveolus. A pulmonary macrophage or neutrophil ingests the bacteria, which begins to multiply. Within a few weeks, the pathogen spreads through regional lymphatics to lymph nodes in the hilum. A few bacilli enter the bloodstream and are spread throughout the body. Approximately 3–12 weeks after infection, a T lymphocyte—mediated inflammatory response facilitates enhanced phagocytosis and killing of intracellular organisms. The inflammatory response corresponds to the time the PPD becomes positive. At this time, a **primary complex** may be visible on the chest radiograph, consisting of a focus of infection in the subpleural area, hilar adenopathy, and a localized pleural effusion.

Clinical and Laboratory Evaluation

History

History focuses on travel and exposure to ill family members or friends. Recent immigrants, homeless children, or individuals who have been exposed to intravenous drug users or HIV-positive persons are at increased risk for tuberculosis.

The clinical manifestations of the disease are diverse and subtle. Multiple foci of infection are sometimes present in children. *M. tuberculosis* may infect the eyes, ears, skin, bone (particularly vertebral bodies), genitourinary tract, and cause intra-abdominal infection. Mothers with untreated tuberculosis during pregnancy transmit infection to the fetus.

Physical Examination

Pertinent findings include weight loss, fever, lymphadenitis, hepatosplenomegaly, abnormalities on neurologic examination, and skin lesions (rare). Lung findings with pulmonary tuberculosis include cough, decreased breath sounds, and dullness to percussion over the affected areas of the lung. Rales are often present.

Tuberculous lymphadenitis (scrofula) is the most common extrapulmonary manifestation. Large, nontender, rubbery, matted anterior cervical or submandibular lymph nodes are evident. Bilateral lymphadenopathy may be present. Signs of acute inflammation such as redness, warmth, erythema, and tenderness are absent. Over time, infected lymph nodes become fluctuant (softer) as nodes become necrotic. Spontaneous drainage and development of a sinus tract may occur.

Children with **miliary tuberculosis** often appear mildly to moderately ill. Fever is present, and hepatosplenomegaly with diffuse lymphadenopathy is apparent.

Diagnosis of tuberculous **meningitis** is often delayed because initial symptoms, including fever, irritability and poor appetite, are nonspecific (stage I). As infection progresses, children develop vomiting, drowsiness, and cranial nerve palsies (stage II). Infants may have a bulging fontanelle, and stiff neck is present in one-third of patients. Severe changes in mental status, seizures, focal neurologic deficits, and involuntary movements eventually develop (stage III).

Laboratory Evaluation

Diagnosis of tuberculosis depends on clinical, radiographic and laboratory findings. A **positive PPD** is indicative of infection. It is important to measure the area of induration (not erythema) in millimeters around the injection site 48–72

TABLE 9.30 Selected Forms of Tuberculosis	
Clinical Form	**Characteristics**
Pulmonary tuberculosis	
• Primary	Asymptomatic, or cough, fever, weight loss
	Chest radiograph looks worse than patient
	Signs of partial bronchial obstruction such as atelectasis may be present
• Progressive primary	May occur in immunosuppressed child
	Enlargement of primary complex, caseation, and cavitation
	Chest radiograph consistent with bronchopneumonia
• Endobronchial tuberculosis	Partial or complete obstruction of bronchus
	Segmental collapse and consolidation
• Reactivation	Classic "adult" form: results from growth of previously dormant bacilli in lung
	Upper lobe disease with cavity
• Pleural	Rare in children < 6 years
	Occurs 6 months after primary infection
	Fever, chest pain
	Chest radiograph shows pleural effusion and primary parenchymal lesion
• Pericardial	Pericardial effusion
Lymphadenitis	Difficult to differentiate from infection with nontuberculous mycobacteria
	Excision of node confirms diagnosis and cures nontuberculous mycobacteria (incisional biopsy may result in chronic drainage; some success with fine needle aspiration)
	Antituberculous therapy required
Miliary tuberculosis	Occurs early after primary infection
	Young children or immunocompromised patients
	Fever, hepatosplenomegaly, lymphadenopathy
	PPD sometimes negative
	Chest radiograph reveals multiple small lesions
	Must exclude meningitis
	Good prognosis with therapy
Meningitis	Occurs early after primary infection
	Diagnosis difficult (40% of children with negative PPD; 25% of children with normal chest radiograph)
	Cerebrospinal fluid
	• Initial polymorphonuclear cell response, usually 50–500 cells/μl
	• Initial diagnosis is often partially treated bacterial meningitis.
	• As illness progresses, mononuclear cells increase, glucose decreases, protein increases

PPD = purified protein derivative.

hours after intradermal injection of 5 tuberculin units of PPD and note it in the medical record. The definition of a positive PPD depends on the age of the child, immune status, and risk factors for exposure (Table 9.31). The PPD may be negative in infants and in children with miliary disease and immunosuppression.

It is necessary to obtain specimens of sputum for AFB smear and culture. In children unable to produce a good sputum sample, specimens of gastric acid are indicated. Gastric aspirates obtained early in the morning before respiratory secretions swallowed during the night pass out of the stomach are sufficient. Samples are collected as children awaken, before they are allowed to eat. Three specimens are obtained on three successive days.

Gastric aspirates are more sensitive than bron-chial alveolar lavage for isolation of *M. tuberculosis;* the organism can also be isolated from urine, tissue, pleural fluid, and CSF (large volumes of CSF are required). Rapid diagnostic tests, including PCR amplification, are currently under investigation and are not used routinely for diagnosis of tuberculosis in children.

Differential Diagnosis

Differential diagnosis of pulmonary tuberculosis includes bacterial or fungal causes of pneumonia such as *S. pneumoniae, S. aureus, M. pneumoniae,* and *C. immitis.* Children with pulmonary tuberculosis typically have less respiratory distress than children with bacterial pneumonia.

Nontuberculous lymphadenitis is similar in

TABLE 9.31	Definition of Positive Mantoux Skin Test*	

Size of Induration (mm)	Interpretation
≥ 15	Positive at any age
≥ 10	Positive if:
	Underlying disease including lymphoma, diabetes mellitus, renal failure, malnutrition, children (< 4 years of age)
	Increased risk of exposure through travel, birth in a country where disease is common, exposure to adults who are migrant farm workers, homelessness, HIV infection, incarceration or use of intravenous drugs
≥ 5	Positive if:
	Close contacts of known or suspected cases
	Children receiving immunosuppressive therapy or with immunosuppressive diseases
	Children with clinical or chest radiograph evidence suspicious for tuberculosis

*Five tuberculin units of purified protein derivative (PPD). Induration is measured 48–72 hours after placement of PPD.
   HIV = human immunodeficiency virus.

presentation to tuberculous lymphadenitis (Table 9.32). Bacterial lymphadenitis is more likely associated with warmth, erythema, and tenderness of the affected node.

The differential diagnosis of tuberculous meningitis includes infection with fungal organisms such as *C. immitis* or partially treated bacterial meningitis.

Management

If tuberculosis is suspected based on exposure, clinical examination, PPD, or chest radiograph, therapy is initiated pending culture results. *M. tuberculosis* grows slowly. Time to isolation and identification ranges from 2 to 10 weeks. Treatment involves the use of medications.

Natural resistance to currently available antituberculous drugs occurs at a fixed rate. Patients with large numbers of bacteria (e.g., with cavitary disease) are more likely to have organisms resistant to at least one antituberculous medication. For this reason, at least two antituberculous medications must be used to effect cure.

Current recommendations for initial treatment of pulmonary disease and lymphadenitis include at least three antituberculous medications (Table 9.33). With extrapulmonary disease, including meningitis, miliary, or bone and joint disease, treatment involves four drugs at first. In the case of suspected drug resistance, it is necessary to add a fourth drug until results of susceptibility testing are known. Drug resistance is considered if the contact source is from Asia, Africa, Latin America,

TABLE 9.32	Selected Nontuberculous Mycobacteria

Organism	Site of Infection
Slow growers (> 7 days for growth)	
Mycobacterium avium-intracellulare	Bronchopulmonary, lymphadenitis, disseminated (HIV-positive)
M. kansasii	Bronchopulmonary, skeletal, skin and soft tissue, disseminated (HIV-positive)
M. szulgai	Bronchopulmonary
M. scrofulaceum	Bronchopulmonary, lymphadenitis, skeletal
M. haemophilum	Skeletal, skin and soft tissue
Intermediate growers (7–10 days of incubation)	
M. marinum	Skin and soft tissue, less often disseminated disease
Rapid growers (< 7 days for growth on agar)	
M. fortuitum	Skin, soft tissue, disseminated, intravascular device
M. chelonae	Skin, soft tissue, disseminated, intravascular device
M. abscessus	Skin, soft tissue, skeletal, disseminated, bronchopulmonary, catheter

HIV = human immunodeficiency virus.

TABLE 9.33	Drugs Commonly Used for Treatment of Childhood Tuberculosis*	

Name	Dose	Side Effects
Isoniazid (INH)	10–15 mg/kg/day (max 300 mg q day)	Elevated transaminases, hepatitis, peripheral neuritis, rash, nausea/diarrhea
Rifampin (RIF)	10–20 mg/kg/day (max 600 mg q day)	Orange urine and secretions, hepatitis, decreased platelets, vomiting
Pyrazinamide (PZA)	20–40 mg/kg/day (max 2 g q day)	Hepatotoxic, hyperuricemia
Streptomycin (SM)	20–40 mg/kg/day IM (max 1 g q day)	Nephrotoxic, rash, vestibular toxicity
Ethambutol (EMB)	15 mg/kg/day (max 2.5 g q day)	Optic neuritis, decreased red/green color discrimination, nausea/diarrhea, rash

Treatment regimens for Drug-Susceptible Tuberculosis[†]
Pulmonary Tuberculosis/Cervical Lymphadenopathy
Three–four drugs (INH/RIF/PZA plus consider SM or EMB) for 2 months, then INH/RIF[††] for 4 months (total duration of therapy = 6 months)
For hilar adenopathy only: (INH/RIF) [total duration of therapy = 9 months]
Meningitis/Miliary Disease/Bone or Joint Disease
Four drugs (INH/RIF/PZA plus SM or EMB) for 2 months, then INH/RIF for 7–10 months (total duration of therapy = 9–12 months)

*Directly observed therapy (DOT) is recommended for treatment of tuberculosis in the United States
[†]If infection with drug-resistant *M. tuberculosis* is a concern, initial therapy with four drugs is given pending susceptibility testing of the organism.
[††]After the initial 2 months of therapy, twice weekly therapy may be appropriate. The dose of drug may be altered if twice weekly dosing is used; refer to recommendations in the American Academy of Pediatrics: Report of the Committee on Infectious Diseases ("Red Book").

or resides in an urban area with a documented high rate of resistance. Previous treatment for tuberculosis and homelessness are additional risk factors for drug-resistant tuberculosis.

Duration of therapy depends on whether the disease is pulmonary or extrapulmonary. Pulmonary disease is typically treated with an intensive short-course therapy for 6 months. If only hilar adenopathy is present, a 9-month regimen with two drugs (isoniazid and rifampin) is acceptable. Treatment of extrapulmonary tuberculosis continues for 9–12 months.

Isoniazid is indicated for children with a positive PPD and no clinical or chest radiographic evidence of disease. Treatment with one drug is adequate because of the small number of tubercle bacilli present. For most infants and children, isoniazid therapy for 9 months prevents subsequent disease.

Children exposed to an infected household member must have a PPD placed. If the PPD is negative, isoniazid is indicated for 3 months until a repeat PPD is placed. Isoniazid is discontinued if the second PPD remains negative. If the initial PPD is positive, it is necessary to perform a complete physical examination and obtain a chest radiograph to look for evidence of disease.

The only vaccine currently available for prevention of tuberculosis is bacille Calmette-Guérin (BCG) vaccine, which is prepared from live attenuated strains of *Mycobacterium bovis*. The vaccine is given worldwide to infants to protect them from miliary or CNS tuberculosis; it has an estimated efficacy of 80%. BCG vaccine is less effective in the prevention of pulmonary tuberculosis. Use of BCG in the United States is not recommended, except in specific circumstances in which infants are at high risk for unavoidable exposure. Children who have received BCG immunization have a characteristic scar at the injection site, and their PPD is often positive. It is not possible to distinguish positivity caused by BCG vaccination from true infection with *M. tuberculosis*. For that reason, it is necessary to evaluate all children with a positive PPD for presence of disease using chest radiography and to give prophylaxis with isoniazid.

LYME DISEASE

The cause of Lyme disease is infection with the spirochete *Borrelia burgdorferi*, which is carried by the disease-transmitting ticks *Ixodes scapularis* (deer tick) in the eastern United States and *Ixodes pacificus* (western black-legged tick) in the western United States. Over 90% of reported cases of Lyme disease occur in 13 states along the mid-Atlantic seaboard and the upper north-central region of the United States.

Principal risk factors for acquiring disease are residence in areas overgrown with tick-infested

TABLE 9.34 Clinical Manifestations of Lyme Disease

	Time After Tick Bite	Symptoms				
		Skin	Constitutional	Musculoskeletal	CNS	Heart
Early localized	3 days–4 weeks	ECM	Fever, malaise, headache, lymphadenopathy	Mylagia/ Arthralgia		
Early disseminated	3–10 weeks	Multiple ECM	Fever, malaise, headache, lymphadenopathy	Arthralgia	Cranial nerve palsies Meningitis Pseudotumor cerebri	Carditis
Late disease	2–12 months		Fatigue	Recurrent arthritis	Subacute encephalopathy Polyradiculoneuropathy	

CNS = central nervous system; ECM = erythema chronicum migrans.

brush as well as occupational or recreational exposure. The estimated risk of *B. burgdorferi* infection after a tick bite in highly endemic areas is 1.4%.

Pathophysiology

Ixodid ticks, which undergo three stages of development (larva, nymph, adult) in a 2-year period, become infected after feeding on small mammals such as the white-footed mouse. Ticks in all stages are capable of causing infection; however, nymphs are most likely to infect humans because they are present in relatively large numbers; are small in size, which allows them to escape detection; and have peak feeding activity coinciding with increased human outdoor activity (spring/summer). Transmission of *B. burgdorferi* requires prolonged tick attachment (> 36–48 hours).

Clinical and Laboratory Evaluation

History and Physical Examination

Clinical manifestations of Lyme disease are divided into three stages: early localized, early disseminated, and late (Table 9.34). The hallmark of early localized disease is a skin rash called **erythema chronicum migrans.** The rash begins as a papule that increases in size over days to weeks to form a large lesion (> 5 cm in diameter). Approximately 60%–80% of infected individuals have erythema chronicum migrans. Constitutional symptoms such as fever, headache, malaise, and lymphadenopathy are sometimes present during the first stage.

Symptoms in the second stage occur as a result of dissemination of the spirochete to multiple organs. Constitutional symptoms, including arthralgia, may persist or recur. Signs and symptoms of meningitis, cranial nerve abnormalities (especially cranial nerve VII), and rarely pseudotumor cerebri may be present. Cardiac abnormalities, including varying degrees of heart block, myopericarditis, and left ventricular failure, occur in 10% of cases.

Pauciarticular arthritis affecting large joints is the most common sign of late disease. Chronic arthritis is more likely among patients with human leukocyte antigen (HLA) types DR-2, DR-3 or DR-4. Late complications of CNS disease are rare in children but include encephalopathy and polyradiculoneuropathy (inflammation of multiple nerves) in adults.

Laboratory Evaluation

It is possible to diagnose Lyme disease clinically if a rash typical of erythema chronicum migrans is present. Serologic tests are used as an adjunct to clinical findings. Testing for antibodies should take place in a reliable reference laboratory. Western immunoblotting is used to confirm positive or equivocal test results. Serology is not recommended for children with only nonspecific symptoms (e.g., fatigue); false-positive results are likely. In addition, such testing is not advisable after tick removal in asymptomatic children.

Management

Treatment of childhood Lyme disease depends on disease stage, nature of symptoms, and extent of organ system involvement. Children who re-

TABLE 9.35	Infectious and Noninfectious Causes of Fever of Unknown Origin	
Infectious Diseases	**Noninfectious Diseases**
Endocarditis	Juvenile rheumatoid arthritis
Liver abscess	Systemic lupus erythematosus
Pyelonephritis	Kawasaki disease
Sinusitis	Malignancy
Pelvic abscess	Familial Mediterranean Fever
Salmonella spp.	Inflammatory bowel disease
Brucella spp.	Drug fever
Mycobacterium tuberculosis	Factitious fever
Bartonella henselae (catscratch disease)	Sarcoidosis
Coxiella burnetii (Q fever)	
Rickettsia rickettsii	
Epstein-Barr virus (infectious mononucleosis)	
Cytomegalovirus	
Malaria	
Toxoplasmosis	

ceive appropriate therapy are unlikely to develop late complications. Antibiotics used include amoxicillin, doxycycline, penicillin, and ceftriaxone.

Prevention of Lyme disease and other tick-transmitted infections involves avoiding exposure to tick-infested areas. If this not possible, clothing that covers arms and legs should be worn, with pants tucked into socks. Clothing, not skin, may be sprayed with permethrin. Diethyltoluamide (DEET)-containing insect repellent is effective when applied to skin, avoiding the face, hands, and abraded areas. It is essential to inspect children daily after possible tick exposure, with particular attention to the head and neck.

FEVER OF UNKNOWN ORIGIN

The diagnosis of fever of unknown origin (FUO) is made when a child presents with a history of fever (≥ 38.3°C) [100.9°F] for 2 weeks or more. Fever without localizing signs for less than 1 week usually results from a self-limited viral infection. The etiology of FUO is variable. Infections are the most common cause in children (30%–40%), with autoimmune disease (7%–10%), malignancy (2%–5%),

---

TABLE 9.36 Insect Vectors of Infectious Diseases

Organism	Vector	Clinical Syndrome	Diagnosis
BACTERIA			
Spirochetes			
Borrelia burgdorferi	Tick	Lyme disease	Screening electroimmunoassay Confirmatory Western blot
Borrelia hermsii	Tick	Relapsing fever	Visualization of spirochete on Wright-, Giemsa-, or acridine orange–stained blood smear Serum antibody test
Gram-negative bacteria			
Francisella tularensis	Tick, deerfly, horsefly	Tularemia	Serology Fluorescent antibody on infected material Culture*
Yersinia pestis	Flea	Plague	Serology Culture
Rickettsia			
Rickettsia rickettsii	Tick	Rocky Mountain spotted fever	Serology, Immunofluorescent stain of skin biopsy
Ehrlichia chaffeensis	Tick	Monocytic ehrlichiosis	Serology PCR Detection of intraleukocytic morulae
Ehrlichia spp.	Tick	Granulocytic ehrlichiosis	Serology PCR Detection of intraleukocytic morulae
VIRUSES			
Coltivirus	Tick	Colorado tick fever	Serology Viral isolation from blood
Arboviruses	Mosquito	Encephalitis†	Serology
PROTOZOA			
Babesia microti	Tick	Babesiosis	Visualization of organism on Giemsa- or Wright-stained smear
Plasmodium spp.	Mosquito	Malaria	Thick and thin blood smears

*Notifiy laboratory that tularemia is suspected so precautions can be taken to avoid infection of laboratory personnel.
†Eastern equine encephalitis, Western equine encephalitis, St. Louis encephalitis, California encephalitis, West Nile Virus encephalitis.
PCR = polymerase chain reaction.

and other (factitious fever, drug fever, sarcoid) in 2% of cases. The cause is never determined in nearly 50% of cases. In most of these, fever resolves spontaneously with no long-term sequelae. Causes may be infectious or noninfectious (Table 9.35.

Clinical and Laboratory Evaluation

History

The diagnosis of FUO is often made by obtaining a thorough history. Important aspects of the history include questions regarding present and past medical history, a complete review of systems, family history of recurrent illness or infection, social history, medications, immunizations, allergies, travel, and animal exposure. Several animal-borne infections may be the cause of the FUO (Tables 9.36 and 9.37). Changes in social behavior and school attendance should be noted.

Physical Examination

☀ Pediatric Pearl

The cause of fever of unknown origin often becomes apparent as symptoms of disease and signs on physical examination evolve over several days.

First, it is necessary to document the existence of fever either in the physician's office or at home, where a parent keeps a daily temperature record. The clinician should educate parents about the proper way to take a temperature. Sometimes hospitalization is necessary to document presence of fever. Second, it is important to note the child's general well-being. Weight loss or poor growth are signs of the existence of a significant medical problem. Third, a complete physical examination is necessary. The clinician should repeat it until the cause of FUO becomes apparent or the fever resolves.

Findings on physical examination may be subtle but guide the diagnostic evaluation. For example, joint pain or swelling suggests infectious or reactive arthritis, collagen vascular disease, or malignancy. A heart murmur leads to the consideration of bacterial endocarditis or acute rheumatic fever. Palpation of a spleen tip is consistent with Epstein-Barr virus infection, endocarditis, or malignancy. A good neurologic examination can reveal abnormalities consistent with a CNS malignancy or brain abscess. Rectal examination may point to a previously unsuspected perirectal abscess or ruptured appendiceal abscess. Findings of eczema or seborrhea suggest immune deficiency or histiocytosis. Careful palpation of bony structures may reveal tenderness consistent with infection or malignancy.

Laboratory Evaluation

The tempo of the diagnostic evaluation for FUO matches the clinical appearance of the child. A child who appears well or mildly ill may benefit from a limited initial evaluation and observation. The ill-appearing child with progressive worsening of symptoms may require hospitalization and multiple diagnostic tests.

TABLE 9.37	Infectious Diseases Associated with Pet Exposure

Animal	Organism	Disease	Clinical Manifestations
Cats	*Bartonella henselae*	Catscratch fever	Fever Lymphadenitis Microabscesses in liver and spleen Bone infection
	Toxoplasma gondii	*Toxoplasmosis*	*Asymptomatic* Mononucleosis-like syndrome Congenital toxoplasmosis
Reptiles	*Salmonella* spp.	Salmonellosis	Diarrhea Bacteremia Local infection (e.g., bone, joint)
Birds	*Chlamydia psittaci*	Psittacosis	Interstitial pneumonia
Dogs	*Toxocara canis*	Visceral larval migrans (immunocompromised)	Lung, liver, eye infection
	Bordetella bronchiseptica		Pneumonia, septicemia, sinusitis
	Leptospira	Leptospirosis	Influenza-like illness or jaundice
	Microsporum canis	Tinea capitis/Tinea corporis	Superficial infection of skin or hair shaft
Rats	*Streptobacillus moniliformis*	Rat-bite fever	Fever, arthritis, arthralgia, rash, endocarditis

Tests ordered are based on findings from the history and physical examination. Useful screening laboratory tests include a CBC; ESR; urinalysis and culture; and serum chemistries, including liver function studies. Chest radiography is useful for showing changes consistent with acute or chronic pulmonary disease, hilar lymphadenopathy, or abnormal heart size or shape. Abdominal ultrasound may reveal an intra-abdominal tumor, appendiceal abscess, liver abscess, or liver and spleen lesions consistent with catscratch disease or abnormalities of the kidneys. Further outpatient evaluation may include a PPD, Monospot, and serology for Epstein-Barr virus, serology for B. henselae, an HIV antibody test or HIV DNA PCR, blood culture, stool for bacterial culture and ova and parasites, serum for antinuclear antibody and rheumatoid factor, or thick and thin blood smears if the travel history is suggestive for malaria.

Diagnostic tests considered include lumbar puncture, CT of the sinuses, repeat blood cultures, echocardiogram, ophthalmologic examination, and bone marrow aspiration. Serologic tests for unusual infection are helpful only if acute and convalescent serum is obtained or if IgM for a specific infectious agent is positive. Nuclear medicine scans are not usually diagnostic unless a probable focus of infection has been identified by history or physical examination.

Management

Empiric oral or parenteral antibiotic therapy is not used in nonimmunocompromised children with FUO unless patients have strong likelihood of bacterial infection or appear very ill. In these circumstances, it is reasonable to begin broad-spectrum antibiotic therapy but only after appropriate cultures have been performed. A trial of nonsteroidal anti-inflammatory drugs (NSAIDs) is recommended if juvenile rheumatoid arthritis is likely. Empiric use of steroids is never appropriate.

If fever persists and outpatient evaluation is not diagnostic, hospitalization is recommended. Observation documents presence and pattern of fever and changes in physical findings. Further diagnostic workup may include evaluation by specialists in infectious disease, rheumatology, or hematology/oncology.

SUGGESTED READINGS

General References
American Academy of Pediatrics, Pickering, LK (ed): 2000 Red Book: Report of the Committee on Infectious Diseases, 25th ed. Elk Grove Village, IL, American Academy of Pediatrics, 2000.

Long SS, Pickering LK, Prober CG (eds): *Principles and Practice of Pediatric Infectious Diseases.* New York, Churchill Livingstone, 1997.
Moyer VA (ed): *Evidence-Based Pediatrics and Child Health.* London, England, BMJ Books, 2000.

Approach to the Evaluation of the Febrile Child
Baker MD: Evaluation and management of infants with fever. *Pediatr Clin North Am* 46(6):1061–72, 1999.
Dowell SF, Marcy SM, Phillips WR, et al: Otitis media—Principles of judicious use of antimicrobial agents. *Pediatrics* 101(1):166–171, 1998.
Hoberman A, Paradise JL: Acute otitis media: Diagnosis and management in the year 2000. *Pediatr Ann* 29(10):609–620, 2000.
Kluger MJ: Fever revisited. *Pediatrics* 90(6):846–850, 1992.
May A, Bauchner H: Fever phobia: The pediatrician's contribution. *Pediatrics* 90(6):851–854, 1992.

Otitis Media
Rosenfeld RM: An evidence-based approach to treating otitis media. *Pediatr Clin North Am* 43(6):1165–1181, 1996.

Pharyngitis
Bisno AL: Acute pharyngitis: Etiology and diagnosis. *Pediatrics* 97(6 Pt 2):949–954, 1996.
Schwartz B, Marcy SM, Phillips WR, et al: Pharyngitis—Principles of judicious use of antimicrobial agents. *Pediatrics;* 101(1):172–174, 1998.

Viral Respiratory Illnesses
Dowell SF, Marcy SM, Phillips WR, et al: Principles of judicious use of antimicrobial agents for pediatric upper respiratory tract infections. *Pediatrics* 101(1): 163–165, 1998.
Hall CB: Respiratory syncytial virus: A continuing culprit and conundrum. *J Pediatr* 135(2 Pt 2):2–7, 1999.
Klassen TP: Croup. A current perspective. *Pediatr Clin North Am* 46(6):1167–1178, 1999.
Stamboulian D, Bonvehi PE, Nacinovich FM, et al: Influenza. *Infect Dis Clin North Am* 14(1):141–166, 2000.

Pneumonia
McCracken GH: Etiology and treatment of pneumonia. *Pediatr Infect Dis J* 19(4):3733–3737, 2000.
Nelson JD: Community-acquired pneumonia in children: Guidelines for treatment. *Pediatr Infect Dis J* 19(3):251–253, 2000.

Central Nervous System Infections
Negrini B, Kelicher KJ, Wald ER: Cerebrospinal fluid findings in aseptic versus bacterial meningitis. *Pediatrics* 105(2):316–319, 2000.
Quagliarello VJ, Scheld WM: Treatment of bacterial meningitis. *N Engl J Med* 336(10):708–716, 1997.
Rajnik M, Ottolini MG: Serious infections of the central nervous system: Encephalitis, meningitis, and brain abscess. *Adolesc Med* 11(2):401–425, 2000.
Sawyer MH: Enterovirus infections: Diagnosis and treatment. *Pediatr Infect Dis J* 18(12):1033–1039, 1999.

Viral and Bacterial Exanthems
Gable EK, Liu G, Morrell DS: Pediatric exanthems. *Prim Care* 27(2):353–369, 2000.
Resnick SD: Staphylococcal toxin-mediated syndromes in childhood. *Semin Dermatol* 11(1):11–18, 1992.

Pediatric Human Immunodeficiency Virus Infection
Working Group on Antiretroviral Therapy and Medical Management of HIV-Infection Children: Guide-

lines for the Use of Antiretroviral Agents in Pediatric HIV infection. December 14, 2001. HIV/AIDS Treatment Information Service Website. (*http://hivatis.org*)

Kaplan JE, Masur H, Holmes KK (eds): Prevention of opportunistic infections in persons infected with HIV. *Clin Infect Dis* 30(Suppl 1):S1–S93, 2000.

Tuberculosis

Starke JR: Tuberculosis in children. *Prim Care* 23(4): 861–881, 1996.

Lyme Disease

Wormser GP, Nadelman RB, Dattwyler RJ, et al: Practice guidelines for the treatment of Lyme disease. *Clin Infect Dis* 31(Suppl 1):S1–S14, 2000.

Chapter 10

Neonatology

Krisa P. Van Meurs and William D. Rhine

PERINATAL AND NEONATAL ASSESSMENT

General Considerations

Neonatology is the subspecialty of pediatrics concerned with sick newborns, and neonatologists strive to understand how fetal development and pathology lead to illness in infants at birth. **Perinatology** is the area of obstetrics concerned with pregnant women and their fetuses, and perinatologists care about the well-being of infants after birth. Use of a common terminology by all practitioners concerned with the care of young infants facilitates effective evaluation and understanding of high-risk fetuses and newborn infants. **Gestational age** is the number of weeks of a pregnancy from the first day of the mother's last menstrual period to the date of birth. **Prematurity** is birth before 37 weeks' gestation; **postmaturity** is any birth after 42 weeks' gestation. The **neonatal period** is 0–28 days after birth.

Pregnancies may be classified as high risk on the basis of two groups of factors: underlying maternal conditions and fetal or obstetric complications.

- **Maternal conditions:** extremes of age; extremes of weight or weight gain; medical disorders, especially diabetes mellitus, hypertension, and congenital heart disease (CHD); use of tobacco, illicit drugs, and excessive alcohol; multiple gestation; history of multiple fetal losses; and delay or avoidance of obstetric care
- **Fetal or obstetric conditions:** premature labor, prolonged rupture of chorionic membranes (> 24 hours), intrauterine growth retardation (IUGR), polyhydramnios (excessive amniotic fluid) or oligohydramnios (decreased amniotic fluid), abnormal fetal position, maternal vaginal bleeding, infection (e.g., chorioamnionitis), and meconium staining of amniotic fluid

Antepartum Testing

Several methods are used to assess fetal health. Clinical markers of fetal well-being include fundal height and fetal movement, and other antepartum tests are available (Table 10.1).

Neonatal Evaluation and Resuscitation

High-risk infants sometimes need assistance in making the transition from fetal to neonatal physiology at the time of delivery. Whenever possible, high-risk deliveries should occur in an environment in which the necessary equipment and appropriately trained personnel are readily available if resuscitation becomes necessary. Preparation is crucial for successful neonatal resuscitation, and communication between the neonatologist and his or her colleagues in obstetrics is often the first step in this preparation.

The **Apgar scoring system** ensures proper evaluation of neonates at the time of delivery (see Table 1.1). Scores are obtained at 1 and 5 minutes after birth. If the score at 5 minutes is less than 7, scores are obtained every 5 minutes thereafter (for 20 minutes after birth) until two scores of greater than 7 are obtained. Skin color (including perfusion) is usually the first factor to be reduced in depressed neonates, followed by respirations, tone, reflexes, and pulse. The usual order of reappearance is pulse, reflexes, color, respirations, and tone.

The Apgar score provides a guideline for the magnitude and duration of cardiopulmonary resuscitation (CPR), if necessary. However, it was not designed to predict neurologic outcome. In fact, most children with abnormal neurologic development have a "good" 5-minute Apgar score of greater than 7, and most children with normal neurologic outcomes have a 5-minute score of less than 7. On the other hand, prolonged depression of Apgar scores (< 4 over 10 minutes) does indicate high risk (> 50%) for death or abnormal neurologic development. Additional markers of potential illness at birth include prematurity and extremes of size—whether **small-for-gestational age (SGA)** or **large-for-gestational age (LGA).**

Initiation of neonatal resuscitation begins with the ABCs of CPR: **airway, breathing,** and **circulation.** Airway management may be initiated by proper head positioning and bag-mask ventilation. If additional oxygenation and ventilation are required, endotracheal intubation may be necessary. If meconium staining of the amniotic fluid is significant, suctioning via an endotracheal tube

TABLE 10.1 Antepartum Tests Used to Assess Fetal Health	
Test	**Use**
Ultrasound studies	Fetal growth, anatomy, and physiologic function; the latter is scored as part of a biophysical profile that includes fetal tone, movement, breathing, heart rate, and amniotic fluid volume; Doppler studies of cord blood flow
Amniocentesis (sampling of amniotic fluid)	Detection of chromosomal abnormalities; estimate of lung maturity
Chorionic villus sampling (first trimester)	Earlier screening for chromosomal or other genetic/metabolic analysis
Percutaneous umbilical blood sampling (ultrasound-guided)	Both diagnostic and therapeutic interventions (e.g., hematocrit measurement, fetal transfusion)
Fetal heart rate monitoring, either at time of delivery or during later part of third trimester: • in absence of contractions (nonstress test) OR • with induction of contractions by oxytocin (stress test)	Fetal well-being
Fetal scalp blood sampling	Measurement of blood gases and determines acidosis during labor

may help clear the airways and prevent **meconium aspiration syndrome (MAS).** Rescue breathing for neonates requires 30–60 breaths/min with adequate pressure, which is demonstrated by good air entry on auscultation or by adequate chest excursion. Circulation is assessed by palpation of the pulse at the brachial artery, in the axilla, or even at the umbilical stump.

In addition to these ABCs, newborns have several unique resuscitation needs. They require **stimulation,** which induces sympathoadrenal-mediated increases in respiratory and cardiac performance; **suctioning,** which removes amniotic fluid from the nasal and oral pharynx and from the lungs; and **drying and warming,** which reduce the oxygen requirements for maintenance of thermoneutrality.

Neonates who are considered ill and in need of further evaluation and therapy should be transferred to a neonatal intensive care unit (NICU). Umbilical vessel cannulation can provide (1) arterial access for blood pressure monitoring and arterial blood gas (ABG) sampling, and (2) venous access for cardiopressor drip administration and estimation of central venous pressure. Laboratory evaluation is based on the clinical picture. A complete blood count (CBC) yields information about hematologic status and possibility of infection. A sepsis workup typically includes blood culture and lumbar puncture. Chest radiography helps distinguish congenital cardiopulmonary disease from infection. However, echocardiography is usually necessary for more definitive diagnosis.

Management of ill newborns includes knowledge of resources available at the treating facility. In the United States, virtually all nurseries participate in a hierarchical referral and education network. **Level 1** nurseries provide basic neonatal care, which may include parenteral antibiotics. **Level 2** nurseries offer more intensive care such as gavage feeds and ventilatory assistance of limited form or duration. **Level 3** nurseries provide the broadest range of neonatal care, including consultation from pediatric subspecialists, advanced respiratory support, and neonatal surgery.

FLUIDS, ELECTROLYTES, AND NUTRITION

Pathophysiology

The maintenance of normal fluid and electrolyte balance may have a positive effect on the outcome of many underlying disease processes. The problems involved in establishing proper fluid and electrolyte administration are commonly encountered in the neonatal period.

Several significant developmental differences in physiology must be taken into account when considering fluid and electrolyte management in the neonatal period. **Total body water** is 85% of birth weight in the third trimester and decreases to 78% at term, compared with 65% in older children (Figure 10.1); more than 50% of the water in term infants is intracellular (Figure 10.2). With growth, there are significant alterations in the bal-

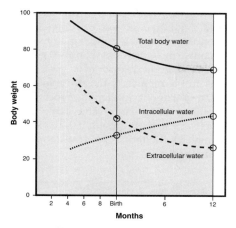

FIGURE 10.1. Changes in body fluid during fetal and neonatal life.

ance between **extracellular fluid (ECF)** and **intracellular fluid (ICF)**. During the first 7–10 days of life, most infants experience a 5%–12% reduction in body weight due to loss of body water, primarily ECF. This reduction in ECF is accompanied by a maturation of renal function. If fluid or electrolyte loading occurs in the first week of life, the ECF compartment may remain expanded, resulting in symptomatic left-to-right shunting through a **patent ductus arteriosus (PDA)**.

The initial goal of fluid and electrolyte therapy is the maintenance of zero balance for fluids and electrolytes, assuming no preexisting deficits or excesses. Over the short term, the positive balance needed for growth can be ignored. The formulation of a reasonable management plan for intake of fluids and electrolytes requires an adequate determination of output in neonates. The four normal sources of fluid loss are **insensible**

water loss (IWL), urine output, sweat, and fecal water loss. IWL, the loss of water through the lungs during respiration and through the skin from evaporation, is greatest in infants of low birth weight and low gestational age because of increased skin permeability, larger body surface area per unit weight, and greater skin blood flow relative to metabolic rate. Other factors that affect IWL are respiratory distress, activity level, environmental factors (e.g., open radiant warmers, phototherapy).

In neonates, who can maximally dilute their urine only to 50 mOsm/L and can concentrate it only to 800 mOsm/L, the intake of water and solutes primarily determines urine volume and osmolality. Sweat losses are almost nonexistent and fecal losses are low in newborns, which makes IWL and urine output the major sources of water loss, except for pathologic losses. Because the neonatal environment can be well controlled, IWL is the most important clinical variable.

Clinical and Laboratory Evaluation

History
Important historical factors include birth weight and gestational age, disease (e.g., respiratory distress, congestive heart failure, hyperbilirubinemia, meningitis, renal failure, gastroschisis), medications (e.g., furosemide, theophylline, indomethacin), fluid and solute therapy, and environmental influences (e.g., phototherapy, open radiant warmers).

Physical Examination
Important physical signs of hydration status include weight increase or decrease and skin turgor. Edema is a sign of overhydration, while a sunken fontanelle and loose skin indicates dehydration.

Laboratory Evaluation
The rate of weight gain should be checked regularly and related to a gestational-age normalized growth curve. In addition, electrolyte levels, urine output, and urine specific gravity should be assessed regularly. Normal urine output should average 1–3 ml/kg/hr. Hypernatremia, a sign of dehydration, is not infrequent in infants who weigh less than 1000 g because of their high skin permeability and increased IWL.

Differential Diagnosis

The differential diagnosis of fluid and electrolyte abnormalities should always include iatrogenic problems (inappropriate fluid or electrolyte therapy or medication side effect). Depending on the

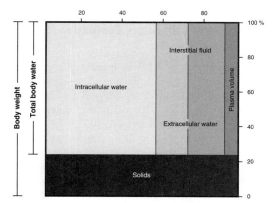

FIGURE 10.2. Percentage distribution of body fluid in term newborns.

specific electrolyte imbalance, other diagnoses may be entertained: hyponatremia [syndrome of inappropriate secretion of antidiuretic hormone (SIADH), heart failure, and hyperglycemia]; hyperkalemia (congenital adrenal hyperplasia); hypochloremia (Bartter syndrome, cystic fibrosis); and hyperchloremia (dehydration).

Management

The goal of therapy is to restore fluid and electrolyte losses and to maintain a normal balance by calculating appropriate maintenance intake. General treatment principles are similar to those used in older children (see Chapter 4). Decisions regarding fluid and electrolyte therapy should be made with the specific disease state in mind (e.g., the need for fluid restriction in heart failure or SIADH).

A weight loss of 5%–12% is expected in the first week after birth and, if not present, suggests probable fluid overload. Fluid management is often more complex in infants who weigh less than 1000 g at birth; weight measurements and serum electrolyte levels usually need to be obtained frequently during the first few days of life. These small, premature infants may have hypernatremic dehydration as the result of inadequate fluid administration or a symptomatic ductus arteriosus due to fluid overload.

Enteral feedings are usually attempted in newborns as soon as feasible. Maternal breast milk is the best choice for infants of all gestational ages; additional supplements provide needed increased calories and electrolytes for premature infants. If breast milk is unavailable or contraindicated, special formulas designed for premature infants are generally appropriate for newborns who weigh less than 1800 g; these formulas provide higher levels of calories, protein, and electrolytes. Newborns who are less than 34 weeks' gestational age lack a well-developed suck-and-swallow reflex. Neonatologists generally recommend beginning gavage feedings in such infants. Newborns who weigh less than 1000 g may require gavage feedings as often as every 2 hours or by continuous nasogastric drip. Feeding volumes and formula concentration should advance slowly because of the risk of feeding intolerance and **necrotizing enterocolitis (NEC)** [see NECROTIZING ENTEROCOLITIS]. The final goal is approximately 120 kcal/kg/day in premature infants and 100 kcal/kg/day in full-term infants.

Infants who do not tolerate optimal nutrition via enteral feedings within several days require **hyperalimentation.** This begins on the second or third day of life, when electrolyte balance has been achieved. A gradual increase in intravenous dextrose concentration of 1–2 mg/kg/min is necessary. Infants who weigh less than 1000 g may not tolerate glucose in excess of 6 mg/kg/min, whereas full-term infants usually tolerate 8–10 mg/kg/min without developing hyperglycemia. The goal is to advance intravenous caloric intake to a level sufficient for growth (80–100 kcal/kg/day) to match intrauterine growth at a comparable gestational age.

RESPIRATORY DISORDERS

RESPIRATORY DISTRESS SYNDROME
Pathophysiology

During fetal development, the lungs pass through a pseudoglandular (7–17 weeks) and canalicular stage (16–25 weeks) and, at about 25 weeks' gestation, enter the terminal sac stage, which lasts until term. Alveolarization occurs mostly postnatally, with some alveoli present beginning at 28 weeks. During this time, two major processes take place. First, pulmonary capillaries begin to grow in approximation with the epithelium, and a gas-exchange surface is created. Second, the epithelial cells differentiate into type I and type II cells. It is the type II cells that produce surfactant. One of the major problems in infants with **respiratory distress syndrome (RDS) [hyaline membrane disease]** is surfactant deficiency, which markedly decreases lung compliance. Diffuse atelectasis results, accompanied by severe **ventilation–perfusion ($\dot{V}/\dot{Q}$) mismatch** and increased work of breathing. Despite advances in understanding the pathophysiology of RDS, specifically the role of surfactant, RDS remains the problem that most frequently affects premature infants.

Clinical and Laboratory Evaluation

History
The prevalence of RDS is inversely correlated with advancing gestational age. Cases of RDS are uncommon at 37 weeks' gestation and beyond, whereas more than 70% of infants between 28 and 30 weeks' gestation have RDS. The critical risk factor is the stage of lung maturity at delivery, not the precise gestational age. Among the numerous factors that may delay lung maturity are maternal diabetes, male sex, second born of twins, and Caucasian race. Several conditions may accelerate lung maturity such as intrauterine growth retardation (IUGR), severe pregnancy-

induced hypertension (PIH), and maternal glucocorticoid administration.

Physical Examination

Within 6 hours of birth, infants with RDS typically exhibit the following clinical signs: tachypnea, retractions, nasal flaring, grunting, and cyanosis. The prominent retractions result from the compliant rib cage in newborns and the generation of high intrathoracic pressures, which are needed to expand the poorly compliant lungs. The typical expiratory grunt, an early feature, is thought to result from partial closure of the glottis during expiration in an attempt to trap air and maintain functional residual capacity. The typical presentation is rarely seen in infants who weigh less than 1000 g at birth, because they are usually intubated immediately in the delivery room.

Pediatric Pearl

Visual inspection of the abdomen is necessary in infants with significant respiratory distress after birth. If the abdomen is scaphoid, the diagnosis is most likely congenital diaphragmatic hernia.

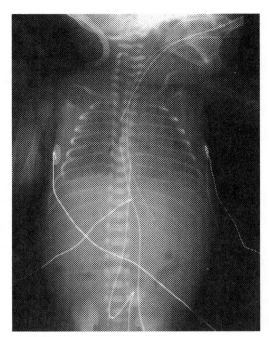

FIGURE 10.3. Chest radiograph of an infant with respiratory distress syndrome.

Laboratory Evaluation

The classic findings of RDS on chest radiograph are low-volume lungs with a **reticulogranular ("ground glass") pattern** and **air bronchograms** (Figure 10.3). It is important to note that RDS cannot be reliably differentiated from neonatal pneumonia by radiographic studies alone.

Differential Diagnosis

The differential diagnosis of respiratory distress in the newborn period includes **pneumonia** and **transient tachypnea of the newborn (TTN)** [Table 10.2]; for a complete differential diagnosis of neonatal respiratory distress, see the table. The lungs are the most common site of infection in neonates; infection may be acquired during the prenatal period, at the time of birth, or early in the neonatal period. In neonatal pneumonia, chest radiographs may vary in appearance; unilateral infiltrates to a diffuse pattern with air bronchograms may be seen. The difficulty in differentiating neonatal pneumonia from RDS has led to the frequent use of antibiotics in infants with RDS.

TTN, which tends to occur in term infants, is the delayed reabsorption of fetal lung fluid. It occurs more commonly after a cesarean section, because the infant's thorax is not subjected to the same pressures as in a vaginal delivery. The symptoms, which usually last between 12 and 72 hours, consist of tachypnea, grunting, nasal flaring, and cyanosis. Because TTN has many overlapping features with RDS and pneumonia, it often presents a diagnostic dilemma. Chest radiography may be helpful diagnostically, because the films show prominent perihilar streaking and fluid in the interlobar fissures (Figure 10.4).

Management

The central goal of management of RDS is the maintenance of adequate gas exchange to allow for normal tissue function and avoidance of the consequences of hypoxemia and hypercapnia. Routinely used therapeutic methods include the following:

- Oxygen therapy with monitoring of blood gases
- Continuous positive airway pressure (CPAP)
- Mechanical ventilation
- Artificial surfactant replacement

Treatment must be provided in such a way as to minimize potential adverse consequences such as pneumothorax, pneumomediastinum, pulmonary interstitial emphysema (PIE), and lung injury with subsequent development of chronic lung disease (CLD).

TABLE 10.2	Neonatal Respiratory Distress

Airway/pulmonary anomalies

Nasal/nasopharyngeal	Choanal atresia
Oral	Macroglossia (Beckwith-Wiedemann syndrome)
	Micrognathia (Pierre Robin syndrome)
Neck	Congenital goiter
	Cystic hygroma
Larynx	Laryngomalacia
	Subglottic stenosis
	Vocal cord paralysis
	Laryngeal web
Trachea	Vascular ring
	Tracheoesophageal fistula
	Bronchial stenosis/atresia
	Tracheomalacia
	Tracheal stenosis/agenesis
Lungs	Pulmonary hypoplasia
	Congenital diaphragmatic hernia
	Congenital lobar emphysema
	Pulmonary sequestration
	Pulmonary lymphangiectasia

Lung disease

Acute	Respiratory distress syndrome (RDS)
	Transient tachypnea of the newborn (TTN)
	Pneumonia
	Aspiration syndromes (e.g., meconium, blood, amniotic fluid)
Chronic	Bronchopulmonary dysplasia (BPD)
	Wilson-Mikity syndrome
Complications	Atelectasis
	Air leak syndrome (e.g., pneumothorax, pneumomediastinum, pneumoperi-cardium, pneumoperitoneum)
	Pulmonary interstitial emphysema (PIE)
	Pulmonary hemorrhage

Nonpulmonary disease

Persistent pulmonary hypertension of the newborn (PPHN)
Metabolic abnormalities (e.g., acidosis, hypothermia)
Congestive heart failure
Central nervous system (CNS) anomalies

MECONIUM ASPIRATION SYNDROME

Pathophysiology

Meconium aspiration syndrome (MAS) is characterized by staining of the amniotic fluid with meconium in association with respiratory distress. Meconium staining complicates 8%–20% of all deliveries but is seen in up to 44% of postdates or other high-risk pregnancies. A leading theory of MAS contends that acute and chronic fetal distress lead to meconium passage in utero; gasping by the fetus or newborn results in aspiration of meconium-stained amniotic fluid into the airway. The exact relationship between meconium staining and fetal distress is still unclear.

The pulmonary problems seen in MAS result from a mixture of complete and partial airway ob-struction by the meconium. The completely obstructed areas become atelectatic, while the partially obstructed airways develop a ball-valve effect, leading to air trapping with overexpansion. Air leaks, including pneumothorax, pneumomediastinum, pneumopericardium, and pneumoperitoneum, are often complications of MAS. Other possible complications are **persistent pulmonary hypertension of the newborn (PPHN)** [see PERSISTENT PULMONARY HYPERTENSION OF THE NEWBORN].

Clinical and Laboratory Evaluation

History

MAS is most common in infants with a history of postmaturity, fetal distress, or meconium staining.

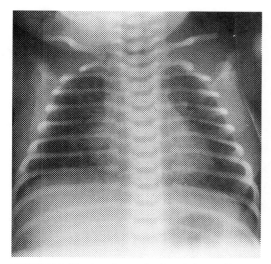

FIGURE 10.4. Chest radiograph of an infant with transient tachypnea of the newborn.

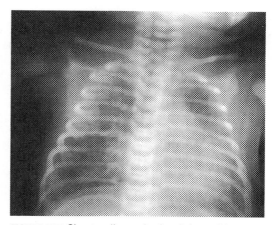

FIGURE 10.5. Chest radiograph of an infant with meconium aspiration syndrome.

Physical Examination

Common features of MAS are meconium staining of the skin and nails, peeling skin, grunting, nasal flaring, retractions, marked tachypnea, and varying degrees of cyanosis.

Laboratory Evaluation

A chest radiograph should be obtained. Coarse, fluffy infiltrates with alternating areas of lucency are commonly visible (Figure 10.5). Air leak phenomena such as pneumothorax or pneumomediastinum and hyperinflation with flattening of the diaphragm are also frequently seen. ABGs identify hypoxemia and hypercarbia.

Differential Diagnosis

Conditions to be considered included blood or amniotic fluid aspiration and pneumonia.

Management

Whenever meconium staining is present, suctioning of the nose and oropharynx after delivery of the head is indicated. This is followed by immediate intubation and suctioning of the trachea after delivery if the meconium is thick or the infant is depressed. Some cases of MAS may not be preventable because of in utero aspiration.

Infants with MAS are at risk for increasing respiratory distress with hypoxemia and hypercarbia, which may also be further complicated by PPHN. Chest physiotherapy and suctioning is one of the many therapeutic technique appropri-

ate for infants with MAS. The following modes of therapy are also used to treat infants with MAS:

- Chest physiotherapy and suctioning
- Transcutaneous oxygen saturation monitoring with generous use of supplemental oxygen to prevent hypoxemia and possible hypoxic pulmonary vasoconstriction, which may result in persistent pulmonary hypertension of the newborn (PPHN)
- ABG monitoring for prompt recognition and treatment of acidosis, hypoxemia, and hypercarbia
- CPAP or mechanical ventilation to maintain normal oxygenation and ventilation
- Sedation or neuromuscular paralysis for infants on high ventilator settings
- Routine administration of antibiotics because of possible occurrence of a secondary bacterial pneumonia

PERSISTENT PULMONARY HYPERTENSION OF THE NEWBORN

Pathophysiology

Persistent pulmonary hypertension of the newborn (PPHN), also known as **persistent fetal circulation,** is the combination of pulmonary hypertension and right-to-left shunting of desaturated blood through fetal pathways [a patent foramen ovale (PFO) or a patent ductus arteriosus (PDA)] in a structurally normal heart. This pathologic process is due to a sustained elevation in pulmonary vascular resistance (PVR) after birth. Normally, the PVR falls rapidly after birth and with the first breath. In contrast, the systemic vascular resistance (SVR) increases rapidly with cord clamping. These events result in functional closure of the PFO and constriction of the PDA with separation of the pulmonary and systemic circulations (see Chapter 13). When PVR exceeds SVR, right-to-left shunting can occur at the PFO or PDA, resulting in systemic hypoxemia. The elevation in PVR may be idiopathic or secondary to MAS, congenital diaphragmatic hernia, hyperviscosity, or sepsis, and other causes. Acute hypoxia and acidosis at birth may cause pulmonary vasoconstriction and an elevation of pulmonary artery pressure.

A morphologic abnormality has also been identified in infants who die of PPHN. Key features are an increase in the thickness of the media of normally muscularized arteries and extension of smooth muscle distally into normally nonmuscularized intra-acinar arteries. This abnormality results in a decrease in the cross-sectional area of the pulmonary vascular bed and an increased resistance to pulmonary blood flow. Experts have speculated that chronic hypoxia in utero may cause these vascular changes.

Clinical and Laboratory Evaluation

History
The occurrence of any condition associated with the various secondary causes of PPHN (MAS, sepsis, congenital diaphragmatic hernia, RDS, hyperviscosity) is relevant to formation of a diagnosis. In utero exposure to prostaglandin synthetase inhibitors (aspirin, indomethacin) may cause premature constriction of the PDA and secondary PPHN.

Physical Examination
No pathognomonic findings are encountered in infants with PPHN other than cyanosis, which may vary in severity.

Laboratory Evaluation
Preductal (right arm) and postductal (umbilical artery or leg) ABGs demonstrate a difference in PaO_2 of more than 10 mm Hg when there is right-to-left ductal (PDA) shunting, but this difference is not present when shunting occurs only at the level of the PFO. Two-dimensional echocardiography with color flow Doppler can demonstrate the right-to-left shunting pattern and rule out any structural heart defects (Figure 10.6).

Differential Diagnosis

Pulmonary processes such as RDS, MAS, congenital diaphragmatic hernia, and pneumonia should be considered. Cyanotic CHD (see Chapter 13) should also be ruled out.

Management

The management of PPHN has changed dramatically with recent medical advances. Modes of treatment include the following:

- Prompt correction of hypoxia and acidosis to reverse pulmonary vasospasm, because they are both potent pulmonary vasoconstrictors
- 100% oxygen administered by hood
- Initiation of intubation and mechanical ventilation if hypoxemia persists
- High-frequency ventilation (often used in term infants with PPHN)
- Volume expansion or administration of inotropic agents such as dopamine or dobutamine to ensure adequate cardiac output

For infants who do not respond to these therapies, additional treatment may be necessary. Clinical trials have found that infants with PPHN benefit from surfactant replacement therapy, probably because the initial lung injury has resulted in an inactivation of surfactant. Two large randomized clinical trials demonstrated the efficacy of inhaled nitric oxide in term infants with hypoxic respiratory failure, and in 1999, the Food and Drug Administration (FDA) approved this agent for such use. If infants fail to improve with the surfactant replacement and inhaled nitric oxide, **extracorporeal membrane oxygenation (ECMO),** a modified form of heart–lung bypass, continues to be successful in most cases.

CHRONIC LUNG DISEASE

Infants are diagnosed with **chronic lung disease (CLD)** if they continue to require oxygen after the age of 28 days and have abnormal chest radiographs. The incidence of CLD, which varies among institutions, is approximately 20%–40% in infants who weigh less than 1500 g at birth. Although artificial surfactant has reduced the mortality associated with RDS, it has not decreased the incidence of CLD.

Pathophysiology

The pathogenesis of CLD involves multiple etiologic factors: immature alveoli, barotrauma resulting from prolonged mechanical ventilation, oxygen toxicity with oxygen radical formation, infection from either prenatally acquired infections, chronic aspiration caused by gastroesophageal reflux, pulmonary edema resulting from volume overload, and PDA.

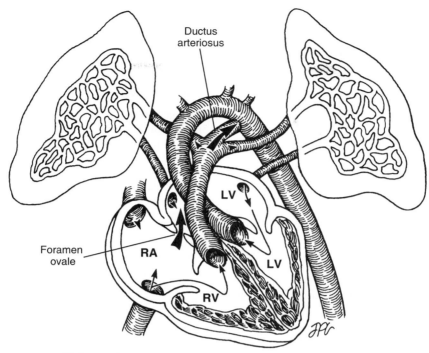

FIGURE 10.6. Right-to-left shunting patterns seen in infants with persistent pulmonary hypertension of the newborn. A shunt at the patent foramen ovale or patent ductus arteriosus may be present. LA = left atrium; LV = left ventricle; RA = right atrium; RV = right ventricle.

Clinical and Laboratory Evaluation

History
Infants commonly have a history that includes prematurity, prolonged mechanical ventilation, the need for high inspired oxygen concentration, infection, or PDA.

Physical Examination
Physical findings include tachypnea, retractions, and failure to thrive.

Laboratory Evaluation
In CLD, ABGs commonly indicate mild-to-moderate hypoxemia and hypercarbia. Pulmonary function tests usually denote increased airway resistance and decreased dynamic lung compliance. Abnormalities apparent on chest radiography vary with the stage of CLD: stage I is indistinguishable from early RDS; stage II shows increased opacification; stage III shows bubbly lucencies, streaky densities, and mild hyperinflation; and stage IV is a nonhomogeneous pattern of hyperinflation mixed with dense streaky areas of atelectasis and collapse (Figure 10.7). The severe forms of CLD have been seen less

commonly in recent years, and a typical progression is no longer evident.

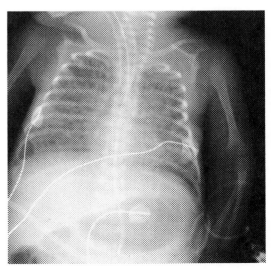

FIGURE 10.7. Chest radiograph of an infant with stage IV bronchopulmonary dysplasia.

Differential Diagnosis

Diagnosis of CLD is made on the basis of clinical history and a typical radiographic appearance. Similar radiographic features can be seen with chronic pulmonary insufficiency of prematurity, Wilson-Mikity syndrome, pulmonary interstitial emphysema (PIE), CHD, and recurrent aspiration pneumonia (Figure 10.8).

Management

Just as the etiology of CLD is multifactorial, its treatment is multifaceted. Restriction of fluid intake is necessary until respiratory status has stabilized, although it is important to provide the calories necessary for adequate growth. Growth problems are common in infants with CLD, and intensive nutritional support is critical. Once infants are extubated, supplemental oxygen keeps the PaO_2 between 60 and 80 mm Hg during sleep, feeding, and other activities to avoid pulmonary hypertension and to provide adequate tissue oxygenation. Ventilator adjustments optimize blood gases and minimize the damaging effects of barotrauma and oxygen toxicity.

Pharmacologic management of CLD includes diuretics (e.g., furosemide or chlorothiazide and spironolactone) to treat excessive interstitial lung fluid; bronchodilators (e.g., nebulized albuterol) to reduce airway resistance; corticosteroids to decrease pulmonary inflammation and increase lung compliance; electrolyte supplements (e.g., sodium chloride, potassium chloride, ammonium chloride) to treat losses secondary to diuretic therapy; and antioxidants (e.g., vitamin A). Infants with

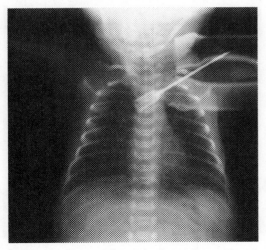

FIGURE 10.8. Chest radiograph of an infant with pulmonary interstitial emphysema.

CLD have lower plasma levels of vitamin A, and supplementation has been shown to reduce the incidence and severity of the disease.

APNEA

Pathophysiology

Apnea, defined as the cessation of respiration for more than 10 seconds, occurs frequently in premature infants; the incidence decreases with increased gestational age. Apnea affects approximately 25% of infants who weigh less than 2500 g at birth and 84% of newborns who weigh less than 1000 g. Experts believe that immaturity of central respiratory control is a key factor in the etiology of apnea of prematurity. Carbon dioxide responsiveness reflective of central chemoreceptor activity is less well developed in premature infants. In addition, hypoxia can result in transient hyperventilation, followed by hypoventilation and apnea. Apnea is more frequent during rapid eye movement (REM) and transitional sleep when the respiratory pattern is irregular.

The presence or absence of upper airway obstruction distinguishes the three types of apnea. **Central apnea** (10%–25% of cases) is characterized by no inspiratory effort, **obstructive apnea** (10%–20% of cases) by airway obstruction with no nasal airflow, and **mixed apnea** (50%–70% of cases), by elements of both types. In contrast, **periodic breathing** is defined as recurrent sequences of cessation of breathing of 5–10 seconds followed by 10–15 seconds of hyperventilation. This breathing pattern is normal in premature infants.

Clinical and Laboratory Evaluation

History

In infants born at more than 34 weeks' gestation, it is important to search for an underlying cause other than prematurity. History of feeding intolerance, vomiting, lethargy, temperature instability, seizures, and maternal history of infection or drug use may indicate an alternate cause of apnea (Figure 10.9).

Physical Examination

Presenting features in apnea may include cyanosis, tachypnea, respiratory distress, congenital anomalies, or neurologic abnormalities such as lethargy, hypotonia, or jitteriness. Bradycardia and, on occasion, cyanosis frequently accompany apnea.

Laboratory Evaluation

Various blood studies (CBC, electrolytes, calcium, magnesium, glucose, drug toxicology screen)

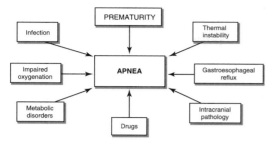

FIGURE 10.9. Specific contributory causes of apnea.

may be useful. Additional tests that may help determine the cause of the apnea include head ultrasound, head computed tomography (CT), genetic consultation, barium swallow or pH probe, and ABG analysis.

Differential Diagnosis

Several conditions may lead to apnea (see Figure 10.9).

Management

Identification of a potential cause of apnea such as hypoxemia, infection, or anemia warrants treatment of the causal condition. Exclusion of other etiologies leads to a diagnosis of idiopathic apnea of prematurity. Methylxanthines (theophylline and caffeine), the pharmacologic agents most widely used to treat apnea, act on the brainstem, producing central stimulation of respiratory drive. Serum levels of theophylline (8–10 $\mu g/ml$) and caffeine (10–20 $\mu g/ml$) are usually therapeutic. Side effects, which are seen with higher levels of theophylline, include tachycardia, irritability, vomiting and other gastrointestinal (GI) signs, and seizures. Apnea that is unresponsive to other therapies may require CPAP or mechanical ventilation.

NEONATAL INFECTIONS

CONGENITAL INFECTIONS

Pathophysiology

Congenital infections may occur any time during pregnancy, labor, and delivery. Transmission may occur through the placenta or may ascend into the amniotic fluid through the vaginal

canal. First-trimester infections may affect virtually any of the developing organ systems and often lead to significant **IUGR.** The acronym **TORCH (to**xoplasmosis, **r**ubella, **c**ytomegalovirus (CMV), and **h**erpes simplex) describes only some of the major causes of intrauterine infection; others include **human immunodeficiency virus (HIV), enterovirus, parvovirus, varicella,** and **syphilis.** Some of these infections as well as viral hepatitis may arise from postpartum exposure through skin contact or via breast milk. The risk of peripartum transmission of herpes simplex is greatest with vaginal delivery in a mother with primary, not recurrent, genital herpes.

Clinical and Laboratory Evaluation

History

It is important to review maternal history carefully. Many severe congenital infections occur unexpectedly; they are often associated with mild, nonspecific illness in the pregnant woman. It is routine to screen most pregnant women for antibody titers against rubella and hepatitis B and occasionally for toxoplasmosis. (Consumption of raw meat or exposure to cat feces increases the risk of toxoplasmosis.) Risk of other congenital infections may have to be inferred. For example, intravenous drug use or history of sexually transmitted diseases increases the risk of viral hepatitis and HIV.

Physical Examination

The effects of congenital infection vary depending on the causative organism and the maternal and fetal hosts. Many affected fetuses are asymptomatic at birth. The most commonly shared sequelae are:

- Growth retardation
- Premature delivery
- Central nervous system (CNS) abnormalities, including microcephaly, intracranial calcifications, and chorioretinitis
- Hepatosplenomegaly, often with accompanying jaundice
- Bruising or petechiae that may accompany thrombocytopenia
- Skin lesions

Infants with congenital viral infections may also present with acute symptomatology such as interstitial pneumonitis, myocarditis, or encephalitis. Clinical findings specific for certain conditions are:

- Congenital rubella syndrome: cataracts, hearing loss, heart lesions, blueberry-muffin spots

(skin lesions associated with extramedullary hematopoiesis)
- Congenital herpes simplex: skin, eye, or mouth lesions or more severe systemic symptoms, including seizures or multiorgan system failure, usually after the first week of life
- Parvovirus B19: possible fetal hemolytic crisis associated with hydrops fetalis

> ## Pediatric Pearl
>
> Infants with hepatosplenomegaly and thrombocytopenia should be evaluated for congenital viral infection.

Laboratory Evaluation

The combination of careful review of maternal history with clinical evaluation of the affected newborn is the best guide to the selection of necessary diagnostic studies. Serologic testing is most helpful for rubella, toxoplasmosis, and herpes infections. However, repeat testing may be necessary because increased levels of immunoglobulin G (IgG) may result from passive transfer of maternal IgG or from neonatal production. IgM, which cannot pass through the placenta from mother to fetus, often is a more reliable indicator of true neonatal infection. Urine cultures are best for demonstrating active CMV infection. Blood, cerebrospinal fluid (CSF), skin lesion cultures, or viral polymerase chain reaction (PCR) testing are usually diagnostic for herpes and enteroviral infections. Specific electroencephalographic (EEG) changes, often accompanied by characteristic neuroradiographic findings on CT scan or magnetic resonance imaging (MRI), result from herpes encephalitis.

Differential Diagnosis

The differential diagnosis depends on the signs and symptoms at presentation. Growth retardation and multiorgan dysfunction may also signify a genetic syndrome or metabolic disease (see Chapter 11).

Management

Unfortunately, management of congenital infection is usually only supportive (e.g., provision of cardiopulmonary assistance or correction of coagulopathy). However, the following modes of treatment may be useful in specific conditions:

- Neonatal herpes infection: antiviral agents acyclovir and vidarabine to reduce mortality and morbidity
- Toxoplasmosis: a regimen of pyrimethamine, sulfadiazine, and folinic acid (neonates); spiramycin (infected pregnant women)
- HIV infection: use of zidovudine in prophylactic treatment of HIV-positive newborns (see Chapter 9)

BACTERIAL INFECTIONS

Pathophysiology

Bacterial infections may be blood-borne, crossing the placenta, or may ascend the vaginal canal, especially after **prolonged rupture of membranes.** The specific pathogen involved depends on maternal colonization. The agents that cause the most common neonatal bacterial infections are group B streptococcus, which colonizes the vagina or cervix of 15%–25% of pregnant women; *Escherichia coli; Staphylococcus aureus;* and *Listeria monocytogenes.* Attack rates vary considerably over time and by geographic area. Other bacterial pathogens (e.g., coagulase-negative staphylococcus, *Klebsiella,* and *Serratia*) are more often associated with nosocomial (hospital-derived) infection, for which premature infants, with their relatively impaired immune function, are at higher risk.

Clinical and Laboratory Evaluation

History

It is important to obtain a complete obstetric history; maternal risk factors for neonatal bacterial sepsis include prolonged or premature rupture of membranes associated with labor, chorioamnionitis, and urinary tract infection. Intrapartum evidence of infection includes otherwise unexplained fetal tachycardia, meconium staining of the amniotic fluid, and perinatal depression. Risk of nosocomial infection increases with extreme prematurity, hyperalimentation administration, prolonged intravascular access, and surgical procedures.

Physical Examination

Septic neonates may initially be asymptomatic, may present later with subtle findings, or may rapidly progress to cardiopulmonary shock. Early findings associated with bacterial infection include temperature instability (more often hypothermia than hyperthermia), tachypnea, labored respirations, and feeding intolerance. Physical findings may include lethargy or irritability, rales if there is an accompanying pneumonia, jaundice, or decreased perfusion. Other dermatologic findings such as petechiae or purpura occur rarely.

Laboratory Evaluation

The approach to laboratory evaluation for potential bacterial sepsis is not standardized, and interpretation of laboratory data may depend on clinical evaluation. A positive blood culture confirms the diagnosis, but a negative blood culture does not rule it out. Small sample volume, the degree of bacteremia, or the inhibition of bacterial growth by antepartum maternal antibiotic administration may cause a negative culture result. White blood cell (WBC) counts may be either lowered or elevated in infected infants, with an increase in the percentage of immature lymphocytes, thrombocytopenia, or abnormal inclusion bodies.

Other tests may prove useful. Chest radiography may show evidence of an accompanying pneumonia. Lumbar puncture rules out meningitis. Urinalysis and culture are usually reserved for evaluation of sepsis occurring several days after birth, because urinary tract infections soon after birth are usually hematogenous in origin and not necessarily a reflection of abnormal urinary structure or function. Antigen detection tests of serum, urine, and CSF lack the sensitivity and specificity to diagnosis neonatal sepsis accurately. Measurement of acute-phase reactants such as C-reactive protein may be useful in both ruling out neonatal sepsis and helping determine the duration of antibiotic therapy.

Differential Diagnosis

The signs and symptoms of bacterial infection are relatively nonspecific. Viral or fungal infection (most commonly by *Candida*), often accompanied by cardiovascular instability, may also occur in neonates. In addition, cardiorespiratory or metabolic disease may manifest with systemic signs similar to infection.

Management

Often, a high degree of suspicion of infection is sufficient to lead to initiation of empiric antibiotic administration without a confirmatory positive blood culture. Therapy is usually started with two drugs: ampicillin and an aminoglycoside (e.g., gentamicin) or a cephalosporin. In cases of nosocomial infection, broader spectrum coverage (vancomycin and a cephalosporin) against more resistant organisms, including coagulase-negative staphylococcus, may be needed. Results of culture and sensitivity tests may later alter the antibiotic choice.

Septic neonates may require significant intensive care support, including intravenous fluid therapy, respiratory support with supplemental oxygen and mechanical ventilation, and cardiovascular support with intravascular colloid volume or cardiopressor drugs such as dopamine. Granulocyte transfusions may be beneficial in septic neonates with profound neutropenia that includes depletion of the bone marrow storage pools. Immunoglobulin therapy has also been used as an adjunctive treatment.

Pediatric Pearl

Infants diagnosed with *E. coli* sepsis should also be evaluated for galactosemia.

HYPERBILIRUBINEMIA

Pathophysiology

Approximately 50% of neonates have visible jaundice. It is necessary to understand bilirubin metabolism to distinguish "physiologic" from "pathologic" jaundice. Bilirubin is a degradation product of hemoglobin and, to a lesser extent, of myoglobin and other "nonheme" proteins. In newborns, the hemoglobin concentration is relatively high (15–18 g/100 ml), and any bruising from birth trauma or other sites of hemorrhage may exacerbate the expected baseline level of hemolysis. Markedly increased erythrocyte destruction may result from Rh or ABO isoimmunization, structural (e.g., hereditary spherocytosis) or metabolic [e.g., glucose-6-phosphate dehydrogenase (G6PD) deficiency] erythrocyte defects, or infection leads to elevated bilirubin.

Bilirubin occurs in two forms: **unconjugated** or **indirect,** most of which is bound to serum albumin; and **conjugated** or **direct,** which usually has one or two glucuronides. The enzyme **glucuronyl transferase** catalyzes bilirubin conjugation in the liver. Glucuronyl transferase activity is low at birth and increases to adult levels in the ensuing days to weeks; prematurity delays this maturation. Conjugated bilirubin is more soluble and excretable in the bile and urine. Bilirubin may also be reabsorbed from the intestines in a process known as **enterohepatic recirculation**. Critically ill newborns often have decreased intestinal motility or may not be receiving enteral feeds, which leads to higher levels of serum bilirubin via increased enterohepatic recirculation. Recent studies have suggested that maternal breast milk may elevate bilirubin levels by enhancing the enterohepatic reabsorption of bilirubin.

Excessive serum unconjugated bilirubin may lead to **bilirubin encephalopathy** or **kernicterus**. In this condition, yellow staining of the pons, basal ganglia, and other cerebellar structures is associated with permanent neurologic injury. Conjugated bilirubin does not cross the blood–brain barrier and is therefore not associated with neurologic injury.

Clinical and Laboratory Evaluation

History
Historical factors may be important in the diagnosis and treatment of hyperbilirubinemia. This condition may be associated with prematurity, sepsis, ethnicity (more prevalent in Asian and American Indian populations), poor enteral intake, dehydration, and breastfeeding.

Physical Examination
Serum bilirubin levels need be only 3–5 mg/dl to cause visible jaundice. The extent of jaundice roughly correlates with the severity of hyperbilirubinemia, with mild hyperbilirubinemia most noticeable in the face and sclerae and with severe hyperbilirubinemia causing a deeper yellow hue throughout the body.

Initial signs and symptoms of kernicterus include altered cry, seizures, obtundation, and opisthotonic (arched back) posturing. The long-term effects of kernicterus include the choreoathetoid form of cerebral palsy, mental retardation, high-tone hearing loss, and gaze palsy.

Laboratory Evaluation
The benchmark measures of hyperbilirubinemia are serum levels of total and direct bilirubin. When direct bilirubin is greater than 1.5 mg/dl and more than 10% of the total bilirubin, a patient is said to have conjugated hyperbilirubinemia. End-tidal carbon monoxide (CO) monitors are now available to measure exhaled CO, which correlates with the degree of hemolysis, because hemoglobin degrades into bilirubin and CO on an equimolar basis. Skin surface photometers, which are being used more frequently to screen a wider population of newborns, assess hyperbilirubinemia qualitatively.

At any given level of hyperbilirubinemia, ABG analysis and serum albumin measurement may help identify neonates at higher risk of brain injury. MRI of the brains of kernicteric patients may demonstrate characteristic changes in the basal ganglia and hippocampus.

A possible hemolytic etiology of hyperbilirubinemia is evaluated by comparing maternal and infant blood and Rh types, Coombs test, and reticulocyte count. Additional laboratory studies may be indicated to rule out other etiologies, including sepsis, hepatic disorders, and metabolic diseases (e.g., G6PD deficiency).

Differential Diagnosis

The differential diagnosis of unconjugated hyperbilirubinemia is extensive (Table 10.3). Several other diseases may cause conjugated hyperbilirubinemia, including extrahepatic biliary obstruction and intrahepatic cholestasis associated with infections, metabolic disorders, or hyperalimentation.

Management

Controversy exists about when to initiate therapeutic measures to lower serum bilirubin because permanent neurologic injury depends on more than serum bilirubin level alone. Serum bilirubin levels of greater than 20 mg/dl in conjunction with significant hemolysis have been found to be associated with kernicterus. Recent data suggest that otherwise healthy term infants may tolerate bilirubin levels up to 25 mg/dl with little, if any, risk of permanent neurologic injury.

Phototherapy, which induces isomerization of bilirubin to a more soluble form that is excreted in the urine, has been the mainstay of treatment. Although it may be initiated when the serum bilirubin level reaches 10–15 mg/dl, it is often started at lower levels in tiny premature neonates and at higher levels in otherwise healthy term infants without hemolysis. **Double-volume exchange transfusion** is reserved for higher levels of bilirubin, because of the attendant risks of catheter placement such as infection and embolic phenomena. Nomograms of normative bilirubin values over time are available for term newborns to help predict which patients may reach levels that might require phototherapy or exchange transfusion.

Other modes of therapy may be effective. Phenobarbital is sometimes used because it enhances bilirubin excretion from the liver. Recently, trials of metalloporphyrins have demonstrated that these agents decrease bilirubin production by competition for heme oxygenase, which catalyzes

TABLE 10.3	Differential Diagnosis of Unconjugated Hyperbilirubinemia

Physiologic jaundice: breast milk jaundice

Hemolytic anemia
- Congenital: hereditary spherocytosis, G6PD deficiency, pyruvate kinase deficiency, galactosemia, hemoglobinopathies
- Acquired: Rh or ABO incompatibility, infection, drugs (e.g., vitamin K)

Polycythemia: chronic fetal hypoxia, maternal–fetal or twin–twin transfusion, delayed cord clamping, maternal diabetes mellitus

Hematoma or hemorrhage: birth trauma, pulmonary hemorrhage, intraventricular hemorrhage (IVH)

Glucuronyl transferase defect
- Congenital: type I (Crigler-Najjar syndrome), type II deficiency, Gilbert syndrome
- Acquired: drugs (e.g., novobiocin), Lucey-Driscoll syndrome

Metabolic disorders: galactosemia, hypothyroidism, maternal diabetes mellitus

Increased enterohepatic circulation: intestinal obstruction, ileus, swallowed blood

Alterations of bilirubin–albumin binding: aspirin, sulfonamides, acidosis

G6PD = glucose-6-phosphate dehydrogenase.

the first step in the breakdown of hemoglobin into bilirubin.

HEMATOLOGIC DISORDERS

ANEMIA (SEE CHAPTER 16)

Pathophysiology

Several changes in red blood cell (RBC) mass occur during the neonatal period. **Fetal hemoglobin,** which makes up 70%–90% of hemoglobin at birth, binds oxygen more tightly, resulting in a shift of the hemoglobin–oxygen dissociation curve to the left. This shift benefits the fetus in utero by facilitating oxygen exchange from maternal to fetal RBCs. However, this feature proves disadvantageous to newborns, because release to the tissues is impaired (Figure 10.10). In utero fetal oxygen saturation is approximately 65%, resulting in high levels of erythropoietin, reticulocyte counts of 3%–7%, and steadily rising hemoglobin levels that reach a mean of 17.5 g/dl at term. After birth, with an oxygen saturation in excess of 95%, erythropoietin levels and reticulocyte counts fall dramatically. The hemoglobin level increases slightly after birth as the result of hemoconcentration, usually returning to birth levels at 1 week and then progressively falling. The postnatal decline is due to the suppression of erythropoietin and expansion of the blood volume.

The usual **physiologic anemia of infancy** occurs in full-term infants at 2–3 months with hemoglobin levels of approximately 9 g/dl. In premature infants, the nadir occurs earlier (4–7 weeks) and is lower (7–8 g/dl). This anemia of prematurity is an exaggeration of the normal physiologic anemia resulting from a smaller RBC mass at birth, shortened RBC survival, more significant blood volume increase caused by growth, and, often, frequent phlebotomy for laboratory analysis. Consumption of iron stores during this period is rapid, and without supplementation, iron deficiency anemia will result.

Clinical and Laboratory Evaluation

History
It is necessary to obtain a complete obstetric history (e.g., for abruptio placentae or cord rupture), a family history (e.g., for anemia, jaundice, gallstones, or splenectomy), as well as consider a history of blood loss, hemolysis, or frequent phlebotomy.

Physical Examination
Physical findings include pallor, tachycardia, tachypnea, hepatosplenomegaly, hypotension, and poor perfusion.

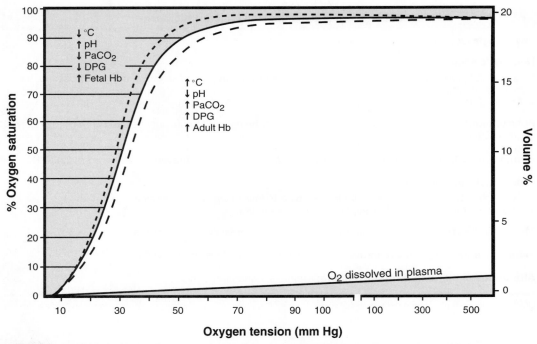

FIGURE 10.10. The oxygen dissociation curve of hemoglobin, which reflects the affinity of hemoglobin for oxygen. With a shift to the left, the affinity for oxygen increases, and less oxygen is released to the tissues. With a shift to the right, the opposite effect occurs. DPG = diphosphoglycerate; Hb = hemoglobin.

Laboratory Evaluation

A CBC, reticulocyte count, blood smear, Coombs test, bilirubin, Apt test, and Kleihauer-Betke test may be useful. In addition, ultrasound of the abdomen and head may help.

Differential Diagnosis

The causes of anemia include blood loss, hemolysis, and reductions in production of blood cells (Table 10.4).

Management

Specific indications for RBC transfusion depend on assessment of an infant's current physiologic status. Replacement of blood lost acutely is generally necessary, whereas replacement of blood drawn for laboratory evaluations is not required. Transfusions consisting of packed RBCs with a hematocrit of 60%–70% are given in aliquots; 10–20 ml/kg is generally tolerated without symptoms of cardiovascular overload. Packed RBC transfusion is necessary for infants with significant cardiorespiratory compromise, who should have hematocrits above 40% to optimize oxygen delivery. Healthy premature infants may tolerate lower

hematocrits but may benefit from transfusion if they exhibit poor weight gain, apnea, persistent tachycardia, or require supplemental oxygen.

POLYCYTHEMIA

Pathophysiology

Polycythemia is defined as a venous hemoglobin exceeding 20 g/dl or a hematocrit of over 65%. As the central hematocrit rises above 65%, blood viscosity increases exponentially, and capillary blood flow is reduced. Infarction and thrombosis may occur in the brain, lungs, intestines, or other organs. The causes of polycythemia include increased erythropoietin in response to tissue hypoxia (e.g., asphyxia) and increased blood volume (e.g., twin–twin transfusion).

Clinical and Laboratory Evaluation

History

Historical factors are important in the diagnosis and treatment of polycythemia. Infants at risk for polycythemia include infants of diabetic mothers, SGA infants, recipients of in utero twin–twin transfusions, and infants with delayed cord clamping. Polycythemia may result in feeding problems,

TABLE 10.4 **Differential Diagnosis of Anemia**

Blood loss
- Obstetric causes
  Abruptio placentae or placenta previa
  Cord rupture or hematoma
  Fetomaternal or fetoplacental bleeding
  Twin–twin transfusion
  Anomalous vessels (e.g., vasa previa, velamentous insertion)
- Neonatal causes
  Iatrogenic (e.g., phlebotomy, surgical bleeding)
  Intracranial bleeding
  Cephalohematoma
  Gastrointestinal hemorrhage
  Rupture of liver or spleen

Hemolysis
- Immune
  Rh, ABO, or minor blood group incompatibility
  Maternal autoimmune disease
  Drug-induced hemolysis
- Nonimmune
  Hereditary RBC disorders
  RBC membrane defects (e.g., spherocytosis, elliptocytosis)
  Metabolic defects (e.g., G6PD, pyruvate kinase)
  Hemoglobinopathies
  Infection
  Disseminated intravascular coagulation (DIC)
  Vitamin E deficiency
  Microangiopathic hemolytic anemia (e.g., cavernous hemangioma)

Diminished production of RBCs
  Anemia of prematurity
  Diamond-Blackfan syndrome
  Congenital leukemia
  Viral infections
  Osteopetrosis

G6PD = glucose-6-phosphate dehydrogenase; RBC = red blood cell.

NEC, hypoglycemia, seizures, renal vein thrombosis, and cerebral infarcts.

Physical Examination

Most infants with polycythemia are asymptomatic. However, tachypnea, congestive heart failure, cyanosis, plethora, jitteriness, hypotonia, lethargy, or jaundice are sometimes evident.

Laboratory Evaluation

A central venous hematocrit of greater than 65% or a hemoglobin of greater than 20 g/dl is indicative of polycythemia.

Management

A partial exchange transfusion is performed to replace blood with crystalloid or colloid. The treatment is simple, but the timing of implementation is controversial. In general, treatment is performed in symptomatic infants with hematocrits greater than 65% and in asymptomatic infants with hematocrits greater than 70%. Intravenous hydration may be given to asymptomatic infants with hematocrits between 60% and 70%.

THROMBOCYTOPENIA

Pathophysiology

Thrombocytopenia is defined as a platelet count of less than $150,000/mm^3$. The steady-state level of platelets in the blood reflects a balance between production and destruction. Platelet production can be evaluated by looking at the megakaryocytes in the bone marrow, while platelet destruction is studied by isotope labeling or by following the platelet count over time. Large platelets seen in the peripheral smear are indicative of increased destruction with young, larger platelets coming from the bone marrow.

Clinical and Laboratory Evaluation

History
Maternal history may be useful. A history of maternal thrombocytopenia, splenectomy, autoimmune disease, drug use, or infection may explain the neonatal thrombocytopenia.

Physical Examination
Physical findings may include petechiae, bruises, hepatosplenomegaly, jaundice, and congenital anomalies.

Laboratory Evaluation
The maternal platelet count should be checked, and if it is normal, platelet typing of the parents is indicated. A CBC, platelet count, prothrombin time, partial thromboplastin time, fibrinogen, and d-dimer are warranted in the infant.

Differential Diagnosis

The differential diagnosis of thrombocytopenia involves decreased platelet production, increased platelet destruction, and disorders of platelet function (Table 10.5).

TABLE 10.5	**Differential Diagnosis of Thrombocytopenia**

Decreased platelet production
    Absent radii syndrome
    Congenital cytomegalovirus and rubella
    Trisomy 13 and 18
    Methylmalonic aciduria, isovaleric acidemia, ketotic hyperglycinemia
    Bone marrow infiltration (osteopetrosis, leukemia, histiocytosis, tumors)
    Megaloblastic anemia (folate or vitamin B_{12} deficiency)
    Wiskott-Aldrich syndrome

Increased platelet destruction
- Immune
    Autoimmune (induction of platelet antibodies by maternal platelets)
    Maternal idiopathic thrombocytopenic purpura (ITP)
    Maternal autoimmune disease
    Drug-induced (digoxin, chlorothiazide, quinidine)
- Isoimmune (induction of platelet antibodies, usually against platelet antigen PI^{A1})
- Nonimmune
    Incidental maternal thrombocytopenia
    Peripheral consumption
        Disseminated intravascular coagulation (DIC)
        Kasabach-Merritt syndrome
        Sepsis
        Drug injury (e.g., thiazides, hydralazine, aspirin)
        Hypersplenism (congenital hepatitis, congenital viral infection)

Disorders of platelet function
    Bernard-Soulier syndrome
    Gray platelet syndrome
    May-Hegglin anomaly

Other conditions
    Thrombocytopenia after exchange transfusion or multiple transfusions

Management

In general, platelet transfusions are appropriate for clinical bleeding and for infants at risk for complications such as intraventricular hemorrhage. The exact platelet count at which prophylactic platelet transfusions are given is controversial and depends on several clinical variables (e.g., gestation age, illness of abnormal severity). Treatment also depends on the specific cause of the thrombocytopenia.

NEUROLOGIC DISORDERS

INTRAVENTRICULAR HEMORRHAGE

Pathophysiology

Intraventricular hemorrhage (IVH) usually starts in the **subependymal germinal matrix.** Bleeding may then extend within the ventricles to the **pos-terior fossa,** which may lead to **obliterative arachnoiditis** and **obstructive hydrocephalus.**

Autopsies of neonates as well as animal models have served as the basis of the neuropathology of IVH. About 15% of patients with IVH have a parenchymal lesion (i.e., hemorrhagic necrosis in periventricular white matter). Two-thirds of IVHs are unilateral; most of the remainder are asymmetric when they are bilateral. IVH is classified using the Papile system as follows: grade 1, subependymal/germinal matrix bleed; grade 2, intraventricular bleed; grade 3, intraventricular bleed with ventriculomegaly; and grade 4, parenchymal hemorrhage.

The etiology of IVH is complex. Experts believe that IVH is not an extension of subependymal hemorrhage but rather a subsequent hemorrhagic venous infarction. Other possible etiologies or exacerbating factors include local potassium concentration, increased intraventricular pressure, and lactic acidosis. **Intravascular factors** implicated in the development of IVH include fluctuating cerebral blood flow, increased cerebral venous pressure, and platelet and coagulation factors (probably not very significant in most cases of IVH, although they may exacerbate any bleeding that is present). **Vascular factors** associated with IVH include tenuous capillary integrity and vulnerability to hypoxic–ischemic injury. **Extravascular factors** that affect IVH include deficient vascular support, fibrinolytic activity, and postnatal decrease in tissue pressure.

Long-term morbidity associated with IVH is quite variable. Minimal, if any, handicap is usually found with grade 1 and 2 bleeds. Grade 3 and 4 hemorrhages are associated with a 50%–100% incidence of motor and mental deficits, including hydrocephalus, cerebral palsy, retardation, and seizure disorders. Neonates with severe IVH involving parenchymal hemorrhage often do not survive. In one study, 40% of infants with localized grade 4 IVH died, and 80% with extensive grade 4 bleeds succumbed.

Clinical and Laboratory Evaluation

History

IVH correlates most significantly with prematurity. In premature infants whose birth weight is less than 1500 g, the incidence of all types of IVH is approximately 30%. Grade 3 and grade 4 disease occurs in about 10% of cases. Cardiorespiratory instability and, to a lesser extent, coagulopathy, are also associated with a higher risk of IVH.

Physical Examination

Physical findings include cardiorespiratory instability, metabolic acidosis, hematocrit decline, a tense anterior fontanelle, and a change in neurologic status. Because these findings are neither very specific nor sensitive indicators of IVH, diagnosis requires neuroradiographic confirmation.

Laboratory Evaluation

Cranial ultrasonography is the most widely used neuroradiographic study for detection of IVH (Figure 10.11). Descriptors of the laterality and magnitude of the IVH are also useful. Head CT and MRI can also be used diagnostically.

Differential Diagnosis

Other neuropathologies that occur in premature infants may accompany IVH or may develop independently. These include periventricular leukomalacia, a symmetric, nonhemorrhagic, ischemic white matter injury with a predilection for periventricular arterial border zones, as well as pon-

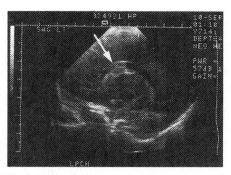

FIGURE 10.11. Head ultrasound showing a grade 3 intraventricular hemorrhage. The *arrow* indicates the location of the hemorrhage within a dilated left lateral ventricle.

tine neuronal necrosis, which is seen in as many as 50% of patients with IVH and also associated with hypoxic–ischemic insult.

Pediatric Pearl

Newborn infants with seizures should be evaluated with a head CT or MRI to rule out congenital anomalies, hemorrhage, or infarct.

Management

Prevention of premature birth is the prenatal intervention most likely to decrease the incidence of IVH. Maternal transport to a center equipped for high-risk obstetrics and neonatology prior to premature delivery may also decrease the likelihood of IVH by provision of optimal labor, delivery, and resuscitation. Recently, studies have found that administration of antenatal steroids to mothers delivering prematurely reduces the incidence and severity of IVH. Other drugs that have been studied to prevent development of IVH in premature at-risk neonates include phenobarbital, indomethacin, ethamsylate (a prostaglandin synthesis inhibitor), and vitamin E. Postnatal interventions aimed at reducing IVH include (1) minimizing cerebral blood flow fluctuations by the use of paralytics or sedation, and (2) closure of the symptomatic PDA.

HYPOXIC–ISCHEMIC INJURY

Pathophysiology

Inadequate blood flow or oxygen delivery to the brain may cause **hypoxic–ischemic encephalopathy (HIE),** a clinical term preferable to the less specific "**perinatal asphyxia.**" Prenatal origins of this hypoxia/ischemia may be maternal, placental, or fetal (Table 10.6). Hypoxic–ischemic injury may also develop any time after birth; for example, it may result from the cardiorespiratory insufficiency that may be seen in severe lung immaturity or with sepsis.

The extent and permanence of brain injury depend on the magnitude and duration of hypoxia and ischemia, as well as host factors such as the degree of prematurity. Partial asphyxia can lead to brain swelling and edema; necrosis of the cerebral cortex, basal ganglia, and thalamus; and alteration of the blood–brain barrier. Total asphyxia is more typically associated with damage to the brainstem and thalamic nuclei.

Cerebral blood flow is normally autoregulated, with an increase in flow seen with elevation of PCO_2, with acidosis, or with decreased PO_2. Loss of cerebral blood flow autoregulation may lead to concomitant IVH. Recently, studies have found that extracellular glutamate is elevated after hypoxia and is associated with neuronal toxicity that can be ameliorated by specific chemical blockers to the membrane channels leading to glutamate release. Usually only a minority of the injury occurs immediately secondary to acute necrosis. The bulk of the CNS injury usually begins with reperfusion and is secondary to apoptotic changes (programmed cell death) over days to weeks; metabolic changes are detectable by magnetic resonance spectroscopy for weeks to months.

TABLE 10.6 Causes of Hypoxic–Ischemic Encephalopathy

Maternal causes
- Decreased maternal PO_2 (from heart or lung disease)
- Decreased uteroplacental blood flow (seen in hypotension)
- Hypertensive disease with vasospasm
- Uterine abnormalities

Placental abnormalities
- Placenta previa
- Vasa previa
- Abruptio placentae
- Cord abnormalities
  Prolapse
  Compression
  Knot formation (may deprive fetus of adequate blood and oxygen)

Fetal origins
- Hemolysis (e.g., from Rh incompatibility)
- Fetal–maternal transfusion
- Twin–twin transfusion

Clinical and Laboratory Evaluation

History
Review of the obstetrical history, particularly potential causes of intrauterine growth retardation, helps identify maternal or placental risk factors for hypoxia and ischemia. Cord pH and fetal heart tracings may also reflect the acidosis that can accompany hypoxia and ischemia.

Physical Examination
Three stages of HIE in neonates have been described: stage 1, mild irritability and hypertonia, associated usually with good outcome; stage 2, hypotonia, and, sometimes, seizures, associated with variable long-term neurologic deficits; and stage 3, prolonged stupor and coma, usually leading to severe permanent neurologic injury. Classification of all HIE-affected newborns is not always straightforward because of individual variation in response to hypoxia and ischemia.

The neurologic examination may be limited or altered by other neonatal diseases or their treatment. Other organ systems are also frequently affected by hypoxic–ischemic insults: the kidneys, by oliguria, proteinuria, and hematuria; the heart, by tricuspid regurgitation and ventricular dysfunction; the lungs, by pulmonary hypertension; the intestines, by ileus or disruption of the brush border enzymes; and the bone marrow, by thrombocytopenia.

Laboratory Evaluation
Several laboratory studies may provide useful information. A lumbar puncture and CSF analysis should rule out an infectious neurologic insult; bloody CSF may suggest an intracranial hemorrhage. Cranial ultrasound may show decreased ventricular size that may accompany the cerebral edema following an acute insult and can rule out associated IVH. In HIE, CT scanning and MRI imaging yield more information; cerebral edema, changes in gray-white differentiation, hemorrhage, and infarcts reflect acute changes. Focal or global atrophy are signs of the more chronic sequelae of HIE. EEG is quite useful in following patients with the disease. Abnormalities range from decreased amplitude with excessive sharp waves, to frank seizures, and finally to the most ominous patterns of burst-suppression or a flat, isoelectric tracing.

Differential Diagnosis

Other neonatal neurologic insults may arise from congenital or neonatal infections, vascular accidents (e.g., subarachnoid hemorrhage), chromosomal or other genetic syndromes, maternal or neonatal drug exposure, and metabolic diseases.

Management

The best management strategy for HIE is prevention of hypoxic and ischemic stresses whenever possible. General supportive care ensures good cardiopulmonary function, glucose and electrolyte balance, and adequate renal function. Anticonvulsant therapy may begin prophylactically or after appreciation of seizures; phenobarbital, benzodiazepines, and phenytoin are the drugs of choice. Postinsult strategies designed to decrease cerebral edema such as head elevation, hyperventilation, fluid restriction, and mannitol or other diuretic use are of equivocal benefit. Hypothermia, either systemic or localized with a head cooling device, is under investigation in prospective, randomized, controlled trials as a potential treatment for HIE, based on data suggesting that hypothermia may ameliorate CNS apoptotic injury. Other experimental therapies under consideration include calcium channel blockers, *N*-methyl-D-aspartate (NMDA) antagonists (e.g., dextromethorphan) and iron chelators (e.g., deferoxamine).

DRUG EXPOSURE

Pathophysiology

Maternal drug exposure may lead to neurologic insult by any of several mechanisms. Drugs such as **alcohol** may have a direct teratogenic effect as seen in **fetal alcohol syndrome,** in which subtle interruption of facial development can occur, especially in the first trimester. **Cocaine** directly affects the fetus through interference with dopamine and norepinephrine uptake at the postsynaptic junction. This neurologic toxicity may not be reversible by cessation of cocaine use. Cocaine may also indirectly influence the fetus through uteroplacental and fetal vasoconstriction and hypoxia; these effects include premature birth, growth retardation, microcephaly, and neurologic insults from infarcts during development. Opiates (e.g., **heroin, methadone**) presumably alter opiate receptors associated with endorphin and enkephalin production. Any of these insults may be complicated by the socioeconomic and lifestyle problems that accompany drug abuse and that increase the likelihood of malnutrition, poor fetal growth, and sexually transmitted infections.

Clinical and Laboratory Evaluation

History

Maternal history is quite unreliable as a measure of recreational drug use. However, a nonthreatening manner on the part of the physician encourages self-reporting. The clinician may infer suspicion of drug use from behavior such as delayed or absent prenatal care. Unexplained placental abruption may raise the possibility of maternal cocaine use.

Pediatric Pearl

Infants born after a placental abruption should be evaluated for intrauterine drug exposure. Cocaine is a known cause of uterine vascular changes that increase the risk of abruptio placentae.

Physical Examination

Prematurity or SGA status may be the only sign of maternal drug use. Craniofacial anomalies, including hypoplastic philtrum, thin upper lip, decreased nose-to-midface length ratio, short palpebral fissures, and a flattened maxillary region are primarily associated with fetal alcohol syndrome. Cardiac, renal, GI, and limb anomalies may also be linked to this condition. Mild facial dysmorphism or microcephaly, as well as limb reduction defects and urinary tract anomalies, may result from cocaine use.

Laboratory Evaluation

Maternal and neonatal drug screening offers insight into only relatively recent maternal drug abuse. Unfortunately, permanent injury from drugs may have occurred months before cessation of the drug habit. Toxicology studies from meconium or hair samples are more likely to demonstrate the presence of drugs even several weeks after last use.

Repeated observation by health care providers using an objective, quantifiable scoring system is the best method for the diagnosis of neonatal abstinence or withdrawal syndrome. Common signs and symptoms of withdrawal may be neurologic, including irritability or seizures; GI, including poor feeding, vomiting, and diarrhea; respiratory; and autonomic, such as altered cry, sneezing, and sweating.

Differential Diagnosis

The signs and symptoms of drug exposure or withdrawal are nonspecific. Neurologic symptoms such as jitteriness or seizures may arise from infectious or metabolic disease. GI symptoms that mimic narcotic withdrawal may also result from anatomic or infectious causes.

Management

Supportive care is appropriate for symptomatic drug-exposed neonates. Severe narcotic withdrawal may necessitate pharmacologic intervention with an agent such as phenobarbital or an opiate such as morphine or methadone, which must be tapered slowly over several weeks. Long-term follow-up, together with parental behavioral modification and support classes, may be of help in achieving optimal developmental potential in drug-exposed infants.

OTHER DISORDERS AND ISSUES

NECROTIZING ENTEROCOLITIS

Pathophysiology

Necrotizing enterocolitis (NEC), the most common serious GI tract disorder seen in the NICU, occurs in 1%–5% of all NICU admissions and has an overall mortality of 20%–40%. Its pathogenesis is unclear but appears to be multifactorial. Characterized by acute intestinal necrosis, NEC may be the final common response of the immature GI tract to multiple damaging insults such as ischemia, infectious agents, enteral feedings, and medications.

Clinical and Laboratory Evaluation

History

History is important in the diagnosis of NEC. Prematurity is the greatest risk factor, although 7%–10% of cases occur in term infants. Suggested risks include perinatal asphyxia, IUGR, polycythemia, exchange transfusion, PDA, and rapid feeding practices. Over 90% of infants who develop NEC have received enteral feedings. Infants present with a history of feeding intolerance, vomiting, and heme-positive or grossly bloody stools.

The mean age of onset of NEC is 10 days. The clinical course of disease varies from a fulminant one with rapidly progressive signs of intestinal necrosis, sepsis, and shock to a more indolent one with gradual onset of abdominal distention, ileus, tenderness, and heme-positive stools. The potential long-term sequelae of NEC include strictures, short bowel syndrome, and failure to thrive.

Physical Examination

Abdominal examination reveals progressive abdominal distention, tenderness, guarding, and, occasionally, abdominal wall erythema. Systemic signs of NEC include lethargy, apnea and bradycardia, irritability, temperature instability, and hypotension/hypoperfusion. In fulminant NEC, metabolic acidosis, respiratory failure, and disseminated intravascular coagulation (DIC) can be seen.

Laboratory Evaluation

Stool, urine, blood, and CSF cultures are necessary in NEC. Conditions seen in NEC include hyponatremia, neutropenia or leukocytosis with a left shift, thrombocytopenia, abnormal coagulation studies, and positive blood or CSF cultures. Other findings consistent with the disease are an abnormal bowel gas pattern suggestive of ileus, bowel wall edema, and a fixed loop. A careful review of serial radiographs is often necessary. **Pneumatosis intestinalis,** which indicates air within the subserosal bowel wall, is pathognomonic (Figure 10.12). Portal or hepatic venous air, associated with an increased mortality rate, is visible in fulminant NEC. A left lateral decubitus or a cross-table lateral film is of help in determining whether intestinal perforation with pneumoperitoneum has occurred.

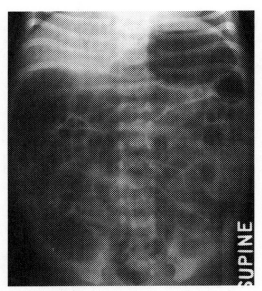

FIGURE 10.12. Abdominal radiograph of a patient with necrotizing enterocolitis.

Differential Diagnosis

The differential diagnosis of NEC includes sepsis or pneumonia with a resultant ileus, other causes of a surgical abdomen such as malrotation, volvulus, perforation, and infectious enterocolitis. Early diagnosis is an important factor in the outcome, and it is important to maintain a high index of suspicion in a susceptible population.

Management

Treatment should be initiated promptly when signs and symptoms suggestive of NEC are present. Because the condition varies in severity from a mild GI disturbance to a fulminant disease, specific treatment should be based on the severity of the clinical manifestations.

- In general, bowel rest with a nasogastric tube to suction is appropriate for infants with suspected NEC.
- If an infant is expected to receive nothing by mouth for a prolonged period, hyperalimentation is initiated.
- Administration of broad-spectrum antibiotics follow the culturing of stool, urine, blood, and CSF. This treatment generally continues for 7–14 days.
- When respiratory distress and shock accompany NEC, infants may require intubation, mechanical ventilation, and ABG monitoring.
- Ongoing blood pressure support may necessitate volume boluses or inotropic agents such as dopamine.
- Necrotic bowel may cause metabolic acidosis and coagulopathy that warrant treatment.
- Surgical intervention may be necessary. The only absolute indication for surgical intervention is pneumoperitoneum. However, pneumoperitoneum is underrecognized radiographically, leading many surgeons to operate when a progressive clinical deterioration occurs despite medical therapy.

FOLLOW-UP OF THE NURSERY GRADUATE

As smaller and sicker infants survive as a result of advances in obstetric and neonatal care, the risk of chronic sequelae rises. Follow-up studies of infants born in the modern era of NICU care in the 1960s document a significant decrease in adverse neurodevelopmental outcomes. More recent studies show a continued decrease in mortality. However, the incidence of adverse neurodevelopmental outcome has remained unchanged, resulting in an increase in the absolute number of impaired survivors. Most NICU survivors are without severe handicaps but require substantial intervention to achieve an optimal outcome. The evidence that educational enrichment during infancy and early childhood might improve the outcome of high-risk infants, especially those from disadvantaged groups, is increasing.

Management of the postdischarge care of NICU graduates may be beyond the skill and expertise of some primary care providers. Thus, a neonatal follow-up program is an important part of every modern NICU, which provides an extension of the specialized care provided in the NICU and eases the transition to the home environment. The areas targeted for monitoring and intervention are growth and nutrition, neurologic development, psychomotor development, and vision and hearing. The central focus is enhancement of the functioning of newborns and families. Some issues that are commonly encountered at and following discharge include growth, CLD, neurodevelopmental assessment, retinopathy of prematurity, and hearing screening.

Growth Retardation

Growth retardation occurs in as many as 50% of very low birth weight (VLBW) infants and is also common in infants with NEC, bronchopulmonary dysplasia, and cardiac disease. NICU graduates may be difficult to feed because of tiring, have problems with regulation of state of arousal, or require the administration of multiple medications. Prolonged inadequate nutrition has a significant effect on brain growth and neurodevelopmental outcome. To promote growth, neonatal nutrition must be optimized. High-calorie formulas are necessary for infants with obvious growth delays. Nutritionists with NICU experience frequently review feeding practices and make recommendations to physicians and parents.

Catch-up growth normally occurs in the first 2–3 years of life. When plotting growth percentiles on standardized charts, correction for gestational age should be made during the first 2 years of life.

Chronic Lung Disease

After discharge, infants with CLD require close monitoring of respiratory status, including visits for drug and electrolyte levels, pulse oximetry, and blood gases. Approximately 50% of infants with CLD require rehospitalization during the first year of life. CLD usually resolves by 2 years of age.

Neurodevelopmental Delay

Infants most at risk for neurodevelopmental problems are those with severe asphyxia, periventricular hemorrhage (grades 3 and 4), meningitis, neonatal seizures, IUGR, CLD, multiple congenital anomalies, and VLBW. Many of these infants have transient neurologic abnormalities such as hypotonia or hypertonia. Identification of major neurologic problems is usually possible in the latter half of the first year of life—earlier if they are severe. Major neurodevelopmental handicaps are generally classified as **cerebral palsy** (spastic diplegia, spastic quadriplegia, spastic hemiplegia, or paresis), hydrocephalus, blindness, seizures, or deafness.

To assess the severity of neurodevelopmental problems, the Bayley Scales of Infant Development, the most common psychomotor evaluation used in high-risk children, is helpful. Usually, the reported percentage of premature infants with abnormal scores is 5%–20%, but recent studies have found abnormal scores at 2 years of age in 37% of infants with birth weights of less than 1000 g. These children have more neurologic dysfunction, lower intelligence quotients, and more behavioral difficulties than other NICU graduates. Even in VLBW children with normal intelligence, subtle neuroperceptual abnormalities that may result in school problems have been documented.

Retinopathy of Prematurity

Retinopathy of prematurity (ROP), a developmental problem of the incompletely vascularized retina that occurs in premature infants, may result in a range of outcomes varying from normal vision to blindness. The normal development of the retina is interrupted. Beginning at 15–18 weeks' gestation, the retinal vessels normally grow outward from the ora serrata. An injury such as hyperoxia or asphyxia may arrest this development. After the initial injury, proliferation of vessel growth in an abnormal fashion may form a ridge of tissue, which may either regress or worsen with the growth of fibrovascular tissue into the vitreous. With contraction of the neovascular tissue, the retina becomes distorted, forming a scar that may result in retinal detachment.

Which infants will experience regression or progression of the retinopathy is unclear, but some investigators have suggested that chronic hypoxia is a risk factor. Regular retinal examination beginning at age 6 weeks is necessary for all infants born before 34 weeks' gestation who were exposed to oxygen. At that time, information is recorded on the location, extent, and severity of retinal changes. Even infants with mild disease have a higher incidence of myopia, strabismus, and amblyopia.

The strongest predictors of ROP have always been gestational age and birth weight. Studies have found that ROP occurs in 66% of all premature infants with birth weights of less than 1250 g, with 6% requiring cryotherapy to prevent retinal detachment. Cryotherapy is proven to reduce the incidence of poor visual outcome. Blindness due to ROP occurs in approximately 1%–2% for infants with birth weights of less than 1000 g.

Sensorineural Hearing Loss

NICU graduates have a substantial risk of sensorineural hearing loss. The numerous risk factors for hearing loss include gestational age less than 35 weeks, hyperbilirubinemia requiring exchange transfusion, ototoxic drugs, congenital viral infections, PPHN, and neurologic injury (e.g., intracranial hemorrhage, seizures, meningitis, or asphyxia). Generally, at-risk infants undergo an auditory brainstem-evoked response a screening test prior to discharge and periodic hearing examinations during the first 2 years of life. The incidence of hearing impairment is approximately 10% in infants with birth weights of less than 1000 g.

SUGGESTED READINGS

American Academy of Pediatrics and American College of Obstetricians and Gynecologists: *Guidelines for Perinatal Care,* 4th ed. Elk Grove Village, IL: American Academy of Pediatrics, 1997.

Cloherty JP, Stark AR (eds): *Manual of Neonatal Care,* 4th ed. Philadelphia: Lippincott Williams & Wilkins, 1998.

Fanaroff AA, Martin RJ (eds): *Neonatal–Perinatal Medicine: Diseases of the Fetus and Infant,* 6th ed. St Louis: Mosby–Year Book, 1996.

Kattwinkel J, American Academy of Pediatrics, and NRP Steering Committee: *Textbook of Neonatal Resuscitation.* Elk Grove Village, IL: American Academy of Pediatrics, 2000.

Klaus MH, Fanaroff AA: *Care of the High-Risk Neonate,* 5th ed. Philadelphia: WB Saunders, 2001.

Remington JS, Klein JO: *Infectious Diseases of the Fetus and Newborn Infant,* 5th ed. Philadelphia: WB Saunders, 2001.

Volpe JJ: *Neurology of the Newborn,* 4th ed. Philadelphia: WB Saunders, 2000.

Chapter 11

Genetics

Robert W. Marion

Clinical genetics, a pediatric subspecialty, poses unique challenges. Because of the generalized nature of most genetic diseases, which affect many organ systems, the clinical geneticist must first be a generalist and then a subspecialist. In addition, contact with children with genetic diseases and congenital malformations can be a daunting experience for students. Individuals with genetic disorders are often very sick and may be disfigured in appearance. Finally, because these disorders often occur in infants born to parents who are about the same age as the medical student, dealing with these families may be psychologically difficult.

Congenital malformations are defined as clinically significant abnormalities in either form or function. Malformations result from a localized error in **morphogenesis,** an event that usually occurs early in the first trimester of pregnancy. Malformations differ from **deformations;** in deformations, early morphogenesis has progressed normally but **environmental factors,** often external to the fetus, disturb the normally developing tissue. Thus, the presence of a malformation such as a cleft palate implies an abnormality that occurred during embryonic life, while a deformation such as congenital dislocation of the hip results from disturbances during the second or third trimester or, in some cases (e.g., dolichocephalic head shape in premature infants), even during early postnatal life. It is important to distinguish between these two conditions for prognostic reasons. Malformations often require aggressive surgical or medical management, while deformations often resolve on their own once the disturbing environmental force has been removed.

A **malformation sequence** occurs when a single malformation, leads to other structural changes as a result of later, related developmental consequences. One example of such a disorder is the **Pierre Robin** malformation sequence, in which a single primary malformation, the failure of growth of the mandible during the first few weeks of gestation (**micrognathia**), results secondarily in a U-shaped **cleft palate** and **glossoptosis** (the presence of a large tongue that falls backwards and obstructs the airway).

A **malformation syndrome,** which is defined as a recognizable pattern of anomalies that results from a single identifiable underlying cause, may involve a series of malformations, malformation sequences, and deformations. For example, in infants with Down syndrome, malformations of the central nervous system (CNS), craniofacies, heart, and limbs all result from the presence of an extra copy of chromosome 21 in every nucleated cell of the body.

An **association** differs from a syndrome because although recognizable patterns of malformations appear repetitively, no common unifying cause of the pattern is yet known. For example, although certain features such as **v**ertebral anomalies, **a**nal atresia, **c**ardiac defects, **t**racheoesophageal fistula, **r**enal anomalies, and **l**imb anomalies (VACTERL) occur more commonly together than would be expected by chance, no single causative agent has been identified.

Only about 50% of all infants in whom multiple congenital anomalies are present ultimately receive a diagnosis of an identifiable etiology or a particular malformation syndrome. Confirmation of a syndromic diagnosis is important for three reasons.

1. Identification of a diagnosis guides the physician during the remainder of the child's evaluation. Knowledge that specific internal malformations may be associated with the identified disorder, as well as information concerning the natural history of the entity, allows the physician to anticipate problems before they become evident.
2. Confirmation of a diagnosis improves communication between the physician and the family. It allows the parents, through a better understanding of the natural history of their child's disorder, to make informed decisions.
3. Confirmation of a diagnosis allows for proper genetic counseling, offering the parents an ac-

curate recurrence risk and the potential for prenatal diagnosis in future pregnancies.

APPROACH TO THE CHILD WITH CONGENITAL MALFORMATIONS

Unfortunately, congenital malformations are not rare in children. Approximately 3% of all infants born in the United States each year have one or more birth defects that are discovered during the neonatal period. This figure is closer to 7%–8% in a population of 1-year-old children, because some malformations such as congenital heart and renal anomalies remain clinically silent during the newborn period, only to manifest themselves later in the first year of life. Finally, it has been estimated that as many as 40%–50% of all admissions to pediatric services are for children with congenital malformations. This section will provide a framework for evaluating children with one or more congenital malformations.

Clinical and Laboratory Evaluation

History

Infants do not begin their life histories at the time of birth. During the 40 weeks of intrauterine life, they have been growing and developing, and a great deal of information can be obtained about

their health through carefully questioning the mother about her pregnancy (Table 11.1).

Physical Examination

While examining the child, the examiner should note all features, both those that appear normal and those that appear abnormal. This review highlights those features in which clues for the diagnosis of congenital malformation syndromes are most likely to be found.

GENERAL APPEARANCE. First, the clinician should carefully measure height and weight and plot the values on appropriate growth curves. This information helps categorize the underlying problem. Growth that is appropriate for age is consistent with the presence of a single gene disorder, a multifactorially inherited condition, or, most commonly, no genetic disease. **Growth retardation,** whether beginning pre- or postnatally, may result from a chromosomal abnormality or exposure to toxic, teratogenic agents. Finally, a larger-than-expected size suggests an **overgrowth syndrome** (e.g., Sotos cerebral gigantism or Beckwith-Wiedemann syndrome), or, in the newborn, a diabetic mother. The practitioner should also assess the child's body habitus. Is the child proportionate? If not, are the arms and legs too short for the head and trunk, implying the presence of a short-

---

TABLE 11.1 **Approach to the Dysmorphic Child: History**

Questions about the parents

How old are they?

How many previous pregnancies did the mother have? Did she have any spontaneous abortions? Was there neonatal demise?

Did the mother work outside the home during the pregnancy? Was she exposed to toxic chemicals?

Does the mother have any underlying medical conditions (e.g., diabetes mellitus, seizure disorder)?

Did the mother take any medications during the pregnancy?

Did the mother smoke cigarettes or use alcohol or other drugs during the pregnancy?

How much weight did the mother gain during the pregnancy?

Questions about the pregnancy

When did quickening occur?

Were fetal movements active (as compared with previous pregnancies)?

Was any special testing performed (e.g., amniocentesis, chorionic villus sampling, sonography)?

Did mother have illnesses (e.g., infections, fever)?

Questions about delivery

Was the infant full term, premature, or postmature?

Was the infant's size normal, large, or small (for gestational age)?

Were there any complications in the delivery room or nursery?

Questions about family history

Does a complete pedigree contain any evidence of past congenital malformations, similar or dissimilar anomalies, neonatal demise, or pregnancy loss?

limbed bone dysplasia such as **achondroplasia**? Are the trunk and head too short for the extremities, suggesting a disorder affecting the vertebrae, such as spondyloepiphyseal dysplasia?

CRANIOFACIES. Careful examination of the craniofacial region is of crucial importance in the diagnosis of many congenital malformation syndromes. The head circumference should be carefully measured and plotted on an appropriate growth curve. It is also important to describe the overall shape of the skull. Is the child normocephalic? Is the head long and thin (dolichocephalic) or short and wide (brachycephalic)? Is the head lopsided (plagiocephalic)?

> ### Pediatric Pearl
>
> It is never helpful to describe a child's face as "funny-looking." The clinician should attempt to carefully describe what makes the facial features unusual.

Next, the examiner should concentrate on the face. An assessment of facial symmetry is essential. Asymmetry may be due to either a deforming process related to the intrauterine position of the fetus or malformations of one side of the face. For purposes of examination, the clinician may divide the infant's face into four regions and evaluate each region separately (Figure 11.1). Assessment of the forehead for both overt prominence (as is the case in **achondroplasia**) or deficiency (described as a sloping appearance, as occurs in children with **primary microcephaly**) is necessary. Examination of the midface, the region extending from the eyebrows to the upper lip and from the outer canthi of the eyes to the commissures of the mouth, is especially important. Assessment of the distance between the eyes (inner canthal distance and interpupillary distance) confirms the presence of **hypotelorism** (eyes that are too close together, suggestive of an associated defect in midline brain formation) or **hypertelorism** (eyes that are too far apart). Measurement of the length of the palpebral fissures (measured from inner canthus to outer canthus) determines whether these structures are short (as in **fetal alcohol syndrome**) or excessively long (as in the Kabuki make-up syndrome).

The obliquity (or slant) of the eyes in either an upward (**Down syndrome**) or a downward (**Treacher Collins syndrome**) direction; the presence of epicanthal folds (Down syndrome or fetal alcohol syndrome); the height of the nasal bridge (flat in Down, fetal alcohol, and other syndromes, and raised in **velocardiofacial syndrome**); the length of the philtrum (which should have a central depression surrounded by two pillars); and the upper vermilion border (the pink part of the lip) should be noted and recorded.

The third portion of the face to be examined, the malar region, extends bilaterally from the ear into the midface. It is essential to evaluate the ears; the clinician should measure their maximal

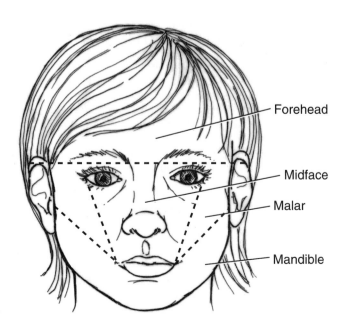

FIGURE 11.1. The four regions of the face.

length and plot the values on a growth curve. It is also necessary to examine the position of the ears; so-called **"low-set" ears** end below a line extended laterally from the outer canthus of the eye. Ears may be low set because they are microtic (unusually small) or because of anomalies of the mandibular region of the face. Description and notation of the architecture of each ear is essential.

The final portion of the face that warrants evaluation is the mandibular region, the area contained between the lower portion of both ears, including the mouth. The mandible should normally be slightly retruded in newborns; when viewed in profile, it should end slightly behind the level of the philtrum and upper lip. If this retrusion is exaggerated, the infant might be affected with micrognathia, a feature of the Pierre Robin malformation sequence.

EXTREMITIES. Anomalies of the extremities are common features of a vast number of congenital malformation syndromes. The pediatrician should conduct a brief examination of all joints. The presence of **single or multiple contractures** suggests either intrinsic neuromuscular dysfunction, as in the case of some forms of **muscular dystrophy**, or external deforming forces. Inability to pronate and supinate the elbow suggests **radioulnar synostosis**, an anomaly that occurs in fetal alcohol syndrome and in some of the X chromosome aneuploidy syndromes.

Close examination of the hands is extremely important. **Polydactyly** (extra digits) most often occurs as an isolated but fairly common autosomal dominant trait, but it can also be a prominent feature of a syndrome such as **trisomy 13.** In contrast, **oligodactyly,** a deficiency in the number of fingers or toes, is a less common finding. It may be part of a more severe limb reduction deficiency disorder, as occurs in patients with **Fanconi syndrome,** or may be secondary to an intrauterine amputation, as is the case in the **amniotic band disruption sequence.** Another disorder of the extremities, **syndactyly** (a joining of two or more digits) is fairly common in a number of syndromes.

GENITALIA. When examining the male genitalia, the clinician should briefly observe the penis and scrotum. If the penis appears short, measurement of penile length is necessary, and the practitioner should plot it on an appropriate growth curve. Ambiguity of the genitalia should suggest the presence of either an endocrinologic disorder such as **congenital adrenal hyperplasia,** a chromosomal disorder such as 45,X/46,XY mosaicism, or an inherited syndrome.

Hypospadias is a common congenital malformation, occurring in approximately 1 in 300 newborn males. This is most often an isolated malformation, but if it occurs in the presence of other anomalies, the possibility that the child is affected with a syndrome warrants consideration.

Laboratory Evaluation

In most children with multiple congenital anomalies, only a limited number of laboratory tests are necessary.

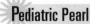

Pediatric Pearl

Karyotype analysis is warranted in any child who has three or more detected abnormalities.

Chromosome analyses are not indicated in the infant with an isolated cleft lip or palate unless other malformations are present. Chromosome analysis involves three types of cells:

1. **Peripheral blood lymphocytes** stimulated to divide by use of mitogenic agents. Because this requires 2–3 days in culture, results are not available for at least 72 hours.
2. **Skin fibroblasts.** Results from fibroblast cultures usually require 2–3 weeks.
3. **Bone marrow cells,** which because they are already rapidly dividing, can be analyzed immediately and yield results within 1 day.

The urgency of the situation dictates the type of cells used. When it is necessary to make critical management decisions, as in a child with features of trisomy 13 or 18, a bone marrow sample may be indicated. In the child with features of trisomy 21 or in whom no clear diagnosis is evident, peripheral blood lymphocytes are usually studied.

Any child with evident multiple external malformations should also have a careful evaluation to rule out the presence of associated internal malformations. Ultrasound evaluations of the head and abdomen are warranted; a chest radiograph, electrocardiogram (ECG), and echocardiogram are indicated in any child with anomalies who has an audible heart murmur or syndrome with a known risk for cardiac anomalies (e.g., Down syndrome).

In addition, specialized testing such as fluorescent in situ hybridization (FISH) or direct DNA testing is necessary in the child suspected of having a syndrome known to be associated with a specific chromosome deletion (e.g., Prader-Willi syndrome, which is associated with deletion of chromosome 15q11.2) or a known single gene defect (e.g., fragile X syndrome, which is associated with a failure to express the FMR1 gene on the X chromosome).

Diagnosis

Although the presence of characteristic findings may sometimes make the definitive diagnosis of a malformation syndrome simple, in the majority of cases no specific diagnosis is immediately evident. Some constellations of findings are rare, and finding a "match" may prove difficult. In many cases, all laboratory tests are normal, and confirmation relies on subjective findings. Clinical geneticists have attempted to resolve this problem by the development of scoring systems, cross-referenced tables of anomalies that allow the development of a differential diagnosis, and computerized diagnostic programs.

Making an accurate diagnosis is important for three reasons. One, it offers an explanation for why the child was born with specific problems. Often, before a diagnosis is made, parents feel that in some way they were directly responsible for their child's problem. Providing a diagnosis often allays this guilt. Two, a correct diagnosis allows the physician to provide anticipatory guidance. Because the natural history of so many disorders is known, the health care provider can perform screening to check for problems known to occur in that condition, and at the same time, often reassure the parent about other complications that have not been reported previously. Three, an accurate diagnosis allows the pediatrician to provide genetic counseling concerning future progeny, when available. In addition, referral for prenatal testing may occur early in subsequent pregnancies.

Once a diagnosis is made, the clinician can provide the family with a wealth of educational material. The World Wide Web has become an important source of such information (Table 11.2). However, because the Web is not subject to editorial control, some of the information is inaccurate or inappropriate. Therefore, it is essential that the clinician screen the sites before encouraging a family to seek Web-based information. A good screening tool is the Web site of the National Organization for Rare Disorders (NORD). Because the field of medical genetics is expanding so rapidly, it is also difficult to remain current regarding the availability of testing for specific conditions. The GeneTests Web site, which provides constantly updated information regarding such testing, has become indispensable.

CHARACTERISTICS OF SOME GENETIC AND CONGENITAL MALFORMATION SYNDROMES

Congenital malformations can be classified into five categories (Table 11.3):

1. Chromosomal disorders, which account for 7% of all anomalies
2. Single gene disorders, which demonstrate Mendelian inheritance patterns and account for another 7% of the total
3. Multifactorially inherited disorders, which result from an interplay of genetic and environmental factors and account for 20% of all congenital anomalies
4. Teratogenically induced disorders, caused by exposure of the conceptus to a toxic environmental agent, accounting for 7%
5. Unknown causes, which presently account for 50% of all malformations

Because so many genetic disorders exist, only a handful of representative conditions will be discussed.

Chromosomal Disorders

The cells of all normal humans contain 46 chromosomes. The chromosomes may be divided into two major types: the 44 autosomes and the two sex chromosomes. Occurring in pairs and numbered from 1 (the largest) to 22 (the smallest), the autosomes are indistinguishable in males and females, who are genetically distinguished on the basis of their complement of sex chromosomes. Males have an X and a Y chromosome, and females have two X chromosomes.

Autosomal Aberrations

The impression that a chromosomal defect is present is strengthened by the presence of a group of cardinal features that are frequently found in such individuals, including:

- Growth retardation, which may begin in utero
- Developmental retardation, which is often profound
- Structural defects of the craniofacies, CNS, and cardiovascular system, as well as other internal organ systems

For each of the common autosomal chromosomal aberration syndromes, a definite pattern of

TABLE 11.2	**World Wide Web Sites With Information About Common Genetic Disorders**

General sites
- Online Mendelian Inheritance in Man (OMIM)

www.ncbi.nlm.nih.gov/omim/searchomim.html

Maintained by McKusick-Nathans Institute for Genetic Medicine at Johns Hopkins University. Each entry contains a bibliography of all articles published in the medical literature about a given condition.
- Gene tests

www.genetests.org

Provides updated information on testing for specific genetic diseases

Patient resources
- National Organization for Rare Disorders (NORD)

www.rarediseases.org

A clearinghouse for information about genetic conditions, which allows clinicians to search its database and find appropriate disease-specific web sites. It provides links to support groups for specific conditions.
- Online Genetic Support Groups Directory

www.mostgene.org

Provides alphabetical list of genetic disorders

Common genetic conditions and their Web sites
- Achondroplasia and other bone dysplasias
  Little People of America (LPA): *www.lpaonline.org*
- Spina bifida and other neural tube defects (information on latex allergy)
  Spina Bifida Association of America (SBAA): *www.sbaa.org*
- Cystic fibrosis
  Cystic Fibrosis Foundation (CFF): *www.cff.org*
- Down syndrome: *www.nas.com/downsyn*
  (There are several good sites, but this is a good place to start.)
- Cleft lip, cleft palate, and other craniofacial disorders
  Wide Smiles (organization name): *www.widesmiles.org*
- Fragile X syndrome
  FRAXA Research Foundation: *www.fraxa.org*
- Marfan syndrome
  National Marfan Foundation: *www.marfan.org*
- Duchenne muscular dystrophy and other forms of muscular dystrophy
  Muscular Dystrophy Association (MDA) USA: *www.mdausa.org*
- Neurofibromatosis
  National Neurofibromatosis Organization: *www.nf.org*
  Although most of the information listed is about neurofibromatosis type 1, there are mention of other forms as well.
- Prader-Willi syndrome
  Prader-Willi Syndrome Association (PWSA): *www.pwsausa.org*
- Velocardiofacial syndrome (DiGeorge syndrome)
  Velocardiofacial Syndrome (VCFS) Education Foundation: *www.vcfsef.org*
- Williams syndrome
  Williams Syndrome Association: *www.williams-syndrome.org*
- Organic/Amino Acidemias
  Organic Acidemia Association (OAA): *www.oaanews.org*
- Mucopolysaccharidoses, including Hunter, Hurler, Morquio, and other mucopolysaccharidoses
  National Mucopolysaccharidosis (MPS) Society: *www.mpssociety.org*

malformations is known to occur. However, although the karyotype may be the same from individual to individual, striking variability in expression may exist.

TRISOMY 21 (DOWN SYNDROME). This disorder, the most common and best known of all cytogenetic aber-

rations, occurs in 1 in every 800 births. Although the cause of the entity is always an extra copy of chromosome 21, the configuration of that extra chromosome is not always the same. In 92.5% of cases, straightforward trisomy 21 occurs. In 4.5% of cases, the extra chromosome is part of a Robertsonian translocation, a rearrangement of chromo-

TABLE 11.3 Classification of Congenital Malformations*

Causes	Number (%)
Single gene mutations	8400 (7.5%)
Chromosomal abnormalities	6720 (6.0%)
Multifactorially inherited conditions	22,400 (20.0%)
Teratogenically induced conditions	7200 (6.5%)
Unknown causes	67,200 (60.0%)

*Total number of births in 1987 was 3,600,00, of which there were 112,000 (3%) infants with malformations.

TABLE 11.4 External Characteristics of Children With Down Syndrome

Craniofacial abnormalities
Hypoplastic midface
Flattened nasal bridge
Eyes
 Upward slanting palpebral fissures
 Epicanthal folds (flaps of skin) covering inner canthi of eyes
 Irides with speckled appearance caused by Brushfield spots
Flat occiput, causing brachycephalic appearance with flattened facial profile
Large tongue, often protruding from mouth
Flattened upper part of helices of ears

Extracranial findings
 Shortening of hands and fingers (brachydactyly) [most striking in fifth finger]
 Simian crease (single crease across palm of hand) [50%]
 Skin usually doughy in consistency
 (Males only) Small penis (often)

somal material in which one chromosome 21 is attached to another chromosome (most commonly chromosome 14). In approximately 3% of cases, mosaicism occurs; there are two separate populations of cells, one with trisomy 21, the other with a normal chromosome complement. Although it is widely believed that individuals with mosaic Down syndrome are more mildly affected, there are wide variations in clinical findings in mosaic individuals.

The diagnosis of Down syndrome is nearly always made in the newborn period. Affected children, who are often of normal birth weight and length, are strikingly hypotonic. This floppiness causes them to feed poorly and to seem less active than other babies. In addition to the hypotonia, several other external and internal characteristics are present (Tables 11. 4 and 11.5). The facial appearance of affected children is striking (Figure 11.2).

Life expectancy figures in individuals with Down syndrome are difficult to cite with confidence. In the past, premature death resulting from infectious diseases such as hepatitis was not uncommon, because many such children were placed in institutions at birth. With better care and with more aggressive treatment of congenital heart defects, it is expected that long-term survival will occur in the majority of children born with Down syndrome.

Although the cause of Down syndrome is well known, the reason for the nondisjunction that leads to trisomy 21 remains a mystery. Down syndrome is commonly associated with advanced maternal age. Exactly why this may lead to aberrant chromosomal development is not understood, but the association has led to the development of a series of prenatal diagnostic techniques that are currently offered to women over 35 years of age, the age at which the risk of bearing a child

TABLE 11.5 Internal Malformations in Children With Down Syndrome

Congenital heart disease (40%)
 Atrioventricular canal
 Ventricular septal defect, atrial septal defect
 Valvular disease
Gastrointestinal defects (10%)
 Duodenal atresia
 Tracheoesophageal fistula
 Annular pancreas
 Imperforate anus
 Hirschsprung disease
Growth retardation (90%)
Developmental retardation (99%)
 Mental retardation (primarily moderate; may range from borderline to profound)
Neurologic defects (99%)
 Hypotonia
 Seizures (10%)
 Presenile dementia (as early as third decade)
Endocrinologic abnormalities
 Hypothyroidism or hyperthyroidism (20%)
 Infertility in males (100%)
Hematologic abnormalities
 Leukemoid reaction during neonatal period
 Leukemia (all types) [risk increased > 20-fold]
Skeletal abnormalities
 Joint hypermobility
 Atlantoaxial instability (10%–15%)
 Osteoarthritis of cervical spine

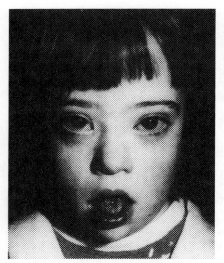

FIGURE 11.2. Facial features of an individual with Down syndrome.

with trisomy 21 is approximately equivalent to the risk introduced by amniocentesis.

There is some misunderstanding about the relationship between Down syndrome and maternal age. Only 25% of all children with Down syndrome are born to women older than 35 years of age. However, only 5% of *all* infants are born to these older women, so their risk of giving birth to a child with Down syndrome increases strikingly. Advanced paternal age appears to have little effect on the risk of trisomic births. In fact, researchers have recently shown that 89% of cases of trisomy 21 appear to result from nondisjunction occurring in either the first or second meiotic division in the ovum.

Because the majority of infants with Down syndrome are born to women younger than 35 years of age (women who are not routinely referred for amniocentesis), biochemical screening tests have been developed to identify those pregnancies most likely to be at risk for chromosomal abnormalities. These tests, most often evaluating four markers (maternal serum α-fetoprotein, unconjugated estriol, inhibin A, and chorionic gonadotropin) allow the development of a risk profile for each woman. These screening tests are not definitive; they simply identify which women are at increased risk for having a child with Down syndrome. Amniocentesis, the more definitive test for identification of fetal chromosomal abnormalities, should be offered to women at increased risk.

After the birth of a child with Down syndrome, the recurrence risk for future pregnancies depends on cytogenetic findings. With trisomy 21, the chance for recurrence based on empiric observation is approximately 1% for subsequent pregnancies (added to the age-specific risk); this risk is not just for Down syndrome but also for trisomy 18 or 13. If a translocation is discovered, it is essential that the karyotype of both parents be ascertained. Approximately two-thirds of the time, it turns out that the translocation has arisen de novo (a spontaneous event; the empiric recurrence risk following such an event is approximately 1%). In one-third of cases, one of the parents has a balanced translocation. This finding is often but not always accompanied by a history of pregnancy wastage. The recurrence risk depends on which parent carries the translocation: If the mother is the carrier, the risk of recurrence is 10%–15%; if the father is the carrier, the recurrence risk is only 2%–5%.

TRISOMY 18 (EDWARDS SYNDROME). Trisomy 18, which occurs in approximately 1 in 5000 live births, is the second most common autosomal trisomy. Unlike Down syndrome, trisomy 18 is almost universally lethal; less than 10% of affected individuals survive until their first birthday. Although survival into adolescence has been documented, such longevity is rare and is associated with severe or profound mental retardation and innumerable medical problems. As a result of the bleak prognosis, once the diagnosis has been confirmed, most authorities favor limiting the use of medical interventions for the prolongation of life.

Children with trisomy 18 have a characteristic appearance: small-for-gestational age, hypertonia, a characteristic facial appearance, and an unusual hand posture. More than 130 additional malformations have been reported. In addition, aberrant gestational timing occurs in trisomy 18. One-third of infants are born prematurely, another one-third are postmature. Information regarding recurrence risk and recommendations for genetic counseling are the same as for Down syndrome.

TRISOMY 13 (PATAU SYNDROME). Trisomy 13, which occurs in about 1 in 10,000 live births, is also nearly always lethal during fetal or early postnatal life. Affected infants have numerous malformations. They are small-for-gestational age and microcephalic. The midline facial anomalies, including cyclopia (single orbit), cebocephaly (single nostril), and clefts of the lip and palate that are often seen, are associated with midline defects of the brain such as alobar holoprosencephaly (failure of the cerebrum to divide into right and left hemispheres, resulting in a single cerebral holosphere). The forehead is sloping, the ears are small and malformed, and microphthalmia (small eyes) or anophthalmia (no eyes) occur. The hands show postaxial polydactyly and abnormal palmar creases, and the feet are malformed, usually with a club foot or rocker bottom deformity. Males have hypospadias and cryptorchidism, and females have hypoplasia of the labia majora. Internally, numerous malformations are encountered, including congenital heart disease, a nearly constant finding. Like the other autosomal trisomies, trisomy 13 is associated with advanced maternal age. Recurrence risk is similar to that of Down syndrome.

DELETION 5P SYNDROME (CRI-DU-CHAT OR CAT'S CRY SYNDROME). The cause of this syndrome is a deletion of part of the short arm of chromosome 5. Beginning in the newborn period and continuing through the first few months of life, children affected with this disorder have a striking cat-like cry that is caused by laryngeal hypoplasia. Other clinical features include low birth weight and postnatal failure to thrive; hypotonia and developmental delay; microcephaly; and craniofacial dysmorphism, including ocular hypertelorism, epicanthal folds, downward obliquity of the palpebral fissures, and low-set malformed ears. Clefting of the lip and palate, congenital heart disease, and other malformations are occasionally seen.

The clinical severity of cri-du-chat syndrome appears to correlate with the size of the deletion: the larger the deletion, the more severe the expression. Most cases arise de novo. When such is the case, the deletion usually occurs in the copy of chromosome 5 inherited from the father. This finding is believed to be due to the phenomenon of imprinting.

Sex Chromosome Aberrations

Unlike the syndromes caused by anomalies of the autosomal chromosomes, sex chromosome abnormalities tend to be subtle and may remain undetected during early life. No generalizations can be made about the phenotype of such individuals; birth weight is frequently normal; external examination usually reveals no anomalies; and except for the genitourinary tract, internal anomalies are often not present. Sex chromosome anomalies are most often detected during the early teenage years because of the failure of

affected individuals to begin puberty at the appropriate time.

☀ Pediatric Pearl

It is important that patients newly diagnosed with Turner syndrome, Klinefelter syndrome, and related disorders receive appropriate and ongoing psychologic counseling for two reasons: (1) the later time of diagnosis and (2) the sensitive nature of the problems caused by such disorders.

TURNER SYNDROME (45,X). The entity now known as Turner syndrome, a relatively mild disorder, occurs in 1 in 5000 live female births. In most cases, it is associated with normal intelligence, lack of significant disabilities, and normal life expectancy. It is not unusual for girls with Turner syndrome to escape detection during the newborn period. About one-third of affected girls are diagnosed at birth, another one-third during childhood as part of an evaluation for short stature, and the final one-third in the teenage years because of failure to develop secondary sex characteristics.

It has become clear that the 45,X karyotype is consistent with two very different phenotypic expressions, one seen prenatally and the other postnatally. Through studies of spontaneous aborted embryos and fetuses, researchers have discovered that 99% of conceptuses with a 45,X karyotype die early in pregnancy as the result of severe hydrops fetalis from lymphatic obstruction. Turner syndrome is the single leading cause of first-trimester spontaneous abortion, accounting for approximately 9% of all early pregnancy losses.

The newborn with Turner syndrome may have a characteristic appearance at birth with webbing of the neck and puffiness of the hands and feet, as well as an unusual facial appearance, a "shield" chest, cubitus valgus, short fourth metacarpals, and spoon-shaped nails. As these girls age, other features become apparent, including short stature and failure to develop secondary sexual characteristics as a result of failure of ovarian development. Internal anomalies are not uncommon in women with Turner syndrome. Cardiac defects, including coarctation of the aorta, aortic valve stenosis, and dissecting aneurysm of the aorta, a life-threatening complication, occur in approximately one-third of patients. Renal anomalies, including horseshoe-shaped kidneys and duplication of the collecting systems, are seen in more than half of affected patients.

Only half of liveborn individuals with Turner syndrome have a 45,X karyotype. Many girls have some variation of 45,X, including mosaicism and deletions of portions of one X chromosome. Although intelligence in women with Turner syndrome is usually normal, specific cognitive problems commonly occur, including defects in spatial perception, perceptual motor organization, and fine motor skills. Women with Turner syndrome are nearly always infertile. Estrogen replacement therapy may induce the development of secondary sexual characteristics, but unassisted reproduction has not been possible.

Recently, in vitro fertilization technology using donor eggs and hormonal therapy has allowed some women with Turner syndrome to bear children. Although assisted reproduction has offered hope of fertility to adult women with this disorder, great care must be taken, and close medical follow-up is essential. Recent evaluation has shown that pregnancy may have an adverse effect on the aorta, hastening the dissection of an aneurysm.

KLINEFELTER SYNDROME (47,XXY). Klinefelter syndrome, which occurs in 1 in 1000 births, represents the most common genetic cause of hypogonadism and infertility in males. Nearly always normal throughout childhood, the male with Klinefelter syndrome usually remains undiagnosed until adolescence. At that time, males with Klinefelter syndrome are often notably tall, with long arms and legs. In addition, gynecomastia is present, and with the passage of time, central obesity occurs. Intelligence is usually normal, but affected individuals are said to manifest features of immaturity.

☀ Pediatric Pearl

The most striking physical feature in adolescents with Klinefelter syndrome is the failure of growth of the testes.

In spite of the appearance of pubic hair and growth of the penis, the testes remain small, nearly prepubertal in volume, and feel soft and "mushy." This finding, in the presence of normal pubic hair distribution, is pathognomonic for this condition.

In men with Klinefelter syndrome, testosterone replacement therapy results in the development of secondary sex characteristics, including deepening of the voice; male body habitus and beard; and libido. Some affected males have additional X chromosome aneuploidy such as 48,XXXY and 49,XXXXY. As a general rule, the more X chromosomes present, the more abnormal the phenotype.

Nearly all men with Klinefelter syndrome are infertile, producing semen that contains few viable sperm. However, as in Turner syndrome, recent advances in assisted reproduction have allowed some affected men to father children. Using intracytoplasmic sperm injection, a spermatozoa obtained through testicular biopsy is injected into an egg, producing fertilization. Thus far, all liveborn children fathered by men with Klinefelter syndrome using this technology have had normal chromosomal complements.

Single Gene Disorders

Humans are diploid organisms, and each gene is represented at its locus within the genome by two copies, one inherited from each parent. Genes, sequences of DNA, provide instructions to the cell to produce specific proteins. Among the 30,000 genes that compose the human genome, an occasional error (known as a mutation) occurs. Under the proper conditions, it may translate into a clinically distinguishable disease state. Such entities, referred to as single gene disorders, are often passed from parent to child over many generations.

In this section, three types of single gene disorders are discussed: autosomal dominantly inherited traits, which are expressed in individuals in whom at least one copy of a specific gene is errant; autosomal recessively inherited traits, in which two copies of the errant gene are necessary for clinical expression to occur; and X-linked recessive traits, in which the abnormal gene resides on an X chromosome.

In the 1960s, Victor McKusick, M.D., began to catalog all reported human conditions caused by single gene mutations. The resulting treatise, *Mendelian Inheritance in Man,* has been constantly updated since then. The catalog is now maintained online (see Table 11.2). In this section, OMIM entry numbers follow the name of each specific condition.

Autosomal Dominant Disorders

For autosomal dominant traits to be clinically significant, only one copy of an abnormal gene is necessary. These disorders are usually passed from affected parent to affected child, who, because they possess one normal and one abnormal gene, are said to be heterozygous. A pedigree of a family in whom an autosomal dominant trait is segregating (running through the family) illustrates certain rules (Table 11.6, Figure 11.3).

TABLE 11.6	Rules of Autosomal Dominant Inheritance

1. The trait appears in every generation.
2. Each child of an affected parent has a 1 in 2 chance of being affected.
3. No children of unaffected parents are affected.
4. Males and females are equally affected.
5. Male-to-male transmission occurs.
6. Traits generally involve mutations in genes that code for regulatory or structural proteins (e.g., collagen) and are associated with normal life spans.

In genetics, as in life in general, rules are made to be broken. Phenomena such as skipped generations and individuals affected with autosomal dominant traits born into families in which no other members appear to be affected are commonly seen. Explanation of these observations involves use of the following terms.

Penetrance describes the frequency with which heterozygous individuals clinically express an errant gene. A mutant gene is said to be 100% penetrant if all heterozygous individuals express the abnormal phenotype. However, many disorders manifest decreased penetrance, with some individuals who are carriers of the mutant gene showing no ill effects. Such a situation would account for so-called "skipped generations."

Unlike penetrance, **expressivity** is the extent to which the clinical features of an autosomal dominant trait are expressed in the heterozygous individual. Mutant genes that show variable expressivity (such as the one that causes neurofibromatosis) result in clinical conditions that range from mild to severe. Thus, an errant gene that is 100% penetrant but is variably expressed shows some effects in all heterozygotes, but those effects may either be extremely mild or life-threatening.

Pleiotropy is defined as multiple, seemingly unrelated clinical effects that are caused by a single mutated gene or gene pair. For example, individuals with **Marfan syndrome** have abnormalities of their skeletal, ophthalmologic, and cardiovascular systems, all of which are clearly the result of a single gene defect; random occurrence of such conditions would be unlikely.

A spontaneous mutation is defined as any permanent inheritable change in the sequence of genomic DNA. If a mutation affects a gene, an individual with an autosomal dominant trait may be born into a family in which no other members are affected with that trait. Spontaneous mutations leading to the appearance of autosomal dominant traits are often associated with increased paternal age ($\geq$ 35 years of age).

ACHONDROPLASIA (OMIM #100800). A defect of cartilage-derived bone, achondroplasia is an autosomal dominant disorder that leads to numerous phenotypic abnormalities, including short stature, macrocephaly, a flat midface with prominent forehead, and rhizomelic ("root of the limb") shortening of the limbs (i.e., the proximal part of the limbs are most strikingly affected). Occurring in approximately 1 in 12,000 births, achondroplasia is the most common bone dysplasia in humans.

The cause of achondroplasia is a mutation in the fibroblast growth factor receptor 3 (FGFR3) gene. Localized to chromosome 4p16, FGFR3 is expressed in early human development in the cartilage growth plates of long bones during endochondral ossification. Eighty percent of cases of achondroplasia are the result of spontaneous mutations. More than 95% of cases of achondroplasia are due to one of only two mutations in the same base pair (site 1138); this site is an extremely active

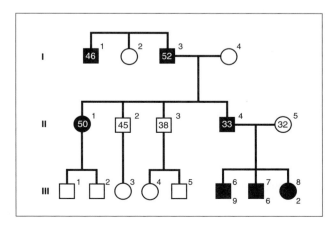

FIGURE 11.3. Pedigree of a family with autosomal dominant familial hypercholesterolemia. Key: □ = male; ○ = female; ■ = affected male; ● = affected female; ■ with *arrow* = proband.

mutational "hot spot" (a region where mutations appear to be more prone to occur).

As the child with achondroplasia grows, numerous related medical and psychologic problems may occur. In infancy, hydrocephalus and central apnea, both resulting from a narrowing of the foramen magnum, may occur. Later in childhood, bowing of the legs as a result of unequal growth of the tibia and fibula, dental malocclusion, and hearing loss from middle ear dysfunction are common. During late childhood and early adolescence, the psychologic effects of the marked shortening of stature are often seen for the first time. In adulthood, neurologic complications such as sciatica, resulting from nerve root compression, are often present. The expected life span of individuals affected with achondroplasia is normal. Although affected persons with achondroplasia usually have normal intelligence, societies have discriminated against them for centuries because of their appearance.

The basis of diagnosis of achondroplasia is the presence of the physical findings described above as well as characteristic radiographic anomalies. Molecular testing should be performed only if the diagnosis is uncertain on clinical or radiologic grounds, or in cases in which prenatal diagnosis through amniocentesis is requested.

NEUROFIBROMATOSIS TYPE 1 (NF-1) [OMIM #162200]. NF-1, a common (1 in 4000 births) autosomal dominant disorder, was originally described by von Recklinghausen in 1882. It was formerly known as "the elephant man's disease," but it is now clear that Joseph Merrick, the so-called Elephant Man, suffered from another disorder, Proteus syndrome. NF-1 is characterized by a large number of separate, seemingly unconnected clinical findings (Table 11.7).

Although the penetrance of NF-1 is high, the expression of the gene is extremely variable. In fact, many individuals who carry the mutated gene go through life unaware of their diagnosis. Most patients manifest only café-au-lait spots (hyperpigmented areas); axillary or inguinal freckling; and small subcutaneous nodules, which represent Schwann cell tumors known as neurofibromas. Ten percent of individuals who carry the gene for NF-1 suffer more severe manifestations, including astrocytomas, optic gliomas and other brain tumors, craniofacial disfigurement, scoliosis, and pseudarthrosis (the presence of a false joint, usually in a long bone).

The staggering array of clinical features represents one of the best examples of pleiotropy known to exist in any autosomal dominant syn-

---

TABLE 11.7 Criteria for Diagnosis of Neurofibromatosis Type 1 (NF-1)*

Café-au-lait spots
    Prepubertal: five or more (> 0.5 cm in diameter)
    Postpubertal: five or more (> 1.5 cm in diameter)
Axillary or inguinal "freckling"
Neurofibromas (dysplastic Schwann cell tumors)
    Two or more neurofibromas *or*
    One or more plexiform neurofibromas
Lisch nodules (pigmented iridal hamartomas)
Optic glioma (one or more neurofibromas of the optic nerve)
    Skeletal manifestations including
    Scoliosis (often rapidly progressive)
    Pseudarthrosis (bowing of a bone due to skeletal defect)
    Bony rarefaction or overgrowth due to presence of plexiform neurofibroma
    Sphenoid wing dysplasia (5%)
Family history of NF-1 in parent or child diagnosed according to above criteria (additional features include developmental delay/learning disability, central nervous system tumors, hypertension)

*To make a diagnosis of NF-1, patients must fulfill at least two of these criteria.

---

drome. Although the explanation of this phenomenon is still not clear, three major scientific breakthroughs have permitted the solution of at least part of the riddle of NF-1.

1. Mapping of the gene responsible for the disorder (in 1987) to the long arm of chromosome 17 (17q11.2)
2. Identification in different families of many different mutations, deletions, and insertions within this gene, providing one clue to the puzzle of the marked variability of clinical expression
3. Identification of the protein responsible for the disorder. Named "neurofibromin," the protein is believed to function as a negative regulator or inhibitor to p21-*ras*, a proto-oncogene. Decreased production of neurofibromin leads to overexpression of this proto-oncogene, presumably causing the features of the disorder.

Molecular techniques for diagnosis of an isolated case of NF-1 are usually not helpful because of the large number of mutations that have been identified in the neurofibromin gene. As in achondroplasia, confirmation of the diagnosis of NF-1 is based on the presence of clinical features (see Table 11.7).

MARFAN SYNDROME (OMIM #154700). This autosomal dominant condition, which occurs in approximately 1 in 10,000 live born infants, is due to a single gene defect that causes abnormalities in several organ systems. Significantly, three systems are most often affected. In the skeletal system, dolichostenomelia (tall, thin body habitus), arachnodactyly (spidery-like fingers and toes), pectus excavatum or carinatum, kyphoscoliosis, and joint laxity occur. In the ophthalmologic system, high myopia and a defect in the suspensory ligament of the lens, which leads to ectopia lentis, cause decreased visual acuity. In the cardiovascular system, a defect in the wall of the aorta leads to progressive dilatation of the ascending aorta, causing aortic insufficiency and, if untreated, ultimately resulting in dissecting aneurysm of the aorta with sudden death.

The fact that these systems are modified has led to the belief that a defect in some element of connective tissue common to these organs is responsible for Marfan syndrome. In the 1990s, a defect in the protein fibrillin 1, an essential element of the myofibrillar array of connective tissue, has been documented in individuals with Marfan syndrome. The gene responsible for coding for this protein is located on the long arm of chromosome 15. Unlike achondroplasia, in which only a handful of mutations occur in the causative gene, Marfan syndrome is associated with many mutations. Virtually every family with a member with Marfan syndrome has a different mutation. As in NF-1, the diagnosis of Marfan syndrome is made based on the presence of characteristic clinical features.

Autosomal Recessive Disorders

Certain disorders follow an autosomal recessive pattern of inheritance. Unlike in autosomal dominant disorders, for an autosomal recessive disorder to be clinically significant, two copies of an abnormal gene must be present. An individual bearing two errant copies of the same gene is said to be **homozygous.** For a homozygous individual to be conceived, both parents must carry at least one copy of the errant gene and are, therefore, **heterozygous.** However, because a single errant copy of the gene is not sufficient to cause clinical abnormalities, heterozygous parents are nearly always asymptomatic. Thus, in most autosomal recessive disorders, the presence of a disease in a child is the first sign that an abnormality is segregating in a family.

The family pedigree in which an autosomal recessive trait is segregating illustrates the rules of autosomal recessive inheritance (Table 11.8; Figure 11.4).

TABLE 11.8	**Rules of Autosomal Recessive Inheritance**

1. The trait appears in siblings, not in their parents or offspring.
2. On average, 25% of siblings of the proband are affected (at the time of conception, each sibling has a 25% chance of being affected).
3. A "normal" sibling of an affected individual has a two-thirds chance of being a carrier (heterozygote).
4. Males and females are equally likely to be affected.
5. Rare traits are likely to be associated with parental consanguinity.
6. Traits generally involve mutations in genes that code for enzymes (e.g., phenylalanine hydroxylase, deficient in phenylketonuria) and are associated with serious illness and shortened life span.

SICKLE CELL DISEASE (OMIM #603903). Sickle cell disease is considered briefly here because of its autosomal recessive pattern of inheritance. (See Chapter 16 for more details.) Much is known about the genetic basis of sickle cell disease, the first human mutation to be elucidated. This mutation, which is caused by a single base substitution in the gene locus on the short arm of chromosome 11, results in the substitution of a valine residue for the glutamic acid residue that normally resides at position 6 in the β globin molecule. This

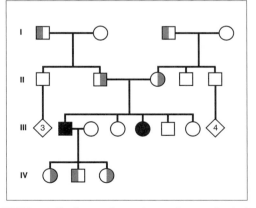

FIGURE 11.4. Pedigree of an autosomal recessive trait. Affected individuals are found in only one generation. Note that both parents of an affected child are obligate heterozygotes (designated by *half-shaded* symbols), as are all of the offspring of a mating between an affected individual and a homozygous normal individual. Key: □ = male; ○ = female; ■ = affected male; ● = affected female; ◧ = heterozygous (carrier) male; ◑ = heterozygous (carrier) female; ◇ = sex not known.

tiny defect leads to instability of the hemoglobin molecule, so that when oxygen saturation decreases, the hemoglobin molecule "collapses." This results in a deformation of the red blood cell (RBC) [sickle shape] and in occlusion of capillaries and smaller arterioles.

Individuals who are heterozygous for the sickle cell disease gene are said to have sickle trait. Such individuals, although clinically normal, have RBCs that sickle when subjected to low oxygen tension in vitro, a phenomenon that has allowed differentiation of these individuals from the rest of the population. The heterozygous state is present in approximately 1 of every 10 African Americans. As a result of this very high heterozygote frequency, the occurrence of newborns with sickle cell disease in this population can be easily predicted using the Hardy-Weinberg equation:

1. The chance of the mating of two individuals with the trait is approximately $1/10 \times 1/10$, or $1/100$.
2. The chance that a child with sickle cell disease will be born to two parents, both of whom have trait, is $1/4$.
3. Thus, the general incidence is $1/100 \times 1/4$, or $1/400$.

As calculated, 1 of every 400 children born to parents of African American heritage will have sickle cell disease. The actual number is very close to the predicted frequency.

The reason that sickle cell disease, which causes such severe symptomatology in the homozygous affected individual, continues to be so prevalent in the population is that autosomal recessive traits depend only on the survival of the heterozygotes. It is not necessary for the gene's survival for homozygotes to reach childbearing age. This has led to a theory explaining why the sickle cell mutation has been maintained at such a high level in the population. If instead of causing harm, a particular gene mutation present in the heterozygous state actually protects the individual in some way, the mutated gene has pressure to remain in the population. The mutation makes the carrier more fit and gives the heterozygote a selective advantage over homozygous unaffected individuals.

The first clue to the fact that sickle trait offered the heterozygote an advantage came from the observations that the sickle gene occurred in highest frequencies in regions where falciparum malaria is common. Epidemiologic studies have shown that heterozygotes are resistant to severe infection from the parasite *Plasmodium falciparum*. In Africa, individuals who have sickle trait become infected as frequently as do people who are free of the trait,

but the former group has fewer complications resulting from the infection; the need for hospitalization is less, and deaths are far fewer. Physiologic studies have determined the reason for this increased survival. In individuals without sickle trait, the malaria parasite uses the RBCs of its host to proceed through its life cycle. In individuals with sickle trait, this process is interrupted, and the spread of the parasite is attenuated.

Sickle cell anemia, like some other autosomal recessive traits, occurs with markedly increased frequency within certain ethnic groups. This distribution pattern has raised the possibility of eradicating the conditions through directed screening programs, genetic counseling, and prenatal diagnosis. This approach has been used in Tay-Sachs disease, a condition that occurs most frequently in individuals of Ashkenazi Jewish background.

ELLIS-VAN CREVELD SYNDROME (OMIM #225500). Although some autosomal recessive traits are relatively common, the majority are rare disorders that occur infrequently in most populations. Ellis-van Creveld syndrome, also called chondroectodermal dysplasia, is one of these conditions. This disorder involves a combination of short stature (with disproportionately shortened extremities), polydactyly, a narrowed thorax, and congenital heart disease with abnormalities of the mouth (thickened frenula, defects in alveolar ridge, and dental anomalies) and the nails (hypoplasia). Recently, researchers found that mutations within the EVS gene on chromosome 4p16.1 cause Ellis-van Creveld syndrome.

In 1964, McKusick discovered multiple cases of Ellis-van Creveld syndrome in an inbred Old Order Amish village in Pennsylvania. A study of trends within the Amish population explained why so many individuals with this disorder were concentrated in such a small area. The Amish tend to isolate themselves within small villages. When, through reproduction, the village becomes too crowded, one or two nuclear families break away from the main group and establish a new community some distance away from the original town. The founders of this new community reproduce, their children marry and, in turn, reproduce, and eventually, the entire village is populated by descendants of the original founder couple. The founders bring with them their "genetic baggage," including the presence of one or more rare autosomal recessive traits carried in the heterozygous state. Through a few generations, the gene frequency of these rare traits increases dramatically, since most people never leave the home village.

X-linked Recessive Disorders

Disorders caused by abnormalities of genes linked to the X chromosome have a distinct and unusual pattern of inheritance known as X-linked recessive. Heterozygous females, who display little or no effects, usually carry these disorders and pass them on to their sons, who are **hemizygous** because they have only one X chromosome. These males usually suffer severe manifestations.

The observation that males can survive with only one copy of the X chromosome while females with one copy (Turner syndrome) have an increased prenatal mortality puzzled geneticists throughout much of the early part of the 20th century. In 1962, Mary Lyon postulated the explanation for this phenomenon. According to the Lyon hypothesis, at a very early stage in development, one of the two X chromosomes in every cell of the female pre-embryo becomes randomly inactivated. Thus, females are essentially mosaics, their bodies composed of two separate cell types, with each bearing a separate, active X chromosome. As the result of "lyonization," when an errant gene is present on one X chromosome, some cells express the abnormality, while others do not. Because inactivation of the X chromosome occurs randomly, it is possible that, by chance, one cell type may predominate over the other. Therefore, some women who carry an abnormal gene on one of their X chromosomes may, because of random inactivation of most of the X chromosomes bearing the normal gene, express symptoms of the disease caused by that abnormal gene.

The pedigree of a family in which an X-linked recessive inherited disorder is segregating illustrates the rules of X-linked recessive inheritance (Table 11.9; Figure 11.5).

DUCHENNE MUSCULAR DYSTROPHY (OMIM #310200). Duchenne muscular dystrophy, the most common form of muscular dystrophy, occurs in 1 in every 3500 boys born in the United States. Among the clinical features of this condition are a "waddling" gait, usually discovered at about 3 years of age and excessive falling (see Chapter 19). In most cases, pseudohypertrophy of the calf muscles is apparent on initial examination, and serum creatine kinase is markedly elevated. Affected boys show a slowly progressive downhill course. Death, usually from cardiopulmonary complications, occurs in the second or third decade.

Although Duchenne muscular dystrophy has long been known to be linked to the X chromosome, characterization of the gene responsible for the condition and the protein that codes for it occurred only in the late 1980s. Using a procedure

TABLE 11.9 Rules of X-linked Recessive Inheritance
1. The incidence of the trait is higher in males than females.
2. The trait is passed from carrier females, who may show mild expression of the gene, to their sons, who are more severely affected.
3. Each son of a carrier female has a 1 in 2 chance of being affected.
4. The trait is transmitted from affected males to all of their daughters. It is never transmitted from father to son.
5. Because the trait can be passed through multiple carrier females, it may "skip" generations.

known as "reverse genetics," researchers identified the protein dystrophin as the component of muscle cells that is deficient in men with this form as well as some other forms of muscular dystrophy. The characterization of dystrophin has led to major advances in both the diagnosis and potential treatment of Duchenne muscular dystrophy.

Mothers and sisters of affected males may or may not be carriers of the abnormal gene. In the past, counseling was offered based on statistical probabilities, which depended on several conditions such as the number of other affected males in the family and the level of creatine kinase in the woman's blood. Fetal sex determination was the only possible method of prenatal diagnosis in

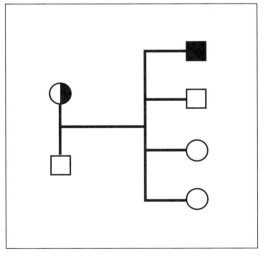

FIGURE 11.5. Pedigree of an X-linked recessive trait. Only male children of carrier females are affected. All girls born to hemizygous fathers are carriers; boys born to these men are never affected. Key: □ = male; ○ = female (noncarrier); ■ = hemizygous affected male; ◑ = heterozygous (carrier) female.

women believed to be carriers. However, because the actual gene defect responsible for Duchenne muscular dystrophy has been discovered, counseling with certainty is now available following testing of many of these female relatives. In addition, once a female has been identified as a carrier, direct prenatal diagnosis of the fetus involves either amniocentesis or chorionic villus sampling. Because of the inheritance pattern, men with Duchenne muscular dystrophy who reproduce cannot have affected children. All daughters born to such men will be obligate carriers (and therefore, are at risk for having sons who are affected), whereas sons, having received the father's Y chromosome, will be completely free of disease.

HEMOPHILIA A. Hemophilia A is the most common hemorrhagic disorder occurring in children. The cause of this condition is a profound deficiency of factor VIII, an essential protein for coagulation. Most boys with classic hemophilia are diagnosed in early childhood after one or more episodes of unexplained bleeding. Because of their inability to clot, boys with hemophilia have recurrent episodes of hemarthrosis (bleeding into joint spaces), that can lead to chronic, painful arthritis. They develop intramuscular hematomas (see Chapter 16). Head trauma is a serious and potentially lethal problem because of the possibility of intracranial bleeding (see Chapter 23).

The genetics of hemophilia is identical to that of Duchenne muscular dystrophy because it is an X-linked recessive disorder. Similarly, the gene responsible for producing factor VIII has been characterized, and direct DNA diagnosis is possible. As with Duchenne muscular dystrophy, the children of males affected with hemophilia are not themselves affected; however, all their daughters will be carriers and, as a result, should receive prenatal diagnosis during pregnancy if they wish. All first-degree relatives of affected males (i.e., mothers, sisters) should routinely have the opportunity to be tested and, if found to be carriers, should also be referred for prenatal diagnosis by either chorionic villus sampling or amniocentesis.

Multifactorially Inherited Disorders

Of the four etiologic categories of congenital or genetic disorders, multifactorial (also known as polygenic) inheritance is by far the most common. Such inheritance is responsible for 20% of all congenital malformations and also plays a role in determining susceptibility to most chronic disorders of adult life, including atherosclerosis and coronary artery disease, cancer, and diabetes. The cause of multifactorial inheritance is an interplay between multiple background genes and the environment in which those genes are expressed. Although multifactorial conditions tend to cluster in families, they do not conform to simple Mendelian patterns of inheritance.

Traits that are inherited in a multifactorial manner show a blending of features known as **continuous variations** (e.g., the bell-shaped distribution in the plot of the height of all medical students in the United States). When a trait such as height is the subject, excessive shortness or tallness is not necessarily considered a pathologic condition. However, for certain traits such as the timing of closure of the neural tube or of fusion of the palatal arches in the midline, distribution at the outer ends of the curve may have serious, life-threatening implications. Two relatively common congenital malformations that demonstrate multifactorial inheritance are discussed here.

Neural Tube Defects

Neural tube defects, consisting of anencephaly, meningocele, and meningomyelocele, are among the most common disabling birth defects that occur in humans. The embryology involved in the closure of the neural tube is well understood. At approximately 18 days after conception, the neural plate begins to involute. At first, an indentation known as the neural groove can be seen, but at 23 days after conception the edges of the neural groove meet to form the beginning of a tube. Over the next few days, this tube "zippers" closed; at the cephalad end, the tube becomes the skull; at the caudal end, the spine. For these structures to form normally, it is essential that complete closure of the tube occur by a specific time (known as the **threshold**). If closure of the cephalad end is not complete, abnormal brain development occurs, with anencephaly, a uniformly lethal condition. If closure of the caudal end is not complete, the child will be born with myelomeningocele (also known as spina bifida).

In 1990, it was estimated that myelomeningocele affected 1 in 1000 liveborn infants in the United States. Anencephaly occurs with a similar frequency, although most of these infants are either stillborn or die in the neonatal period. Multiple factors, both genetic and nongenetic, dictate the speed with which the neural tube closes. Evidence for this comes from the following observations:

- Neural tube defects show ethnic differences in frequency. Far more common in the British

Isles, they are much less common in Asia; in Ireland, the incidence is 1 in 250. These ethnic differences suggest a genetic component.

- Couples from the British Isles who come to the United States have a risk intermediate between the risks in the United Kingdom and in the United States, suggesting an environmental component.
- The occurrence of neural tube defects exhibits seasonality. Affected infants are more likely to be born during the late fall and early winter, again suggesting an environmental component.
- Periconceptual supplementation with folic acid has now conclusively been shown to significantly decrease the risk of having a child with a neural tube defect. This nutritional influence suggests yet another environmental component.
- Parents who have one child with a neural tube defect are 20–40 times more likely to have a second affected child. This provides further evidence of a genetic component.

Children with myelomeningocele have an assortment of medical and surgical problems. They require neurosurgical procedures in the newborn period to close the spinal defect and, in as many as 90% of cases, placement of a ventriculoperitoneal shunt is necessary to alleviate obstructive hydrocephalus. Children with shunts require ongoing neurosurgical surveillance to evaluate for shunt obstruction. In 85% of patients, neurogenic bowel and bladder occurs as a result of the level of the spinal lesion; close supervision by both a urologist (who manages the bladder through clean intermittent catheterization) and a gastroenterologist is required. Numerous orthopedic problems occur, including joint contractures, clubfoot deformity, scoliosis, and paraparesis. Management by an orthopedic surgeon, in conjunction with a physiatrist and orthotist, is necessary. The pediatrician provides routine health care maintenance and coordinates the care provided by the numerous other members of the multidisciplinary team of health care professionals.

Because of the elevated recurrence risk associated with neural tube defects, prenatal diagnosis consisting of amniocentesis, α-fetoprotein screening, and sonography should be offered to the family. In recent years, researchers have demonstrated conclusively that folic acid reduces the risk of having either a first or subsequent child with a neural tube defect. Because the effect occurs only if folic acid supplementation begins at least 2 months before conception, the U.S. Department of Health and Human Services now recommends that all women of childbearing age take 0.4 mg of folic

acid per day. Women who have had a previous child with a neural tube defect are at increased risk of recurrence, so they should take a higher dose of folic acid. It is recommended that first-degree female relatives of an individual with a neural tube defect take 4 mg of folic acid per day, beginning at least 2 months before planned conception. By following these recommendations, women may reduce the risk of bearing a child with a neural tube defect by up to 70%.

Pediatric Pearl

In recent years, clinicians have realized that an allergy to latex products develops in virtually all children with myelomeningocele. Before 1980, this allergy was almost unknown, but it has led to life-threatening complications due to anaphylaxis in affected patients. The Spina Bifida Association of America recommends that the use of latex products be avoided in all patients with neural tube defects.

Hypertrophic Pyloric Stenosis

Hypertrophic pyloric stenosis is a disorder of historic importance in that it was the disease for which the multifactorial threshold model was actually developed. Although it originates in fetal life, because of its pathophysiology, hypertrophic pyloric stenosis is a condition that is usually not diagnosed until late in the first month after birth. Hypertrophy of the muscles of the pylorus leads to obstruction of the flow of partially digested food from the stomach into the first section of the duodenum. Vomiting becomes progressively worse and becomes projectile in nature (see Chapter 25). At presentation, the child is usually dehydrated, has a significant electrolyte imbalance (hypochloremic alkalosis), and is extremely sick and irritable.

To the geneticist, the two most interesting features of hypertrophic pyloric stenosis are its sex distribution and its empirically derived risk of recurrence. Pyloric stenosis is five times more common in boys (5/1000) than in girls. Furthermore, the recurrence risk is very different for males and females, with children born to affected women at much higher risk than those born to affected men. Assuming that the threshold for developing pyloric stenosis is lower for males than for females explains the observed sex distribution. Not only would more males be affected, but also the females who did have the disorder would be more severely affected. The more severely affected the parent, the higher the recurrence risk, thus explaining the observed data.

Teratogenically Induced Disorders

Defined as a chemical or environmental agent that has the potential to damage embryonic tissue primordia and resulting in one or more congenital malformations, teratogens are responsible for approximately 6.5% of all birth defects. Knowledge of these agents and their effect on the developing embryo or fetus is important for two reasons. One, this frequency is probably falsely low because of underreporting. As time passes, more is known about the effects of environmental agents on development, and it is likely that this frequency will significantly increase. Two, and perhaps more importantly, congenital malformations caused by teratogenic agents are all potentially preventable.

The first evidence that physical agents had the potential to harm developing humans came from Australia in 1941. N. McAllister Gregg, an ophthalmologist, noted a sharp increase in the number of infants born with congenital cataracts. On examining these children further, he noted a distinct pattern of abnormalities including sensorineural deafness, microcephaly with developmental delay, and congenital heart disease. By reviewing the pregnancy records, he discovered that all affected infants had been born to women who had been infected with German measles during their pregnancies. Rubella was the first known teratogen.

For nearly 20 years, people believed that most physical agents could not damage the developing human; viral agents might be a special case. This changed dramatically in 1960 when Pfeiffer and Kostellow reported the cases of two German children with phocomelia, a severe limb defect. Within a few months, an epidemic of phocomelia gripped Germany and other European countries. Epidemiologic evaluation soon uncovered the putative cause. Mothers of nearly all affected infants had been treated with thalidomide, a potent sedative and antiemetic, during early pregnancy. Before authorities withdrew the drug from the market, malformations occurred in 7000 European and Australian infants. [Because of Food and Drug Administration (FDA) regulations, the drug was never marketed in the United States.] The thalidomide saga opened the floodgates. Soon, physicians were attempting to attribute every observed malformation to some drug that had been administered to the mother during pregnancy. The truth probably lies somewhere in between.

Teratogenically induced disorders can be divided into three major groups: (1) those due to maternal factors, (2) those due to exposure to drugs and chemicals, and (3) those due to environmental agents.

Maternal Factors

From the time of Gregg's initial observation regarding the effects of the rubella virus, it has been known that the presence of maternal illness can have lethal or devastating effects on the conceptus. These illnesses may be further broken down into two categories: maternal infections and other maternal illnesses.

MATERNAL INFECTIONS. Some common infectious agents have harmful effects on the conceptus (Table 11.10). The effect each of these infectious agents has on the developing embryo or fetus is related to the timing of infection; generally, the earlier the infection, the more devastating the effects.

MATERNAL ILLNESS (OTHER THAN INFECTIONS). The conceptus is sensitive to a number of maternal metabolic disturbances. It is important to note that in most cases, strict control of the underlying metabolic abnormality in the mother will serve to protect the fetus. Two examples are maternal diabetes mellitus and maternal phenylketonuria (PKU).

Approximately 10% of infants of diabetic mothers are born with an abnormality in form or function that is detectable in the neonatal period. Malformations include the caudal regression sequence (a severe defect characterized by absence of the sacrum, defects of the lower limbs, imperforate anus, and abnormalities of the genitourinary tract) and the VACTERL association. The presence and severity of anomalies appears to be directly related to the degree of glycemic control during the first trimester of pregnancy.

PKU, an inborn error of metabolism caused by a deficiency of phenylalanine hydroxylase, has become a relatively innocuous disease as a result of a combination of neonatal screening and the institution of special diets. In the past, the tendency has been to limit intake of phenylalanine in affected individuals until late childhood, when liberalization of the diet has occurred. However, it was noted that offspring of women with PKU were at significant risk for mental retardation, microcephaly, and congenital heart disease. In the late 1980s, physicians began to return women in their childbearing years to low phenylalanine diets and found that if this

TABLE 11.10	Selected Infectious Teratogenic Agents
Agent	**Congenital Malformations**
Rubella	CNS (microcephaly, MR)
	Eye (cataracts, glaucoma)
	Deafness
	Cardiac (VSD, ASD, PDA)
	Growth deficiency
	Bone dysplasia
	Other conditions
Cytomegalovirus	CNS (microcephaly, MR, calcifications)
	Eye (bicophthalmia, blindness)
	Deafness
	Miscarriage
Toxoplasma gondii	CNS (microcephaly, calcifications, MR)
	Eye (microphthalmia, chorioretinitis)
	Miscarriage
Herpes simplex	CNS (microcephaly, MR)
	Eye (microphthalmia, retinal dysplasia)
Varicella	CNS (microcephaly, MR)
	Eye (cataracts, microphthalmia)
	Limb deficiency
	Cicatricial skin lesions
Human immunodeficiency virus	CNS (microcephaly, calcifications, MR)
	Eye (prominent eyes, blue sclerae)
	Characteristic facies
	Immunodeficiency

ASD = atrial septal defect; CNS = central nervous system; MR = mental retardation; PDA = patent ductus arteriosus; VSD = ventral septal defect.

change was instituted before the start of pregnancy, the fetus was at little or no increased risk for these anomalies.

Drugs and Chemicals

This category of teratogens has special significance because, to some extent, use of these agents by pregnant women is often regulated by their physicians. Therefore, it is essential for the physician to have a clear understanding of agents that can cause birth defects.

NONPRESCRIPTION DRUGS. This group of drugs includes alcohol, cocaine, heroin, and marijuana. Also considered as part of this group are caffeine and nicotine, agents that are believed not to have teratogenic potential. The teratogenic effects of two nonprescription agents, alcohol and cocaine, are discussed.

Features of **fetal alcohol syndrome** include prenatal and postnatal growth deficiency, microcephaly with developmental delay, various skeletal and cardiac anomalies, and a characteristic facial appearance. The full-blown syndrome occurs in 3–5/1000 children, making fetal alco-

hol syndrome the most common teratogenic syndrome encountered in humans. It is estimated that a pregnant woman has to drink at least 6 ounces of alcohol each day during the pregnancy to cause full-blown fetal alcohol syndrome. If alcohol ingestion begins after the first trimester (following the completion of organogenesis), the child is likely to have few of the physical features of fetal alcohol syndrome but is at significant risk for the developmental and behavioral consequences of fetal alcohol exposure. This latter condition, termed fetal alcohol effects, is much more common than fetal alcohol syndrome and affects 20%–30% of infants of alcoholic women. Therefore, alcohol is a behavioral teratogen as well as a structural teratogen.

More recently, attention has focused on the effects of other drugs of abuse on the developing embryo. A spectrum of anomalies has been observed in some offspring of women using cocaine, including intracranial hemorrhages leading to developmental disabilities and microcephaly, intestinal atresias, limb reduction defects, and striking urinary tract anomalies such as the "prune belly syndrome." The cause of these anomalies appears to be vascular disruption resulting from the vasoconstrictive effects of the drug occurring at critical times of gestation.

PRESCRIPTION DRUGS. These agents are important because their use is recommended by a physician. Thalidomide was the first prescription drug known to cause malformations. The effects of three other drugs, hydantoin, warfarin, and *cis*-retinoic acid, are described in this section.

Features of **fetal hydantoin syndrome** include a characteristic facies, mild mental retardation, and hypoplasia of the distal phalanges of the fingers and toes, with tiny or absent nails a striking characteristic of the disorder. In recent years, the pathogenetic mechanism responsible for the malformations has been described and appears to be related to the level of epoxide hydrolase, an enzyme in the mother's circulation, which is responsible for the breakdown of a metabolite of hydantoin. The risk of the syndrome is low; less than 10% of exposed embryos have features of the disorder.

Warfarin is also known to cause malformations. Deep vein thrombosis is a relatively common complication of pregnancy. The use of anticoagulant medication is critical to prevent pulmonary embolism, and warfarin is the oral medication most commonly used to treat this condition. In 1966, a pattern of malformations was described, including hypoplasia of the nasal bridge with upper airway obstruction, stippled calcification in the epiphyses of numerous bones, and mental retardation. The pathogenesis of these defects is unclear. Warfarin is contraindicated in pregnancy.

cis-**Retinoic acid,** a vitamin A congener, is an effective agent in the treatment of cystic acne. In the early 1980s, clinicians found that this drug was a potent teratogen. Up to 70% of pregnancies in which women received *cis*-retinoic acid during the first trimester were abnormal. Some ended in miscarriage, others ended in the birth of a child with what has become known as the Accutane embryopathy, a pattern of anomalies including severe craniofacial disorders (abnormalities of the skull, ears, eyes, nose and palate), cardiac defects, and the DiGeorge malformation sequence (hypoparathyroidism, T-cell deficiency).

Environmental Agents

In contrast to prescription and street drugs, exposure to chemicals and agents in the environment is not easily controllable. Some environmental agents clearly do *not* cause birth defects. Contrary to media reports, there is no convincing evidence that exposure to video display terminals, electromagnetic fields, caffeine, or inhaled cigarette smoke can induce malformations in fetuses. Two agents, radiation and methylmercury, are known to cause problems. They are described in this section.

RADIATION. From the experience in the Japanese cities of Hiroshima and Nagasaki, it became clear that radiation exposure during fetal life can have lethal or devastating consequences. In addition to a significantly higher rate of spontaneous abortion than normal, pregnancies exposed to high doses of radiation resulted in the birth of children with microcephaly, mental retardation, and skeletal malformations. The dose of ionizing radiation needed to induce these anomalies is more than 5 rads and probably closer to 25 rads. In contrast, the radiation dose used in diagnostic radiology examinations is extremely low, with most exposures in the range of a few millirads. Therefore, diagnostic radiologic procedures are probably safe in pregnancy.

METHYLMERCURY. An inadvertent spill of methylmercury into the water supply in the city of Minamata, Japan, in the 1960s led to an outbreak of congenital malformations in infants who were gestating during that period. These children were born with neurologic aberrations that included developmental retardation, cerebral palsy–like movement disorders, and, in some cases, blindness. This entity has raised concern about the possibility of abnormalities in the offspring of women who, because of diets rich in mercury-contaminated fish, ingest large amounts of this element.

SUGGESTED READINGS*

General Reference

Gelehrter TD, Collins FS, Ginsburg TF: *Principles of Medical Genetics,* 2nd ed. Baltimore, Williams & Wilkins, 1998.

Nussbaum RL, McInnes RR, Willard H: *Thompson & Thompson's Genetics in Medicine,* 6th ed. Philadelphia, WB Saunders, 2001.

Specific Conditions

Buyse ML (ed): *Birth Defects Encyclopedia.* Cambridge, MA, Blackwell Scientific Publications, 1990.

Jones KL: *Smith's Recognizable Patterns of Human Malformations,* 5th ed. Philadelphia, WB Saunders, 1997.

The Human Factor

Marion RW: The boy who felt no pain. Boston, Addison-Wesley, 1990.

See Table 11.2 for information about on-line references.

Chapter 12

Developmental Disabilities

Maris D. Rosenberg and
D. Rani C. Kathirithamby

Monitoring children's development is a critical aspect of pediatric health care maintenance. The pediatrician who suspects developmental problems in a child whose parents have not expressed concerns must be prepared to help the family gain access to evaluation services and obtain appropriate intervention. Early intervention has the potential to affect both the child's developmental outcome and the family's functioning. This chapter discusses developmental screening and the presentation of developmental disabilities. It focuses on three developmental disabilities that manifest in infancy/early childhood: mental retardation, cerebral palsy, and autism; in addition, it highlights learning disability, which becomes evident during the school-age years.

ROLE OF DEVELOPMENTAL SCREENING

In a 1994 statement, the Committee on Children with Disabilities of the American Academy of Pediatrics (AAP) discussed the importance of monitoring children's development over time. Such **developmental surveillance** implies obtaining a careful history of a particular child's attainment of developmental milestones, close observation of the child, and attention to parents' questions and concerns. While all children deserve careful monitoring, those with risk factors for developmental disability merit closer scrutiny (Table 12.1). In fact, some children may qualify for intervention services based solely on the presence of risk factors. Public Law 99–457 (1986), reauthorized as PL 102–119 (Individuals with Disabilities Education Act, 1991), mandates the early identification and treatment of children who either manifest or are at risk for developmental disabilities.

Screening instruments enable the pediatrician to monitor children's developmental progress over time more objectively. It should be emphasized that screening procedures are not diagnostic for particular developmental disabilities and do not determine precise level of functioning. However, they are the first step in recognizing a potential problem and obtaining further diagnostic evaluation. The widely used Denver Developmental Screening Test (DENVER II) is a sensitive tool that identifies children who may suffer from developmental delays (see Figure 2.1). Comparing children's performance on the four parts of the DENVER II—language, fine motor–adaptive, gross motor, and personal–social—also provides a quick overview of the child's general development. Other useful screening instruments are also available (Table 12.2).

Familiarization with developmental milestones is essential for proper developmental surveillance. While the timing of acquisition of particular skills varies from child to child, the pattern of development tends to remain the same. Using a tool such as the DENVER II helps the pediatrician appreciate the normal sequence of development and the age range in which acquisition of specific skills can be expected to occur. For example, independent walking tends to occur by 15 months of age in 90% of the children in the DENVER II standardization sample, with 25% of children walking by 11 months of age.

PRESENTATION OF DEVELOPMENTAL DISABILITIES

Developmental disabilities present in an age- related manner. They manifest during the first year of life as motor delays, during the toddler and preschool years as language delays, and during school years as learning problems.

Pediatric Pearl

Generally, the earlier the occurrence of the developmental disability, the more severe the condition.

TABLE 12.1 Risk Factors for Disability in Children

Neonatal Factors

Birth weight < 1501 g
Gestational age < 33 weeks
CNS insult or abnormality
Maternal prenatal alcohol abuse
Maternal phenylketonuria (PKU)
Abnormalities in muscle tone
Hyperbilirubinemia (< 20 mg/dl)
Hypoglycemia (< 20 mg/dl)
Growth deficiency/nutritional problems
Perinatally/congenitally transmitted infection
Stay in neonatal intensive care unit of < 10 days
Maternal prenatal abuse of illicit substances
Prenatal exposure to certain therapeutic drugs with known potential developmental implications
Asphyxia (Apgar score at 5 minutes of < 3)
Suspected hearing impairment
Suspected vision impairment
Inborn metabolic disorder

Postneonatal and Early Childhood Factors

Serious illness/traumatic injury with implications for CNS
Human immunodeficiency virus (HIV) infection
Congenital malformations
Parental/caregiver concern about developmental status

Other Possible Factors

Lack of prenatal care
Parental substance abuse
No well-child care by age 6 months
Significant delay in immunizations
Elevated blood lead levels (> 19 mEq/dl)
Growth deficiency/nutritional problems
Chronicity of serious otitis media (continuous for minimum of 3 months)
Parental developmental disability/mental illness
Other circumstances that the clinician believes place the child at developmental risk

---

CNS = central nervous system.

From the time of birth until the age of 1 year, the pace of motor development is rapid and proceeds in a predictable manner. Attainment of gross motor milestones depends on the symmetrical development of muscle tone and strength, which progresses cranially to caudally. In addition, motor development depends on the extinguishing of primitive reflexes and the emergence of postural reactions. Thus, the development of head control, ability to roll over, independent sitting, and walking all occur in sequence at approximately 3 months, 4 months, 6 months, and 12 months of age, respectively. Deviations in development at this early stage tend to present as motor milestone delays and may signify a neuromuscular, genetic/metabolic, infectious, or other abnormality. A careful medical evaluation is essential to determine the cause of developmental delay.

As children enter their second year, the development of communication becomes a sensitive indicator of overall development. The act of pointing or gesturing to express desires or indicate interest is a critical milestone that should be present by 1 year of age. Children's single word vocabulary increases through the second year, with the emergence of two-word combinations by 2 years of age and three-word combinations by 3 years of age. Clarity of speech also improves; 50%–75% of children's speech becoming intelligible to strangers between 2 and 3 years of age. The quality and symbolism of children's play is also a valuable indicator of cognitive and linguistic development. Even with uncooperative children, watching them at play may yield a good deal of information.

First and foremost, the evaluation of language delay in children must involve a thorough hearing

TABLE 12.2 **Screening and Assessment Instruments Used in Children**

Method	Author(s)	Age/grade	Administration Time (minutes)	Description
Ages & Stages Questionnaires (11)	Bickel, Squires, and Mounts (1995)	4–48 months (2–4-month intervals)	10–15	Assesses communication, fine motor, problem-solving, and personal–social skills
Brigance Preschool Screen for 3- and 4-year-olds	Brigance (1985)	3–4 years	12	Screens behavior, motor, language, number concept, and visual–perceptual skills
Child Development Review (parent questionnaire)	Ireton (1994)	18 months–5 years	10	Includes 6 open-ended questions and 26-item problem list Screens social self-help, gross motor, fine motor, and language areas of development
Clinical Linguistic and Auditory Milestones Scale (CLAMS)	Capute et al (1986)	1 month–3 years	10	Tests expressive and receptive language
DENVER II Screening Exam	Frankenburg (1989)	1 month–6 years	15–30	Requires observation and parental report
Early Language Milestone Scale (2nd edition)	Coplan (1993)	1–36 months		Assesses language in format similar to DENVER II
Einstein Assessment of School-Related Skills	Gottesman and Cerullo (1988, 1996)	Kindergarten–grade 5	7–10	Identifies children at risk for learning difficulties

assessment. Developmentally appropriate instruments are available to objectively measure thresholds for critical frequencies for speech development. It is not enough to wave a rattle or clap the hands and judge a child's response. Electrophysiologic (e.g., evoked potentials) and otoacoustic techniques are available for children who are untestable using behavioral methods (e.g., visual reinforcement audiometry, play audiometry). The pediatrician can use these as early as the newborn period in the evaluation of at-risk children. The National Institutes of Health (NIH) Consensus Conference (1993) established criteria for hearing screening in children. Children who meet high-risk criteria for hearing loss should undergo screening so that it is possible to identify them before they develop a language delay.

Once the clinician determines that hearing is normal, she should try to discover whether the language delay appears to be part of a more global problem (e.g., cognitive delay), or whether it is isolated in the domain of speech and language. Language delay in the preschool years is a classic manifestation of mental retardation, but coexisting delays in fine motor–adaptive and personal–social skills may not be obvious until careful developmental screening has been completed. This is particularly true in children who are more mildly impaired. Other children may appear to have a limited ability to socialize and relate to others in addition to their delays in spoken language. These children may be manifesting autistic spectrum disorders. Conversely, many children do appear to exhibit delays that are limited to language. In such cases it is important to determine the degree to which receptive skills, expressive skills, and speech articulation are affected. These issues are critical in implementing intervention strategies that assist affected children in their communication development.

MENTAL RETARDATION

Mental retardation refers to significantly subaverage intellectual functioning that exists concurrently with related limitations in adaptive skills. About 3% of the general population functions in the range of mental retardation. Onset must occur before the age of 18 years.

The definition of mental retardation also implies deficits in adaptive functioning. Mental retardation may be associated with other disabilities (e.g., cerebral palsy, autistic speech disorders), and the varying degrees of severity of mental retardation affect the prognosis for ultimate functioning. Adaptive functioning refers to the ability of an individual to care for himself and to function in his family or community as appropriate for age and sociocultural background. In 1992, the American Association on Mental Retardation (AAMR) revised the formal definition of mental retardation to reflect the different levels of support needed for daily functioning. The definition specifies that the adaptive deficits exist in two or more areas such as communication, home living, community use, health and safety, self-care, social skills, and self-direction and functional academics. Such deficits are documented using standardized instruments such as the Vineland Social Maturity Scale or the AAMR Adaptive Behavior Scale.

Mentally retarded children present as children who are functioning below age expectancy across all domains. In other words, they seem like younger children. The AAMR definition of mental retardation no longer uses degree of severity in classification, but other classification systems, including that of the *Diagnostic and Statistical Manual of Mental Disorders,* 4th edition (text revision) [DSM IV-TR], specify ranges of functioning that are helpful in anticipating intervention needs, rate of progress, and ultimate prognosis.

Mild retardation, which affects about 85% of individuals with mental retardation, is characterized by intelligence quotients (IQs) [developmental age divided by chronologic age] in the range of 50–70; the exact number varies with the standard deviation of the test being used. These children tend to present during the preschool years, often with no stigmatizing physical features. Academically, they tend to achieve up to a sixth grade level. Adults with mild mental retardation can live independently, hold jobs, and raise children. They may require assistance in more complex tasks such as negotiating public transportation and arranging budgets, schedules, and they may need help coping during periods of stress.

Moderate retardation affects about 10% of the mentally retarded population. Children functioning in this range are likely to present in the toddler or early preschool years. These individuals are unlikely to progress beyond a second grade level academically. With training, they may attend to self-care needs and can work, usually in supervised settings.

Severe and profound retardation encompasses the remaining 4%–5% of the portion of the population who is mentally retarded. Children functioning in this range are likely to present with developmental delays in infancy. An identifiable medical etiology may be apparent on workup, with probable stigmatizing features and associated disabilities such as cerebral palsy, seizure disorders, or sensory deficits. These individuals have little or no potential for independent living.

Psychological Assessment

It is necessary to document the subaverage intellectual functioning of mental retardation using culturally, linguistically, and developmentally appropriate standardized psychological tests. Such methods of assessment yield measures such as IQ. An IQ score of two or more standard deviations below the mean (generally ≤ 70) satisfies this criterion for diagnosis of mental retardation. Examples of standardized tests commonly used in children are the Wechsler Intelligence Scale for Children (WISC-3) and the Stanford-Binet Intelligence Scale.

Results of psychological tests reliably obtained after 2½ of age are generally predictive of an individual's level of functioning and can be used as a basis for educational planning. Although assessment tools for infants and younger children are available (e.g., Bayley Scales of Infant Development), they do not yield results considered predictive of later functioning.

Clinical and Laboratory Evaluation

Medical evaluation of children with mental retardation must involve a search for the cause of the condition. The many different conditions that cause mental retardation all involve insult to the developing central nervous system (CNS) [Table 12.3].

History

A careful prenatal, perinatal, and early medical history may suggest risk factors for developmental disability or events associated with CNS injury that might result in mental retardation.

TABLE 12.3 **Possible Contributing Factors in the Pathogenesis of Mental Retardation**

Preconceptual Disorders

Single gene abnormalities (e.g., inborn errors of metabolism, neurocutaneous disorders)
Chromosomal abnormalities (e.g., X-linked disorders, translocations, fragile syndrome)
Mitochondrial abnormalities
Polygenic familial syndromes

Early Embryonic Disruptions

Chromosomal disorders (e.g., trisomies, mosaics)
Infections (e.g., CMV, rubella, toxoplasmosis, HIV)
Teratogens (e.g., alcohol, radiation)
Placental dysfunction
Congenital CNS malformations (idiopathic)

Fetal Brain Insults

Infections (e.g., HIV, toxoplasmosis, CMV, herpes simplex)
Toxins (e.g., alcohol, cocaine, lead, maternal phenylketonuria, maternal tobacco smoking)
Placental insufficiency/intrauterine malnutrition

Perinatal Difficulties

Extreme prematurity
Hypoxic–ischemic injury
Intracranial hemorrhage
Metabolic disorders (e.g., hypoglycemia, hyperbilirubinemia)
Infections (e.g., herpes simplex, bacterial meningitis)

Postnatal Brain Insults

Infections (e.g., encephalitis, meningitis)
Trauma (e.g., severe head injury)
Asphyxia (e.g., near-drowning, prolonged apnea, suffocation)
Metabolic disorders (e.g., hypoglycemia, hypernatremia)
Toxins (e.g., lead)
Intracranial hemorrhage
Malnutrition

Postnatal Experiential Disruptions

Poverty and family disorganization
Dysfunctional infant–caregiver interaction
Parental psychopathology
Parental substance abuse

CMV = cytomegalovirus; CNS = central nervous system; HIV = human immunodeficiency virus.

Family history must also be taken into account to uncover any potential genetic cause.

The age and manner of presentation of mental retardation are important to note, because they provide clues to the severity of the condition. The more severe the retardation, the earlier developmental delays are likely to manifest themselves. The greater the severity, the more likely the presence of associated stigmatizing features or medical findings that bring the child to professional attention. Severe, profound mental retardation tends to affect all socioeconomic classes relatively equally. The milder forms tend to occur more in social classes in which psychosocial or environ-mental stressors may contribute to the etiology of the condition.

Physical Examination

Careful physical and neurologic examination may reveal stigmata (suggestive of a genetic syndrome) [e.g., fetal alcohol syndrome, Down syndrome] or neurologic abnormalities that should guide further medical workup.

Laboratory Evaluation

Laboratory assessment is indicated only when history or examination results suggest a particular etiology. The indiscriminate performance of laboratory or radiologic screening is not cost effective, because it is impossible to determine the precise cause in the majority of cases.

Management

In discussions of the results of evaluation with parents, the clinician must carefully explain the meaning of the term "mental retardation." Parents may associate negative stereotypes involving behavioral and other stigmatizing conditions with the diagnosis of mental retardation. Without proper explanation, parents of mildly retarded youngsters may picture their child becoming wheelchair-dependent or otherwise severely impaired. Furthermore, parents who may not understand the difference between cognitive delay and emotional disturbance may believe that their child suffers from the latter condition. The pediatrician may be tempted to use other terminology such as "developmental delay," and while this may be more palatable, he must be careful to use the same diagnostic terminology that will be used in accessing services for the child. It is preferable for parents to hear the appropriate terminology, properly explained, rather than to see the diagnosis on paper for the first time without the benefit of the pediatrician's support.

The pediatrician is in a position to serve as advisor and advocate for the child with mental retardation and her family. Early on, the pediatrician must help the family access appropriate evaluation for the child and provide support and information as the family navigates through an often frightening and complicated process. The pediatrician must remain available to counsel and support the parents once a diagnosis has been reached and intervention services are accessed. Monitoring a child's progress is critical throughout the pediatric years. Any deterioration in functioning or progress that exceeds that predicted for a child's level of retardation suggests possible confounding factors and mandates reevaluation. The pediatrician should bear in mind that each child, no matter what her level of functioning, can reach a certain potential, albeit at a slower rate than normal. The physician should help parents and other family members keep this realistically in mind while attempting to preserve optimum functioning of the family as a whole.

CEREBRAL PALSY

Cerebral palsy is a disorder of movement and posture that continues to be the most frequent childhood motor disability. The incidence of cerebral palsy has remained constant at a rate of 2–3/1000 live births during the last four decades.

Pathophysiology

Cerebral palsy results from a nonprogressive lesion, an injury sustained during the period of brain growth, or a developmental deficit of the brain. Although motor deficits are the essential diagnostic feature of cerebral palsy, associated deficits resulting from the central nervous system (CNS) pathology may occur. The brain lesions that lead to cerebral palsy may occur during the prenatal, perinatal, and postnatal periods. The most common causes of cerebral palsy are prenatal (Table 12.4). There are three major types of cerebral palsy: **spastic, dyskinetic,** and **mixed** (Table 12.5). Rare types of cerebral palsy include atonic and rigid types.

Clinical and Laboratory Evaluation

History

The history should include a detailed prenatal, perinatal, and developmental history; family history; medical history; feeding history; and a re-

---

TABLE 12.4 Risk Factors Associated With Cerebral Palsy

Prenatal
Congenital malformations
Social and economic factors
Maternal intrauterine infection
Reproductive insufficiency
Toxic or teratogenic agents
Maternal mental retardation, seizures, hyperthyroidism
Multiple births
Placental complication
Abdominal trauma

Neonatal
Prematurity: < 32 weeks' gestation
Birth weight < 2500 g
Growth retardation
Abnormal presentation
Intracranial hemorrhage
Infection
Bradycardia and hypoxia
Seizures
Hyperbilirubinemia

Postnatal
Trauma
Infection
Intracranial Hemorrhage
Coagulopathy

TABLE 12.5 Classification of Cerebral Palsy

Type/Subtype	Involvement/Characteristics
Spastic (most common)	
Spastic diplegia	Both legs
Spastic quadriparesis	Both arms and legs, but more severe in lower extremities
Spastic triplegia	Both lower legs and one arm
Spastic hemiparesis	One side of body, arm and leg (more involvement in arm)
Spastic monoplegia	One limb, usually mild, and very often a misdiagnosed hemiplegia
Dyskinetic	
Athetosis	Slow writhing movements of the face and distal extremities
Dystonia	Rhythmic twisting movements of trunk and proximal limbs with changes in muscle tone
Chorea (uncommon)	Rapid irregular jerky movements of face and extremities
Mixed	
Spastic athetoid	Spasticity and athetoid movements
Spastic ataxic	Unsteadiness, nystagmus, dyskinetic and uncoordinated movements

view of systems. Early symptoms and signs that should arouse suspicion of cerebral palsy are delayed motor development and abnormal muscle tone, along with posture and movement patterns.

Physical Examination

The physical examination should consist of a general examination (head circumference, height, and weight), an assessment of the musculoskeletal system (range of motion of major joints, leg length, spine assessment), and a neurologic examination (alertness, cranial nerves, muscle tone, posture reflexes). Gait, mobility, functional, and developmental assessments are also important. During the course of the examination, the clinician should remember that several medical conditions are associated with cerebral palsy (Table 12.6).

Laboratory Evaluation

Laboratory studies, neurodiagnostic imaging, visual auditory evoked potentials, electroencephalograms (EEGs), and electrophysiologic studies

TABLE 12.6 Medical Conditions Associated With Cerebral Palsy

Mental retardation
Seizures
Hydrocephalus
Speech and communication disorders
Swallowing problems
Vision impairment
Hearing impairment
Learning disabilities
Behavior disabilities
Dental abnormalities

may be appropriate. Blood and urine samples should be obtained to rule out metabolic and genetic diseases. Other tests include thyroid function, chromosomes, organic and amino acids, lactate and pyruvate when appropriate.

Neuroimaging studies [magnetic resonance imaging (MRI), computed tomography (CT), and cranial ultrasound] are necessary to rule out intracranial hemorrhages, congenital malformations, and periventricular leukomalacia. Evoked potentials may provide information regarding the integrity of visual and auditory pathways.

Clinical Course

The clinical course of cerebral palsy is diverse depending on type, severity, and clinical manifestations. Clinical findings at the time of diagnosis may change over the years due to growth and development or due to therapeutic intervention or lack of it. Initially, children may be hypotonic; later, they may become hypertonic or dyskinetic. Secondary adverse musculoskeletal effects due to muscle imbalance, abnormal posture, and abnormal muscle tone affect the functional outcome and tend to occur earlier in children with moderate-to-severe disability.

In **spastic hemiparesis,** children may have significant loss of function in the affected hand if sensory impairment is present in addition to the weakness and/or spasticity. This can lead to contractures and growth disturbances in the affected limb. However, most affected children can be independent in self-care, with adaptive utensils for bimanual fine motor skills. Almost all children with hemiplegia walk; they may need orthosis to support a weak limb or to stretch tight muscles.

In **spastic diplegia,** children may have impaired hand function at the onset. With therapeutic exercises and functional training, they usually achieve independence in activities of daily living. With intensive physical therapy and the use of orthotic devices, walkers, and crutches, standing and walking may be possible. For long-distance mobility, wheelchairs may be necessary. Spasticity may lead to contractures of major joints and abnormalities of posture and gait. Orthopedic deformities may require surgical intervention.

In **spastic quadriparesis,** children have varying degrees of severity in motor deficits, which directly influence the acquisition of motor skills and functional independence. Persistent increased muscle tone in the extremities may cause hip dislocation, pain, and scoliosis, especially in nonambulatory children. Associated deficits such as mental retardation, seizures, hearing and visual impairments, and oromotor deficits may further compromise the acquisition of functional skills. Of children with spastic quadriparesis, 25% have minimal or no functional limitations in activities of daily living, 50% have moderate involvement and need assistance in self-care and mobility, and the remaining 25% have severe deficits and require total care.

Pediatric Pearl

Mental retardation is the most serious associated deficit in cerebral palsy, with an overall incidence of 30%–50%. It is one of the main factors that preclude independent living skills in adults with cerebral palsy.

In **dyskinetic cerebral palsy,** children have prolonged hypotonia and persistent primitive reflexes. Between 18 months and 2 years of age they develop athetoid movements in their distal extremities, which progress to dystonic movements with growth and maturation. Upper extremities are more involved than the lower extremities. About 50% of children walk independently, often after 3 years of age, and they develop upper extremity control adequate for self-care activities. Scoliosis may occur later in life.

Prediction of long-term outcome in cerebral palsy in the first few years of life is difficult. The outcome is determined by the severity of the motor deficits, presence of associated deficits (see Table 12.6), and effect of intervention. Overall, 75% of children with cerebral palsy walk either in-

dependently or with assistance. Failure to achieve independent sitting by 2 years of age and the persistence of primitive reflexes at 18 months of age has been shown to herald a poor prognosis for walking in children with cerebral palsy. The presence of mental retardation, seizure disorders, and severe motor disability render functional independence less likely in adults.

Pediatric Pearl

Good prognostic indicators of independent walking are independent sitting by 2 years of age, and suppression of obligatory primitive reflexes by 18 months of age.

Differential Diagnosis

Because motor control is acquired gradually during the first year of life, it is difficult to recognize motor deficits at birth or in the child's first few months of life, unless the abnormalities are significant. As the neuromuscular deficit and the abnormal movement patterns continue to evolve, the diagnosis can be usually confirmed at the end of the first year. In mild cases the diagnosis may be overlooked until much later when the abnormalities in walking and significant developmental delays are noted.

Management

Management of cerebral palsy involves treatment of motor disabilities, treatment of associated deficits (see Table 12.6), promotion of good physical and emotional health, family support, appropriate educational and vocational services, integration into the community, and prevention or minimizing potential complications. Once the diagnostic workup is complete, the clinician should develop a therapeutic plan. In many instances, it is not possible to establish a definitive diagnosis of cerebral palsy with certainty when the symptoms and signs are mild. As the child grows, the motor deficits and delays may become more apparent. However, the intervention must be initiated when there is evidence of motor delays or abnormalities of muscle tone. The primary goals of intervention are to maximize functional skills, foster independence, and prevent or minimize complications. Periodic evaluation and assessment of physical growth and nutrition is essential, and appropriate educational placement with classroom adaptation to compensate for the disability and counseling for emotional and social adjustment is imperative.

The treatment of motor deficits involves various types of therapeutic systems. No one method is suitable for all children, and therefore, development of individualized therapeutic regimens depending on age and the extent of involvement is necessary. Important components of therapy include stretching of tight muscles, maintaining and improving range of motion in joints, and strengthening weak muscles. In infants and young children these essential components are achieved by placing the children in different positions to encourage the use of spastic muscle groups or through age appropriate play and by use of adaptive toys and games. In addition to strengthening and stretching exercises, physical therapy involves training of postural and motor control to achieve age-appropriate developmental skills. Occupational therapy promotes achievement of self-care skills and fine motor skills. Speech and language pathologists encourage activities to improve oral motor functions such as feeding, swallowing, and articulation.

Orthotic Devices

Orthoses are used as an adjunct to physical and occupational therapy to maintain range of motion of joints, provide support in weightbearing or walking when the muscles are weak, or improve function such as in hand splints to assist in feeding. Orthoses may be necessary following surgery to maintain the surgical correction. Therapists may fabricate them using low-density plastic materials such as Aquaplast; usually, these devices are quite inexpensive and need frequent changing as children grow. Custom-fabricated orthoses made of laminated plastic or polypropylene are quite expensive. Periodic evaluation is necessary to ensure proper fit and assess the need for continued use.

Durable Medical Equipment

Durable medical equipment refers to devices used to achieve self-care, mobility, communication, vocational skills, and recreational activities in cases where attainment of these skills may not be otherwise possible. An adapted bath chair may assist parents in bathing a child with poor head and trunk control who is unable to sit. An adapted stroller or a wheelchair can help transport a child to school. A walker or crutches can assist a child who has impaired balance to walk. When choosing equipment, it is important to consider the functional goals, prognosis, patient and family needs, and cost effectiveness. Periodic evaluation is important, and as the result of

children's growth and achievement of functional skills, repair and replacement of the devices may be necessary.

Early Intervention

These family-focused services, which are part of a multidisciplinary approach to the treatment of cerebral palsy, help establish effective parenting skills and improved infant–caregiver interactions. Services can be either home-based or center-based. Parents receive instructions concerning handling and positioning as well as on feeding techniques. Trained physical, occupational, and speech therapists provide the teaching. The goal is to promote normal movement patterns and to enable young children with limited motor abilities to explore their environment. Families also receive psychosocial support to improve parents' coping abilities. Early intervention programs provide services until the child's third birthday. At that time, referrals to preschool programs for continuation of services are available if needed.

Orthopedic Surgery

Well-timed use of orthopedic procedures can improve function and prevent or correct deformities in children with cerebral palsy. Affected children usually do not have orthopedic problems at birth, but they develop deformities and limitations in range of motion due to spastic muscle imbalance and deforming forces. Prior to surgery it is essential that clear-cut goals and expectation for surgery are established and postoperative management is organized. Postoperative management usually includes physical therapy for range of motion, strengthening, gait training, and use of orthoses and casts to maintain surgical correction.

Several neurosurgical procedures have been used in the treatment of spasticity. Selective dorsal rhizotomy of L2–L5 spinal rootlets followed by intensive physical therapy has been successful in decreasing spasticity. In children who are ambulatory, postoperative gait analysis has shown an increase in stride length and an improvement in hip and knee range of motion. In nonambulatory children, decreasing spasticity by selective dorsal rhizotomy has resulted in easier management by caregivers and an improvement in optimal positioning thereby preventing decubiti and deformities.

Asymmetric muscle imbalance, poor posture, spastic muscles, and joint contractions all contribute to the development of spinal curvature. Serial radiographs should be taken at regular intervals to monitor the spine. Curves up to 20° necessitate physical therapy for stretching of tight muscles and careful monitoring. Curves between 20°–40° require use of a spinal orthosis in conjunction with stretching exercises and proper positioning to delay or control the rate of progression of the spinal curve during growth. When scoliosis is progressive in spite of adequate use of orthoses or when the curve is greater than 40°, surgery is indicated. Progression of the curvature appears to be greater in children who are nonambulatory.

Spastic muscles of the hip can cause pelvic obliquity, decreased sitting balance, and gait deviations in children who are ambulatory. Deformities of the knees can cause crouch posture when standing and can interfere with sitting and walking.

Deformities due to spastic muscle imbalance of the calf muscles result in equinus deformity of ankles and toe walking. Surgery for correction of deformities of the lower extremities involves lengthening of tight muscles, tendon transfers, osteotomies, or arthrodesis in older individuals. Postoperative management includes immobilization in a cast for 6–8 weeks followed by use of orthoses and gait training as needed.

Deformities of the upper extremities are due to dynamic muscle imbalance, spasticity, and contractures. Goals of treatment are to improve function and appearance. Prior to surgery, it is important to do a botulinum toxin A neuromuscular block of selected muscles to assess the effect. Postoperative intensive rehabilitation and use of casting as well as dynamic splints are important. Commonly used procedures include tendon lengthening of elbows, tendon lengthening of thumb, Z-plasty of first web space, and tendon transfer to improve supination and wrist extension.

Medical Management

An integral part of management of motor disabilities includes treatment of abnormal muscle tone. Many modalities are available, including therapeutic heat, cold, biofeedback, and functional and therapeutic electrical stimulation. Although studies have shown that these treatments are effective in decreasing spasticity, the effects are of short duration and few validated studies are available.

Intramuscular blocks using botulinum neurotoxin A (Botox) reduce spasticity for 3–6 months when administered to selected spastic muscles. This treatment improves range of motion and decreases deformities, and it has proved especially useful in management of spastic triceps surae muscles in toe walking. Following the procedure, it is important to use an orthosis to maintain the range of motion and to continue physical therapy to increase the muscle strength and motor control.

Frequently used **oral antispastic medications** are benzodiazepines, tizanidine, dantrolene sodium, and baclofen, which decrease the muscle tone but do not necessarily improve function. When used in large doses in treatment of moderate-to-severe spasticity, side effects that preclude long-term use include weakness, fatigue, and drowsiness.

In addition, baclofen may be administered via a programmable pump that has been surgically implanted in the anterior abdominal wall and connected with a catheter to the spinal canal (intrathecal). This technique results in improved function and reduced spasticity. Long-term efficacy in children with cerebral palsy has not been established. The advantages of this procedure include easy administration of the medication directly into the spinal canal with an ability to use very low doses to achieve the desired effects. The disadvantages are the prohibitive cost of the equipment and medication as well as possible infection, cerebrospinal fluid (CSF) leaks, and kinking of the catheter.

AUTISTIC SPECTRUM DISORDERS

Autism refers to a developmental disorder affecting communication, socialization, and range of activities and interests. It is not one single disorder but the extreme end of a spectrum that encompasses a wide variation in behavioral phenotype. This spectrum is termed the **pervasive developmental disorders (PDDs).** The DSM IV-TR lists diagnostic criteria for autistic disorder (Table 12.7). Other PDDs include Asperger syndrome, Rett syndrome, childhood disintegrative disorder, and PDD not otherwise specified, which all involve varying combinations of diagnostic criteria.

Autism implies a severe impairment in reciprocal social interaction. Awareness of existence, thoughts, or feelings of others may be markedly impaired. Children may seem to be "in their own world," showing little or no interest in social relationships. They may not seek to share pleasurable or painful experiences. Displays of affection may appear inappropriate in context. Eye contact may be limited but is not necessarily absent.

Communication is significantly impaired, with total lack of spoken language or atypical use of language. Comprehension is also severely affected. Autistic children may be unable to follow even simple verbal directions. They may communicate their desires by grabbing their caregiver's hand to point to an object. Children who do speak have severely impaired social rules of language, **prag-**

TABLE 12.7 Diagnostic Criteria for Autistic Disorder

Total of six (or more) items from (1), (2), and (3), with at least two from (1) and one each from (2) and (3):

1. Qualitative impairment in social interaction, as manifested by at least two of the following:
   a. Marked impairment in the use of multiple nonverbal behaviors such as eye-to-eye gaze, facial expression, body postures, and gestures to regulate social interaction
   b. Failure to develop peer relationships appropriate to developmental level
   c. Lack of spontaneous seeking to share enjoyment, interests, or achievements with other people (e.g., lack of showing, bringing, or pointing out objects of interest)
   d. Lack of social emotional reciprocity

2. Qualitative impairments in communication as manifested by at least one of the following:
   a. Delay in, or total lack of, the development of spoken language (not accompanied by an attempt to compensate through alternative modes of communication such as gesture or mime)
   b. In individuals with adequate speech, marked impairment in the ability to initiate or sustain a conversation with others
   c. Stereotyped and repetitive use of language or idiosyncratic language
   d. Lack of varied, spontaneous make-believe play or social imitative play appropriate to developmental level

3. Restricted repetitive and stereotyped patterns of behavior, interests, and activities, as manifested by at least one of the following:
   a. Preoccupation with one or more stereotyped and restricted patterns of interest that is abnormal either in intensity or focus
   b. Apparently inflexible adherence to specific, nonfunctional routines or rituals
   c. Stereotyped and repetitive motor mannerisms (e.g., hand or finger flapping or twisting, complex whole-body movements)
   d. Persistent preoccupation with parts of objects

Delays or abnormal functioning in at least one of the following areas, with onset prior to 3 years of age: (1) social interaction, (2) language as used in social communication, or (3) symbolic or imaginative play

Not better accounted for by Rett disorder or childhood disintegrative disorder

matics, which compromise or prevent the ability to engage in conversation. Language may be idiosyncratic, consisting of utterances of abnormal intonation, rate, or rhythm. **Echolalia,** the repetition of what was heard immediately or sometime in the past, may be prominent. Autistic children may repeat television commercials or favorite songs, or may appear to be reciting monologues or scripts. Play lacks symbolism and is often repetitive and devoid of imagination.

Autistic children may exhibit atypical patterns of behavior, interests, and activities, showing intense attachment to a particular object such as a piece of string or a magazine page. Insistence on routines or rituals is seen. Autistic children may engage in a variety of self-stimulatory behaviors such as rocking in place, spinning in circles, or flapping hands. Interruption of these patterns of behavior may cause severe distress. Temper tantrums, hyperactivity, self-injurious behaviors, aggression, and destructiveness are common.

Estimates suggest that autistic disorders occur in 2–5 individuals per 10,000 population, with a male-to-female ratio of 4:1.

Pathophysiology

Autism has no single known cause. A definite etiology is evident in only 10%–20% of cases. Genetics may play a role; 90% of monozygotic (identical) twins, but only 10% of dizygotic (fraternal) twins or siblings tend to be diagnosed on the same spectrum. Syndromes such as fragile X syndrome or tuberous sclerosis have been implicated but no definite association has been found.

Psychological Assessment

The intelligence of autistic children most often tests in the mental retardation range. However, the language and social deficits that define the autistic disorders make it difficult to obtain an accurate estimate of an individual's intellectual potential using standardized psychological tests. Underlying cognitive level contributes significantly to the behavioral phenotype. Autistic individuals may have uneven cognitive profiles. Some autistic children with higher functioning may display unusual abilities or talents, amass facts about obscure subjects, or have unusually keen memories. Individuals functioning in the severe to profound ranges of mental retardation may be labeled autistic when in fact their remoteness is due to significant cognitive impairment.

Clinical and Laboratory Evaluation

History
Children with autism generally present in the preschool years with histories of delayed speech and language development. There may be descriptions, often in retrospect, of remoteness or unusual placidity during infancy. As toddlers, autistic children may seem unusually independent. Approximately one-third of parents report that their child's language or social skills appeared normal and then seemed to have regressed somewhere between 18–24 months of age. This phenomenon of autistic regression is currently under study. The physician should question parents of all children on the autistic spectrum about regression. It is also essential to take a careful family and past medical history. Neurologic referral without delay is necessary for children with a positive history of regression.

Physical Examination
Physical and neurologic examination is indicated, as it is for all children with developmental delay. For example, the presence of dysmorphic features consistent with genetic syndromes, neurocutaneous disorders, or other neurologic abnormalities is noteworthy.

Laboratory Evaluation
The examiner should order laboratory tests only when a particular medical condition is suspected.

Differential Diagnosis

Autistic disorder must be differentiated from other disorders on the PDD spectrum. **Asperger disorder** involves impaired socialization without delay in language development or significant cognitive delay. **Rett syndrome** affects only girls, who manifest severe cognitive delays after a period of apparently normal development, slowing of brain growth and hand mannerisms. **Childhood disintegrative disorder** involves severe cognitive and social regression in children who were developing normally in the first 2 years of life. **PDD not otherwise specified** is the diagnostic terminology reserved for those individuals manifesting at least two diagnostic criteria on the PDD spectrum but not those for specific disorders. In addition, an acquired epileptic aphasia, **Landau-Kleffer syndrome,** may have the same presenting features as autism and responds to antiepileptic treatment.

Management

There is no cure for autism. The most effective intervention is individualized education aimed at promoting communication and socialization while minimizing negative behaviors. Programs using **applied behavioral analysis** involve intensive individual instruction in a highly structured setting. Psychotropic medications can be beneficial in achieving behavioral control. Prognosis is generally determined by underlying cognitive potential, degree of communication impairment, and associated behavioral profile. Ultimate functioning in autism ranges from complete lack of communication skills and dependence on others to independent living and attainment of advanced educational degrees.

Parents of autistic children frequently receive promises of dramatic results from unconventional, inadequately studied interventions that may be time-intensive, costly, and offer little but false hopes. It is the pediatrician's responsibility to assist parents in gathering information and objectively interpreting what is known about new and unorthodox therapies. As with mental retardation and other developmental disabilities, the pediatrician should serve as a source of information and support, guiding families in accessing services, monitoring their children's progress, and anticipating needs of children and families.

LEARNING DISABILITIES

Learning disabilities refers to a broad range of disorders that cause difficulties in academic achievement well beyond those expected given an individual's level of intellectual functioning. The National Joint Committee on Learning Disabilities defines learning disabilities as

> a heterogeneous group of disorders manifested by significant difficulties in acquisition and use of listening, speaking, reading, writing, reasoning, or mathematical abilities, or of social skills. These disorders are intrinsic to the

individual, presumed to be due to central nervous system dysfunction, and may occur across the life span. Problems in self-regulatory behaviors, social perception, and social interaction may exist with learning disabilities but do not by themselves constitute a learning disability. Although learning disabilities may occur concomitantly with other handicapping conditions (for example sensory impairment, mental retardation, serious emotional disturbance) or with extrinsic influences (such as cultural differences, insufficient or inappropriate instruction), they are not the result of those conditions or influences.

Learning disabilities affect an estimated 2%–10% of children and adults, with a male-to-female ratio of approximately 4:1. The prevalence varies depending on the precise definition of the disability. Associated problems include perinatal injury, neurologic conditions, and chronic illness or genetic predisposition, but it is often impossible to account for a particular learning disability.

Clinical and Laboratory Evaluation

History
Children with learning disabilities often present with difficulties learning to read. Many have difficulty in associating letter symbols with sounds, and blending sounds into words. These difficulties with **phonemic awareness,** which are often seen in children who have histories of language delays, are broadly termed **language-based learning disabilities.** After children have mastered basic phonics, language-based learning disabilities may affect children's comprehension of what they have read. Still other children have difficulty recognizing symbols or visually decoding written words. Such nonverbal or perceptually based learning disabilities also have profound implications for academic achievement. Learning problems may also result from difficulties with memory or attention. Inattention associated with attention deficit hyperactivity disorder can be a primary cause of academic failure or can be secondary to a student's inability to process the information presented in the classroom.

Children with learning disabilities may be puzzling to their parents and teachers. They are smart children who have trouble learning, who seem competent in other aspects of their lives; however, they perform poorly in school. Their parents may conclude that they are not working to their full potential (i.e., they are lazy). Such children may fidget, daydream, or "act out" because of long-standing difficulties keeping up with the pace of classwork. Thus, they begin to

feel or may actually be labeled as "bad" as well as "stupid." Negative self-esteem is inevitably associated with learning disabilities.

Physical Examination
A physical examination should be performed to rule out chronic medical conditions that might predispose to problems with attention or ability to focus in the classroom. Hearing and vision screening and neurologic examination must be completed. Episodes of staring, for examples, either observed or reported, merit consideration of possible absence seizures.

Laboratory Evaluation
As is the case with other developmental disabilities, no routine laboratory assessment is indicated. Tests should be ordered only to confirm or rule out the clinical suspicion of contributory medical conditions.

Management
Careful multidisciplinary assessment is necessary in order to diagnose a learning disability. A standardized psychological assessment first documents cognitive potential. It is necessary to distinguish children with learning disabilities from "slow learners"—children whose intelligence falls in the borderline range (IQ that is one standard deviation below the mean). While the pace of learning of borderline IQ children is somewhat slow, no one single area of deficit, such as in language, memory or perceptual skills, is identifiable. Educational evaluation should then pinpoint areas of strength and weakness, academic strategies, and areas that need remediation. Additional components of the evaluation such as speech and language, occupational therapy, and psychosocial assessments, should be considered based on a child's particular problem.

Since 1975, Public Law 94–142 (Education for All Handicapped Children Act, renamed the Individuals with Disabilities Education Act in 1991) has mandated that all school-age children with a suspected disability receive evaluation and appropriate intervention services in the least restrictive environment. Multidisciplinary evaluation results in the formulation of an individual education plan (IEP), which delineates individual goals and implementation strategies. Under the law, parents have the right to be full participants in the educational planning for their children.

Although the pediatrician does not play the primary role in the diagnosis or management of learning disabilities, parents who are frustrated with their child's poor performance in school may consult the physician. Parents may mistakenly attribute school failure to behavioral issues or to factors that they perceive are under the child's control. Raising the possibility of a learning disability can be the first step in advocating for proper evaluation and securing services aimed at helping the child learn.

SUGGESTED READINGS

Abbott R, Johann-Murphy M, Shiminsky-Maher T, et al: Selective dorsal rhizotomy: Outcome and complications in treating spastic cerebral palsy. *Neurosurgery* 33:851, 1993.

Albright AL: Intrathecal baclofen in cerebral palsy movement disorders. *J Child Neurol* 11:529, 1996.

American Academy of Pediatrics Committee on Children with Disabilities: Pediatric services for infants and children with special needs. *Pediatrics* 92:163, 1993.

American Academy of Pediatrics Committee on Children with Disabilities: Screening infants and young children for developmental disabilities. *Pediatrics* 93:863–865, 1994.

American Academy of Neurology and the Child Neurology Society, Practice Parameter: Screening and diagnosis of autism: Report of the quality standards subcommittee. *Neurology* 55:468–479, 2000.

American Association on Mental Retardation: *Mental Retardation: Definition, Classification and Systems of Supports.* Washington, DC, 1992.

American Psychiatric Association: *Diagnostic and Statistical Manual of Mental Disorders,* 4th ed. (text revision). Washington, DC, American Psychiatric Press, 2000.

Bayley N: *Bayley Scales of Infant Development,* 2nd ed. San Antonio, Psychological Corporation, 1993.

Frankenburg W, et al: *Denver II Training Manual.* Denver, Denver Developmental Materials, 1990.

Individuals with Disabilities Education Act PL 101–476, Title 20, USC 1400 et seq, US Stat at large 104 (Part 2), 1103–1151 (October 30, 1990).

Korman LA, Mooney JF, Smith BP, et al: Management of spasticity in cerebral palsy with botulinum A toxin. *J Ped Orthop* 14:299–303, 1994.

Lambert N, et al: *AAMR Adaptive Behavior Scales Revised School Edition,* Austin, TX, Pro-ed, 1993.

Mathew DJ, Stempien LM: Orthopedic management of the disabled child. In *Basic Clinical Rehabilitation Medicine.* Edited by Sinaki M. St. Louis, Mosby, 1993.

Miller F, Bachrach SJ: *Cerebral Palsy. A Complete Guide to Caregiving.* Baltimore, Johns Hopkins University Press, 1995.

National Institutes of Health Consensus Development Conference: *Early Identification of Hearing Impairment in Infants and Children.* Washington, DC, National Institutes of Health, 1993.

Sparrow S, et al: *Vineland Adaptive Behavior Scales,* Circle Pines, MN, American Guidance Service, 1984.

Thorndike R, et al: *Guide for Administration and Scoring the Stanford Binet Intelligence Scale,* 4th ed. Chicago, Riverside Publishing, 1984.

Wechsler D: *Manual for the Wechsler Intelligence Scale for Children,* 3rd ed. San Antonio, Psychological Corporation, 1991.

Chapter 13

Cardiology

Daniel Bernstein

CONGENITAL HEART DISEASE

Congenital structural defects are the most common cause of cardiovascular morbidity and mortality in children, unlike in adults, where diseases of the myocardium itself (e.g., ischemic cardiomyopathy secondary to coronary atherosclerosis) make up the largest portion of clinical cardiology practice. Other significant causes of cardiovascular disease in children include cardiovascular dysfunction associated with systemic illness, arrhythmia, and acquired heart disease. Congenital heart disease is present in 8/1000 newborns; 50% of these are of sufficient severity to warrant cardiac catheterization or surgery in the first year of life.

Pathophysiology

Not all congenital lesions present with symptoms immediately at birth. Knowledge of the cardiovascular adaptations during the transition from fetal to extrauterine life is important in understanding the clinical presentation and pathophysiology of congenital heart lesions.

The **fetal circulation** places the right and left ventricles in a parallel circuit as opposed to the series circuit of the newborn or adult (Figure 13.1). In the fetus, the placenta provides gas and metabolite exchange. Three structures are important for maintaining this parallel circuit: the **ductus arteriosus**, the **foramen ovale,** and the **ductus venosus.** Venous return from the upper body enters the right atrium, the right ventricle, and then exits the heart via the pulmonary artery (see Figure 13.1A). Only 3%–5% of right ventricular outflow enters the lungs. Because there is no gas exchange in the lungs, the pulmonary circulation is vasoconstricted. Instead, the majority of right ventricular blood supplies the descending aorta via the ductus arteriosus (right-to-left shunt). Forty percent of fetal cardiac output goes to the placenta via the two umbilical arteries. Oxygenated blood from the placenta then returns to the fetus via the umbilical vein, entering the fetal inferior vena cava via the ductus venosus. This oxygen-enriched blood is selectively routed toward the left atrium by the eustachian valve, located at the inferior vena caval–right atrial junction, and the flap of the foramen ovale. This blood then traverses the mitral valve, enters the left ventricle, and is ejected into the ascending aorta.

At birth, the mechanical expansion of the lungs combined with the increase in arterial PO_2 decrease pulmonary vascular resistance dramatically. Right ventricular outflow now flows entirely into the low resistance pulmonary circulation (see Figure 13.1B). Because the pulmonary vascular resistance is now lower than systemic resistance, the shunt through the ductus arteriosus reverses (left-to-right shunt).

Over the course of several days the high arterial PO_2 constricts the ductus arteriosus. The increased pulmonary blood flow returning to the left atrium increases left atrial volume and pressure sufficiently to functionally close the foramen ovale. The removal of the placenta from the circulation also leads to closure of the ductus venosus. Thus, within several days, an almost total transition from a parallel (fetal) to a series (adult) circulation is completed. When congenital structural cardiac defects are superimposed on these dramatic physiologic changes, they often impede this smooth transition and increase the burden on the newborn myocardium. Finally, because the ductus arteriosus and foramen ovale do not close completely at birth, they may remain patent in certain congenital cardiac lesions. These structures may either provide a lifesaving pathway for blood to bypass a congenital defect (e.g., in pulmonary atresia, coarctation of the aorta, or transposition of the great vessels) or may present an additional stress to the circulation [patent ductus arteriosus (PDA) or persistent fetal circulation associated with pulmonary hypertension].

Clinical and Laboratory Evaluation

History
The cardiac history should always begin with a careful review of the pregnancy, including exposure to potential teratogens as well as maternal history of infections or gestational diabetes, which

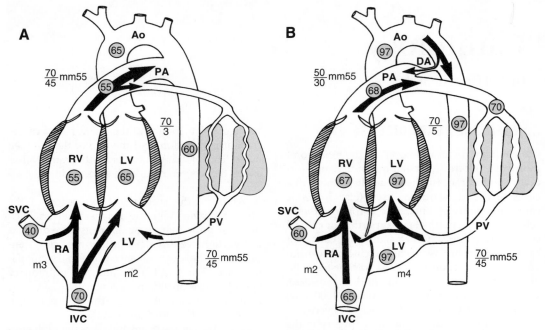

FIGURE 13.1. Transition of the fetal to the newborn circulation. (*A*) fetal circulation; (*B*) early postnatal circulation.

can cause hypertrophic cardiomyopathy. A review of the perinatal period should focus on the Apgar scores, the occurrence of cyanosis or respiratory distress, and prematurity. If cardiac symptoms were present in infancy, it is necessary to enquire when symptoms began, because the timing of presentation can provide a clue as to the specific cardiac condition.

The symptoms of congestive heart failure are age-specific. In infants, **feeding difficulties** are common; feeding represents a significant stress for infants with congenital heart lesions. These problems may be manifest as falling asleep halfway through a feed, sweating with feeds, or frequent gastroesophageal reflux. Other symptoms and signs include rapid breathing, nasal flaring, periorbital or flank edema, irritability and chest retractions. Cyanosis often goes unrecognized by parents, especially in newborns, unless it is severe.

In older children, the early stages of congestive heart failure may be manifested by difficulty in keeping up with peers during physical activities, by requiring a nap after coming home from school, and by poor growth. In older children and adolescents, complaints of anorexia, nausea, and abdominal pain are often more common than respiratory distress. Other frequent complaints include unusual weight gain and pedal edema.

Pediatric Pearl

Abdominal distress is one of the more common symptoms of congestive heart failure in older children and adolescents.

Physical Examination

GENERAL EVALUATION. The comprehensive cardiac examination begins before the clinician ever touches the patient. A novice examiner may place undue emphasis on cardiac murmurs; however, evaluation of the significance of a murmur is best performed in the context of the rest of the physical examination. Often other signs such as the quality of the pulses, the presence or absence of growth retardation, the splitting of the second heart sound, or the presence of a ventricular heave allow the clinician to establish a specific cardiac diagnosis. With practice, not only will the examiner be able to diagnose a specific heart lesion, but the severity as well [e.g., the size of a ventricular septal defect (VSD) or the severity of aortic stenosis].

The examination should begin with a general assessment of the patient, with particular attention to the presence of **cyanosis, abnormalities of growth and development** (including head circumference in infants), **vital signs** (including both upper and lower extremity blood pressures), **quality of peripheral perfusion,** and evidence of **respiratory distress**. Cyanosis is usually best detected by examination of the nail beds, tongue, and mucous membranes (**central cyanosis**). Cyanosis is often incorrectly diagnosed in young infants because the color of the hands or feet is affected by cold (**acrocyanosis**).

Examination of the chest for equality of breath sounds and absence of **adventitious sounds** or **rales,** which could indicate pulmonary edema, is necessary. Many infants and young children who manifest **wheezing,** rather than rales, as a sign of pulmonary edema are often initially misdiagnosed as having bronchiolitis or asthma. The cardiac etiology comes to light once a chest radiograph reveals cardiomegaly.

The presence and degree of **hepatosplenomegaly** is worth noting, although in infants and younger children, the abdominal examination should occur after the chest is auscultated (for obvious reasons). **Edema** is evident in dependent regions: in infants, in the periorbital region and over the flanks; in older children, in the lower extremities.

Palpation of the **peripheral pulses** is necessary in all extremities, with radial and femoral pulses felt simultaneously. Normally the femoral pulse should occur immediately before the radial pulse. However, in children with **coarctation of the aorta,** blood flow to the descending aorta may derive predominantly through collateral vessels. This results in the femoral pulse being delayed until after the radial pulse, known as a **radial–femoral delay**. This is a very sensitive indicator for the presence of coarctation.

The quality of the pulses can also yield important information regarding the severity of congenital heart lesions. For example, as aortic stenosis becomes more severe, both the amplitude and rate of rise of the pulse becomes diminished. Pulses may also be weak in patients with left ventricular dysfunction such as in dilated cardiomyopathy or in any condition that results in diminished cardiac output. Irregular pulses are a sign of arrhythmia.

CARDIAC EXAMINATION. The cardiac examination consists of three components: inspection, palpation, and auscultation. It begins with visual inspection of the precordium for evidence of a sternal or left precordial bulge, indicating chronic right or left ventricular enlargement. This is often best accomplished by standing at the foot of the examination table, with the patient lying supine. In children, the **point of maximal impulse** can usually be visualized directly.

The next step in the cardiac evaluation is palpation of the precordium for **thrills or heaves**. An increased impulse below the sternum or along the left sternal border is usually associated with right ventricular hypertrophy or enlargement, whereas left ventricular enlargement is manifested by an increased and laterally displaced point of maximal impulse. Palpation of the precordium for thrills should take place next. Thrills at the lower left sternal border are usually associated with a VSD, those at the upper left sternal border with pulmonary outflow tract stenosis, and those at the upper right sternal border with aortic outflow tract stenosis. Palpation of the suprasternal notch for thrills should also occur. Because the aortic arch lies directly under the notch, the presence of a thrill in this location may detect even mild degrees of left ventricular outflow tract stenosis (e.g., bicuspid aortic valve). Although palpation of a carotid thrill may be useful in older children, this examination is difficult in infants.

Only after the above elements are completed should the clinician begin an examination for heart sounds and murmurs. It is helpful to warm the stethoscope briefly by rubbing it between your hands, especially when examining infants.

The examiner should first turn attention to auscultation of the heart sounds. The **first heart sound** (S_1), which may be split in some children, is best auscultated at the lower left sternal border or apex. The first heart sound may be muffled in conditions that result in decreased compliance of the left ventricle such as moderate-to-severe **aortic stenosis** or the **cardiomyopathies**.

The **second heart sound** (S_2) is heard best at the upper left and right sternal borders. Normally, it is physiologically split into aortic and pulmonic components, with the pulmonic component varying with respirations (Figure 13.2). With inspiration, there is a decrease in intrathoracic pressure and an increased return of blood to the right atrium. There is also a concomitant slight decrease in pulmonary venous return to the left atrium. The increased volume of blood flowing across the right ventricular outflow tract results in the pulmonary valve closing later in the cardiac cycle, which is heard as an increase in the splitting of S_2.

The quality of S_2 is quite important in the diagnosis of congenital heart disease. A single second sound may indicate absence or severe steno-

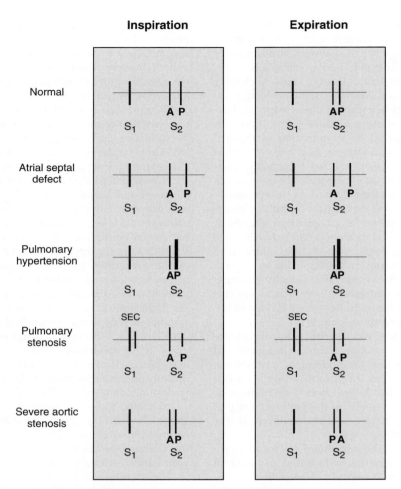

FIGURE 13.2. Variation of the heart sounds with respiration. S_1 = first heart sound due to closure of the mitral and tricuspid valves, S_2 = second heart sound due to closure of the aortic (A) and pulmonary (P) valves, SEC = systolic ejection click.

sis of one of the semilunar valves (**aortic or pulmonary stenosis or atresia**). A single second sound may also be audible in **transposition of the great vessels**. If systemic or pulmonary artery pressures are elevated, that component of S_2 is increased. Thus, in evaluating patients for the presence of **pulmonary hypertension,** careful examination for the presence of a loud pulmonary component of S_2 is vital.

The splitting of S_2 also varies with congenital heart lesions (see Figure 13.2), the most common of which is the **atrial septal defect (ASD)**. Here S_2 is widely split and fixed in its splitting; that is, it does not vary with respirations. This results from the increased blood flow across the pul-

monary valve (due to the left-to-right shunt) through all phases of the respiratory cycle and equilibration of pressures between the two atria. A widely split S_2 may also be heard in patients with **right bundle branch block** due to delayed activation of right ventricular contraction.

Ejection clicks are audible immediately following S_1 and are usually associated with mild-to-moderate degrees of stenosis of the aortic or pulmonary valve. Gallops (S_3 or S_4) are ventricular filling sounds. Many normal children have an S_3 gallop, whereas an S_4 is usually pathologic. Rubs are a sign of pericardial effusion, although with large effusions the rub may disappear and the heart sounds become muffled.

CARDIAC MURMURS. The subject of childhood murmurs could fill a complete book [Zuberbuhler's book is excellent (see SUGGESTED READINGS)]. Here are some basic physiologic concepts. The common congenital heart lesions can be differentiated by the quality of the heart murmurs they produce. (Tables 13.1 and 13.2).

To best appreciate the basics of heart murmurs, it is necessary to understand their relationship to the cardiac cycle (Figure 13.3). Murmurs may be heard in either systole or diastole alone, as two separate murmurs during both phases of the cardiac cycle (to-and-fro murmur), or continuously (Figure 13.4). The early phase of cardiac contraction (immediately after S_1 [i.e., closure of the tricuspid and mitral valves)] is known as **isovolumic contraction,** because in this phase there is no egress of blood from a normal ventricle. Once the ventricular pressure rises to equal pulmonary arterial or aortic pressure, the appropriate semilunar valve opens, and the **ejection** phase of systole begins. It is important to note that a heart murmur that begins with isovolumic contraction (immediately after S_1) must involve egress of blood from the ventricle through a defect of some sort [either a VSD or via regurgitation of one of the atrioventricular (AV) valves], because at this point in the cardiac cycle, the aortic and pulmonic valves are still closed. Similarly, murmurs related to abnormal flow across the ventricular outflow tracts must begin during the ejection phase of systole, and there is a short space between S_1 and the murmur. If S_1 is easily audible in the presence of a systolic murmur, it is likely that the murmur is an ejection murmur.

It is essential to evaluate murmurs for several features, all of which aid in assessing not only the type of congenital heart lesion but also the severity. The **"shape"** of the murmur is determined by whether it is heard uniformly through a portion of the cardiac cycle (e.g., **pan or holosystolic**), rises and falls (**crescendo-decrescendo**) or falls only (**decrescendo**) [see Figure 13.4]. The **length** of the murmur in the cardiac cycle is often a good indication of severity. For example, as pulmonic stenosis worsens, the time it takes for the volume of blood to leave the right ventricle lengthens, and thus the murmur becomes longer.

The **loudness** of the murmur is related to the pressure difference across the area that the blood flows. In ASDs, where the pressure across the two atria is either equal or low (0–5 mm Hg), no murmur is audible due to the defect itself, but a flow murmur is heard across the right ventricular outflow tract due to the increased volume of pulmonary blood flow. In valvar stenosis, the more severe the stenosis, the greater the pressure drop across the valve and thus the louder the murmur. The **tonal quality** of the murmur is also affected by pressure differences. Blowing murmurs are of low frequency and usually associated with low pressure differences such as across a large "nonrestrictive" VSD (large enough so that right ventricular pressure is equal to left ventricular pressure) or in tricuspid regurgitation (the difference between right ventricular and right atrial pressure is usually low). Harsh murmurs are of high frequency and usually heard best with the diaphragm. They are associated with high pressure differences such as in a small "restrictive" VSD (where the right ventricular pressure is much lower then left ventricular pressure), in more severe degrees of valvar stenosis, and in mitral regurgitation (because the difference between left ventricular and left atrial pressure is usually high).

INNOCENT MURMURS. Innocent or functional murmurs are common in children, with a reported prevalence between 5% and 90%, depending on the population studied and the methods used. The job of the pediatrician and pediatric cardiologist is to distinguish the approximately 2%–7% of these murmurs that represent organic heart disease and avoid labeling normal children with cardiac diagnoses.

The most important steps in differentiating an innocent from an organic murmur include obtaining a history demonstrating an absence of cardiac symptoms, documenting normal growth and development, and noting the absence of other abnormalities on examination (e.g., heaves, thrills, abnormal heart sounds, alterations in the pulses, or cyanosis). If any of these factors is positive, the murmur must be considered organic until proven otherwise. If these factors are all negative, several features of the murmur itself can be used to confirm its innocent nature (Table 13.3).

Laboratory Evaluation

The comprehensive evaluation of the pediatric electrocardiogram (ECG) is beyond the scope of this chapter. However, **several aspects of the pe-**

TABLE 13.1 Physical Findings in Common Acyanotic Congenital Heart Lesions

Congenital Lesion	Palpation	Cardiac Auscultation	ECG	Chest Radiograph
Left-to-right shunts				
Atrial septal defect (ASD)	RV impulse	Fixed, widely split S_2 Systolic ejection murmur ULSB Middiastolic rumble LLSB	Normal; occasionally RSR' in right precordial leads Normal or LVH; RVH if large	Large RA, LA, RV, PA Increased pulmonary markings
Ventricular septal defect (VSD)	LV impulse Thrill LLSB	±Widely split S_2 Holosystolic (or crescendo–decrescendo) murmur LLSB Middiastolic rumble apex	Normal or LVH; RVH if large	Large LA, LV, PA Increased pulmonary markings
AV septal defect (AV canal)	RV impulse ± LV impulse	± Loud S_1 Holosystolic murmur LLSB Soft ejection murmur ULSB Middiastolic rumble LLSB or apex	Superior, counterclockwise axis	Large RA, LA, RV, LV Increased pulmonary markings
Patent ductus arteriosus (PDA)	LV impulse Bounding pulses	Continuous murmur ULSB and subclavicular area	Normal or LVH	Large LA, LV
Obstructive lesions				
Pulmonic stenosis (PS)	RV impulse Thrill ULSB	Systolic ejection click (mild PS) Soft P_2 Systolic ejection murmur ULSB	RVH	Uptilt of cardiac apex (RVH)
Aortic stenosis (AS)	LV impulse Decreased pulses Thrill URSB, SSN, carotids	Systolic ejection click (mild AS) Soft A_2 Systolic ejection murmur URSB and MLSB	LVH	Dilated ascending aorta
Coarctation of the aorta (CoAo)	Decreased and delayed pulses in lower compared with upper extremities	Systolic ejection click (bicuspid aortic valve) Systolic or continuous murmur LSB and left subscapular area	RVH, LVH	Collateral arteries (rib notching) Inverted-3 sign Increased pulmonary markings

ECG = electrocardiogram; LA = left atrium; LSB = left sternal border; LV = left ventricle (ventricular); LVH = left ventricular hypertrophy; MLSB = middle left sternal border; PA = pulmonary artery; RA = right atrium; RV = right ventricle (ventricular); RVH = right ventricular hypertrophy; SSN = suprasternal notch; ULSB = upper left sternal border; URSB = upper right sternal border.

TABLE 13.2 Physical Findings in Common Cyanotic Congenital Heart Lesions

Congenital Lesion	Palpation	Cardiac Auscultation	ECG	Chest Radiograph
Lesions with decreased pulmonary blood flow				
Critical pulmonic stenosis	RV impulse	Single S_2 ± Systolic ejection murmur ULSB Continuous murmur ULSB (PDA or bronchial collaterals)	RVH	Decreased pulmonary flow
Tetralogy of Fallot	RV impulse ± Thrill ULSB	Loud, single S_2 Harsh systolic ejection murmur ULSB and MLSB	RVH, RAD	Decreased pulmonary flow "Boot-shaped" heart Right aortic arch (25%)
Tricuspid atresia	LV impulse	Narrowly split S_2, soft P_2 Harsh systolic murmur LSB	LVH, left superior axis	Decreased pulmonary markings Round cardiac silhouette
Ebstein anomaly of tricuspid valve		Triple or quadruple heart sounds Soft, holosystolic murmur LLSB	RAE, prolonged P-R, bundle-branch block, preexcitation	Massive RA enlargement, globular cardiac silhouette
Lesions with increased pulmonary blood flow				
Transposition of the great arteries		Loud A_2, soft or absent P_2 ± Soft systolic ejection murmur MLSB	Normal in newborn period Later RVH, RAD	Normal in newborn; increased pulmonary markings afterwards, egg-shaped heart Narrow mediastinum

(continued)

TABLE 13.2 Physical Findings in Common Cyanotic Congenital Heart Lesions *(Continued)*

Congenital Lesion	Palpation	Cardiac Auscultation	ECG	Chest Radiograph
Truncus arteriosus	RV impulse LV impulse Systolic ejection click MLSB	Loud single S_2 Harsh systolic murmur MLSB Continuous murmur—lungs	RVH, LVH pulmonary markings	Cardiac enlargement, increased Right aortic arch (25%)
Hypoplastic left heart (HLHS)	RV impulse Poor perfusion Poor peripheral pulses	± Soft midsystolic murmur LSB ± Middiastolic rumble LLSB	RAH, RVH	Cardiac enlargement, increased pulmonary markings, ± pulmonary venous obstruction
Total anomalous pulmonary venous return (TAPVR)	RV impulse	Gallop rhythm Soft systolic ejection murmur LSB Middiastolic rumble LLSB	RVH, RAH	Unobstructed: cardiac enlarge- ment and increased pulmonary markings Obstructed: diffuse, hazy, reticulated pulmonary markings

ECG = electrocardiogram; LA = left atrium; LLSB = lower left sternal border; LSB = left sternal border; LV = left ventricle (ventricular); LVH = left ventricular hypertrophy; MLSB = middle left sternal border; PA = pulmonary artery; RA = right atrium; RAD = right axis deviation; RAE = right atrial enlargement; RV = right ventricle (ventricular); RVH = right ventricular hypertrophy; SSN = suprasternal notch; ULSB = upper left sternal border; URSB = upper right sternal border.

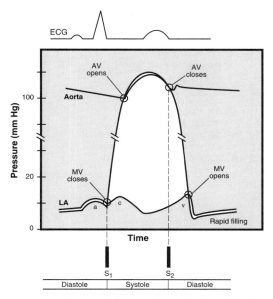

FIGURE 13.3. Events of the cardiac cycle. Systole is divided into two phases: isovolemic contraction and ejection. Diastole is divided into three phases: isovolemic relaxation, rapid ventricular filling, and atrial contraction. a = atrial contraction, c = ventricular contraction, v = atrial filling, AV = aortic valve, LA = left atrial, LV = left ventricular, MV = mitral valve.

diatric ECG are different from the adult ECG and deserve special mention.

Interpretation of the ECG should begin with assessment of heart rate and regularity of rhythm. Heart rate is high in infancy and gradually decreases with increasing age, so it is necessary to diagnose tachycardia or bradycardia by referring to normal values for age. Assessment of whether the rhythm is sinus includes the following criteria: P wave before every QRS, normal PR interval, and normal P-wave axis (P wave upright in leads I and aVF). An abnormal P-wave axis may indicate an ectopic atrial focus, atrial inversion (associated with congenital heart disease), or a junctional beat with retrograde P-wave conduction. It is important to examine the P wave for the presence of right atrial enlargement (P wave > 2.5 mm in lead II and aVR) or left atrial enlargement (notched or biphasic P waves in leads V_1–V_2).

Next comes measurement of ECG intervals and durations [PR, QRS, and QTc (QT corrected for heart rate = QT/$\sqrt{RR}$)]. To note abnormalities, it is necessary to compare the values with normal intervals based on age and, in the case of

the PR interval, heart rate. An abnormally long QRS complex indicates either right or left bundle branch block; in the presence of this, ventricular hypertrophy is difficult to interpret.

By noting which lead is nearly isoelectric and finding the lead orthogonal to it, it is possible to assess the axis. Examination of voltages in the precordial leads is next; leads V_1 and V_5–V_6 are compared with normal values for age. Finally, examination of ST and T waves for depressions, elevations, and polarity occurs; T-wave polarity is very age dependent. In the fetal circulation, both right and left ventricles are pumping against systemic pressure so that the right ventricular wall is relatively thick in the immediate perinatal period. Thus, most newborns have right axis deviation and increased right ventricular forces compared with older children. In the first 24 hours of life, a QR may be present in V_1 and the axis may be as rightward as 205 degrees. One of the most common pitfalls in interpreting newborn ECGs is the false reading of right ventricular hypertrophy.

The T wave in lead V_1 is an important indicator of right ventricular hypertrophy in children. In the immediate newborn period, the T wave is positive in V_1, becoming inverted at approximately 6 days of age. Up until the age of approximately 6 years, the T wave in V_1 should remain inverted, and in many children, it remains inverted until the teenage years. However, if the T wave is positive in V_1 between the ages of 6 days and 6 years, it strongly suggests right ventricular hypertrophy, even in the absence of specific voltage criteria. This is another common error in interpreting pediatric ECGs.

As part of the initial evaluation, the chest radiograph (both frontal and lateral views) may be valuable in making the diagnosis of congenital heart disease. A transcutaneous oxygen saturation measurement or arterial blood gases may easily confirm cyanosis. To differentiate pulmonary-based cyanosis from cardiac-based cyanosis, it is usually necessary to have the patient breathe 100% oxygen for several minutes and remeasure the arterial blood gases (hyperoxia test). If the etiology is pulmonary, the arterial PO_2 should increase to at least above 150 mm Hg, whereas the PO_2 will not increase as dramatically if the etiology is cardiac. Two-dimensional echocardiography, magnetic resonance imaging (MRI), and computed tomography (CT) are useful for determining cardiac structure. Pulsed, continuous-wave, and color-flow Doppler echocardiography help assess blood flows and pressure gradients.

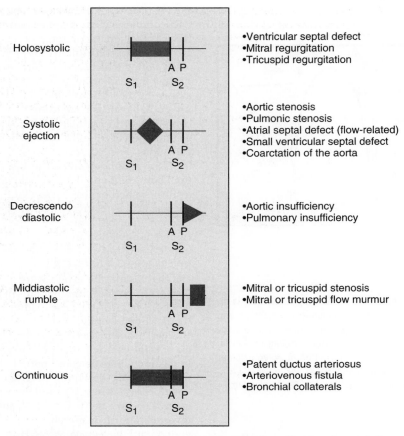

FIGURE 13.4. Timing and shape of cardiac murmurs. S_1 = first heart sound; S_2 = second heart sound, with aortic (A) and pulmonary (P) components.

Differential Diagnosis

Congenital cardiac defects can be classified into two major groups based on the presence or absence of cyanosis (Figure 13.5). The chest radiograph can then be used to further refine the diagnosis based on whether the pulmonary vascular markings show evidence of increased, normal, or decreased pulmonary circulation (Figures 13.6 and 13.7).

Acyanotic Congenital Heart Lesions

This group of congenital lesions can be divided by physiologic principles into those that induce a **volume load** on the heart (most commonly due to a left-to-right shunt but may also result from AV valve regurgitation or abnormalities of the myocardium itself—the cardiomyopathies) and those that induce a **pressure load** on the heart

(subvalvar, valvar, or great vessel stenoses). The chest radiograph is a useful tool for differentiating between these two major categories, because heart size and pulmonary vascular markings are usually both increased in the left-to-right shunt lesions.

VOLUME LESIONS. The most common lesions in this group are the left-to-right shunts: **ASD, VSD, AV septal defect (AV canal or endocardial cushion defect), and PDA.** The common pathophysiologic denominator in this group of lesions is a communication between the left and right sides of the circulation and the shunting of fully oxygenated blood back into the lungs. The direction and magnitude of a shunt across a defect such as a large VSD depends on the relative pulmonary and systemic pressures and vascular resistances. Although pulmonary vascular resis-

TABLE 13.3 Qualities of Innocent Murmurs in Children

Murmur	Characteristics	Differential Diagnosis
Still's murmur	Low-pitch systolic ejection murmur Best heard at mid-left sternal border with minimal radiation Not greater than grade III Vibratory or musical in quality Decreases with change in position (e.g., standing, lying prone)	Small ventral septal defect (usually harsher, possible thrill) Mild pulmonic stenosis (radiates more to lungs, right ventricular impulse, ejection click) Atrial septal defect (fixed split second heart sound); IHSS (increased left ventricular impulse)
Branch pulmonary stenosis	Usually heard in neonatal period Soft systolic ejection murmur at upper left sternal border radiating and often louder in lung fields (important to listen in both axillae) Disappears within first few months of life	Mild pulmonic stenosis (increased right ventricular impulse, systolic ejection click) Atrial septal defect (fixed split second heart sound)
Innocent pulmonary murmur	Soft systolic ejection murmur at upper left sternal border Blowing, nonmusical Higher pitched than Still's murmur Often accentuated by fever or anemia Often present in pectus excavatum	Mild pulmonic stenosis (increased right ventricular impulse, systolic ejection click) Atrial septal defect (fixed split second heart sound)
Venous hum	Medium-pitched, soft blowing continuous murmur at upper right sternal border and infraclavicular area	

IHSS = idiopathic hypertrophic subaortic stenosis.

tance falls dramatically at birth, it remains moderately elevated for several weeks before declining to normal adult levels. Thus, in a lesion such as a large VSD, there may be little shunting or symptoms in the first week of life, and it is not unusual that a murmur is not heard in the newborn nursery.

As pulmonary resistance drops over the first month of life, the left-to-right shunt increases, and so does the intensity of the murmur and the symptoms. This is true for other left-to-right shunt lesions such as AV septal defect and PDA as well.

The increased volume of blood in the lungs is quantitated by pediatric cardiologists as the **pulmonary-to-systemic blood flow ratio** or **Qp:Qs**. A 3:1 shunt implies three times the normal pulmonary blood flow. This increase in pulmonary blood flow decreases pulmonary compliance and increases the work of breathing. Fluid leaks into the interstitium or alveoli causing pulmonary edema and the common symptoms: tachypnea, chest retractions, nasal flaring, poor feeding, and wheezing (see Table 13.1).

To maintain a left ventricular output, which is now several times normal (although most of this output is ineffective, because it returns to the lungs), heart rate and stroke volume must increase, mediated by an increase in sympathetic stimulation. The increased work of breathing and the increase in circulating catecholamines lead to an elevation in total body oxygen requirements, taxing the oxygen delivery capability of the circulation. Thus, common symptoms include tachycardia, sweating, irritability, and failure to thrive.

While isolated valvular regurgitant lesions are less common, AV valve regurgitation is often a feature of complete AV septal (AV canal) defects. The combination of left-to-right shunt and valve regurgitation increases the volume load on the heart and usually leads to earlier presentation and more severe symptomatology.

Unlike the left-to-right shunts, the **cardiomyopathies** (see CARDIOMYOPATHIES) cause heart failure directly due to diminished cardiac muscle function. This leads to increased atrial and ventricular filling pressures as well as pulmonary edema secondary to increased capillary pressure.

OBSTRUCTIVE LESIONS. The most common obstructive lesions are **valvar pulmonic stenosis, valvar aortic stenosis,** and **coarctation of the aorta.** The

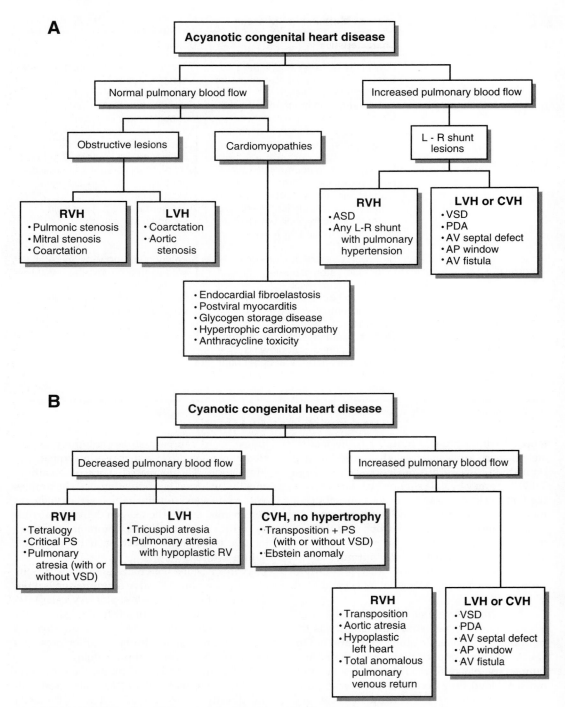

FIGURE 13.5. Classification of congenital heart disease. Determination of pulmonary blood flow is made by chest radiograph; Determination of hypertrophy is made by electrocardiogram (ECG). AP window = aortopulmonary window; ASD = atrial septal defect; AV septal defect = atrioventricular septal defect; AV fistula = arteriovenous fistula; CVH = combined ventricular hypertrophy; L-R = left-to-right; LVH = left ventricular hypertrophy; PDA = patent ductus arteriosus; PS = pulmonary stenosis; RV = right ventricle; RVH = right ventricular hypertrophy; VSD = ventricular septal defect.

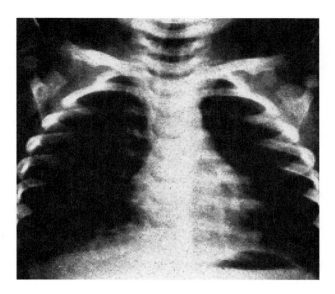

FIGURE 13.6. Normal chest radiograph.

common pathophysiologic denominator of these lesions is that, unless the stenosis is severe, cardiac output is maintained; thus, in children, symptoms of heart failure are often not present. This compensation is accomplished by a marked increase in cardiac wall thickness (hypertrophy). Subtle radiographic changes in the cardiac silhouette (as compared to the volume lesions) may detect hypertrophy. However, the 12-lead ECG is best for detection of left or right ventricular hypertrophy.

Severe pulmonic stenosis in the newborn period (**critical pulmonic stenosis**) often leads to right-sided cardiac failure (hepatomegaly, peripheral edema) and to right-to-left shunting across a patent foramen ovale or ASD; therefore, it is often classified as a cyanotic heart lesion. The pulmonary vascular markings on the chest radiograph are normal or decreased. and the ECG shows right ventricular hypertrophy. Severe aortic stenosis in the newborn period (**critical aortic stenosis**) presents with diminished pulses in all extremities and signs of left-sided heart failure (pulmonary edema), right-sided failure (hepatomegaly, peripheral edema), often progressing to total circulatory collapse. If the ductus arteriosus is still open, the oxygen saturation may be decreased; aortic blood flow may be supplied by a right-to-left ductal shunt. The ECG reveals left ventricular hypertrophy.

Coarctation of the aorta may present solely with a systolic murmur and with diminished pulses in the lower compared with the upper extremities. Thus, it is important to always palpate

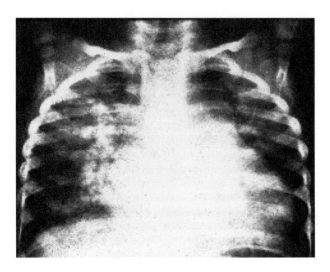

FIGURE 13.7. Chest radiograph in a patient with a large ventricular septal defect showing cardiomegaly and increased pulmonary vascular markings.

both the femoral and either the brachial or radial pulses simultaneously during a routine screening examination of any infant or child. A coarctation may be localized to the area of the descending aorta immediately opposite the ductus arteriosus (**juxtaductal coarctation**). In the first few days or weeks of life, the ductus arteriosus may remain partially patent and serves as a conduit for blood flow to partially bypass the obstruction at the level of the coarctation. Affected infants often become symptomatic when the ductus finally closes. In more severe forms, coarctation involves hypoplasia of the transverse aortic arch, in which case it presents with a more significant obstruction to blood flow and usually causes heart failure and signs of poor perfusion in the neonatal period. In coarctation, especially in infancy, the ECG often shows a combination of both right and left ventricular hypertrophy.

Cyanotic Congenital Heart Lesions

This group of congenital heart lesions can be divided by physiologic principles into those associated with decreased pulmonary blood flow (e.g., **tetralogy of Fallot, pulmonary atresia with intact septum, tricuspid atresia, total anomalous pulmonary venous return with obstruction**) and those associated with increased pulmonary blood flow (**transposition of the great arteries, single ventricle, truncus arteriosus, total anomalous pulmonary venous return without obstruction**). The chest radiograph is again an important primary initial diagnostic tool for differentiating between these two major categories (Figures 13.8 and 13.9).

CYANOTIC LESIONS WITH DECREASED PULMONARY BLOOD FLOW. Two basic pathophysiologic elements underlie all of these lesions. First is an obstruction to pulmonary blood flow at some level (tricuspid valve, subpulmonary muscle bundles, pulmonary valve, main or branch pulmonary arteries). Second is a means by which deoxygenated blood can flow right-to-left to enter the systemic circulation (patent foramen ovale, ASD, or VSD). It is important to remember that even with severe pulmonic stenosis, systemic desaturation does not occur unless there is right-to-left shunting at some level.

Tricuspid atresia involves the right-to-left shunting of deoxygenated blood across either a

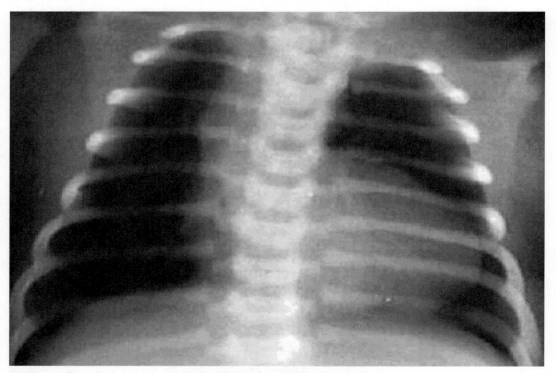

FIGURE 13.8. Chest radiograph in a patient with tetralogy of Fallot. The cardiac apex is tilted upward, signifying right ventricular enlargement; the left upper mediastinal shadow is narrowed due to hypoplasia of the main pulmonary artery segment; and the pulmonary vascular markings are decreased. This is the typical "boot shape" appearance of tetralogy of Fallot.

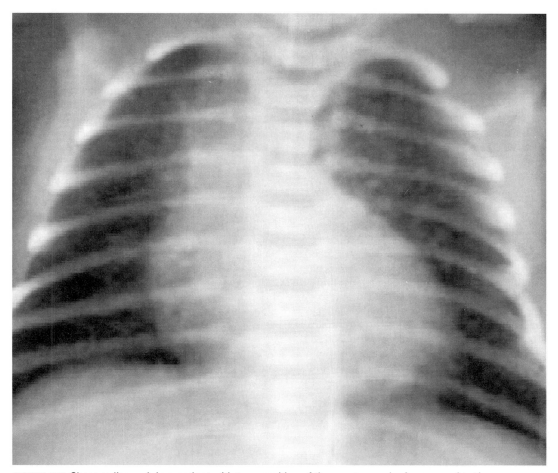

FIGURE 13.9. Chest radiograph in a patient with transposition of the great vessels. As opposed to the patient with tetralogy of Fallot (see Figure 13.8), it is easy to appreciate that this cyanotic patient has increased pulmonary vascular markings.

patent foramen or ASD to the left atrium, where it mixes with pulmonary venous return and enters the left ventricle. Blood enters the lungs either from the right ventricle (via a VSD) or through a PDA.

Tetralogy of Fallot is a constellation of anatomic findings (subvalvar, valvar, or supravalvar pulmonic stenosis, VSD, aorta overriding the VSD, right ventricular hypertrophy). Deoxygenated blood shunts right-to-left across the VSD into the overriding ascending aorta. In these lesions, the degree of clinical cyanosis depends on the degree of obstruction to pulmonary blood flow. If the obstruction is mild, cyanosis may not be present at rest but only with stress (hypercyanotic episodes known as "Tet spells"). If the obstruction is severe, pulmonary flow may be totally dependent on the patency of the ductus arteriosus. These infants present with profound cyanosis in the newborn period and require pharmacologic treatment (**prostaglandin E$_1$**) to maintain ductal patency until surgical intervention.

CYANOTIC LESIONS WITH INCREASED PULMONARY BLOOD FLOW. Although pulmonary blood flow is more than adequate, only a small portion of this oxygenated blood can enter the systemic circulation because of the defect. **Transposition of the great arteries** is the most common lesion in this group. In transposition of the great arteries, the aorta arises from the right ventricle and the pulmonary artery from the left ventricle. Deoxygenated blood from the body returns to the right side of the heart and is pumped directly back to the body again. Oxygenated blood from the lungs returns to the left side of the heart and is pumped back into the lungs. If not for the persistence of fetal pathways such as the foramen ovale and ductus arteriosus, this lesion would not be compatible with life. These pathways allow for some degree of both left-to-right and right-to-left mixing of oxygenated and deoxygenated blood until surgical intervention takes place.

Cardiac lesions leading to a **single or common ventricle** are known as **total mixing lesions,** because deoxygenated systemic venous blood and oxygenated pulmonary venous blood usually mix totally in the heart, resulting in equal oxygen saturations in the pulmonary artery and aorta. Unless pulmonary stenosis is present, pulmonary blood flow is torrential, and affected infants usually present with both mild cyanosis and heart failure. If pulmonary stenosis is present, then pulmonary blood flow is limited, and these infants usually present with more profound cyanosis without heart failure. **Truncus arteriosus** also results in total mixing of systemic and pulmonary venous blood; however, mixing occurs at the great vessel level.

One additional common lesion, **total anomalous pulmonary venous return with obstruction,** causes cyanosis and the appearance of pulmonary edema on chest radiograph. However, this finding is actually secondary to obstruction to blood flowing out of the lungs at the level of the pulmonary veins rather than to an increased volume of pulmonary blood flow. In contrast, **total anomalous pulmonary venous return without obstruction** results in increased pulmonary blood flow and cyanosis due to total mixing of systemic venous and pulmonary venous blood at the level of the right atrium.

Management

Congestive Heart Failure

Congestive heart failure in the pediatric age group may be associated with left-to-right shunt lesions and pulmonary overcirculation, to primary or secondary cardiomyopathies, or to arrhythmias such as supraventricular tachycardia (SVT). The ultimate management of congestive heart failure is directed at correcting the underlying cause. However, initial management strategies are aimed at lessening the symptoms of tachypnea, edema, and failure to thrive as well as improving the ability of the heart to maintain adequate systemic oxygen delivery. The therapeutic measures useful for treating congestive heart failure are directed toward improving myocardial contractile function, decreasing preload and afterload, and improving the balance between systemic oxygen consumption and oxygen delivery (Table 13.4).

Cyanosis

CYANOTIC CONGENITAL HEART DISEASE IN THE NEWBORN. The management of most forms of cyanotic congenital heart disease is surgical, whether a palliative shunt procedure or anatomic repair. However, in the initial hours or days after birth and while awaiting further diagnostic evaluation such as cardiac catheterization, an infusion of **prostaglandin E$_1$** usually stabilizes the patient by keeping the ductus arteriosus patent pharmacologically. In lesions associated with decreased pulmonary blood flow, the ductus supplements pulmonary flow and may even be its only source (e.g., in pulmonary atresia). In the transposition group of lesions, the patent ductus allows mixing of oxygenated and deoxygenated blood between the right and left sides of the heart. In patients with transposition of the great arteries, a balloon-tipped catheter, introduced via the femoral vein at the time of cardiac catheterization, is used to improve the amount of mixing at atrial level by ripping a large hole in the atrial septum (**Rashkind atrial septostomy**).

HYPERCYANOTIC SPELLS IN TETRALOGY OF FALLOT. **Hypercyanotic spells ("Tet spells")** are manifested by a marked increase in the level of cyanosis associated with agitation, crying, and hyperpnea. They may progress to loss of consciousness and may rarely lead to seizures, stroke, or death. Precipitating factors include either an increase in oxygen demands, a decrease in systemic vascular resistance, a decrease in systemic venous return, or spasm of the infundibular subpulmonary muscle. Treatment of hypercyanotic spells involves the following steps, which should be implemented in sequential order: comfort, placement in a knee–chest position to increase systemic venous return and increase peripheral vascular resistance, subcutaneous or intravenous morphine sulfate, the β-adrenergic blocker propranolol, or intravenous methoxamine or phenylephrine to increase systemic vascular resistance.

Techniques in the Management of Congestive Heart Failure in Children

Therapy	Mechanism/Advantages	Disadvantages
General supportive measures		
Bed rest	Reduces oxygen consumption	Increases risk of deep vein thrombosis, pulmonary atelectasis
Oxygen	Improves systemic oxygenation in presence of pulmonary edema	May cause pulmonary vasodilation and increase left-to-right shunting
Salt and water restriction	Decreases edema and congestion	Often limits caloric intake and contributes to failure to thrive
Transfusion	Increases oxygen–carrying capacity Reduces left-to-right shunt	Risk of infection
Diuretics		
Furosemide	Ascending loop of Henle	Hypokalemia, hyponatremia
Chlorothiazide	Distal tubule	Hypokalemia, hyponatremia
Aldactone	Aldosterone antagonist	K^+ sparing
Positive inotropic agents		
Digitalis	Inhibits Na^+–K^+-ATPase and increases intracellular Ca^{2+}	Increases myocardial oxygen consumption
Dopamine	Acts at cardiac β-adrenergic receptor to increase contractility and heart rate; at low doses, acts at renal dopamine receptor to increase renal blood flow	At high doses, acts on peripheral α-adrenergic receptor to increase afterload Potentially arrhythmogenic
Dobutamine	Acts at cardiac β-adrenergic receptor to increase contractility and heart rate; acts on peripheral β-adrenergic receptors to reduce afterload	
Amrinone, Milrinone	Phosphodiesterase inhibitor; synergistic with β-adrenergic receptor agonists	
Afterload reducing agents		
Hydralazine	Direct arteriolar vasodilator	Hypotension
Prazosin	Peripheral α-adrenergic blocker	Hypotension; reduced preload
Captopril	Angiotensin-converting enzyme inhibitor; does not cause reflex stimulation of renin	
Nitroprusside	Arterial and venous vasodilator	Intravenous only

CARDIAC DYSRHYTHMIAS

Pathophysiology

The cardiac conduction system is comprised of a group of specialized cells with unique depolarization properties (Figure 13.10). The **SA node,** located at the superior vena caval–right atrial junction, controls heart rate; it is modulated by both sympathetic and parasympathetic (vagal) input. Depolarization spreads from the SA node through atrial myocardium to the **AV node,** located at the junction of the atria and ventricles near the mouth of the coronary sinus. The specialized cells of the AV node slow conduction, thus allowing an appropriate interval between atrial and ventricular contraction. During rapid atrial dysrhythmias, the AV node prevents conduction of every atrial beat, resulting in varying degrees of block, and protects the patient from a low cardiac output due to a rapid ventricular rate.

From the AV node, impulses travel to the ventricles via the **bundle of His,** located immediately posterior and inferior to the membranous portion of the ventricular septum. This location renders this portion of the conduction system vulnerable to damage during surgical repair of congenital heart lesions such as VSDs. From the bundle of His arise the **right and left bundle**

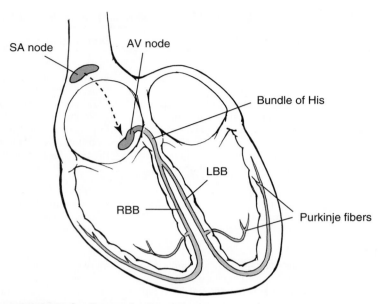

FIGURE 13.10. Cardiac conduction system.

branches leading finally to the **Purkinje fibers** that terminate in the subendocardium.

All cardiac cells are potentially capable of firing spontaneously. The orderly flow of impulses through the normal conduction system is thus dependent on higher foci (e.g., SA node) firing more rapidly than lower foci (e.g., ventricular cells), resulting in suppression of the more slowly firing cells. This property (called **overdrive suppression**) can be utilized clinically to treat certain dysrhythmias.

Anatomic abnormalities of the specialized conduction system are responsible for many of the common pediatric dysrhythmias. **Heart block** may be due to damage of the AV node or bundle of His due to inflammation (maternal systemic lupus erythematosus, rheumatic fever), medications (digoxin), or surgical trauma. **SVT** may be due to the presence of a congenital accessory conduction pathway, leading to abnormal impulse conduction between atria and ventricles (see ATRIAL DYSRHYTHMIAS); to increased automaticity (spontaneous firing) of an ectopic atrial pacemaker, or to intra-atrial reentry. In children, **ventricular tachycardia** often results from a global insult to the myocardium that renders individual ventricular cells irritable (hypoxia, electrolyte imbalances, myocarditis, drugs); a genetic abnormality in cardiac structure (hypertrophic cardiomyopathy) or ion channel function (long QT syndrome); or abnormal hemodynamics from palliated congenital heart disease (e.g., tetralogy of Fallot, single ventricle).

Clinical and Laboratory Evaluation

History
When evaluating a patient with a dysrhythmia, the clinician must first assess the degree of the patient's stability. If blood pressure and perfusion are abnormal, only minimal historical information is obtained before treatment is initiated: duration of symptoms, prior history of dysrhythmias or congenital heart disease, and exposure to medications or drugs.

Physical Examination
Assessment of the patient's general clinical status begins with the standard ABCs of emergency care: evaluation of the **a**irway, **b**reathing, and **c**irculation. The cardiac evaluation includes the patient's color (pale, cyanotic), peripheral perfusion, pulses, and blood pressure. In patients with a tachyarrhythmia, it may be difficult to evaluate heart murmurs, although a gallop rhythm is often audible. A thoracotomy or sternotomy scar is a clue that the patient has had prior surgery for correction of a congenital heart lesion.

Laboratory Evaluation
The most important laboratory tests are the 12-lead ECG and a long (2-minute) rhythm strip (usually lead II). A full 12-lead ECG should always supplement a single lead tracing from a monitor in the diagnosis of arrhythmia, because it is not possible to evaluate the true morphology

of the various waves and complexes using a single lead.

Pediatric Pearl

Common artifacts in a full 12-lead ECG are apparent because of their frequency: electrical artifacts are usually 60 cycles/second, and respirator artifacts occur at the rate at which the ventilator is set.

In the presence of ventricular dysrhythmias, it is necessary to obtain a "stat" blood sample for evaluation of electrolytes, calcium, and magnesium, as well as assessment of the patient's oxygenation (transcutaneous oximetry or arterial blood gas).

Differential Diagnosis and Management

An algorithmic approach is useful in the diagnosis of pediatric dysrhythmias (Figure 13.11). Characteristic ECG tracings are typical of the more common dysrhythmias (Figure 13.12). A brief discussion of these dysrhythmias follows.

Sinus Rhythms

Sinus arrhythmia, which is common in children, is a cyclic variation in heart rate associated with respirations. Usually the heart rate increases with inspiration and slows with expiration. The ECG is otherwise totally normal. The younger the child, the more pronounced the sinus arrhythmia.

Sinus tachycardia is also quite common in children and occurs as a result of stress (e.g., fever or dehydration) or pathologic conditions (e.g., congestive heart failure, anemia, hyperthyroidism). Some medications (e.g., certain cold preparations and β-agonists used for asthma) can cause sinus tachycardia. It is possible to differentiate sinus tachycardia from **SVT** based on several findings (Table 13.5).

Sinus bradycardia may occur during sleep, when it may be a normal finding. It is not uncommon for a sleeping child to have a heart rate less than 80 beats/min, although the heart rate will increase appropriately when the child is disturbed. Competitive athletes may also have a resting sinus bradycardia. Pathologic causes of bradycardia include hypothyroidism, increased intracranial pressure, hypothermia, hyperkalemia, and digitalis overdose.

Atrial Dysrhythmias

Premature atrial contractions (PACs) result from the firing of an ectopic focus in the atrium. PACs, which can be seen in many normal children, are one of the most common dysrhythmias in the newborn period. Although PACs are usually conducted, they will not be conducted if they occur too early in the cardiac cycle; the AV node is still refractory (**blocked PACs**). It is possible to differentiate PACs from **premature ventricular contractions (PVCs)** based on several ECG characteristics (Table 13.6). Isolated PACs do not require treatment. Frequent PACs in newborns usually resolve by 1 month of age.

Supraventricular tachycardia (SVT) can be divided into two major categories based on etiology: a **reentrant pathway (preexcitation syndrome)** or an atrial **ectopic focus.** Preexcitation is more common and is usually due to an **accessory pathway** or **bypass tract** that leads to accelerated conduction between atria and ventricle. In patients with **Wolff-Parkinson-White syndrome,** an abnormal myocardial bridge, called a bundle of Kent, lies between one of the atria and one of the ventricles. Cardiac impulses travel anterograde (from atrium to ventricle) through the bundle of Kent, which does not have the built-in time delay of the AV node. This leads to a shortened PR interval, and, because one of the ventricles is excited before the other, the QRS complex is widened (**delta wave on the 12-lead ECG**). Other preexcitation syndromes exist, including the **Lown-Ganong-Levine** syndrome, in which the PR interval is short but the QRS complex is normal, and AV nodal reentry.

Pediatric Pearl

Examination of the T wave may reveal slight irregularities from one beat to the next that could represent a hidden P wave, thus indicating SVT or atrial flutter.

Patients with SVT typically present with heart rates of 200–300 beats/min (see Table 13.5). In children, atrial rates as fast as 300 beats/min may be conducted 1:1 to the ventricles. Most initial episodes of SVT occur in the first 4 months of life; however, SVT may develop at any age. Infants often present with irritability, tiredness, and decreased feeding, and occasionally with overt signs of congestive heart failure (sweating, labored respirations, and decreased perfusion leading to shock). However, in the absence of heart disease, patients with SVT can often tolerate the dysrhythmia for 12–24 hours before these signs of

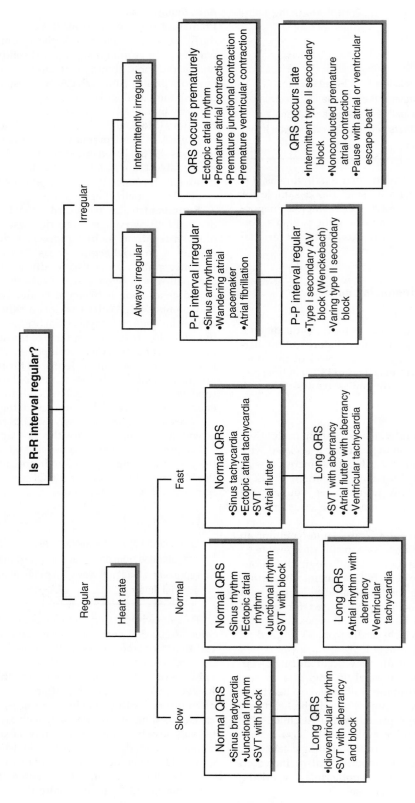

FIGURE 13.11. Approach to the diagnostic evaluation of the pediatric patient with a dysrhythmia. AV = atrioventricular; SVT = supraventricular tachycardia.

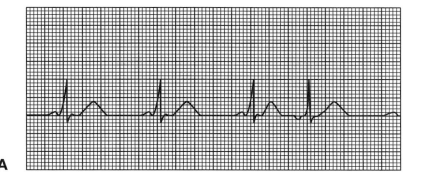

A

B

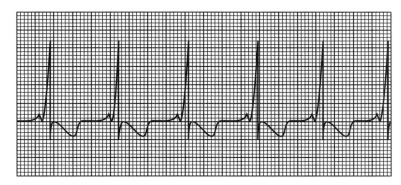

C

FIGURE 13.12. Common pediatric dysrhythmias. (*A*) premature atrial contraction; (*B*) supraventricular tachycardia; (*C*) Wolff-Parkinson-White syndrome; *(continued)*

heart failure intervene. Older children may complain of palpitations and dizziness.

The treatment of the SVTs involves several measures (Table 13.7). For patients who are stable, vagal maneuvers or pharmacologic management with antiarrhythmic drugs are the treatments of choice. However, for patients who have signs of decreased perfusion and shock, **synchronized DC cardioversion** is warranted.

After the initial episode has resolved, infants and children are usually treated for 6–12 months with antiarrhythmic agents such as digitalis (except in Wolff-Parkinson-White syndrome) or the β-blocker propranolol. Each of these drugs has its particular benefits and side effects that might limit treatment. Occasionally, use of more than one drug is necessary to maintain normal sinus rhythm. A trial without medications is appropri-

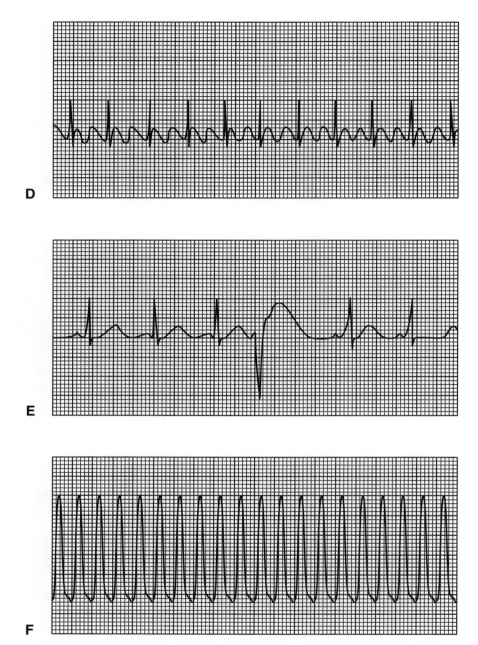

FIGURE 13.12. (*CONTINUED*) (*D*) atrial flutter; (*E*) premature ventricular contraction; (*F*) ventricular tachycardia; *(continued)*

ate in patients who are tachycardia-free for 6–12 months. **Radiofrequency catheter ablation,** which allows patients to be medication-free, is the recommended treatment option for children whose SVT is resistant to medications and for older children with Wolff-Parkinson-White syndrome.

Atrial flutter (intra-atrial reentry tachycardia) and **atrial fibrillation** are less common in children and usually encountered in the setting of congenital heart disease. If AV conduction is 1:1, symptoms of heart failure may rapidly develop. Often the AV node blocks extremely rapid

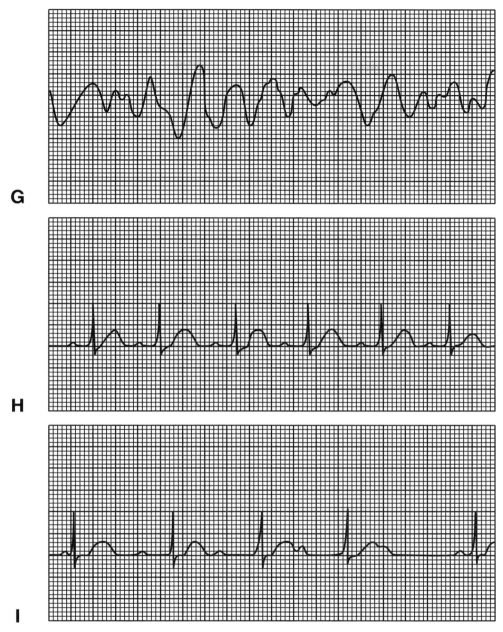

FIGURE 13.12. (*CONTINUED*) (*G*) ventricular fibrillation; (*H*) first-degree AV block; (*I*) second-degree atrioventricular (AV) block, Mobitz type I; *(continued)*

conduction, and the atrial:ventricular rate is 2:1 or 3:1. The initial treatment of choice for either of these dysrhythmias is synchronized DC cardioversion followed by initiation of antiarrhythmic medication.

Ventricular Dysrhythmias

Premature ventricular contractions (PVCs) are often encountered in children hospitalized for other reasons such as patients in the pediatric intensive care unit (ICU) for trauma, infections,

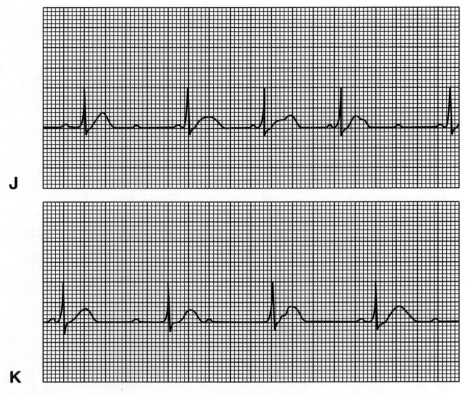

FIGURE 13.12. (*CONTINUED*) (*J*) second-degree AV block, Mobitz type II; (*K*) third-degree AV block.

postoperative monitoring or in those undergoing routine surgical procedures during anesthetic induction or recovery. For a comparison of PVCs and PACs on the basis of ECG findings, see Table 13.6. PVCs are usually considered benign when they occur singly, arise from a single ectopic focus (have the same morphology and axis), when the coupling interval (time between the previous normal QRS complex and the premature beat) is constant, and when there is no underlying heart disease (Table 13.8). Unifocal PVCs usually disappear if the patient exercises. Malignant PVCs warrant further evaluation and often require treatment.

Malignant PVCs and ventricular tachycardia often occur secondary to another abnormality

TABLE 13.5	**Sinus Tachycardia Compared With Supraventricular Tachycardia**	
	Sinus Tachycardia	**Supraventricular Tachycardia**
Heart rate (beats/min)	Usually < 200	Usually > 220
Heart rate variability	Present	Usually absent
History	Fever, dehydration, acute blood loss	Irritability, lethargy, poor feeding, tachypnea, sweating
Physical examination	Infectious source of fever; decreased skin turgor; absence of hepatomegaly; clear lung fields; source of acute blood loss	Signs of congestive heart failure: rales, hepatomegaly, respiratory distress, poor perfusion
Chest radiograph	Normal or small heart size; pneumonia as source of fever	Possible cardiomegaly or pulmonary edema

TABLE 13.6 **Premature Atrial Complexes (PACs) Compared With Premature Ventricular Complexes (PVCs)**

	PACs	PVCs
QRS timing	Premature	Premature
QRS duration	Usually normal; occasionally prolonged	Prolonged
QRS morphology	Usually the same as sinus rhythm QRS complexes	Different from sinus rhythm QRS complexes
ST-T abnormalities	Rare	More common
P wave	Usually precedes QRS complex	None; occasionally will follow QRS complex
Fusion beats	None	May be present
Compensatory pause	Not usually (but not reliable)	Usually (but not reliable)

such as an electrolyte disturbance, hypoxia, or medication or drug (Table 13.9). Thus, the mainstay of treatment for any ventricular dysrhythmia is correction of the underlying abnormality. No pharmacologic agent is totally effective in treating ventricular dysrhythmias unless the underlying cause is also corrected. Other causes include myocarditis and a genetic predisposition (long QT syndrome, hypertrophic cardiomyopathy).

Ventricular tachycardia (VT) is defined as the occurrence of three or more PVCs in a row. When the ventricular rate is slow, patients may be minimally symptomatic. However, when ventricular rates are fast, cardiogenic shock rapidly ensues. Because of the possibility of degeneration into **ventricular fibrillation,** emergent treatment is necessary for all ventricular tachycardias. To confuse matters, with VT, the ECG may show P waves (with either retrograde conduction or AV dissociation), and with some SVTs, it may show aberrant conduction and thus wide QRS complexes. However, clinicians should almost always assume that children with a wide complex tachycardia have VT and treat them appropriately (Table 13.10). When VT is seen in children who have one of the congenital long QT syndromes (**Romano-Ward** or **Jervell-Lange-Nielsen**), the ECG morphology is an undulating wavy line alternating both above

and below an imaginary baseline (**torsade de pointes**).

Pediatric Pearl

It is important to search for underlying causes of PVCs or VT in pediatric patients (e.g., electrolyte abnormalities, hypoxia). Antiarrhythmic agents may not be completely effective unless these provoking factors are resolved.

Ventricular fibrillation (VF) manifests with absent pulses and shock. Immediate cardiopulmonary resuscitation is necessary. The ECG shows either a coarse or fine wavy line without recognizable QRS complexes. The treatment for VF is DC cardioversion and, as with VT, correction of the underlying cause (e.g., hypoxemia, electrolyte disturbance).

Conduction Disorders

First-degree AV block occurs when the PR interval is greater than normal values for both age and heart rate. First-degree block may occur in the presence of some congenital heart lesions (corrected transposition of the great arteries) and with myocarditis or rheumatic fever. Although first-degree AV block usually does not warrant treatment, it does require follow-up monitoring

TABLE 13.7 **Treatment of Supraventricular Tachycardia**

1. Vagal maneuvers (carotid massage, immerse face in ice water)
2. Adenosine 0.05–0.2 mg/kg by rapid IV push
3. Verapamil 0.1–0.2 mg/kg slowly IV (contraindicated in children < 1 year of age); have IV calcium ready
4. Propranolol 0.01–0.1 mg/kg IV slowly (used less often)
5. Digitalis (total digitalizing dose 20–40 μg/kg, depending on age)
6. Overdrive pacing (transesophageal or transvenous)
7. Synchronized DC cardioversion (0.25–2.0 watt-sec/kg) if patient is unstable

DC = direct current; IV = intravenous.

TABLE 13.8 **Benign Versus Malignant Premature Ventricular Complexes (PVCs)**

	Benign PVCs	Malignant PVCs
Heart disease	Not usual	Often seen with congenital or ischemic heart disease
Coupling interval	Fixed	Variable
Baseline QT interval	Usually normal	May be prolonged
Focality of PVCs	Unifocal	Multifocal
R on T	Absent	Present
Response to exercise	Suppresses PVCs	Increases PVCs
Couplets or runs	None	May be present

for worsening block. The PR interval is usually slightly prolonged with digitalis treatment; this is not necessarily a sign of digitalis toxicity.

Second-degree AV block may be of two forms: Mobitz type I (Wenckebach) and type II. In **Mobitz type I,** there is progressive prolongation of the PR interval until a dropped QRS occurs. Thus, patients may have 2:1, 3:2, or 4:3 AV block. In **Mobitz type II,** QRS complexes are dropped in varying ratios (e.g., 2:1, 3:1, 3:2). Both of these dysrhythmias require cardiologic evaluation and may be an indication for a pacemaker.

Third-degree AV block or **complete AV dissociation** occurs when the atria and ventricles beat independently and there is not a regular relationship between the P waves and QRS complexes on ECG. This condition may occur congenitally (especially in newborns whose mothers have systemic lupus erythematosus), in association with underlying congenital heart disease (most commonly in corrected transposition of the great ar-

TABLE 13.9 **Causes of Premature Ventricular Complexes (PVCs)**

Blood gas and electrolyte abnormalities
  Hypoxia
  Acidosis
  Hypokalemia
  Hyperkalemia
Myocardial factors
  Acute myocarditis
  Rheumatic fever
  Myocardial ischemia
  After open heart surgery
Drugs and toxins
  Digitalis
  Any antiarrhythmic drug
  Anesthetic agents
  Sympathomimetic agents
  Phenothiazines
  Cocaine
  Caffeine
  Nicotine

teries), or after surgical repair of congenital heart disease (most commonly in VSDs, AV septal defects, or mitral or aortic valve replacement). If the heart rate is adequate to maintain a reasonable cardiac output, children are asymptomatic and treatment may not be indicated. However, if the heart rate is slow enough to result in symptoms such as exercise intolerance or syncope, pacemaker implantation is indicated. Additional patients requiring consideration for pacemaker implantation are asymptomatic infants with heart rates less than 50 beats/min and any child with long (> 3 second) pauses.

INFECTIVE ENDOCARDITIS

The incidence of infective endocarditis in children with congenital heart disease is approximately 1.5 cases per 1000 patient-years. Given the serious morbidity and high mortality associated with endocarditis, prevention is a mainstay of treatment of children with congenital heart disease.

Pathophysiology

In the presence of congenital heart disease, turbulent blood flow causes damage to endothelial surfaces, allowing the deposition of fibrin and platelets. Within these tiny sterile thrombi, circulating bacteria initially adhere and then grow, partially protected from the cleansing action of laminar blood flow. Bacteria such as **streptococci** that produce glycoproteins are more easily adherent to these lesions, thus explaining their prevalence as causative agents. Lesions of infective endocarditis most usually occur on the downstream side of a lesion such as on the aortic surface of a stenotic aortic valve or on the right ventricular surface of a VSD. High velocity lesions that produce more turbulence (e.g., small VSDs) are more susceptible to endocarditis than low velocity lesions such as ASDs.

TABLE 13.10 Treatment of Premature Ventricular Complexes (PVCs) and Ventricular Tachycardia

1. Treatment of underlying causes
2. Lidocaine 1 mg/kg IV bolus followed by 0.5–1.5 mg/kg/hr drip
3. Procainamide 1 mg/kg IV (may be repeated in 5 min)
4. Bretylium 5 mg/kg IV
5. If heart rate is slow: atropine 0.01–0.02 mg/kg IV
6. Overdrive atrial or ventricular pacing
7. If patient is hemodynamically unstable; synchronized DC cardioversion (0.5–1.5 watt-sec/kg)

DC = direct current; IV = intravenous.

After correction of most congenital heart defects, the risk of endocarditis decreases. However, patients with prosthetic valves or artificial conduits such as Blalock-Taussig shunts may have increased susceptibility to infective endocarditis. Patients with rheumatic heart disease are also at risk.

Clinical and Laboratory Evaluation

History
A history of congenital or rheumatic heart disease is present in almost all patients with infective endocarditis. It is often possible to identify a source of infection such as a recent dental or surgical procedure, abscess, or significant trauma. Indwelling urinary or intravenous catheters also put patients at risk. Persistent fever, anorexia and weight loss, malaise, myalgias, arthralgias, and worsening congestive heart failure may be presenting symptoms.

Physical Examination
A new or changing heart murmur may be audible. Splenomegaly is present in 60%–70% of patients, and peripheral embolization of bacteria may cause petechiae, splinter hemorrhages, or small infarcts. Other skin manifestations are the result of circulating antibody–antigen complexes and include Osler nodes (painful red nodules on the fingers or toes), Janeway lesions (painless hemorrhagic lesions on the palms and soles) and Roth spots (retinal hemorrhages).

Laboratory Evaluation
Blood cultures demonstrate the specific organism, most often **streptococci** or **staphylococci,** although any bacterial strain may be involved. Gram-negative bacilli or enterococci are more common after genitourinary instrumentation or infection. *Candida albicans* is encountered in patients who develop endocarditis after open heart surgery, especially those with prosthetic valves. Additional laboratory findings include a mild leukocytosis, elevated erythrocyte sedimentation rate (ESR); anemia; and, quite commonly, microscopic hematuria. Echocardiography, if positive, is often diagnostic; however, a negative echocardiogram, especially in younger children, does not eliminate the possibility of endocarditis.

Management

The primary strategy for management of infective endocarditis is prevention.

Prophylaxis for Subacute Bacterial Endocarditis
It is in the outpatient clinic that the real fight against subacute bacterial endocarditis (SBE) takes place through **prevention**. The clinician should inform the parents of children with congenital heart lesions about the risks of SBE as soon as the diagnosis is made and give them a card with the American Heart Association (AHA) recommendations for prophylaxis. If the diagnosis is made in infancy, the greatest potential risk occurs during surgical procedures, perhaps to correct other congenital anomalies, especially genitourinary. As soon as children reach the age when dental visits begin, it is necessary to reacquaint parents with SBE precautions and reissue a prophylaxis card (Figure 13.13).

Treatment
The decision to initiate therapy before blood culture confirmation depends on the severity of the illness. In subacute cases, it may be appropriate to withhold antibiotics for a few days awaiting culture results. However, if clinical features are highly suggestive of infective endocarditis or if the patient is seriously ill, treatment usually involves a broad-spectrum antibiotic that covers the most likely infective agents.

Once the organism is positively identified, specific antibiotic therapy can begin, usually a

---

Name: _____

needs protection from
BACTERIAL ENDOCARDITIS
because of an existing
HEART CONDITION

Diagnosis: _____

Prescribed by: _____

Date: _____

This wallet card is to be given to patients by their physician. Healthcare professionals, please see back of card for reference to the complete statement.

Prophylactic Regimens for Dental, Oral, Respiratory Tract, or Esophageal Procedures. (Follow-up dose no longer recommended.) Total children's dose should not exceed adult dose.

I. **Standard general prophylaxis for patients at risk:**
    Amoxicillin: Adults, 2.0 g (children, 50 mg/kg) given orally one hour before procedure.

II. **Unable to take oral medications:**
    Ampicillin: Adults, 2.0 g (children, 50 mg/kg) given IM or IV within 30 minutes before procedure.

III. **Amoxicillin/ampicillin/penicillin-allergic patients:**
    Clindamycin: Adults, 600 mg (children, 20 mg/kg) given orally one hour before procedure.
    -OR-
    Cephalexin* or Cefadroxil*: Adults, 2.0 g (children, 50 mg/kg) orally one hour before procedure.
    -OR-
    Azithromycin or Clarithromycin: Adults, 500 mg (children, 15 mg/kg) orally one hour before procedure.

IV. **Amoxicillin/ampicillin/penicillin-allergic patients unable to take oral medications:**
    Clindamycin: Adults, 600 mg (children, 20 mg/kg) IV within 30 minutes before procedure.
    -OR-
    Cefazolin: Adults, 1.0 g (children, 25 mg/kg) IM or IV within 30 minutes before procedure.

---

*Cephalosporins should not be used in patients with immediate-type hypersensitivity reaction to penicillins.

Prophylactic Regimens for Genitourinary/Gastrointestinal Procedures. Total children's dose should not exceed adult dose.

I. **High-risk patients:**
    Ampicillin plus gentamicin: Ampicillin (adults, 2.0 g; children, 50 mg/kg) **plus** gentamicin 1.5 mg/kg (for both adults and children, not to exceed 120 mg) IM or IV within 30 minutes before starting procedure. 6 hours later, ampicillin (adults, 1 g; children, 25 mg/kg) IM or IV, or amoxicillin (adults, 1.0 g; children, 25 mg/kg) orally.

II. **High-risk patients allergic to ampicillin/amoxicillin:**
    Vancomycin plus gentamicin: Vancomycin (adults, 1.0 g; children, 20 mg/kg) IV over 1–2 hours **plus** gentamicin 1.5 mg/kg (for both adults and children, not to exceed 120 mg) IM or IV. Complete injection/infusion within 30 minutes before starting procedure.

III. **Moderate-risk patients:**
    Amoxicillin: Adults, 2.0 g (children, 50 mg/kg) orally one hour before procedure.
    -OR-
    Ampicillin: Adults, 2.0 g (children, 50 mg/kg) IM or IV within 30 minutes before starting procedure.

IV. **Moderate-risk patients allergic to ampicillin/amoxicillin:**
    Vancomycin: Adults, 1.0 g (children, 20 mg/kg) over 1–2 hours. Complete infusion within 30 minutes of starting the procedure.

NOTE: For patients already taking an antibiotic, or for other special situations, please refer to the full statement referenced below.

Adapted from *Prevention of Bacterial Endocarditis: Recommendations by the American Heart Association* by the Committee on Rheumatic Fever, Endocarditis, and Kawasaki Disease. *JAMA* 1997;277:1794–1801. *Circulation.* July 1, 1997 (in press). (Also excerpted in *JADA.* 1997 [in press]). ©1997, American Medical Association.

Healthcare Professionals — Please refer to these recommendations (endorsed by the American Dental Association and American Society for Gastrointestinal Endoscopy) for more complete information as to which patients and which procedures need prophylaxis.

The Council on Dental Therapeutics of the American Dental Association has approved this statement as it relates to dentistry.

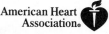

Fighting Heart Disease and Stroke

National Center
7272 Greenville Avenue
Dallas, TX 75231-4596

♻ printed on recycled paper

78-1005
5-99
97 04 25 A

FIGURE 13.13. Recommendations of the American Heart Association for prophylaxis against subacute bacterial endocarditis.

4–6-week parenteral course. Surgical management is reserved for resistant (usually fungal) organisms or those cases in which a vegetation affects function of a prosthetic heart valve. Despite recent advances in antimicrobial management, the mortality rate of infective endocarditis is still as high as 25%.

CARDIOMYOPATHIES

Pathophysiology

Diseases of the myocardium can be divided based on their etiology into infectious, metabolic, infiltrative, ischemic, and primary myopathic causes (Table 13.11). Myocarditis, the most common cause of myocardial disease, is an acute inflammation most often caused by a viral infection. Many viruses have been identified as etiologic agents; however, **adenovirus** and **coxsackie B virus** are by far the most common in children. In earlier years, it was often impossible to identify a specific viral agent, because peripheral serum titers were often nondiagnostic. More recent studies utilizing the polymerase chain reaction to analyze myocardial biopsy specimens have increased the ability to identify specific viral agents. Biopsy specimens reveal an acute inflammatory infiltrate and evidence of myocyte necrosis, often replaced later by fibrous scar tissue.

Common metabolic causes of myocardial dysfunction include electrolyte abnormalities such as hypocalcemia and hypomagnesemia, hypoglycemia, and hypothyroidism. Rarer causes relate to deficiencies of a specific nutrient, an inborn error of metabolism, or are secondary to a toxin (see Table 13.11). Infiltrative myocardial diseases also occur with inborn errors of metabolism such as the abnormal glycogen deposition associated with

---

TABLE 13.11 **Causes of Diseases of the Myocardium**

Infectious diseases

Viral myocarditis
  Adenovirus, Coxsackievirus (most common)
  Mumps, measles, rubella, echovirus, cytomegalovirus, HIV, arbovirus, poliovirus
Nonviral myocarditis
  Toxoplasma gondii, Mycoplasma pneumoniae, rickettsiae, *Chlamydia trachomatis,* diphtheria toxin,
    Trypanosoma cruzi (Chagas disease)
Immunologic myocarditis
  Acute rheumatic fever
  Kawasaki syndrome

Metabolic diseases

Electrolyte abnormalities
  Hypocalcemia, hypomagnesemia, hypokalemia, hyperkalemia, hypoglycemia
Endocrine abnormalities
  Infants of diabetic mothers, hypothyroidism, pheochromocytoma
Drugs and toxins
  Alcohol, cocaine, adriamycin, chloroquine, ipecac, radiation
Vitamin and trace metal deficiencies [thiamine (beriberi), selenium (Keshan disease), carnitine, taurine]

Infiltrative diseases

Glycogen storage diseases (Pompe)
Glycolipid disease (Fabry)
Hemochromatosis (in patients receiving multiple transfusions)
Mucopolysaccharidoses
Cystinosis
Amyloidosis
Sarcoidosis
Neoplasms [lymphoma, rhabdomyoma (seen in tuberous sclerosis)]

Ischemic diseases

Anomalous left coronary artery
Congenital coronary artery stenosis
Coronary cameral fistula
Accelerated atherosclerosis (familial hyperlipidemias)
Kawasaki disease
Postoperative arterial switch procedure

Primary myopathic diseases

Idiopathic dilated cardiomyopathy
Hypertrophic cardiomyopathy (IHSS)
Endocardial fibroelastosis
Muscular dystrophies (Duchenne, Becker)
Friedreich ataxia

HIV = human immunodeficiency virus; IHSS = idiopathic hypertrophic subaortic stenosis.

type II (Pompe) glycogen storage disease. Ischemic heart disease is uncommon in children; however, it may occur with congenital abnormalities of the coronary arteries (e.g., anomalous origin of the left coronary artery from the pulmonary artery), in homozygous hyperlipidemias, and in postoperative patients after repair of complex congenital heart disease.

With use of new tools in molecular genetics and genomics, many cardiomyopathies formerly considered idiopathic are now being recognized as resulting from specific gene defects. Hypertrophic cardiomyopathy [also known as idiopathic hypertrophic subaortic stenosis (IHSS)] is one of the more common genetic causes of primary myocardial disease in children. In addition, infants born to diabetic mothers may develop a transient hypertrophic cardiomyopathy, which resolves over a period of several months.

Cardiomyopathies can also be divided based on their physiology into dilated, hypertrophic, and restrictive subtypes. In dilated cardiomyopathy, the left ventricular end-diastolic volume is increased, and the ventricular wall is proportionally thin. The primary physiologic derangement is a decrease in systolic function (contraction). In contrast, in hypertrophic cardiomyopathy, the end-diastolic volume is decreased and the ventricular wall is thickened, either eccentrically or concentrically. The primary physiologic derangement involves diastolic function (relaxation), although if the subaortic muscle is thick enough to cause obstruction, changes in systolic function may also occur. In restrictive cardiomyopathy, the ventricular volume is normal to mildly decreased, and the wall thickness is normal or minimally increased. The primary physiologic derangement involves diastolic function due to extremely poor compliance (distensibility) of the ventricular chamber. The atria are typically markedly enlarged.

Clinical and Laboratory Evaluation

History

Children with myocarditis may present with either a rapid onset (more common in infants) or a more insidious onset (more common in older children) of symptoms of congestive heart failure. They may have a history of an upper respiratory tract infection or gastroenteritis within the previous month. Younger children may display evidence of decreased activity, irritability, or feeding intolerance. Older children may complain of difficulty breathing, chronic cough, easy fatigability, abdominal symptoms, dyspnea on exertion, orthopnea, or recent weight gain.

In patients with metabolic myopathies, presentation is usually more insidious, although occasionally a family history of a specific metabolic disorder raises the index of suspicion and leads to an earlier diagnosis. Many patients may have been followed for weeks or months with a diagnosis of upper respiratory tract infection, pneumonia, or asthma. Occasionally, patients with hypertrophic or restrictive cardiomyopathy are first diagnosed when they present with syncope, or even with "missed sudden death," secondary to arrhythmia.

Physical Examination

General physical signs of congestive heart failure are similar to those described in the section on congenital heart defects (see CONGENITAL HEART DISEASE). Findings include tachypnea, subcostal retractions, wheezes or rales, hepatosplenomegaly, and poor peripheral perfusion and pulses. Edema occurs around the eyes and on the back in infants and in the lower extremities in older children and adolescents. The cardiac examination may reveal diminished heart sounds, an increased cardiac impulse, a gallop rhythm, and often a holosystolic murmur of mitral or tricuspid insufficiency due to dilatation of one or both of the semilunar valve rings. The presence of a rub suggests pericardial involvement. Hepatomegaly is common.

Laboratory Evaluation

The chest radiograph is the best laboratory test for evaluation of cardiac chamber enlargement and the presence of pulmonary edema. The ECG is the best test for evaluation of chamber hypertrophy. In myocarditis, the ECG may show low voltage QRS complexes, ST-segment depression, and various degrees of heart block and other dysrhythmias. The hypertrophic myopathies demonstrate either isolated left or biventricular hypertrophy, and signs of ischemia or strain (e.g., T-wave inversion in lead V_6) may be evident. Some of the metabolic or infiltrative myopathies have distinctive ECG patterns such as the short PR interval and hypertrophy pattern associated with Pompe disease. In suspected viral myocarditis, serum viral titers are only rarely diagnostic. A myocardial biopsy, performed transvenously in the cardiac catheterization laboratory, yields a specific diagnosis in many cases.

Differential Diagnosis

The differential diagnosis of acute myocardial dysfunction includes all of the conditions listed in Table 13.11. Endocardial biopsy sometimes allows a definitive diagnosis, but it often shows only fibrosis and compensatory hypertrophy of remaining myocardial cells. These cases lead to a diagnosis of **idiopathic dilated cardiomyopathy**. Polymerase chain reaction analysis, usually performed in a research laboratory, has recategorized many of these "idiopathic" cases as the chronic stage of postviral myocarditis.

Management

The treatment of acute myocarditis involves supportive therapy with diuretics, low-dose digitalis (the inflamed myocardium is more sensitive to the arrhythmogenic effects of digitalis), and in cases of hemodynamic decompensation, intravenous inotropic agents (e.g., dopamine, dobutamine, milrinone) or afterload-reducing drugs (e.g., nitroprusside, captopril). Specific anti-inflammatory therapy with corticosteroids or other immunosuppressives or intravenous immune globulin (IVIG) is still controversial. For patients who do not respond to intravenous inotropes, several methods of artifical circulatory support are available, including extracorporeal membrane oxygenation (ECMO) and left ventricular assist devices (LVADs). Cardiac transplantation is the only specific treatment available for children with the more severe forms of dilated or restrictive cardiomyopathy. Currently, the 1-year and 5-year survival rates for pediatric heart transplant recipients are 80% and 68%, respectively.

For children with hypertrophic cardiomyopathy, surgical resection of subaortic muscle, antiarrhythmics (e.g., amiodarone) or an implantable cardiodefibrillator (ICD) may reduce the risk of sudden death secondary to ventricular arrhythmias. Transplantation is an option in the most severe cases.

RHEUMATIC HEART DISEASE

Improvement in public hygiene and standards of living, combined with the routine antibiotic treatment of streptococcal pharyngitis, has resulted in a marked decrease in the incidence of rheumatic fever in the United States. However, rheumatic fever is still a major public health problem in many developing countries. A worrisome resurgence of rheumatic fever began in the United States in the mid-1980s; the exact reasons for this are unknown.

Pathophysiology

Acute rheumatic fever is associated with an infection (usually of the pharynx) with **group A β-hemolytic streptococci** that triggers an abnormal immune response in genetically susceptible individuals. In these individuals, B lymphocytes are sensitized by streptococcal antigens, leading to the formation of antistreptococcal antibodies. Immune complexes form that cross-react with antigens present on cardiac muscle, leading to inflammation and both myocardial and valvular disease.

Pathologic changes occur not only in the heart but in connective tissue and in perivascular tissue. The characteristic pathologic lesion is the **Aschoff body,** consisting of an inflammatory focus surrounding disrupted connective tissue fibers. The initial acute attack leads to a **pancarditis** (involvement of pericardium, myocardium, and endocardium). Initial attacks of rheumatic fever result in valve thickening (**verrucous valvulitis**), leading to regurgitation, most frequently of the mitral and aortic valves. Pathologic changes also occur in the joints (**arthritis**), skin (**subcutaneous nodules, erythema marginatum**), and central nervous system (CNS) [**chorea**]. In the heart, recurrent attacks result in repeated scarring of the affected valves, usually resulting in the development of mitral stenosis.

Clinical and Laboratory Evaluation

History

Patients may present with a history of a recent episode of untreated or partially treated pharyngitis, although this history is variable. A complaint of **migratory polyarthritis,** usually affecting large joints with transient erythema and effusions, is often the major presenting symptom. Symptoms of **congestive heart failure** are less common. **Sydenham chorea** is also a less common presentation of acute rheumatic fever. The chorea consists of sudden abnormal movements of the extremities but may develop insidiously as clumsiness or deteriorating school performance. Muscle weakness and behavioral disturbances are common. A history of previous episodes of acute rheumatic fever is very significant, as recurrence risks are high (5%–50% higher than in the nonaffected population).

Physical Examination

The physical examination should focus on detection of **arthritis** (joint swelling, redness, warmth, and pain) as opposed to **arthralgias** (pain alone). The cardiac examination may be notable for a friction rub secondary to a pericardial effusion, a gallop rhythm, or a new heart murmur of mitral regurgitation (holosystolic) or aortic regurgitation (decrescendo diastolic). The classical skin lesions are 0.5–1.0-cm, painless, **subcutaneous nodules** on the extensor surfaces of the hands, feet, scalp, or vertebra. The typical rash is **erythema marginatum,** although it occurs in only about 10% of patients, and consists of an evanescent erythematous macule with a clear center and serpiginous outline. Erythema marginatum is predominantly truncal, is also migratory, and is usually nonpruritic.

Laboratory Evaluation

The standard laboratory evaluation shows elevation of several acute phase reactants, including ESR and C-reactive protein; however, these findings are very nonspecific. A rising titer of antistreptococcal antibodies (antistreptolysin O antibodies, anti-DNAse B, antihyaluronidase) is very important in making the diagnosis. Culture of group A β-streptococci from the pharynx is also important.

The ECG may show a prolonged PR interval or first-degree heart block. The chest radiograph reveals cardiac enlargement in patients with active carditis and pulmonary edema in patients with congestive heart failure.

Differential Diagnosis

The diagnosis of acute rheumatic fever may be difficult, because most patients do not present with all of the textbook criteria. The AHA has guidelines for the diagnosis of rheumatic fever, known as the modified Jones criteria (Table 13.12). The differential diagnosis often includes several of the rheumatic diseases of childhood, such as rheumatoid arthritis and systemic lupus erythematosus (see Chapter 21).

Management

Treatment involves eradication of the streptococcal infection with penicillin. Benzathine penicillin G given as an intramuscular injection of 0.6–1.2 million units is the most effective, because compliance is ensured. Anti-inflammatory agents such as aspirin, which are begun at 30–60 mg/kg/day in four divided doses, are continued depending on the individual's response, usually for 2–6 weeks. Corticosteroids are rarely used, although they may be beneficial in the treatment of patients with severe carditis and congestive heart failure. For patients in heart failure, other treatment modalities are used as needed (see Table 13.4). Clinicians no longer require strict bed rest. However, they still recommend a modified and gradual ambulatory program during the acute phase of the illness.

An important concept in rheumatic fever treatment is the prevention of future episodes. Once affected, children are at high risk for recurrent attacks and continue to receive penicillin prophylaxis. This involves either twice-daily penicillin G (250,000 units) or parenteral benzathine penicillin G (1.2 million units) given intramuscularly every 4 weeks. The latter is preferred, because compliance problems are fewer.

KAWASAKI DISEASE

First described in 1967 in Japan, **Kawasaki disease** (also known as **mucocutaneous lymph node syndrome**) is a generalized vasculitis of unknown etiology. It is currently one of the leading causes of acquired heart disease in children. Although initial reports of Kawasaki disease were confined to

---

TABLE 13.12 **Modified Jones Criteria for Diagnosis of Acute Rheumatic Fever***

Major manifestations

1. Carditis (cardiomegaly, heart murmur, pericarditis, congestive heart failure)
2. Polyarthritis
3. Erythema marginatum
4. Subcutaneous nodules
5. Chorea

Minor manifestations

1. History of previous episode of rheumatic fever
2. Arthralgias
3. Fever
4. Increased acute phase reactants (ESR, C-reactive protein, WBC count, anemia)
5. ECG changes (increase PR or QT intervals)

---

*The presence of two major or one major and two minor manifestations combined with evidence of recent streptococcal infection (positive throat culture, elevated antistreptolysin O titer, history of scarlet fever) are highly indicative of diagnosis of rheumatic fever.

ECG = electrocardiogram; ESR = erythrocyte sedimentation rate; WBC = white blood cell.

Asia, the disease has now been described worldwide. It occurs in both endemic and epidemic patterns. Epidemics have usually taken place during the winter or spring. In the United States, the prevalence is approximately 9 cases per 100,000 children less than 5 years of age, with 80% of cases in children younger than 8 years of age. Kawasaki disease is more prevalent in children of Asian ancestry.

Pathophysiology

Coronary artery disease is present in 20% of untreated patients with Kawasaki disease. In untreated patients, there are four pathologic stages.

- **Stage 1** (first 2 weeks): An acute vasculitis, involving predominantly the coronary arteries, is present. A pancarditis with inflammatory changes in the cardiac conduction system accompanies the vasculitis.
- **Stage 2** (2–4 weeks after onset): The coronary vasculitis persists, and coronary artery aneurysms may occur. In some cases, thrombosis in the aneurysms may occur, with obstruction of coronary blood flow.
- **Stage 3** (4–8 weeks): Coronary inflammation begins to subside, although aneurysms may still be present. The myocardial inflammation is almost resolved.
- **Stage 4** (> 8 weeks after onset): Scar formation and calcification of the coronary arteries, stenosis and recanalization of the coronary lumen, and myocardial fibrosis occur. Other arteries may be involved and, rarely, peripheral arterial involvement may be severe enough to cause gangrenous changes in the extremities.

Clinical and Laboratory Evaluation

History and Physical Examination

Clinically, Kawasaki disease has three distinct phases: acute, subacute, and chronic. The acute febrile phase with typical skin and mucous membrane manifestations lasts up to 2 weeks (Table 13.13). The subacute phase is characterized by milder clinical disease and thrombocytosis, during which time coronary aneurysms may develop. This phase may last from the second to the fourth week of illness. The chronic phase, during which symptoms and laboratory abnormalities resolve, lasts up to 2 months after onset. During the acute phase, diagnosis is based on fulfilling five of six major criteria.

Additional clinical features may be present. Such symptoms include arthralgia or arthritis, cough, rhinorrhea, pneumonia, abdominal pain, diarrhea, jaundice, irritability, aseptic meningitis, and carditis.

The cardiac examination may be significant for the presence of a gallop rhythm. A flow murmur may be heard secondary to the high fever and mild anemia. A pericardial friction rub or distant heart sounds may indicate the presence of a pericardial effusion, which occurs in one-third of patients. Rarely, murmurs of mitral or aortic regurgitation are present when the carditis is severe.

Laboratory Evaluation

A complete blood count (CBC) shows an elevated white blood cell (WBC) count and mild anemia. During the early acute phase, the platelet count is normal but becomes elevated during the second and third weeks of the disease. The ESR and other

---

TABLE 13.13 **Diagnostic Criteria for Kawasaki Disease***

Fever	Usually high, persisting for at least 5 days and lasting up to 3 weeks
Conjunctivitis	Bilateral, painless, beginning within 2 days of the fever and lasting up to 3–5 weeks; absence of exudate
Rash	Polymorphous, most commonly urticarial, with large, raised, erythematous plaques on both trunk and extremities; occasionally scarlatiniform in nature
Changes in hands and feet	Begins with erythema and swelling during first 10 days; followed by peeling of skin starting near nails, at 10–14 days after disease onset
Mucous membrane erythema	Including pharyngitis, dry, fissured lips, and "strawberry tongue"
Cervical lymphadenopathy	Often unilateral, nonpurulent, at least 1.5 cm in diameter; occurring within 3 days after onset of fever and lasting 2–3 weeks

*Fever and at least four of the remaining five features must be present to make the diagnosis of Kawasaki disease. However, in the presence of coronary aneurysms, diagnosis can be established with fewer than four features.

acute phase reactants are elevated. Urinalysis reveals sterile pyuria and proteinuria. If a lumbar puncture is performed, spinal fluid examination finds mild pleocytosis with normal glucose and protein levels. Abdominal ultrasound may show hydrops of the gallbladder.

The ECG may be normal or may show prolonged PR or QT intervals, low voltages, ST-T wave changes, or dysrhythmia. During the subacute phase, signs of coronary ischemia or infarction may be present (abnormal Q waves or ST segments). Clinicians usually obtain an echocardiogram at the time of initial diagnosis to establish a baseline with which subsequent studies can be compared and to detect a pericardial effusion. Occasionally, this initial echocardiogram reveals early coronary aneurysms. A repeat echocardiogram is then appropriate 3–4 weeks after onset; it demonstrates coronary aneurysms, if present. If no aneurysms are evident at this time, a final follow-up echocardiogram at 6–8 weeks and another several months later are usually warranted.

Differential Diagnosis

Several infectious diseases may present with symptoms and signs similar to those of Kawasaki disease, including measles, scarlet fever, staphylococcal scalded skin syndrome, toxic shock syndrome, and Rocky Mountain spotted fever (see Chapter 9). Other disorders worthy of consideration in the differential diagnosis include allergic drug reactions, Stevens-Johnson syndrome, myocarditis, rheumatic diseases such as juvenile rheumatoid arthritis, and mercury poisoning.

Management

Initial therapy of Kawasaki disease is directed at reducing inflammation and preventing development of coronary artery aneurysms. Chronic therapy is directed at preventing coronary artery thrombosis. When the diagnosis is first established, intravenous gamma globulin, given as 2 g/kg as a single infusion over 12 hours, is appropriate. Alternatively, a dosage of 400 mg/kg/day, infused over 2 hours for a total of 4 days may be used. If administered within the first 10 days of the onset of disease, gamma globulin has been shown to significantly decrease the risk of aneurysm formation.

During the acute phase, aspirin is also given at 80–100 mg/kg/day orally four times daily. Aspirin reduces systemic symptoms and also decreases the risk of aneurysm formation. When patients become afebrile, they continue to take aspirin at a lower dose of 3–5 mg/kg given once daily. Discontinuation of low-dose aspirin is appropriate 6–8 weeks after the onset of illness, unless coronary aneurysms are present. Patients with documented aneurysms should continue to take low-dose aspirin indefinitely. Patients with giant aneurysms or those who present with coronary thrombosis may require systemic anticoagulation with heparin or warfarin.

Long-term management of patients with aneurysms depends on assessment of the patient's risk, as determined by the site and size of the coronary aneurysms. Follow-up of these patients with ECGs and echocardiograms at 6–12-month intervals are appropriate. Coronary angiography is warranted if these noninvasive tests are abnormal. Exercise stress testing is used to screen for coronary insufficiency and to guide recommendations regarding participation in sports activities.

CHEST PAIN

Chest pain is a very common complaint in general pediatrics. It ranks just behind headache and abdominal pain in frequency and becomes a more common problem in older children and adolescents.

Pathophysiology

The causes of chest pain are varied, ranging from musculoskeletal problems to functional causes. They are not all thoracic (Tables 13.14 and 13.15).

Clinical and Laboratory Evaluation

History

A careful and detailed history is critical to the proper evaluation of chest pain in children; often physical findings and laboratory studies are not helpful. The examiner should be careful to acknowledge the patient's and parents' concerns and not try to rush the diagnosis, because the success of chest pain relief often depends on the ability of the physician to reassure the family regarding the usually benign nature of the problem. The focus of attention should be on the location, duration and quality of the pain, and in particular whether it is pleuritic in nature. Inciting circumstances and whether the pain occurs at rest or wakes the patient from sleep are important historical items. The coexistence of **palpitations** is suggestive of a dysrhythmia as the cause of the chest pain, although emotion-induced chest pain is often associated with tachycardia.

TABLE 13.14 Common Thoracic Causes of Chest Pain in Children

Etiology	Description	Evaluation
Costochondritis	History of an upper respiratory tract infection or vigorous exercise; pain is often unilateral	Pain is reproduced by palpation or movement of arm
Tietze syndrome	Pain is intermittent but increased by coughing or movement	Unilateral swelling at sternoclavicular or sternochondral junction
Muscle strain	History of vigorous exertion or excessive weight lifting	Tenderness on palpation and on movement
Stress fracture	Often sports-related (tennis, rowing, football)	Tenderness on palpation and on movement; chest radiograph
Tussive trauma	Chronic cough; history of allergies or chronic illness	Reproduction with coughing
Herpes zoster (shingles)	Pain and burning along intercostal lines; vesicular rash	Tender to palpation along course of nerve

In addition, the physician should note the quality of interactions between child and family members and search for possible hidden agen-

TABLE 13.15 Non–Chest Wall Causes of Chest Pain In Children

Pulmonary
Asthma
Bronchitis
Tracheitis
Pneumonia
Foreign body
Pneumothorax
Pleuritis
Pleurodynia (Devil's grip)
Irritation of the diaphragm from intra-abdominal sources

Cardiac
Dysrhythmia
Mitral valve prolapse
Aortic stenosis
Hypertrophic cardiomyopathy (IHSS) with obstruction
Myocarditis
Pericarditis
Coronary artery anomalies
   Congenital
   Aneurysms (after Kawasaki disease)
Angina secondary to sickle cell crisis

Gastrointestinal
Esophagitis and gastroesophageal reflux
Achalasia
Foreign body
Esophageal spasm

Other
Scoliosis and other spinal deformities
Psychogenic (anxiety, hyperventilation syndrome)

das or secondary gain. Often the pain is a manifestation of a fear (e.g., fear of dying in a child who has recently lost a friend or relative). Determining whether children have missed school and whether the pain occurs on weekends as well as school days is important.

Physical Examination
Inspection of the chest for signs of trauma, congenital abnormalities, or alterations in respirations is important. Examination of the back should include an evaluation for scoliosis. Palpation of all areas of the chest wall determines whether the pain is musculoskeletal in origin and whether cardiac signs (heave, thrill) are present. Careful auscultation detects pulmonary abnormalities (adventitious sounds, decreased breath sounds) as well as cardiac abnormalities.

Laboratory Evaluation
It is important to keep laboratory studies to an absolute minimum unless specific findings point to an organic cause, which requires further evaluation (e.g., rib fracture, pneumonia, pericardial rub).

Differential Diagnosis

Thoracic conditions are by far the most common causes of chest pain (see Table 13.14). A variety of other conditions may also result in chest pain (see Table 13.15). Cardiac disease rarely causes chest pain in children, but cardiac conditions that lead to such pain are usually severe. Congenital aortic stenosis or other forms of left ventricular outflow tract obstruction, mitral valve prolapse, or dysrhythmia may be present; diagnosis using cardiac auscultation is easy. Coronary artery problems are quite rare in children; however, if they are suspected, diagnosis is usually possible after careful examination of the ECG.

Management

Management of chest pain in children and adolescents depends on the suspected cause. For thoracic conditions, analgesics and anti-inflammatory agents are usually curative. For suspected cardiac conditions, further evaluation may include ECG, echocardiography, and either treadmill or bicycle exercise stress testing. Once a specific cardiac diagnosis has been established, treatment may take place. Interventions may include surgery or valvuloplasty (for aortic stenosis), surgery or angiography (for coronary artery anomalies), or prohibition or physical activities (for cardiomyopathies).

SYNCOPE

Pathophysiology

Syncope is defined as a temporary loss of consciousness and postural tone. Causes of syncope include cardiovascular, CNS, and metabolic disorders as well as reactions to cardioactive drugs. These disorders may lead to a loss of consciousness due to a primary decrease in cerebral perfusion, to a global decrease in cardiac output, to an abnormality in peripheral vascular tone, or to a decrease in cerebral substrate delivery. Cerebral blood flow is normally autoregulated (i.e., it remains relatively constant despite wide fluctuations in blood pressure). Thus, systemic arterial blood pressure must fall precipitously in order for cerebral perfusion to decrease. Although some causes of syncope are intrinsically benign, they are dangerous because of the risk associated with the loss of consciousness during activities such as driving. Other causes may be intrinsically dangerous and can lead to cerebral ischemia or death.

Clinical and Laboratory Evaluation

History

More ominous causes of syncope are often associated with a history of congenital or acquired cardiac disease or other systemic illnesses. A history of Kawasaki disease may be present in patients with syncope due to coronary artery disease. A family history of sudden death or congenital deafness may be found in patients with the long QT syndrome.

When **prodromal** symptoms such as dizziness, pallor, nausea, or hyperventilation occur, **vasovagal syncope** (the common faint) is more likely (see SYNCOPE, DIFFERENTIAL DIAGNOSIS). There may also be a history of an **inciting event** such as fright or stress. In contrast, if there is no prior warning, or if palpitations or chest pain occur, a cardiac etiology is more likely. Syncope occurring after exercise is often a sign of a left heart obstructive lesion (e.g., aortic stenosis). The **duration of unconsciousness** is important but may be difficult to assess; nonprofessional observers may exaggerate the length of the event. Vasovagal faints are usually brief (< 1 minute), whereas longer periods of unconsciousness are potentially more ominous. A history of **multiple episodes** is another indication for concern. Inquiries concerning whether there was any associated tonic–clonic activity, abnormal eye movements, or incontinence that could indicate a seizure disorder are appropriate.

Physical Examination

Careful measurements of heart rate and blood pressure, both in the supine and standing positions, are appropriate. Repeat measurements after the patient has remained standing for 10–15 minutes are necessary. Physical examination findings are especially useful in determining a cardiac etiology; patients with congenital heart disease have diagnostic murmurs such as the systolic ejection murmur of aortic stenosis (see Tables 13.1 and 13.2). Other cardiac findings such as the midsystolic click of mitral valve prolapse may be subtle, and cardiac disease may even be silent (e.g., in coronary artery anomalies). The presence of a midline or thoracotomy scar makes it likely that a patient has undergone an intracardiac surgical repair. In this circumstance, suspicion of an arrhythmogenic cause (either bradycardia or tachycardia) is heightened.

Laboratory Evaluation

The history and physical examination findings should guide the initial laboratory evaluation. If a simple vasovagal faint is suspected, minimal evaluation is necessary. Initial evaluation should include an ECG and measurement of serum glucose, calcium, and electrolytes. If a seizure disorder is suspected, a complete neurologic examination and electroencephalography (EEG) are indicated, and possibly a head CT scan or MRI.

Evaluation of patients with a suspected cardiac or arrhythmogenic etiology may include 24-hour Holter or transtelephonic ECG (cardiobeeper) recording, echocardiogram, treadmill exercise test,

TABLE 13.16 Differential Diagnosis of Syncope in Children

Etiology	Provocation	Prodrome	Duration	Associated Illnesses	Recurrence Risk
Vasovagal	Stress, fright	Dizziness, nausea, sweating	Brief ($<$ 1 min)	None	Rare
Cardiac	Exercise	None, palpitations, chest pain	Several minutes	Congenital heart disease	Yes
Arrhythmogenic	None except fright or surprise in long QT syndrome	None, palpitations	Several minutes	None, congenital heart disease after repair	Yes
Orthostatic	Getting up from bed	None	Brief	Fluid or blood loss, pregnancy	Yes
Seizure disorders	None	None, aura	Variable	None, neurologic disorder	Frequent
Hypoglycemia	Fasting	Weakness, dizziness	Variable (may be prolonged if untreated)	Diabetes	Yes
Vagovagal	Intubation, nasogastric tube, instrumentation	None, dizziness	Brief	None	Occasional
Hysterical	In front of other people, absence of injury	None	Variable	Psychosocial problems	Yes

tilt table testing, and cardiac catheterization with electrophysiologic study.

Differential Diagnosis (Table 13.16)

Vasovagal syncope (common faint) is the result of the interruption of normal central vasomotor tone, leading to arteriolar vasodilation, hypotension, and decreased cerebral perfusion pressure. It is often associated with stimuli such as anxiety, fright, or surprise, and it may be more common after a period of fasting.

Cardiac syncope is most commonly associated with heart lesions that cause obstruction to left-sided blood flow (mitral or aortic stenosis, hypertrophic cardiomyopathy). Syncope may develop in association with severe hypercyanotic spells in patients with right-sided obstructive lesions (e.g., tetralogy of Fallot) [see CONGENITAL HEART DISEASE]. Dizziness or syncope may also occur in patients with low cardiac output due to primary cardiomyopathies. Rarer causes of cardiac syncope in children include intracardiac tumors and coronary artery abnormalities.

Arrhythmogenic syncope may occur in the presence or absence of structural heart disease. In patients with normal hearts, congenital **long QT syndrome** (Romano-Ward syndrome) is one cause. When associated with congenital deafness, it is known as the Jervell-Lange-Nielsen syndrome. Affected patients often present with a history of a sudden fright- or startle-inducing syncope, which occurs secondary to a form of ventricular tachycardia known as **torsade de pointes**. Patients with one of the **preexcitation syndromes** (e.g., Wolff-Parkinson-White syndrome) may have syncope associated with episodes of rapid SVT with one-to-one atrioventricular conduction.

In patients with abnormal hearts, mitral valve prolapse, hypertrophic cardiomyopathy, and arrhythmogenic right ventricular dysplasia are associated with ventricular tachycardia. Ebstein anomaly and corrected transposition are associated with SVT. Patients who have undergone intracardiac repair of congenital heart lesions may be predisposed to the development of heart block (VSD, AV septal defect), ventricular tachyarrhythmias (tetralogy of Fallot), or sick sinus syndrome (atrial repair of transposition of the great vessels).

Orthostatic syncope develops secondary to failure of one of the vascular compensatory responses to postural change, resulting in a decrease in blood pressure and in cerebral perfusion. This form of syncope occurs in conditions that decrease blood volume (dehydration, blood loss), in association with peripheral neuropathies, after prolonged bed rest, and during pregnancy. Antihypertensive medications are another cause of orthostatic syncope.

Vagovagal syncope occurs when vagal stimulation causes severe bradycardia. The excessive vagal tone may be related to tracheal intubation, placement of a nasogastric tube or other instrumentation, or may be secondary to distension of a viscera. When associated with urination, particularly in adolescent males, it is called **micturition syncope**. When severe enough to be disabling, the syndrome is known as **vagotonia**.

Noncardiac causes of syncope include seizure disorders, migraine headaches, hypoglycemia, hypoxemia (especially due to **breath-holding spells** in younger children), and hyperventilation. **Hysterical syncope,** which may occur in older children and adolescents, is remarkable for absence of alterations in heart rate and blood pressure. It is very rare for patients with hysterical syncope to injure themselves during an attack. Drug abuse, especially with crack cocaine, may lead to syncope secondary to cardiac arrhythmias.

Management

Patients with vasovagal syncope rarely require medical intervention. In severe cases, increasing intravascular volume by increasing salt and water intake can be helpful. In patients with cardiac syncope, repair of the primary cardiac lesion, if possible, is usually curative. In arrhythmogenic syncope due to tachyarrhythmias, treatment consists of antiarrhythmic medications or catheter ablation if an accessory pathway is the inciting mechanism. In syncope due to bradycardia or heart block, treatment may require insertion of a pacemaker. If syncope is drug-induced, reduction in the dose or switching to another medication may be curative. Patients with severe vagotonia may require placement of a pacemaker, salt and water loading, and antivagal medications such as atropine.

HYPERTENSION (see Chapter 20, HYPERTENSION AND HYPERTENSIVE EMERGENCIES)

SUGGESTED READINGS
Congenital Heart Disease
Baldwin HS, Artman M: Recent advances in cardiovascular development: Promise for the future. *Cardiovasc Res* 40:456–468, 1998.

Becker AE, Anderson RH: Atrioventricular septal defects: What's in a name? *J Thorac Cardiovasc Surg* 83:461, 1982.

Bernstein D: Cardiovascular System. In: *Nelson Textbook of Pediatrics,* 16th ed. Edited by Behrman WE, Kliegman RM, Arvin A. Philadelphia, WB Saunders, 2000.

Bove EL: Current status of staged reconstruction for hypoplastic left heart syndrome. *Pediatr Cardiol* 19: 308–315, 1998.

Brennan P, Young ID: Congenital heart malformations: Aetiology and associations. *Semin Neonatol* 6:17–25, 2001.

Dunbar-Masterson C, Wypij D, Bellinger DC, et al: General health status of children with D-transposition of the great arteries after the arterial switch operation. *Circulation* 104(suppl 1):I138–42, 2001.

Freedom RM, Hamilton R, Yoo SJ: The Fontan procedure: Analysis of cohorts and late complications. *Cardiol Young* 10:307–31, 2000.

Galioto FM: Physical activity for children with cardiac disease. In *The Science and Practice of Pediatric Cardiology.* Edited by Garson A, Bricker JT, Fisher DJ, et al. Baltimore: Williams & Wilkins, 1998, pp 2585–2592.

Garson A: *The Electrocardiogram in Infants and Children: A Systematic Approach.* Philadelphia, Lea & Febiger, 1983.

Garson A, Bricker JT, McNamara DG: *The Science and Practice of Pediatric Cardiology.* Baltimore, Williams & Wilkins, 1998.

Goldmuntz E: The epidemiology and genetics of congenital heart disease. *Clin Perinatol* 28:1–10, 2001.

Ing FF, Starc TJ, Griffiths SP, et al: Early diagnosis of coarctation of the aorta in children: A continuing dilemma. *Pediatrics* 98:378, 1996.

Keane JF, Driscoll DJ, Gersony WM, et al: Second natural history study of congenital heart defects: Results of treatment of patients with aortic valvar stenosis. *Circulation* 87(suppl 2):I16, 1993.

Latson LA: Per-catheter ASD closure. *Pediatr Cardiol* 19:86–93, 1998.

Lister G, Pitt BR: Cardiopulmonary interactions in the infant with congenital heart disease. *Clin Chest Med* 4:219, 1983.

McCrindle BW, Shaffer KM, Kan JS, et al: Cardinal clinical signs in the differentiation of heart murmurs in children. *Arch Pediatr Adolesc Med* 150:169, 1996.

Murphy Jr DJ: Atrioventricular canal defects. *Curr Treat Options Cardiovasc Med* 1:323–334, 1999.

Parry AJ, McElhinney DB, Kung GC, et al: Elective primary repair of acyanotic tetralogy of Fallot in early infancy: Overall outcome and impact on the pulmonary valve. *J Am Coll Cardiol* 36:2279–2283, 2000.

Pelech AN: The cardiac murmur. When to refer? *Pediatr Clin North Am* 45(1):107, 1998.

Reddy VM, McElhinney DB, Sagrado T, et al: Results of 102 cases of complete repair of congenital heart defects in patients weighing 700 to 2500 grams. *J Thorac Cardiovasc Surg* 117:324–331, 1999.

Rudolph AM: *Congenital Diseases of the Heart: Clinical-Physiological Considerations,* 2nd ed. New York, Futura Publishing, 2001.

Swenson JM, Fischer DR, Miller SA, et al: Are chest radiographs and electrocardiograms still valuable in evaluating new pediatric patients with heart murmurs or chest pain? *Pediatrics* 99:1, 1997.

Wilson DI, Burn J, Scambler P, et al: DiGeorge syndrome: Part of CATCH 22. *J Med Genet* 30:852, 1993.

Zuberbuhler JR: *Clinical Diagnosis in Pediatric Cardiology.* Edinburgh, Churchill Livingstone, 1981.

Cardiac Dysrhythmias

Fried MD: Advances in the diagnosis and therapy of syncope and palpitations in children. *Curr Opin Pediatr* 6:368, 1994.

Kugler JD, Danford DA: Management of infants, children, and adolescents with paroxysmal supraventricular tachycardia. *J Pediatr* 129:324, 1996.

Liberthson RR: Sudden death from cardiac causes in children and young adults. *N Engl J Med* 334:1039, 1996.

Ralston MA, Knilans TK, Hannon DW, et al: Use of adenosine for diagnosis and treatment of tachyarrhythmias in pediatric patients. *J Pediatr* 124:139, 1994.

Risser WL, Anderson SJ, Bolduc SP, et al: Cardiac dysrhythmias and sports. *Pediatrics* 95:786, 1995.

Van Hare GF: Indications for radiofrequency ablation in the pediatric population. *J Cardiovasc Electrophysiol* 8:952, 1997.

Zareba W, Moss AJ, Schwartz PJ, et al, and the International Long-QT Syndrome Registry Research Group: Influence of genotype on the clinical course of the long-QT syndrome. *N Engl J Med* 339:960, 1998.

Zimetbaum P, Josephson ME: Evaluation of patients with palpitations. *N Engl J Med* 338:1369, 1998.

Infective Endocarditis

Bayer AS, Bolger AF, Taubert KA, et al: Diagnosis and management of infective endocarditis and its complications. *Circulation* 98: 2936–2948, 1998.

Dajani AS, Taubert KA, Wilson W, et al: Prevention of bacterial endocarditis. Recommendations by the American Heart Association. *JAMA* 277:1794, 1997.

Milazzo AS Jr, Li JS: Bacterial endocarditis in infants and children. *Pediatr Infect Dis J* 20: 799–801, 2001.

Cardiomyopathies

Batra AS, Lewis AB: Acute myocarditis. *Curr Opin Pediatr* 13(3):234–9, 2001.

Burch M, Runciman M: Dilated cardiomyopathy. *Arch Dis Child* 74:479, 1996.

Chen SC, Balfour IC, Jureidini S: Clinical spectrum of restrictive cardiomyopathy in children. *J Heart Lung Transplant* 20(1):90–92, 2001.

Levi D, Alejos J: Diagnosis and treatment of pediatric viral myocarditis. *Curr Opin Cardiol* 16(2):77–83, 2001.

Roberts R, Sigwart U: New concepts in hypertrophic cardiomyopathies, Part I. *Circulation* 104(17):2113–2116, 2001.

Roberts R, Sigwart U: New concepts in hypertrophic cardiomyopathies, Part II. *Circulation* 104(18):2249–2252, 2001.

Schonberger J, Seidman CE: Many roads lead to a broken heart: The genetics of dilated cardiomyopathy. *Am J Hum Genet* 69(2):249–260, 2001.

Rheumatic Heart Disease

Dajani AS, Bisno AL, Chung KJ, et al: Prevention of rheumatic fever: A statement for health professionals by the Committee on Rheumatic Fever, Endocarditis, and Kawasaki Disease of the Council on Cardiovascular Disease in the Young, the American Heart Association. *Pediatr Infect Dis J* 8:263, 1989.

Stollerman GH: Rheumatic fever in the 21st century. *Clin Infect Dis* 33:806–814, 2001.

Veasy LG, Wiedmeier SE, Orsmond GS, et al: Resurgence of acute rheumatic fever in the intermountain area of the United States. *N Engl J Med* 316:421, 1987.

Kawasaki Disease

Dajani AS, Taubert KA, Gerber MA, et al: Diagnosis and therapy of Kawasaki disease in children. *Circulation* 87: 1776–1780, 1993.

Dajani AS, Taubert KA, Takahashi M, et al: Guidelines for long-term management of patients with Kawasaki disease. *Circulation* 89: 916–922, 1994.

Chest Pain

Gutgesell HP, Barst RJ, Humes RA, et al: Common cardiovascular problems in the young: Part I. Murmurs, chest pain, syncope and irregular rhythms. *Am Fam Physician* 56(7):1825–1830, 1997.

Swenson JM, Fischer DR, Miller SA, et al: Are chest radiographs and electrocardiograms still valuable in evaluating new pediatric patients with heart murmurs or chest pain? *Pediatrics* 99:1, 1997.

Talner NS, Carboni MP: Chest pain in the adolescent and young adult. *Cardiol Rev* 8(1):49–56, 2000.

Syncope

Gutgesell HP, Barst RJ, Humes RA, et al: Common cardiovascular problems in the young: Part I. Murmurs, chest pain, syncope and irregular rhythms. *Am Fam Physician* 56(7):1825–1830, 1997.

Kapoor WN: Evaluation and management of the patient with syncope. *JAMA* 268:2553–2560, 1992.

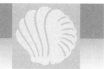

Chapter 14

Endocrinology and Disorders of Growth

Henry Anhalt, Kathryn L. Eckert, and
Ron G. Rosenfeld

The endocrine and nervous systems are responsible for regulating the body's metabolic activities. These two systems, which interact on several levels, combine to form a well-regulated unit that maintains and controls endocrine function. The three anatomic divisions of the endocrine system that are dealt with in this chapter are the **hypothalamus, pituitary gland,** and **cells of target organs**.

Two further divisions of the pituitary gland are the **posterior pituitary** and the **anterior pituitary**. The posterior pituitary **(neurohypophysis)** contains two primary hormones: **vasopressin** [antidiuretic hormone (ADH)] and **oxytocin**. Increased vasopressin secretion is regulated by high plasma osmolality and low circulating blood volume, resulting in water retention. Oxytocin plays a role in uterine contractions and ejection of milk.

The anterior pituitary contains **growth hormone** (GH); **adrenocorticotropic hormone** (ACTH); **thyroid-stimulating hormone** (TSH); **prolactin;** and the gonadotropic hormones, **luteinizing hormone** (LH) and **follicle-stimulating hormone** (FSH). These hormones act on other endocrine glands or directly on specific target cells in the body, affecting growth and maintenance of body functions. Most anterior pituitary hormones are under negative feedback control from their target organs. Negative feedback begins with the secretion of a releasing hormone by the hypothalamus, which signals the pituitary gland to secrete its stimulatory hormone. The stimulatory hormone causes subsequent release by the target organ of the final hormone, which then exhibits negative feedback control on the hypothalamus, diminishing release of the relevant releasing hormone.

The thyroid system is an example of this mechanism (Figure 14.1). The hypothalamus releases thyrotropin-releasing hormone (TRH), which causes release of TSH and subsequent stimulation of the thyroid gland to secrete thyroxine. Thyroxine exerts negative feedback on the hypothalamus and inhibits TRH release.

SHORT STATURE

Short stature is the most common cause of referral to the pediatric endocrinologist. Several intricate processes involving genetic potential, environmental influences, and the hormonal milieu to which the skeletal system is exposed determine growth and, therefore, final adult height. The major mechanism by which linear growth occurs is the lengthening of the skeletal system; insulin-like growth factor I (IGF-I), a small polypeptide secreted by the liver and other tissues, mediates this process. In turn, this peptide is under the control of GH released by the anterior pituitary gland. A thin plate of cartilage, the epiphyseal plate, is juxtaposed between the epiphysis and metaphysis of the long bones, and as long as it remains cartilaginous and not ossified, growth continues. Although IGF-I mediates growth, insulin, thyroid hormone, GH, proper nutritional intake, and appropriate psychosocial environment are all essential for proper growth.

Devices that can accurately and reproducibly measure recumbent length in infants and erect height in older children should be available to physicians who are evaluating children for growth. One formula that is often helpful in determining the genetic influence on growth is the calculation of midparental height. For males, the formula is:

$$\frac{[FH + (MH + 13)]}{2}$$

For females, the formula is

$$\frac{[(FH—13) + MH]}{2}$$

In both equations, FH is the father's height in centimeters and MH is the mother's height in centimeters.

Determination of the midparental height as part of the initial evaluation of a child with short stature allows for an approximate prediction of ex-

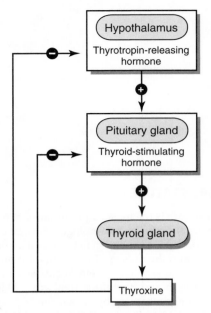

FIGURE 14.1. Thyroid hormone release as an example of positive and negative feedback loops.

pected adult height. Any growth pattern that significantly deviates from midparental height warrants close monitoring; it may indicate pathology.

Growth rates are equally important in assessing children's growth. Standardized growth charts are readily available for both sexes and are invaluable in making this assessment (see Figures 2.3 through 2.7). Normal linear growth is approximately 16–17 cm in the first 6 months of life and 8 cm in the next 6 months of life. Children usually grow at least 10 cm in the second year of life and at least 5–6 cm per year between the fourth and tenth years of life. The presence of any chronic systemic illness may interfere with normal growth.

Pediatric Pearl

Short parents generally have short children. It is always appropriate to evaluate midparental heights before embarking on costly evaluations.

Clinical and Laboratory Evaluation

History

When evaluating children for short stature, it is essential to obtain a careful prenatal and perinatal history. The clinician should pay particular attention to birth weight, length, and mode of delivery. Perinatal asphyxia or hypoxia may explain the later development of short stature, resulting from infarction of part or all of the pituitary gland. The presence of neonatal hypoglycemia or persistent jaundice may provide an additional clue to the presence of hypopituitarism, which may present as either isolated growth hormone deficiency or multiple pituitary hormone deficiency. It is necessary to rule out chronic illness or a history of neoplasm by a careful review of systems [e.g., the presence of headache in patients with central nervous system (CNS) disorders].

Obtaining a careful family medical history is of equal importance. Parental and sibling heights and the timing of onset of secondary sexual characteristics in parents and siblings help understand the contribution that genetic makeup may have. Often, parents note that affected children are not growing as well as their siblings or classmates; therefore, sibling heights and growth patterns are crucial in the evaluative process.

Physical Examination

A careful physical examination is necessary. Accurate measurement of height, weight, and head circumference (in infants) is essential. If the parents are available, measurement of their heights is also necessary. It is important to obtain vital signs, and the clinician should pay particular attention to blood pressure and pulse rate.

In addition, dysmorphic features are worthy of note; short stature may be part of a syndrome. A careful systematic physical examination is warranted to rule out chronic illness. Palpation of the thyroid gland is necessary to rule out goiter or the presence of nodules and associated hypothyroidism or hyperthyroidism. Examination of the genitalia is a crucial part of the examination, and Tanner staging to evaluate sexual maturity is appropriate in all patients (see Figures 3.1 through 3.3). Congenital conditions involving the axial skeleton can cause short stature, and a measurement of arm span, sitting height, and body proportions is helpful in diagnosis. For example, a normal arm span for age with a markedly abnormal height is expected in skeletal dysplasias involving the axial skeleton only. Similarly, it is necessary to obtain an upper:lower body ratio to rule out bony dysplasias of the skeleton that cause dwarfism associated with a short trunk. Weight: height ratios also provide clues regarding the etiology of growth failure. In genetic causes of growth failure (i.e., syndromes), patients are usually normal weight for height, whereas in conditions such as malnutrition, systemic illness, and failure to thrive, patients often have "fallen off" their weight curve prior to evidencing linear growth deceleration.

Laboratory Evaluation

Laboratory evaluation should begin only after performance of a complete physical examination and recording of all abnormal findings. As a general rule, only those children who have demonstrated deceleration of growth or growth rates that are abnormal for their peer group or are more than two standard deviations below the mean for height warrant further investigation. The laboratory workup (Table 14.1) should fit the physical findings and pertinent details of the review of systems. The evaluation of bone age is an index of skeletal maturation. In addition, the evaluation of any girl with unexplained short stature should include a chromosomal analysis to rule out Turner syndrome or Turner mosaicism; in the latter condition, many of the physical stigmata may be absent.

Differential Diagnosis (Table 14.2)

If the complete blood count (CBC), erythrocyte sedimentation rate (ESR), or urinalysis is abnormal, it is necessary to seek an occult illness that accounts for the child's short stature (e.g., inflammatory bowel disease). However, if these values are normal, the IGF-I and insulin-like growth factor–binding protein-3 (IGFBP-3) are low, and bone age is delayed relative to chronologic age, then investigation of GH deficiency is warranted. **Constitutional delay of growth and puberty** is an essential consideration with short stature, a strong parental history of delayed puberty, delayed dentition, and delayed bone age accompanied by a normal growth rate. This condition represents a normal variation, and the clinician should reassure families that once puberty ensues, the child will undergo catch-up growth. A careful history and physical examination, a period of observation, plus a bone age determination are usually sufficient for diagnosis.

TABLE 14.1 **Initial Screening Laboratory Evaluation in Patients With Short Stature**

Insulin-like growth factor-I (IGF-I)
Insulin-like growth factor–binding protein-3 (IGFBP-3)
Complete blood count (CBC)
Erythrocyte sedimentation rate (ESR)
Urinalysis
Serum electrolytes
Bone age
Thyroxine (T$_4$)
Thyroid-stimulating hormone (TSH)

TABLE 14.2 **Differential Diagnosis of Short Stature**

Normal variants
  Normal variant constitutional delay
  Normal variant short stature

Abnormal conditions
  Psychosocial
  Endocrine
    Growth hormone deficiency
    Hypothyroidism
    Cushing disease
    Panhypopituitarism
    Growth hormone insensitivity
  Chronic disease
    Cardiovascular
    Gastrointestinal
    Pulmonary
    Renal
    Hematologic
    Diabetes
  Skeletal
    Osteochondrodysplasia
    Rickets
    Pseudohypoparathyroidism
  Chromosomal abnormalities
    Turner syndrome
    Trisomy 21
  Intrauterine growth retardation
    Placental insufficiency
    Teratogens (e.g., fetal alcohol syndrome)

IGF-I and IGFBP-3, despite being sensitive indicators of GH deficiency, may not be entirely specific. Random serum GH levels are unreliable in diagnosing GH deficiency because GH is normally released in a pulsatile fashion. Therefore, a number of tests have been designed to diagnose GH deficiency by either measuring serum GH during exercise and sleep (when GH is expected to rise) or utilizing known pharmacologic provocative agents for the release of GH (Table 14.3). Many endocrinologists perform a brief stimulation test with oral clonidine, followed by sequential formal testing with two other intravenous pharmacologic agents, usually arginine and insulin, when indicated. Any GH value above 10 ng/ml is considered evidence of appropriate GH secretion to a provocative stimulus. However, if the child "fails" the clonidine stimulus and the arginine–insulin test, the child may be a candidate for GH treatment.

Despite the use of these tests for over 30 years to diagnose GH deficiency, the testing should be abandoned and replaced with critical assessments of growth data, bone age, midparental

TABLE 14.3 Provocative Tests for the Diagnosis of Growth Hormone Deficiency

Exercise
Dopamine
Sleep
Clonidine
Arginine
Insulin
Glucagon
Propranolol

heights, and growth factors for many reasons (Table 14.4). Before initiation of treatment with GH in children with GH deficiency, a magnetic resonance imaging (MRI) scan of the brain is warranted to ensure that an intracranial mass involving the pituitary gland, most commonly a craniopharyngioma, is not missed.

Management

A pediatric endocrinologist skilled in teaching patients and their families how to inject and care for the medication usually initiates GH therapy using recombinant DNA-derived human GH. The initial dose varies from 0.025 to 0.1 mg/kg/day, given as a subcutaneous injection in rotating sites on the skin. Currently, the cost of GH therapy is approximately $10,000–$20,000 a year.

Some potential risks are associated with GH therapy. Local reactions to the injection, such as pain and bruising at the injection site, are generally minor. Slipped capital femoral epiphysis, a condition seen in children during periods of rapid growth, has been attributed in some cases to GH treatment, but it may also occur in untreated GH and thyroid deficiency. Leukemia is also a concern. It has been suggested that patients who receive GH are at greater risk for developing leukemia, but worldwide surveillance

TABLE 14.4 Reasons to Abandon Growth Hormone Provocative Testing

1. Testing does not mimic endogenous growth hormone secretion
2. Arbitrary definitions of subnormal response to stimuli
3. Variation in measured growth hormone across different laboratories
4. Expense, discomfort, and risks of provocative testing
5. Poor reproducibility of the tests
6. Results vary with age and sex steroid status

data suggest that patients without underlying risk factors for malignancy who receive GH are at no greater risk than the general population. Creutzfeldt-Jakob disease, a uniformly fatal disease caused by an as yet unidentified slow virus or prion, was seen in patients who were treated before 1985 with GH of cadaveric pituitary origin. However, no cases of this disease have been reported in those patients treated exclusively with recombinant DNA-derived human GH. Glucose intolerance is another theoretical side effect of GH therapy. One normal physiologic effect of GH is increasing blood sugar in response to hypoglycemia. In conditions of GH excess (e.g., acromegaly), hyperglycemia may occur; thus, it is prudent to consider iatrogenic diabetes mellitus (DM) in those treated patients who present with the typical signs and symptoms of polyuria and polydipsia. Fortunately, this has been a rare problem in GH recipients. Antibodies to GH have been detected in patients treated with GH but are generally of little clinical significance.

Currently, GH therapy has a number of other indications, some approved and others experimental. GH has been approved by the Food and Drug Administration (FDA) to accelerate growth and increase final height of patients with GH deficiency in childhood and adulthood, Turner syndrome, chronic renal failure, intrauterine growth retardation, and Prader-Willi syndrome. In patients with hypophosphatemic rickets, an X-linked disorder of renal tubular phosphate transport, GH is being used in an attempt to increase final adult height. The use of GH to stimulate growth in normal (non-GH deficient), short children remains controversial.

ABNORMALITIES OF PUBERTY

The timing of the events of puberty are slightly different in boys and girls and vary widely among regions and ethnic groups. In boys, the onset of pubertal changes before 9 years of age is considered precocious and after 14 years of age, delayed. In girls, the onset of pubertal changes before 8 years of age is considered precocious and after 13 years of age is considered delayed (see Chapter 3, Adolescent Medicine).

Pathophysiology

Complex interactions between the hypothalamus, pituitary gland, adrenal glands, and gonads control the events of normal puberty. Inhibition of gonadotropin-releasing hormone (GnRH) secretion from the hypothalamus begins to diminish as the prepubertal dip in growth velocity occurs. This results in an increase in both the frequency and the amplitude of GnRH secretion, sensitizing the pituitary to further GnRH release and causing increased secretion of FSH and LH. FSH and LH then stimulate the gonads to produce sex steroid hormones. Estrogen and testosterone cause an increase in somatic growth and development of secondary sexual characteristics and provide an appropriate hormonal milieu for reproduction. The onset of adrenal androgen steroidogenesis (adrenarche) occurs approximately 1–2 years before the onset of true puberty, with true puberty defined by a rise in gonadotropins (FSH, LH) and gonadal sex steroids. The adrenal androgens dehydroepiandrosterone (DHEA) and dehydroepiandrosterone sulfate (DHEAS) are responsible for the development of pubic hair; axillary hair; body odor; and, in the case of males, facial hair.

PUBERTAL DELAY

Pubertal delay is subclassified based broadly on the level of gonadotropins. Elevated gonadotropins or **hypergonadotropic hypogonadism** is due to gonadal failure, while low gonadotropins or **hypogonadotropic hypogonadism** is due to inadequate stimulation of the gonads. Delayed puberty is a far more common complaint in males than in females.

Clinical and Laboratory Evaluation

History and Physical Examination
Patients with **constitutional delay of puberty** often have a strong family history of delayed puberty. Usually, these patients are short with a moderately delayed bone age and a history of growth deceleration since late infancy. Patients with **Kallmann syndrome** complain of hyposmia or anosmia (altered sense of smell) resulting from hypoplastic or absent olfactory nerves. Patients with a history of brain tumor and resection or radiotherapy may develop gonadotropin deficiency as an isolated phenomenon or as part of complete **hypopituitarism**. A history of visual field changes, headache, personality changes, or any sign of raised intracranial pressure may herald discovery of a brain tumor or an infiltrative process. A careful review of systems and physical examination should exclude chronic systemic illness. **Septo-optic dysplasia** can be diagnosed by an abnormal MRI scan of the brain, and patients usually have associated midline defects such as cleft or high-arched palate, hypertelorism or visual disturbances, and midline facial

hypoplasia. Boys with hypogonadism present with prepubertal testes (< 3 ml in volume) and immature facies.

Patients with **Klinefelter syndrome** may have a history of behavioral disorders and evidence of adrenarche, although with small testicles and gynecomastia. Male patients with **gonadal dysgenesis** may have no palpable testes, but in females this presents a much greater diagnostic problem. Recent weight loss and psychologic disturbances may provide the evidence of an eating disorder such as **anorexia nervosa,** particularly in female adolescents or strenuously trained athletes. In female patients with delayed puberty and short stature, **Turner syndrome** or **Turner mosaicism** warrants consideration, even in the absence of the typical stigmata: history of neonatal lymphedema, frequent otitis media, low hairline, high-arched palate, low posteriorly rotated ears, numerous pigmented nevi, cubitus valgus, and dystrophic hyperconvex nails.

Laboratory Evaluation
Initial workup involves evaluation of bone age, gonadotropins, electrolytes, liver and renal function tests, thyroid function tests, serum testosterone in boys and estradiol in girls, and karyotype. If there is biochemical evidence of gonadotropin deficiency, a cranial MRI scan is warranted. In boys, if there is evidence of elevated gonadotropins, adrenarche, and no testicular enlargement, it is necessary to obtain a karyotype to rule out Klinefelter syndrome (47,XXY). In girls, pelvic ultrasound can be performed to delineate the anatomy of the uterus and ovaries.

Differential Diagnosis (Tables 14.5 and 14.6)

Management

The treatment of pubertal delay depends on the etiology of the delay and whether this is a temporary phenomenon, as in constitutional delay of growth and puberty, or a permanent phenomenon, as in gonadal dysgenesis.

Boys with constitutional delay of puberty are often ridiculed by their classmates for the lack of secondary sexual characteristics. If a constitutionally delayed male patient is older than 14 years of age and is concerned about the lack of sexual development and short stature, the recommended treatment is a short course of testosterone therapy consisting of four injections of testosterone enanthate 100–200 mg IM at 3-week

TABLE 14.5 Differential Diagnosis of Hypogonadotropic and Hypergonadotropic Hypogonadism in Boys

Hypogonadotropic hypogonadism
  Constitutional delay of puberty
  Gonadotropin deficiency
    Idiopathic
    X-linked
    Septo-optic dysplasia
    Kallmann syndrome
    Chronic illness
    Brain tumors
    Infiltrative process

Hypergonadotropic hypogonadism
  Gonadal dysgenesis
    Klinefelter syndrome
  Gonadal failure

intervals. This regimen is usually sufficient to induce secondary sexual characteristics without compromising final adult height. Another benefit from this regimen is the concept of "jump-starting" or priming the pituitary in patients with constitutional delay of puberty to begin producing pubertal levels of gonadotropins. This usually occurs within 6 months to a year after the short course of testosterone. If there is a failure of induction of spontaneous puberty within a year after testosterone therapy, a second, more prolonged course of testosterone or permanent testosterone therapy should be considered. However, before reinstituting testosterone therapy, it is essential to seek a cause for the continued delay in pubertal development aggressively.

One of the more difficult diagnostic dilemmas is discriminating between permanent hypogonadotropic hypogonadism and constitutional delay of puberty, which resemble each other clini-

TABLE 14.6 Differential Diagnosis of Hypogonadotropic and Hypergonadotropic Hypogonadism in Girls

Hypogonadotropic hypogonadism
  Gonadotropin deficiency
  Anorexia nervosa
  Athletes
  Chronic illness

Hypergonadotropic hypogonadism
  Gonadal dysgenesis
    Turner syndrome
  Gonadal failure

cally, radiographically, and biochemically. Often, clinicians resign themselves to adopting a wait-and-see approach.

In boys with hypergonadotropic hypogonadism, testosterone therapy is the treatment of choice. The usual adult dose is 200–300 mg testosterone IM every 2–4 weeks. Side effects include fluid retention, mood swings, and priapism.

In girls with gonadotropin deficiency, the clinician should seek a reversible cause and provide treatment. However, if the condition is due to permanent gonadotropin deficiency or hypergonadotropic hypogonadism, as in Turner syndrome, treatment with estrogen and a progestational agent should start between 12 and 14 years of age, depending on the patient's stature. Conjugated estrogen is usually started at a low dose (0.3 mg) and increased to a more physiologic dose (0.625 mg). After this dose is tolerated for approximately 6 months to 1 year, progestational steroid hormones are added on days 17–26 of the cycle, and then both estrogen and progesterone are discontinued for 5 days to allow withdrawal bleeding. Common side effects of female sex steroids are breast swelling, nausea, bloating, and fluid retention.

PRECOCIOUS PUBERTY

As previously described, sexual precocity is defined as the onset of pubertal changes in boys prior to 9 years of age and in girls prior to 8 years of age. This condition can be further subdivided into **isosexual** or **heterosexual precocious puberty**. The development of pubertal changes consistent with the genotype of the patient is considered isosexual, and the development of pubertal changes discordant with the patient's genotype (e.g., breast enlargement in a male) is considered heterosexual. Central precocious puberty is due to stimulation of the gonads by pituitary gonadotropins. Premature production of sex steroids without evidence of pituitary gonadotropin stimulation defines peripheral precocious puberty. Precocious puberty, in contrast to constitutional delay of puberty, is a far more common complaint in females than in males.

Clinical and Laboratory Evaluation

History
Important points in the history include the recent onset of rapid growth, behavioral disturbances, body odor, and vaginal discharge or bleeding. In addition, a careful review of systems could uncover a history of CNS malformation,

trauma, tumor, or poorly treated congenital adrenal hyperplasia (CAH). In adolescent males, inquiry about the use of androgens, estrogens, or marijuana, which may help explain gynecomastia, is warranted. Family history of a similar problem may point to the diagnosis of **familial precocious puberty**. Careful analysis of growth rates may indicate the presence of a growth spurt consistent with true precocious puberty.

Physical Examination

When examining children with precocious puberty, it is important to distinguish between **"true precocious puberty"** and that due to peripheral causes, known as **"pseudoprecocious puberty."** Several clinical characteristics help distinguish among the causes of early puberty in females (Table 14.7).

Visual field and careful neurologic examinations are necessary to rule out the presence of an intracranial process. Palpation of the testicles may reveal enlargement, indicating trophic effects from pituitary gonadotropins, or asymmetry, indicating the presence of a tumor. If both testes are prepubertal in size in a boy with precocious onset of secondary sexual characteristics, the diagnostic evaluation should be directed toward an adrenal etiology. A thorough examination of the skin is warranted, looking for the presence of **café au lait spots,** as would be seen in cases of **McCune-Albright syndrome** or **neurofibromatosis,** as well as in cases of acne or hirsutism. Careful Tanner staging (see Figures 3.1 through 3.3) is necessary as part of the initial physical examination and as a useful adjunct in following patients with precocious puberty.

Laboratory Evaluation

Measurement of random serum gonadotropins is of limited clinical use because the hormones are released in a pulsatile fashion; thus, if sampling occurs at a physiologic nadir, the results may not truly reflect the status of pituitary maturation. In true (or central) precocious puberty, a pelvic ultrasound may show enlargement of the uterus and adnexa.

Serum testosterone and adrenal androgens, if elevated, may suggest precocious adrenarche or a tumor in the adrenal gland or testes as the cause of precocious puberty. An ACTH stimulation test can rule out late-onset CAH. Hypothyroidism or hyperthyroidism may cause either delayed or accelerated puberty; thus, a serum TSH and thyroxine (T_4) are necessary.

If, after preliminary evaluation, **central precocious puberty** is suspected, an intravenous or subcutaneous GnRH test is warranted. This test detects activation of the hypothalamic–pituitary axis by stimulating the pituitary gland with the tropic hormone GnRH. If the pituitary has never been exposed to endogenous GnRH, then a small rise in LH would be expected in response to exogenous GnRH. However, if the pituitary had been exposed to endogenous GnRH before, there is a brisk rise in LH, indicating that the pituitary had been "primed." An increase in LH level above 5 ng/ml is evidence of an activated pituitary gland and diagnostic of true precocious puberty. A cranial MRI scan is then necessary to rule out any anomaly or tumor that could be responsible for precocious puberty.

However, if there is no biochemical evidence of central precocious puberty, then a more careful search for peripheral causes of precocious puberty is warranted. The presence of ovarian cysts on pelvic ultrasound combined with an elevated serum estradiol may indicate estradiol-producing ovarian cysts. Production of estradiol from these cysts may fluctuate, leading to waxing and waning of symptoms.

Differential Diagnosis (Table 14.8)

Management

Irrespective of the cause, true precocious puberty causes advanced somatic growth and skeletal maturation. Thus, patients tend to be tall initially but

---

TABLE 14.7 **Clinical Characteristics of Precocious Puberty in Females**

	Premature Thelarche	Exogenous Estrogen (Pseudoprecocious Puberty)	True Precocious Puberty
Breast development	Advanced	Marked	Marked
Growth velocity	Normal	Normal/advanced	Accelerated
Bone age	Normal	Normal/advanced	Advanced
Serum estradiol	Prepubertal	Prepubertal	Pubertal
GnRH test	Prepubertal	Suppressed	Pubertal or adult

GnRH = gonadotropin-releasing hormone.

TABLE 14.8 Differential Diagnosis of Isosexual versus Heterosexual Pubertal Changes in Patients With Precocious Puberty

MALE

Isosexual
    Central
        Familial
        Central nervous system disease
            Hamartoma
            Postirradiation
            After chronic exposure to androgens
            Poorly controlled or late-onset congenital adrenal hyperplasia
    Peripheral
        Testicular tumor
        Testotoxicosis (gonadotropin-independent puberty)
        Adrenal rest tumor
        Congenital adrenal hyperplasia
Heterosexual
    Estrogenization
        Adrenal adenoma or carcinoma
        Teratoma
    Marijuana use

FEMALE

Isosexual
    Central
        Familial
        Central nervous system disease
            Hamartoma
            Postirradiation
            After chronic exposure to androgens
            Poorly controlled or late-onset congenital adrenal hyperplasia
    Peripheral
        Granulosa cell tumor
        McCune-Albright syndrome
Heterosexual
    Androgenization
        Congenital adrenal hyperplasia
            21-OH deficiency
            11-OH deficiency
        Androgen-producing tumors
            Adrenal adenoma or carcinoma
            Teratoma
        Polycystic ovary disease
        Exposure to exogenous androgens

---

stop growing earlier than their peers, paradoxically ending up as shorter adults. A compromised final adult height, combined with the psychologic risks of early puberty and menarche years before a patient's peer group, justify treatment.

By far the most common cause of central precocious puberty, especially in girls, is idiopathic. The mainstay of treatment of true precocious puberty is monthly administration of GnRH, a pituitary gonadotropin agonist, which effectively binds all the receptors at the level of the pituitary in such a way as to inhibit gonadotropin secretion.

In cases in which the cause of precocious puberty is peripheral, determination of the underlying cause and its treatment are necessary. It is noteworthy that in cases of androgen excess, such as poorly treated 21-hydroxylase deficiency, central precocious puberty may eventually develop after years of peripheral precocious puberty as a result of chronically elevated serum androgens.

Therefore, good control with glucocorticoids is necessary to suppress the formation of excess adrenal androgens.

Patients with benign conditions such as **idiopathic premature thelarche and adrenarche** usually require only reassurance and close follow-up.

McCune-Albright syndrome, a G protein abnormality of intracellular signaling, and **testotoxicosis,** a condition in which the testes produce testosterone independent of stimulation from the gonadotropins, are prototypes for gonadotropin-independent precocious puberty. Patients with gonadotropin-independent isosexual precocious puberty are best treated with pharmacologic agents that inhibit sex steroid formation or those that bind to receptors, thus blocking hormonal action.

An important adjunct to therapy is psychologic counseling for the patient and family.

ADRENAL DISORDERS

CONGENITAL ADRENAL HYPERPLASIA (CAH)

CAH includes a group of disorders that are characterized by a deficiency of an enzyme necessary for the synthesis of cortisol. A deficiency of one of these enzymes leads to hyperfunction and hyperplasia of the adrenal glands.

Pathophysiology

The adrenal gland is comprised of the cortex, which produces adrenal steroids, and the medulla, which secretes catecholamines. The cortex is divided into three layers. The **zona glomerulosa,** the outermost layer, secretes **mineralocorticoids,** and the **zona fasciculata** and **zona reticularis** secrete **glucocorticoids** and **androgens**.

Androgens and glucocorticoids are under the control of the pituitary and hypothalamus, with negative feedback control. The hypothalamus secretes **corticotropin-releasing factor,** which stimulates release of **ACTH** from the anterior pituitary gland. This, in turn, stimulates the adrenal cortex to produce and secrete cortisol. Cortisol exerts a negative feedback on the hypothalamus, causing a decrease in corticotropin-releasing factor release.

In contrast to the glucocorticoids, the secretion of the mineralocorticoids is not governed by ACTH. Instead, the **renin–angiotensin system,** along with serum sodium and potassium, governs the release of the mineralocorticoids (Figure 14.2).

Three pathways in the adrenal gland interact to form cortisol, aldosterone, and testosterone as their final products (Figure 14.3). The initial substrate is cholesterol. At each step, an enzyme must be present for production of the end product. When an enzyme is reduced or absent, buildup of the immediate precursor occurs, leading to varying hormonal effects that are manifest as both metabolic disturbances and genital abnormalities. Each enzyme deficiency has classical clinical features (Table 14.9).

The most common enzyme deficiency is **21-hydroxylase deficiency.** This condition, which accounts for approximately 95% of cases of CAH, is inherited as an autosomal recessive trait. Of those individuals affected, 50%–75% have salt-wasting of varying degrees as a result of insufficient production of aldosterone. Because the enzyme deficiency leads to altered production of cortisol, negative feedback to the hypothalamus is removed, and ACTH production increases. This results in stimulation of the adrenal gland and shunting of the adrenal steroid pathway toward production of androgens, resulting in virilized females and normal-appearing males at birth.

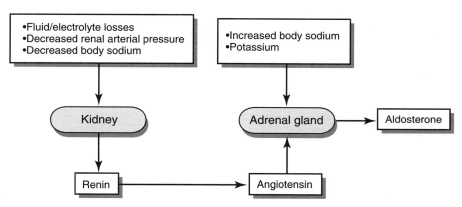

FIGURE 14.2. Regulation of mineralocorticoid secretion.

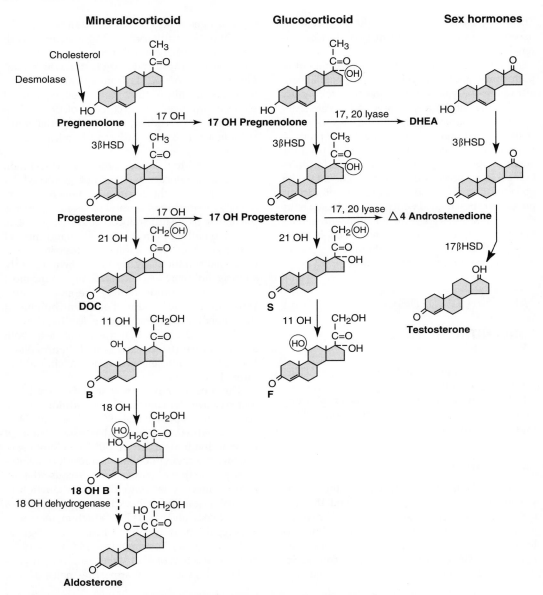

FIGURE 14.3. Pathways of adrenal hormones. DHEA = dehydroepiandrosterone; DOC = deoxycorticosterone; 3βHSD = 3β-hydroxysteroid dehydrogenase; 17bβHSD = 17β-hydroxysteroid dehydrogenase.

In male infants, the disorder is usually not diagnosed until several weeks after birth, when patients present with evidence of salt-wasting, including vomiting and dehydration. In female infants, the disorder may be diagnosed shortly after birth because of the presence of ambiguous genitalia. However, in female newborns with complete virilization, the diagnosis may be missed at birth if infants are mistakenly believed to be cryptorchid males. In the non–salt-losing variety of 21-hydroxylase deficiency, diagnosis may be delayed for several years, depending on the severity of the defect.

Clinical and Laboratory Evaluation

History

In male infants, diagnosis of the salt-losing variety of 21-hydroxylase deficiency typically occurs within the first few weeks of life. Often, infants may have a history of vomiting, diarrhea, failure to gain weight, and lethargy. The diagnosis of

TABLE 14.9	Clinical Features of Syndromes of Adrenal Enzyme Deficiency				

Enzyme Deficiency	Current Nomenclature	Ambiguous Genitalia*	Postnatal Virilization*	Salt-Wasting	Other Symptoms
21-Hydroxylase (classic form—early onset)	P450 c21	F: virilized M: normal	F: virilized M: premature adrenarche	Yes	May present with salt-losing crisis
21-Hydroxylase (nonclassic—late onset)	P450 c21	F: clitoromegaly M: normal	F: virilized M: premature adrenarche	No	
11 β-Hydroxylase	P450 c11	F: virilized M: normal	F: virilized M: premature adrenarche	No	Hypertension
3β-OH steroid dehydrogenase (classic)	3β-HSD	F: virilized M: incomplete, masculinization	F: virilized M: incomplete	Yes	
3β-OH steroid dehydrogenase (nonclassic)	3β-HSD	None	F: virilized M: incomplete	No	
17α-Hydroxylase	P450 c17	F: normal M: incomplete masculinization	F: none M: incomplete	No	Hypertension Primary amenorrhea Delayed puberty
20,22-Desmolase	P450 scc	F: normal M: incomplete masculinization	F: none M: incomplete	Yes	Lethal if deficiency complete

* F = female; M = male.
  3β-HSD = 3β-hydroxysteroid dehydrogenase.

pyloric stenosis frequently has been entertained in these patients before the diagnosis of CAH is made. In female infants, virilization of the genitalia typically leads to the diagnosis of CAH in the neonatal period.

The presentation of other adrenal enzyme deficiencies varies with the specific enzyme defect (see Table 14.9). In contrast, in the non–salt-wasting variety of 21-hydroxylase deficiency, the diagnosis may not be made for several years. Typically, male patients present with tall stature and premature adrenarche (penile enlargement and pubic hair), but enlargement of the testicles is noticeably absent, suggesting adrenal origin of the increased levels of androgens. Female patients may present with tall stature, clitoral enlargement, premature adrenarche (pubic or axillary hair), acne, hirsutism, and menstrual abnormalities.

Physical Examination

The genital examination may be normal in male patients with 21-hydroxylase deficiency, although hyperpigmentation of the scrotum and nipples may be present. The genitalia of female patients may be only mildly virilized with enlargement of the clitoris or may be completely virilized with

scrotal rugae and penile urethra. Of notable importance in these masculinized females is the absence of testicles.

If the diagnosis is delayed, patients may present with salt-losing crisis. When salt-losing crisis occurs, hypotension, tachycardia, dehydration, and shock are usually present.

Pediatric Pearl

In evaluation of children with ambiguous genitalia, it is important to remember that the presence of palpable gonads in the labial folds almost always indicates a chromosomal male child.

Laboratory Evaluation

In infants with ambiguous genitalia caused by 21-hydroxylase deficiency, chromosomal analysis is necessary. A pelvic ultrasound, urethrogram, and a vaginogram may be necessary to determine the presence of female internal genitalia and the location of the urethra. Serum 17-hydroxyprogesterone and renin levels are elevated ($10\times$–$1000\times$ normal). Hyponatremia (< 130 mEq/L), hyperkalemia (> 5.5 mEq/L), and metabolic acidosis are also present. Signs of metabolic acidosis, which typically are noted by 2–6 weeks of age, may be severe.

In other forms of CAH, laboratory data vary with the specific enzyme deficiency. Levels of the precursor steroid immediately before the enzyme deficiency are typically elevated, whereas levels of products after the defect are very low. Standards for adrenal hormone ratios are available and are invaluable in confirming the diagnosis. At times, laboratory data may be ambiguous, and an ACTH (Cortrosyn) stimulation test may be of use in delineating the defect.

Differential Diagnosis

On initial presentation, the diagnosis of an adrenal disorder may be confused with septic shock, pyloric stenosis, or severe dehydration. However, after serum electrolytes are obtained and reveal the presence of hyponatremia and hyperkalemia, the diagnosis typically is straightforward. The process of differentiating among the various types of CAH, congenital adrenal hypoplasia, and Addison disease then involves analyzing the results of the adrenal steroid profiles and ACTH levels.

Pediatric Pearl

Male infants who present with failure to thrive, hypotension, vomiting, and dehydration between birth and 8 weeks of age warrant evaluation for CAH.

Management

Initial management involves restoring intravascular volume and serum sodium and potassium values using 0.5 normal saline. After blood has been drawn for diagnostic studies, replacement medications should begin. With suspected CAH, clinicians should not delay treatment while they await the results of adrenal hormone studies. Mineralocorticoid replacement therapy consists of fludrocortisone (Florinef) 0.1–0.3 mg/day PO. In an emergency, hydrocortisone should be given at a dose of 50–100 mg/m^2 IV or IM, with subsequent doses of 50–100 mg/m^2/day divided into four doses given until the patient recovers. After serum electrolytes stabilize, the steroid doses may be reduced.

Other steps are appropriate in the medical management of adrenal hyperplasia after initial stabilization (Table 14.10). The family should re-

---

TABLE 14.10 **Medical Management of Congenital Adrenal Hyperplasia**

1. Hydrocortisone 15–20 mg/m^2/day in three doses
2. Fludrocortisone 0.05–0.2 mg/day in one to two doses
3. Monitoring of serum 17-hydroxyprogesterone and renin every 3 months
4. Close monitoring of growth rate and pubertal status
5. With illness (e.g., fever, otitis media) triple glucocorticoids
6. With surgery, trauma, or severe stress, increase glucocorticoids to 100 mg/m^2/day
7. Medic-Alert bracelet

---

ceive an emergency kit containing injectable hydrocortisone to administer to the patient in the case of severe stress, trauma, or inability to take oral hydrocortisone.

The presence of hypertension implies overtreatment with fludrocortisone. Close monitoring of growth velocity is appropriate. In the absence of adequate treatment, growth velocity increases and rapid skeletal maturation occurs. If chronic undertreatment occurs, final adult height may be impaired as a result of premature fusion of the epiphyses. Conversely, if overtreatment occurs, growth velocity declines and skeletal age does not progress at a normal rate.

Replacement therapy of mineralocorticoids and glucocorticoids should be continued throughout adult life. This is particularly important in females, in whom fertility may be impaired if CAH is not properly controlled. In addition, control during pregnancy is crucial in preventing virilization of a female fetus.

Surgery often plays a role in the treatment of females with CAH. Those patients with severely virilized external genitalia often need clitoral reduction, relocation of the urethra, and vaginoplasty. Timing of surgery should be individualized. Males generally require no surgical intervention unless inadequate virilization has occurred.

Through the use of amniocentesis, prenatal diagnosis of 21-hydroxylase deficiency is now possible when an index case has been diagnosed in a family. Human leukocyte antigen (HLA) typing, with use of restriction fragment length polymorphism or polymerase chain reaction, also may be used to identify affected fetuses early in pregnancy by comparing parents' and affected siblings' genotype with the fetal genotype. 17-Hydroxyprogesterone is very elevated when measured in the amniotic fluid of a fetus affected with 21-hydroxylase deficiency. Both amniocentesis and HLA typing may help determine whether a fetus is affected, so that early treatment may ensue, thereby decreasing the likelihood of virilization of an affected female fetus. Dexamethasone is given to the pregnant mother throughout the pregnancy unless the fetus is a male or is proved to be a female not affected with 21-hydroxylase deficiency.

ADRENAL INSUFFICIENCY

Pathophysiology

Adrenal insufficiency is characterized by decreased production of glucocorticoids and mineralocorticoids. This disorder, which is rare in children, has several causes (Table 14.11). The most common cause is autoimmune adrenalitis or idiopathic adrenal insufficiency, representing approximately 80% of cases of adrenal insufficiency. In the past, tuberculosis was a common cause of adrenal insufficiency, but this is rare today.

Clinical and Laboratory Evaluation

History
Children with chronic adrenal insufficiency present with symptoms of weakness, fatigue, anorexia, abdominal pain, weight loss, nausea, vomiting, diarrhea, dehydration, and increased skin pigmentation (resulting from elevated ACTH levels). In cases of polyglandular autoimmune syndrome, other symptoms such as mucocutaneous candidiasis may also occur. In cases of congenital adrenal hypoplasia, infants present with vomiting, diarrhea, dehydration, and shock.

Physical Examination
Physical examination reveals abnormal pigmentation of the skin, particularly in the palmar, axillary, and groin creases, as well as in the buccal

TABLE 14.11 Causes of Adrenal Insufficiency

Autoimmune ("idiopathic")
Iatrogenic (chronic corticosteroid therapy)
Tuberculosis
Polyglandular autoimmune syndromes types I and II
ACTH unresponsiveness
ACTH deficiency
Adrenoleukodystrophy
Congenital adrenal hypoplasia
Infiltrative (fungal infection, malignancy, hemorrhage, hemochromatosis)

ACTH = adrenocorticotropic hormone.

mucosa, nipples, and areas that have formed scars as a result of trauma since the onset of ACTH excess. Blood pressure may vary, depending on the stage of the disease. In addition, signs of dehydration are typically present. Height and weight are usually below average.

Pediatric Pearl
A tan all over without a tan line may indicate high ACTH levels associated with primary adrenal insufficiency.

Laboratory Evaluation
Initial laboratory tests reveal:

* Hyponatremia
* Hyperkalemia
* Hypoglycemia
* Elevated blood urea nitrogen (BUN)/creatinine
* CBC: eosinophilia, lymphocytosis
* Elevated serum ACTH (except in secondary adrenal insufficiency)
* Low cortisol level (< 5 mg/dl)
* Blunted cortisol response to synthetic ACTH (Cortrosyn) stimulation test (cortisol < 20 mg/dl)

Adrenal antibodies may be present, along with other signs of autoimmunity (thyroid, parathyroid, islet cell antibodies). A computed tomography (CT) scan may show enlargement of the adrenals in the case of tuberculosis or hemorrhage. Adrenal calcifications may be seen when adrenal hemorrhage has occurred in the past.

Differential Diagnosis

In most cases of adrenal insufficiency, the diagnosis is obvious, particularly when children present with shock, hyperpigmentation, hyponatremia, and hyperkalemia. However, in some cases, the differential diagnosis includes gastrointestinal (GI) disorders, sepsis, and drug or toxin ingestion.
The **polyglandular autoimmune syndromes** occur in both familial and sporadic forms. Type I disease usually occurs early in life and is associated with mucocutaneous candidiasis, hypoparathyroidism, and insulin-dependent DM or thyroid deficiency. In addition, pernicious anemia, chronic active hepatitis, alopecia, malabsorption, and gonadal failure may be present. Type 2 disease is associated with insulin-dependent DM or thyroid deficiency.

ACTH unresponsiveness is a familial form of adrenal insufficiency characterized by a defect of the ACTH receptor on the adrenal gland. Glucocorticoid production is low or absent, whereas mineralocorticoid secretion is preserved.

ACTH deficiency may be an isolated hormonal deficiency or may be seen with evidence of panhypopituitarism.

Adrenoleukodystrophy is an X-linked recessive disorder that manifests as adrenal insufficiency and progressive CNS demyelination, resulting in blindness, deafness, dementia, quadriparesis, and death. Initial symptoms usually occur in the second half of the first decade of life.

Congenital adrenal hypoplasia causes severe salt-wasting in the neonatal period. It may be differentiated from CAH by the absence of increased virilization and a low serum 17-hydroxyprogesterone. This form of adrenal insufficiency occurs in an X-linked form or as an autosomal recessive disorder. In addition, associated CNS defects may also occur.

Infiltrative causes of adrenal insufficiency include hemorrhage, which may be associated with birth trauma, and meningococcemia (Waterhouse-Friderichsen syndrome).

Management

Treatment of adrenal insufficiency includes replacement of glucocorticoids and mineralocorticoids (Table 14.12). Adequacy of glucocorticoid treatment is monitored by normal growth, reduced hyperpigmentation, normalization of vital signs, normal glucose, and suppressed ACTH levels. The adequacy of mineralocorticoid replacement is monitored by normalization of electrolytes and plasma renin levels.

Patients should wear a Medic-Alert bracelet at all times, stating their dependence on glucocorticoids. In addition, the family should receive an emergency kit containing injectable hydrocortisone.

AMBIGUOUS GENITALIA

Rapid evaluation of neonates with ambiguous genitalia is necessary to determine the appropriate sex for rearing.

Pathophysiology

Normal sexual differentiation in the fetus begins with an undifferentiated gonad. In XY males, the presence of testicular differentiating factor, located on the Y chromosome, causes the formation of a fetal testis. The testis then produces testosterone under the influence of placental chorionic gonadotropin, as well as Müllerian-inhibiting factor, which causes the regression of the Müllerian ducts. Conversion of testosterone to dihydrotestosterone and appropriate end-organ response to androgens are also essential in the development of normal male genitalia. Defects at any of these points can lead to ambiguous genitalia. In females, with the presence of normal XX chromosomes and the absence of testicular differentiating factor and Müllerian-inhibiting factor, the Müllerian ducts remain and form female internal genitalia. Normal female external genitalia form unless abnormal androgenic influences occur (CAH or exogenous androgens).

Clinical and Laboratory Evaluation

History and Physical Examination

Ambiguous genitalia is often detected in the early neonatal period when hypospadias, undescended testicles, or varying degrees of virilization of the phallus and labioscrotal folds are present. However, unless the clinician conducts a careful physical examination, paying attention to the presence or absence of testicles and the size of the phallus, it is possible to miss the diagnosis until later in the neonatal period or even as late as adolescence.

To determine the etiology of ambiguous genitalia, the first step involves checking for the presence of testicles. It is also essential to evaluate the degree of hypospadias, labioscrotal fusion, urogenital sinus, and the size of phallus. Normal values of phallus size are important to assess. In full-term infants, the mean stretched penile length is 3.5 cm. Stretched penile length of less than 2 cm is considered to be a microphallus. The clitoral length should not be longer than 1.5 cm.

TABLE 14.12 **Medical Management of Adrenal Insufficiency**

1. Hydrocortisone 12–15 mg/m^2/day
2. Fludrocortisone .05–.3 mg/day
3. Close monitoring of growth rate and pubertal status
4. With illness (e.g., fever, otitis media) triple glucocorticoids
5. With surgery, trauma, severe stress increase glucocorticoids to 100 mg/m^2/day
6. Medic-Alert bracelet

Laboratory Evaluation

Useful laboratory studies include:

- Adrenal steroid levels
- Electrolyte analysis
- Chromosomal analysis. Determination of the karyotype directs the laboratory evaluation (Figure 14.4).
- Ultrasound analysis or MRI to evaluate presence and location of gonads, uterus, and vagina
- Dye contrast studies to determine the location and structure of the urogenital sinus and other internal structures

Differential Diagnosis

The differential diagnosis of ambiguous genitalia may be broken down into three separate categories (Table 14.13). In **true hermaphroditism,** both male and female gonadal tissue are present but may or may not be functional; the karyotype is XX in 80% of patients and XY in 10%. In **female pseudohermaphroditism,** female gonads are present, with ambiguous genitalia; the karyotype is usually XX. In **male pseudohermaphroditism,** testicular tissue is present; the karyotype may be XY, XX, or XO/XY.

Management

Psychosocial support, along with medical management, is crucial in helping families deal with ambiguous genitalia and related issues. In female pseudohermaphrodites with CAH, management consists of replacement of glucocorticoids and mineralocorticoids if indicated by adrenal testing. In addition, surgical reconstruction of the clitoris and vagina is usually recommended. In those patients with maternal androgen exposure and se-

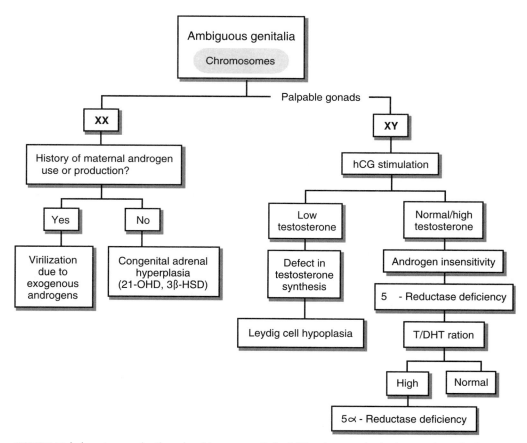

FIGURE 14.4. Laboratory evaluation of ambiguous genitalia. hCG = human chorionic gonadotropin; 3β-HSD = 3β-hydroxysteroid dehydrogenase defect; 21-OHD = 21-hydroxylase deficiency; T/DHT = ratio of testosterone to dihydrotestosterone.

TABLE 14.13 Causes of Ambiguous Genitalia

True hermaphroditism

Female pseudohermaphroditism
  Maternal ingestion or production of androgens
  Congenital adrenal hyperplasia

Male pseudohermaphroditism
  Defects of testicular differentiation and development
    XX male syndrome
    Mixed gonadal dysgenesis
    Persistent Müllerian duct syndrome
  Defects of testosterone synthesis
    Congenital adrenal hyperplasia (17-OHD, 3β-HSD, cholesterol desmolase deficiency)
    17,20-Desmolase deficiency
    17-Hydroxysteroid deficiency
    Leydig cell hypoplasia
  Defects of testosterone metabolism
    Androgen insensitivity syndrome, incomplete or complete

3β-HSD = 3β-hydroxysteroid dehydrogenase; 17-OHD = 17-hydroxylase deficiency.

vere virilization, no treatment other than surgical reconstruction may be required. However, several clinicians in the field of intersex disorders are currently reexamining and challenging these recommendations. Experts have suggested that the affected children themselves be allowed to participate in the decision-making process.

In males with adrenal defects causing decreased testosterone production, therapy is dictated by the degree of masculinization. In those with completely feminized external genitalia, patients should be raised as females, and the gonads should be removed to reduce the risk of malignant degeneration. This recommendation has also come under criticism from patient advocacy groups within the intersex community who recommend delaying genital altering therapy (i.e., surgery) until affected children are old enough to participate in their own care. In those with masculinized genitalia, a short course of testosterone injections in the neonatal period is indicated to enlarge the size of the phallus. Glucocorticoid and mineralocorticoid replacement are also indicated in the presence of CAH.

In cases of complete androgen insensitivity (phenotype: normal female), patients should be raised as females, and the gonads should be removed. In partial androgen insensitivity (with sexual ambiguity), testosterone injections should be used to assess the response in the neonatal period to determine the optimal sex of rearing. Patients with Leydig cell hypoplasia should be assessed in the same manner.

Male children with 5α-reductase deficiency may present with completely feminized genitalia

(in which case they may be raised as females with removal of the gonads) or partially masculinized genitalia. During puberty and adulthood, the production and the secretion of testosterone increase significantly and allow for masculinization of the genitalia despite a persistence of 5α-reductase deficiency.

CUSHING SYNDROME

Cushing syndrome refers to a state of increased cortisol secretion. In children, iatrogenic administration of cortisol is the most common cause of this condition. Cushing syndrome occurs more commonly in females than in males, regardless of age.

Pathophysiology

Hypercortisolism is rare in children; when it occurs before 7 years of age, it typically implies the presence of an adrenal tumor. In contrast, after 7 years of age, most cases are due to increased ACTH secretion. In some cases, an ACTH-secreting pituitary tumor may be found; rarely, a nonendocrine tumor may secrete ACTH or an ACTH-like substance that causes adrenal hyperplasia.

Clinical and Laboratory Evaluation

History
Patients with excessive cortisol secretion typically present with one or more of the following characteristics: obesity, short stature, delayed puberty,

hyperpigmentation, hirsutism, easy bruisability, and muscular weakness. Rarely, children may present with polyuria, polydipsia (resulting from glucocorticoid excess causing hyperglycemia), or personality changes.

Physical Examination

Obesity with a centripetal fat distribution is present, with accumulation in the face, neck, trunk, and abdomen, together with a wasted appearance of the extremities. The typical facial appearance is "moon facies," with chubby cheeks and double chin. In addition, a "buffalo hump" resulting from an increased fat pad in the supraclavicular and dorsocervical region may be evident. Short stature and delayed puberty may also occur; short stature may be the only presenting symptom in some children. Hyperpigmentation may occur with ACTH excess. Excessive hair growth is also commonly seen in children with Cushing syndrome. If the adrenal tumor is producing androgens as well as glucocorticoids, virilization may be apparent.

Laboratory Evaluation

Laboratory studies may indicate:

* Fasting hyperglycemia
* Normal sodium and normal or low potassium
* Hypercalciuria with normal serum calcium and phosphorous
* Hyperinsulinemia
* Elevation of plasma lipoproteins
* CBC: leukocytosis and lymphopenia
* ACTH level: high with primary pituitary pathology, low with primary adrenal pathology

A 24-hour urine collection for free cortisol and creatinine reveals elevated cortisol level (normal: 7–25 μg/g creatinine for prepubertal children). An overnight dexamethasone suppression test (20 μg/kg up to a maximum of 1 mg) at 11:00 P.M. with serum cortisol obtained at 8:00 A.M. (normal suppressed cortisol < 5 μg/dl).

If these tests reveal increased secretion of cortisol, a prolonged dexamethasone suppression test is warranted. A CT or MRI scan to assess the presence of a pituitary or adrenal tumor is necessary, based on the results of the above tests and with the patient's age taken into account (< 7 years means the tumor is more likely of adrenal origin).

Differential Diagnosis

The differential diagnosis for the constellation of symptoms seen with cortisol excess includes exogenous glucocorticoid ingestion and exogenous obesity. Obtaining a complete history usually rules out exogenous steroids; however, ACTH stimulation may be necessary to confirm suppression of the adrenal glands in the presence of physical signs of glucocorticoid excess.

Patients with exogenous obesity typically have normal cortisol values and a history of increased nutritional intake or decreased activity level. In addition, patients with exogenous obesity typically have normal or tall stature.

Pediatric Pearl

Overweight children with short stature warrant careful evaluation for the presence of endocrine dysfunction (hypothyroidism, Cushing syndrome, GH deficiency). Overweight children with tall stature *do not* have Cushing syndrome.

Management

In the case of excessive pituitary ACTH release, management includes transsphenoidal microsurgery, with a remission rate of 85%–95%. Irradiation of the pituitary gland has also been successful in 80% of patients. However, the risk of hypopituitarism is high after irradiation. During and after surgery, glucocorticoid replacement is essential. Postoperatively, hypoadrenalism may continue for several years, requiring replacement. Treatment of adrenal gland tumors consists of surgical removal with replacement of glucocorticoids until the remaining adrenal gland is functioning normally.

DISORDERS OF WATER BALANCE

Water balance is governed by the action of **ADH,** which is regulated by changes in serum osmolality and intravascular volume (Figure 14.5). Alterations in serum osmolality are detected by osmoreceptors that reside in the supraoptic and paraventricular nuclei of the neurohypophysis. The osmoreceptors respond to changes in osmolality as small as 2% and cause alterations in the secretion of ADH and **angiotensin II**. In addition, baroreceptors located in the atria and carotid bodies respond to changes in intravascular volume with subsequent alterations in ADH secretion and thirst. Negative feedback mechanisms include the oropharyngeal reflex, which inhibits further thirst as well as ADH release. **Atrial natriuretic factor** also plays a role in negative feedback. ADH exerts its effect in the kidney at the level of the collecting

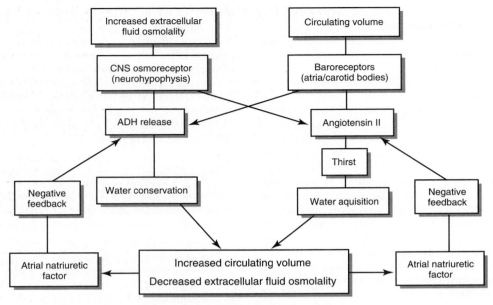

FIGURE 14.5 Regulation of antidiuretic hormone (ADH) secretion. CNS = central nervous system.

duct. In the presence of ADH, the collecting duct becomes more permeable and allows an increase in intravascular volume, with subsequent decline in urine volume.

The disorders of water metabolism can be broken down into **hyponatremic** and **hypernatremic** states (Table 14.14).

DIABETES INSIPIDUS

Pathophysiology

Diabetes insipidus, the traditional name for the condition in which individuals pass large volumes of tasteless (nonsweet) urine, is the inability to concentrate the urine. The etiology may be lack of ADH secretion **(central diabetes insipidus)** or decreased responsiveness of the collecting duct to ADH **(nephrogenic diabetes insipidus)**.

Clinical and Laboratory Evaluation

History

Symptoms of diabetes insipidus in children include polyuria, nocturia, and enuresis in a previously toilet-trained child; clear urine (including first morning urine); poor weight gain; thirst with preference for iced water; and irritability when fluids are withheld. If the diabetes insipidus is due to the presence of a hypothalamic

TABLE 14.14 Disorders of Water Metabolism	
Causes of Hypernatremia	**Causes of Hyponatremia**
Hypervolemic (excess of body Na)	Hypervolemic (edema)
Iatrogenic (error in infant formula preparation)	Congestive heart failure
Salt poisoning	Nephrotic syndrome
Hypovolemic (total body water deficiency)	Cirrhosis
Insufficient intake	Hypovolemic (total body Na decreased)
Excessive loss	Hemorrhage
Renal (diabetes insipidus)	Diarrhea
Gastrointestinal (diarrhea/vomiting)	Diuretics
Burns	Adrenal insufficiency
	Euvolemic (syndrome of inappropriate secretion of antidiuretic hormone)

or pituitary tumor, strabismus, double vision, poor growth, precocious puberty, headache, and vomiting may be present. The severity of symptoms varies, depending on the etiology of the diabetes insipidus as well as on the preservation of thirst, diet, extent of ADH deficiency, and kidney function.

In **familial vasopressin-sensitive diabetes insipidus,** a family history reveals other members with symptoms of polyuria and polydipsia. Typically, symptoms do not occur until after infancy. MRI or CT scans of affected individuals have not shown any abnormalities in the hypothalamic or pituitary area. In addition, studies have shown that affected individuals are capable of vasopressin secretion, leading to the theory of an inherited defect in osmoreceptors. Autosomal dominant inheritance and X-linked inheritance have been described.

Nephrogenic diabetes insipidus is transmitted as an X-linked disorder. Symptoms usually develop within the first 3 weeks of life, although typically the diagnosis is delayed. A history of failure to thrive, vomiting, irritability, constipation, and intermittent fevers is commonly obtained. However, by the time of diagnosis, children are usually severely dehydrated and malnourished.

Physical Examination

In infants, hyperthermia, rapid weight loss, and vascular collapse may be seen. In addition, vomiting, constipation, and growth failure may be present. In older children, weight loss, mild dehydration, and distention of the bladder occur. In the presence of a tumor, signs of increased intracranial pressure may be present, as well as visual field deficits, blindness, and optic atrophy.

Laboratory Evaluation

Laboratory studies reveal:

- Serum sodium usually greater than 140 mEq/L
- Urine osmolality inappropriately dilute in the presence of serum hypertonicity (serum osmolality > 280 mOsm/kg). A water deprivation test reveals the excretion of a dilute urine with osmolality less than plasma osmolality, a rise in the serum sodium of more than 145 mEq/L, a serum osmolality of more than 290 mOsm/kg, and a weight loss of 3%–5%.

Administration of ADH, or its analog, DDAVP, results in increased urine osmolality. MRI of the pituitary/hypothalamus is warranted to evaluate for the presence of tumor, histiocytosis X, or empty sella syndrome. In addition, other laboratory studies to evaluate function of other pituitary hormones (e.g., thyroid hormone, IGF-I) are appropriate.

Patients with nephrogenic diabetes insipidus present with hypernatremia, serum hypertonicity, elevated uric acid concentrations, and dilute urine despite the presence of high intrinsic ADH levels. After exogenous vasopressin administration, a dilute urine and serum hypertonicity continue to be present.

Differential Diagnosis (Table 14.15)

A careful history, including family history of failure to thrive, polyuria, and polydipsia, and the previously described laboratory tests usually reveal the specific etiology. Patients with neurologic changes or evidence of other hormonal deficiency or excess should be evaluated for the presence of a pituitary tumor. In addition, patients who present with diabetes insipidus, otorrhea, or bone pain should raise suspicions of histiocytosis X.

Management

The goal of treatment of diabetes insipidus is achievement of normal growth and weight gain and avoidance of hypertonic dehydration. The

---

TABLE 14.15 **Differential Diagnosis of Diabetes Insipidus**

Central diabetes insipidus
    Vasopressin deficiency
Physiologic suppression of vasopressin secretion
    Psychogenic polydipsia
    Organic polydipsia (hypothalamic disease)
    Drug-induced polydipsia
Reduced renal responsiveness to vasopressin
    Genetic (nephrogenic diabetes insipidus,
        medullary cystic disease)
Pharmacologic
    Lithium
    Diuretics
Osmotic diuresis
    Diabetes mellitus
Electrolyte disturbance
    Hypercalcemia
    Hypokalemia
Renal disease
    Postobstructive diuresis
    Renal tubular acidosis
    Sickle cell disease
Hemodynamic
    Hyperthyroidism

management of central diabetes insipidus involves hormonal replacement with DDAVP, a synthetic analog of arginine vasopressin. The usual dose for children is 2.5–10 μg intranasally once or twice daily. Subcutaneous or intravenous administration at one-tenth the intranasal dose is also possible. In patients with an intact thirst mechanism, the clinician may adjust the dosage as needed to maintain normal serum osmolality and sodium. In patients lacking an intact thirst mechanism, specific fluid requirements must be met in addition to the vasopressin replacement.

Treatment for nephrogenic diabetes insipidus requires high water intake with frequent feedings. Restriction of sodium and salt intake is warranted to prevent enhancement of water loss. Studies have shown that the diuretic chlorothiazide is effective in maintaining serum sodium between 132 and 137 mEq/L, as long as dietary intake of sodium is restricted. Side effects of this therapy include increased serum uric acid and hypokalemia. Indomethacin also has proven effectiveness in the treatment of nephrogenic diabetes insipidus; this agent enhances proximal tubular reabsorption of the glomerular filtrate.

SYNDROME OF INAPPROPRIATE SECRETION OF ANTIDIURETIC HORMONE (SIADH)

Pathophysiology

SIADH is characterized by excessive secretion of vasopressin despite the presence of hyponatremia and the absence of osmotic or nonosmotic stimuli. It occurs in several diseases, usually of the brain or lung, and during therapy with several drugs (Table 14.16).

Clinical and Laboratory Evaluation

History

Patients with SIADH may present with weight gain, weakness, anorexia, nausea and vomiting, personality changes, or lethargy. In severe cases, convulsions and coma may occur as a result of hypotonicity of the serum. In addition, symptoms of an underlying disease (e.g., pneumonia, intracranial process, malignancy) may be present.

The clinician should elicit a complete medication history to rule out drug-induced SIADH. Medications known to stimulate ADH release include clofibrate, chlorpropamide, thiazides, carbamazepine, phenothiazines, vincristine, and cyclophosphamide.

TABLE 14.16 Conditions Associated with Syndromes of Inappropriate Secretion of Antidiuretic Hormone in Children
Pulmonary diseases
Asthma
Pneumonia (viral, bacterial, or fungal)
Pneumothorax
Positive pressure breathing
Acute respiratory failure
Tuberculosis
Central nervous system disorders
Meningitis, encephalitis
Guillain-Barré syndrome
Head trauma
Brain abscess
Brain tumors
Hydrocephalus
Neonatal hypoxia
Respiratory distress syndrome
Aplasia of corpus callosum
Acute intermittent porphyria
General surgery
Drugs
Vasopressin
Desmopressin
Oxytocin
Vinca alkaloids
Cyclophosphamide
Carbamazepine
Clofibrate
Tricyclic antidepressants
Monoamine oxidase inhibitors

Physical Examination

In cases of mild hyponatremia, the physical examination may be completely normal; however, in severe cases patients may be lethargic, comatose, or convulsing. It is worth noting the presence or absence of hypotension, tachycardia, and pitting edema. In the presence of these signs, SIADH is unlikely, and it is necessary to consider a more extensive differential diagnosis.

Laboratory Evaluation

Laboratory studies reveal:

- Serum sodium levels less than 135 mEq/L
- Serum osmolality less than 270 mOsm
- Urine sodium usually increased [fractional excretion of sodium (FE_{Na}) > 1%], with FENa calculated by the following formula:

$$FE_{Na} = \frac{[Urine\ Na/serum\ Na]}{[Urine\ Cr/serum\ Cr]}$$

- Urine osmolality greater than 100 mOsm/kg

- Normal serum BUN/creatinine and uric acid levels
- Elevated serum arginine vasopressin

The use of other laboratory tests depends on the clinician's suspicions of possible underlying etiologies of SIADH (i.e., tumor, meningitis).

Differential Diagnosis

The differential diagnosis of hypotonic hyponatremia involves either excessive water ingestion or decreased water excretion (Table 14.17). First it is necessary to confirm the presence of hypotonicity because falsely lowered sodium values may occur in the presence of hyperglycemia, hyperlipidemia, and other agents that cause an artifactually low serum sodium. In these instances, the serum osmolality is normal or high, whereas in hyponatremia associated with SIADH, it is low (generally < 270 mOsm/kg). Exclusion of disorders other than SIADH is possible based on the history and physical examination. Other laboratory data may be necessary to rule out hypothyroidism or cortisol deficiency.

Management

The management of SIADH should include treatment of the underlying disorder if present. Therapy then is directed at *slowly* raising the serum sodium level (0.5–1.0 mEq/L/hr) to prevent the neurologic complication of central pontine myelinolysis. Fluid restriction cause a steady rise in

---

TABLE 14.17 **Differential Diagnosis of Hypotonic Hyponatremia**

Excessive water ingestion
Decreased water excretion
   Decreased solute delivery to diluting segment
      Starvation
   AVP excess
      SIADH
      Drug-induced AVP secretion
   AVP excess with decreased distal solute
   delivery
      Congestive heart failure
      Cirrhosis of the liver
      Nephrotic syndrome
      Cortisol deficiency
      Hypothyroidism
      Diuretic use
      Renal failure

AVP = arginine vasopressin (ADH); SIADH = syndrome of inappropriate (secretion of) antidiuretic hormone.

---

serum sodium and osmolality, as well as weight loss. Generally, fluid restriction to 50%–75% of maintenance requirements is effective. If hyponatremic seizures occur, it is necessary to give 3% saline (5 ml/kg) slowly until the seizures stop.

Drug therapy to induce vasopressin resistance has been effective in adults but should not be used in children. Medical personnel should be alert to the underlying disorders known to cause SIADH so that earlier diagnosis and treatment may occur (see Table 14.16).

DIABETES MELLITUS

Pathophysiology

Diabetes mellitus (DM) is best described as a disorder of metabolism of carbohydrate, fat, and protein, leading to calorie wastage and accompanied by long-term sequelae involving the heart, eyes, kidneys, and the nervous system. As is true with many of the chronic diseases seen in the pediatric population, psychosocial issues complicate the disease process even further. **Type 1 DM** (juvenile-onset diabetes), the most common form of diabetes in the pediatric population, affects approximately 1–2 children per 1000. Type 1 DM is a state of relative **insulin deficiency** in which individuals are prone to ketosis. In comparison, rarer forms of childhood DM such as the most common form of maturity-onset diabetes of youth (MODY) and classic type 2 DM are states of **insulin resistance**.

Proinsulin, the precursor to insulin, is synthesized in the beta cells of the pancreas as a single coiled protein consisting of two chains: A and B, which are connected by a connecting or C peptide and held together by disulfide bonds (Figure 14.6). When insulin is released systemically, the 31–amino acid C peptide is cleaved from the molecule to form active insulin. The amount of insulin released is dependent on input from the autonomic nervous system, level of caloric intake, exercise, and hormonal influences. GH, glucagon, glucocorticoids, and estrogens all stimulate insulin release; however, they also antagonize the effect of insulin in peripheral tissues.

Insulin acts primarily to drive glucose rapidly into the cell to provide fuel for cellular metabolism in almost all cells in the body, but especially in the liver, muscles, and fat. Insulin inhibits gluconeogenesis and promotes the conversion of liver glucose into fatty acids. Insulin deficiency stimulates excess production of the ketone bodies acetone and β-hydroxybutyrate, which can cause severe metabolic acidosis and even death.

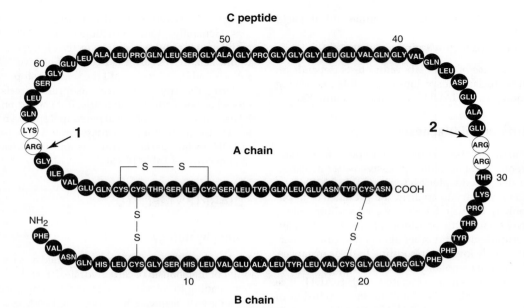

FIGURE 14.6 Proinsulin. *Arrows 1* and *2* indicate the two sites of cleavage that yield insulin and C peptide.

Peak age of onset of type 1 DM is usually 9 years of age. Ninety percent of these patients are positive for either the DR3 or DR4 human leukocyte antigen (HLA), but the HLA type is insufficient to account for all the new cases of DM. It is theorized that a combination of genetic predisposition and antigenemia provoking an autoimmune response that attacks and destroys the beta cells is responsible for subsequent insulinopenia ("double hit" theory) [Figure 14.7]. The predilection for an exaggerated autoimmune response is implicated in the increased incidence of thyroiditis in patients with type 1 DM.

Approximately 15%–30% of children with new onset of insulin-dependent diabetes present initially in **diabetic ketoacidosis** (DKA). This situation is most commonly seen in children younger than 5 years of age. DKA occurs when there is a

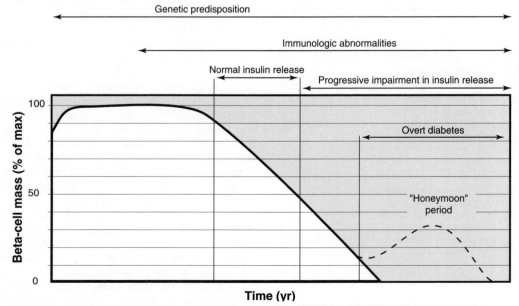

FIGURE 14.7. Proposed scheme of natural history of beta-cell defect in diabetes. Overt diabetes becomes manifest only after destruction of 80%–90% of cell reserve.

decrease in insulin action, as well as an increase in the production of counterregulatory hormones such as epinephrine, norepinephrine, glucagon, cortisol, and GH, all of which have effects opposite to those of insulin.

In children previously diagnosed with insulin-dependent DM, the inciting factor may be infection or vomiting. When children are ill, the cellular glucose requirement increases, and subsequently, the need for insulin also rises. In part, this increased requirement is due to the increased production of counterregulatory hormones associated with illness. Although baseline insulin production in these children may be just barely adequate, there may be a relative lack of insulin action under these conditions of increased glucose needs. Glucose cannot be utilized by cells, and energy production from other substrates must ensue (Figure 14.8).

In addition to the hyperglycemia and ketosis in DKA, electrolyte disturbances, dehydration, and metabolic acidosis are usually present. When the blood glucose exceeds the renal threshold for reabsorption, glycosuria occurs. The osmotic diuresis that results from glycosuria causes fluid and electrolyte losses, leading to low levels of serum sodium, potassium, and phosphate. Other mechanisms of fluid loss in DKA aside from fluid loss resulting from osmotic diuresis include vomiting and the hyperventilation that is a response to the acidosis. Patients with DKA can rapidly lose as much as 7%–10% of their body weight through these mechanisms.

Clinical and Laboratory Evaluation

History

Most patients previously diagnosed with insulin-dependent diabetes and with good glucose control on their current insulin regimen give a history of some inciting illness such as gastroenteritis or a cold, which lead to increasing blood glucose levels. With continued hyperglycemia and stress, polyuria and polydipsia occur. Patients frequently complain of abdominal pain and headache, which are due to the ketonemia. In addition, alterations in consciousness, altered respiratory patterns, air hunger, and acetone breath may be present. In those patients not previously diagnosed with diabetes, the history may include a period of polyuria, polydipsia, polyphagia, bed-wetting in previously toilet-trained children, and weight loss, with progression of the severity of these symptoms eventually leading to DKA.

Physical Examination

The physical examination of patients with DKA may reveal all or some of the following features:

- **HEENT:** Dry mucous membranes, papilledema (if cerebral edema is present), lymphadenopathy, signs of infection (i.e., an injected oropharynx), and acetone breath
- **Cardiovascular:** Orthostatic hypotension, thready pulses, tachycardia, and heart murmur due to dehydration and underlying illness. In the presence of increased intracranial pres-

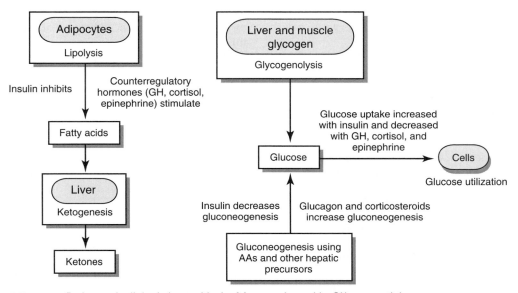

FIGURE 14.8. Pathways in diabetic ketoacidosis. AAs = amino acids; GH = growth hormone.

sure, Cushing triad (altered respiratory pattern, bradycardia, and hypertension) may be present.

- **Pulmonary:** Kussmaul breathing (deep, rapid)
- **Abdomen:** Abdominal pain, decreased bowel sounds
- **Skin:** Decreased turgor
- **Neurologic:** Altered mental status (obtundation, combativeness, coma), signs of increased intracranial pressure (papilledema, dilated, unresponsive pupils)

Laboratory Evaluation

DIABETIC KETOACIDOSIS. Laboratory studies reveal:

- Blood glucose level usually greater than 300 mg/dl
- Ketonemia (ketones positive at > 1:2 dilution of serum)
- Acidosis (bicarbonate < 15 mEq/L and pH ≤ 7.30)
- Sodium may be low, normal, or high, depending on the glucose level and state of hydration. Low sodium is due to renal loss as well as dilutional effects from the osmotic actions of elevated intravascular glucose. Serum sodium decreases by 1.6 mEq/L for every 100-mg/dl increment in blood glucose over 100 mg/dl.
- Low phosphorus
- Increased serum osmolarity
- Elevated BUN
- Normal or high creatinine
- Increased anion gap
- Arterial blood gas [metabolic acidosis (low bicarbonate, low PCO_2, pH < 7.30) varying with the severity of illness]
- Elevated white blood cell (WBC) count with shift to the left
- Ketonuria, glucosuria

DIABETES MELLITUS. Follow-up every 3–4 months, with examination and an HbA_{1c} level, is usually appropriate. Because glucose nonenzymatically glycosylates many proteins in the body, including the hemoglobin molecule, measurement of HbA_{1c} represents a time-honored method of determining control over the previous 1–2 months, as opposed to the instant in time represented by a random blood glucose sample. In general, attempt to achieve as low a value as possible (7%–9%) without risking severe life-threatening hypoglycemia.

Patients with type 1 DM have a high incidence of autoimmune thyroid disease, and thyroid function tests are necessary on a yearly basis. Beginning 3–5 years after diagnosis, an ophthalmology examination and a urinalysis are recommended on a yearly basis to screen for retinopathy and nephropathy, respectively. Patients with proteinuria (> 150 μg/min) are at significant risk for the development of nephrosclerosis and progressive renal failure.

Differential Diagnosis

The diagnosis of DKA, once it is considered, is relatively easy to make. The differential diagnosis of metabolic acidosis in children is relatively limited (Table 14.18). Patients with normal or high urine output despite signs of dehydration, recurrent vomiting, and abdominal pain warrant evaluation for the presence of diabetes.

Management

Diabetic Ketoacidosis

The management of DKA includes very close monitoring of the patient, usually in a pediatric intensive care unit (see Chapter 24). Monitoring of the patient should include constant observation, at least until the anion gap normalizes, arterial pH is greater than 7.25, and serum bicarbonate has begun to rise. Use of a cardiorespiratory monitor is warranted until the patient's metabolic status has normalized.

Admission laboratories should include the following: serum glucose, electrolytes, phosphate, calcium, BUN, creatinine, serum acetone, CBC with differential, and urinalysis. In addition, an arterial blood gas is necessary in patients with altered level of consciousness, abnormal respiratory pattern, or serum bicarbonate of less than 15 mEq/L.

When an infection is suspected, appropriate cultures are warranted. Subsequent laboratory data should include:

- Anion gap calculation every 2 hours
- Blood glucose level every hour (more frequently when adjusting the insulin drip)

TABLE 14.18 **Differential Diagnosis of Metabolic Acidosis in Children**

Lactic acidosis (ischemia, sepsis)
Diabetic ketoacidosis (DKA)
Severe diarrhea
Renal failure and uremia
Organic acidurias
Ingestions (methanol, ethylene glycol, acetone)
Salicylate poisoning (late)
Nonketotic hyperosmolar coma

- Serum electrolytes every 2 hours (more frequently under the following conditions:

1. Initial potassium: < 5 mEq/L or > 6.5 mEq/L
2. No administration of parenteral potassium
3. KCl infusion: > 40 mEq/L/hr or > 0.5 mEq/kg/hr
4. Bicarbonate infusion
5. Significant hyperosmolarity

- Urine ketones every void
- Serum calcium level when giving bicarbonate or phosphate

Fluid resuscitation varies with the individual patient and the severity of illness. Accurate intake and output records are essential and may require placement of a urinary catheter to follow the urine output closely. In addition, twice-daily weights help determine fluid status. Patients who are vomiting or hyperventilating or who have an altered level of consciousness should have nothing by mouth until their status improves. Typically, patients with DKA are 5%–10% dehydrated. If available, weights from before the onset of DKA help determine the degree of dehydration. In addition, serum osmolality can be used to estimate percent dehydration, calculated using the following formula:

$$[Na^+ \times 2] + \left[\frac{\text{blood glucose (mg/dl)}}{18} \right] + \left[\frac{\text{BUN (mg/dl)}}{2.8} \right]$$

The percent increase of the patient's osmolality over normal (275–290 mOsm/kg) reflects the degree of dehydration.

Fluid resuscitation should be provided by intravenous solutions (Table 14.19). Initial fluids should not contain glucose. When the blood glucose level falls to less than 250 mg/dl, glucose can then be added to the intravenous fluids.

It is essential to calculate the sodium content of the resuscitation fluid based on body deficits, dehydration, and ongoing losses (see Chapter 4). In patients with DKA, the use of separate intravenous solutions for maintenance and deficit replacement, urine replacement, and administration of insulin is easier and allows easy adjustment to keep up with changing conditions of ongoing loss.

Insuline administration in patients with DKA should occur by continuous intravenous infusion of regular insulin. The initial rate is 0.05–0.1 units/kg/hr, which may be increased, depending on severity of acidosis and hyperglycemia. The aim is an approximate 50–100 mg/dl/hr decline in blood glucose and a 0.5 mEq/L/hr rise in bicarbonate.

TABLE 14.19 **Fluid Resuscitation for Diabetic Ketoacidosis***

Initial
- Treat hypovolemic shock by replenishing intravascular volume with normal saline at 10–20 ml/kg.
- An arterial line should be placed for close monitoring of blood, gases, glucose, and electrolytes—only in critically ill children.

Subsequent
- Replace remaining deficit by correcting half of the deficit in the first 16–24 hours and the remaining deficit over the next 24 hours. 0.5 normal saline with KCl 40 mEq/L typically is used. In the presence of fever, hyperventilation, or vomiting, additional losses must be replaced.
- Replace urine loss.

---

*Avoid fluid replacement in excess of 4 L/m²/day because of the risk of cerebral edema.

If these values are not attained, the infusion of insulin can be adjusted. When the serum glucose nears 250 mg/dl, dextrose should be added to the intravenous fluid at a concentration of approximately 3 g dextrose/unit of insulin. The rate of dextrose or insulin infusion should be altered to keep the blood glucose at approximately 200 mg/dl. The minimum rate of insulin infusion is 0.025–0.05 units/kg/hr. With a lower rate, the acidosis may worsen because intracellular glucose is not adequate, and further lipolysis, glycogenolysis, and ketosis may occur.

When the blood glucose is in the range of 200–250 mg/dl, serum ketones are cleared, and the anion gap is normal, subcutaneous insulin injections may be started, and the insulin drip discontinued.

In general, bicarbonate by rapid infusion or bolus is not given unless the acidosis is severe and is not responsive to fluids and insulin infusion because the blood–brain barrier is freely permeable to carbon dioxide, whereas bicarbonate equilibrates in the cerebrospinal fluid (CSF) slowly. Thus, large doses of bicarbonate may cause a paradoxical fall in cerebrospinal pH, resulting in cerebral blood vessel dilatation and an increase in intracranial volume, which may cause apnea, coma, or death. If bicarbonate is administered, 1 mEq/kg may be given in a diluted fashion over an hour under constant supervision.

Potassium requirements generally are higher than usual in patients with DKA because of increased urinary losses secondary to acidosis and osmotic diuresis. The addition of KCl (20–40 mEq/L) to intravenous fluids usually is sufficient to replace the body deficit of potassium.

Diabetes Mellitus

The rationale behind treating DM is to normalize glucose metabolism and avoid or delay the long-term complications associated with insulin deficiency. Neuropathy, nephropathy, retinopathy, and cardiomyopathy are just a few of the known complications of DM. Clearly, prevention is the most cost-effective way of dealing with these conditions. Recent studies have suggested that better glucose control is strongly associated with a more favorable prognosis; thus, optimizing insulin therapy is of major importance.

Several insulin preparations are available. Human insulin is available in long-, short-, and intermediate-acting strengths. Therapy is geared to maintain blood glucose values within the range of 80–150 mg/dl, with the occurrence of as few hypoglycemic episodes as possible.

Pediatric Pearl

It is important to note that seeking too tight control may place patients at risk for significant life-threatening hypoglycemia.

Management of most patients involves a combination of short- and long-acting insulin preparations (Table 14.20). The usual total daily dose is approximately 0.5–1.0 units/kg, divided into two-thirds at breakfast and one-third at dinner. This regimen is further subdivided into two-thirds intermediate-acting and one-third short-acting preparations. These recommendations are only an approximate guide; each patient's therapy is individualized. It is expected that patients will monitor both their blood sugar levels three to four times daily using the fingerstick method and their urine for the presence of ketones when they become hyperglycemic or sick.

Although most newly diagnosed patients can be managed as outpatients, some clinicians rec-ommend initial hospitalization to facilitate a multidisciplinary approach. Professional participants should include social workers, nutritionists, nurses, and pediatricians.

Other approaches for optimizing diabetes control include different insulin delivery systems such as the subcutaneous insulin pump and oral or inhaled forms of insulin. The insulin pump, a device worn externally and programmed by the patient, ensures a continuous flow of insulin without the presence of a feedback mechanism and allows maximal flexibility in dietary consumption of carbohydrates. Researchers are also examining fetal pancreatic tissue as a possible candidate for transplantation and designing more sophisticated and noninvasive devices to monitor blood glucose values.

DISORDERS OF THE THYROID GLAND

Pathophysiology

One of the major actions of the thyroid gland is to concentrate exogenous iodide in the body and to convert it into a hormonally active form that is then released to exert its effect on peripheral tissues. Biosynthesis of the active hormone occurs through a number of steps (Figure 14.9). Active transport of iodide into the thyroid gland leads to oxidation of the iodide and iodination of the tyrosyl residues within the thyroglobulin, followed by coupling of the iodotyrosines to form the active compounds thyroxine (T_4) and triiodothyronine (T_3). The active transport of iodide allows sufficient concentration of iodide in the gland despite meager dietary intake. Through this mechanism, thyroid hormone is coupled to its specific binding protein, thyroglobulin, which forms the bulk of the colloid found within the thyroid follicle. Endocytosis of the iodinated thyroglobulin from the stores of colloid and subsequent pinocytosis into the thyroid follicular cell are the first

TABLE 14.20 Insulin Preparations		
Type	**Onset of Action**	**Duration of Action (hr)**
Humalog (very short acting)	5–10 min	2–4
Regular, Novolog (very short acting)	0.5–2 hr	3–6
NPH, lente (intermediate acting)	3–6 hr	12–20
Ultralente (long acting)	6–12 hr	18–36
Lantus (extremely long acting)	1–2 hr	24 hr +

NPH = neutral protamine Hagedorn (insulin).

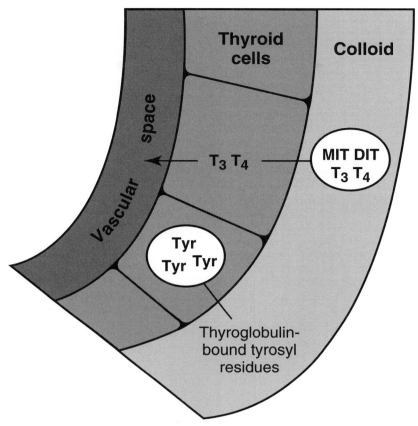

FIGURE 14.9. Biosynthesis of thyroid hormone. Oxidized iodide combines with thyroglobulin-bound tyrosyl (Tyr) residues to form monoiodotyrosine (MIT), diiodotyrosine (DIT), triiodothyronine (T_3), and thyroxine (T_4). Endocytosis, followed by proteolysis of the thyroglobulin molecule by lysosomes, releases T_3, T_4, DIT, and MIT. MIT and DIT are then deiodinated, and the iodide is reutilized, while T_4 and T_3 are released into the systemic circulation.

steps in the release of thyroid hormone into the periphery. Hydrolysis of the thyroglobulin molecule occurs with subsequent release of free T_4 and free T_3 into the peripheral circulation.

Regulation of the release of thyroid hormone into the periphery takes place by a complex system of feedback loops (Figure 14.10). Thyroid-stimulating hormone (TSH) from the pituitary binds to its specific receptor on the surface of the thyroid follicular cell, stimulating an increase in 3′,5′-cyclic adenosine monophosphate (cAMP). This causes the gland to enlarge and initiates a number of processes within the thyroid hormone biosynthetic pathway, ultimately causing an increase in thyroid hormone release. Thyroid-releasing hormone (TRH), a tripeptide produced in the hypothalamus, is transported to cells in the anterior pituitary that produce TSH via the pituitary portal vascular system. TRH synthesis, which increases in response to decreasing body temperature and decreased serum levels of T_4 and T_3, diminishes via negative feedback resulting from increased levels of T_3. TSH increases in response to increasing concentrations of TRH and low levels of T_4 and T_3. Production of T_4 occurs only in the thyroid gland, whereas manufacture of T_3 takes place not only in the thyroid gland but also in many cells in the periphery by monodeiodination of T_4. T_3 has approximately four times the biologic potency and ten times the affinity for nuclear thyroid receptors of T_4.

The more important biologic actions of thyroid hormone, which are many, include increased amino acid turnover, calorigenesis, thermogenesis, augmentation of the β-adrenergic system, and increased growth. Thyroid hormone is also essen-

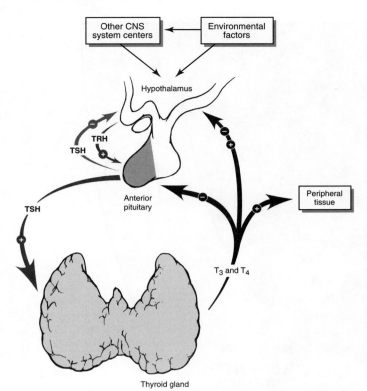

FIGURE 14.10. Feedback loops involved in regulation of thyroid hormone release. CNS = central nervous system; T3 = triiodothyronine; T4 = thyroxine; TRH = thyrotropin-releasing hormone; TSH = thyroid-stimulating hormone.

tial for neonatal brain growth, as evidenced by the development of mental retardation in untreated patients with primary congenital hypothyroidism.

Hypothyroidism

Hypothyroidism can be divided into two large categories, **congenital** and **acquired**. The congenital form can be further subdivided into **primary** (aplasia or hypoplasia of the thyroid gland; common), **secondary** (TSH deficiency; rare), and **tertiary** (TRH deficiency; rarest).

The incidence of primary congenital hypothyroidism is approximately 1 in 3500–5000 live births. The signs and symptoms of congenital hypothyroidism are insidious. The seriousness of the long-term effects of the condition, if left undetected (mental retardation), has resulted in the development of sensitive neonatal screening programs to avoid preventable retardation. Since the inception of these programs in the late 1970s, the incidence of complications from untreated primary congenital hypothyroidism has decreased significantly.

In the acquired form of hypothyroidism, an autoimmune phenomenon with lymphocytic infiltration of the thyroid gland is most common. However, any process that leads to destruction of the thyroid gland ultimately leads to hypothyroidism.

Hyperthyroidism

Hyperthyroidism may be due to either local or diffuse overproduction of thyroid hormone. In children, hyperthyroidism is almost always due to **Graves disease**. In this condition, the thyroid gland autonomously produces large amounts of T_4 and T_3. Graves disease generally results from an autoimmune phenomenon in which antibodies directed at the TSH receptor on the surface of the follicular cells bind and stimulate production of thyroid hormone.

It is now believed that both autoimmune lymphocytic infiltration of the thyroid gland with subsequent hypothyroidism **(Hashimoto thyroiditis)** and **Graves disease** may both be part of a continuum of autoimmune thyroid diseases. Indeed, it is not uncommon to find patients with one form of autoimmune thyroid disease who have a strong family history of the other type of autoimmune thyroid disease.

Clinical and Laboratory Evaluation

History

Patients with classic untreated **congenital hypothyroidism** often present 6–12 weeks after birth with a typical appearance, characterized by a thickened, protuberant tongue, hoarse cry, muscle hypotonia, umbilical hernia, constipation, bradycardia, and prolonged indirect hyperbilirubinemia. These signs are often subtle and easily missed. Although screening for congenital hypothyroidism is now almost universal in the United States, certain methodologic flaws with the testing, which are beyond the scope of this chapter, do exist. Thus, when encountering children with suspicious signs or symptoms, the physician must always keep this diagnosis in mind.

Older infants and children with **acquired hypothyroidism** may present with growth failure, bone age retardation, and delayed or precocious puberty. Other signs of **hypothyroidism** include decreased appetite, lethargy, constipation, dry skin and hair, and prolonged tendon reflex relaxation time. Acquired hypothyroidism is often difficult to diagnose on clinical grounds, because the signs and symptoms are often insidious.

Patients with **hyperthyroidism** may complain of heat intolerance, nervousness, palpitations, increased appetite, proximal muscle weakness, difficulty sleeping, inattention, and emotional lability. Physical signs may include weight loss, tremor, shortened deep tendon reflex relaxation time, and a hyperdynamic precordium. The classic ophthalmopathy of Graves disease is less frequently seen in the pediatric age group, in contrast to adults. However, it is not uncommon to see lid lag and an unusual stare, which are due to the effect of excessive thyroid hormone on the sympathetic nervous system.

Physical Examination

When inspecting the thyroid gland, the physician should look for any asymmetry. The space between the sternocleidomastoid muscle and trachea should be symmetrical. The clinician should stand behind the patient, extend the neck slightly while palpating the thyroid gland, and note the size, texture, presence of nodules, and presence of pain. It is necessary to ask the patient to swallow and feel the gland as it rises with swallowing. In addition, it is appropriate to feel the cricoid cartilage; the isthmus of the thyroid should be directly beneath this. Documentation of the presence of a bruit in an enlarged gland is also warranted.

Laboratory Evaluation

The cornerstone of laboratory diagnosis of disorders of the thyroid gland relies on the use of sensitive serum TSH assays and T_4 levels. Today, almost all neonates born in the United States are screened for a variety of diseases, including phenylketonuria and hypothyroidism, before discharge from the hospital. Blood, most often obtained by a heel stick, is subsequently blotted on filter paper. In California, for example, T_4 is initially assayed, and the lowest 10% of T_4 serum samples are then assayed for elevated TSH values. Providing there is an intact hypothalamic–pituitary axis, elevation in TSH represents a state of inadequate thyroid hormone production. Conversely, the suppression of TSH represents a state of thyroid hormone excess, either endogenous or exogenous. In some cases, patients who have clinical signs of hyperthyroidism but who have normal levels of TSH and T_4 may have isolated elevations of T_3, so-called T_3 toxicosis.

Growth failure may be the only manifestation of hypothyroidism. Therefore, it may be necessary to obtain thyroid function tests on all patients referred for short stature or disorders of sexual maturation.

It is necessary to obtain antithyroglobulin and antimicrosomal antibodies in patients with a goiter as part of the evaluation of autoimmune thyroiditis. Ultrasonography may be necessary when there is a question as to the presence of nodules. Fine needle aspiration is an extremely useful technique in evaluating solitary nodules for the presence of malignancy, a rare phenomenon in children.

Pediatric Pearl

Usually a TSH and total T_4 are sufficient to make a diagnosis of hyper- or hypothyroidism.

Differential Diagnosis

The differential diagnosis of abnormal thyroid function involves a number of conditions (Table 14.21). Most children with acquired hypothyroidism have autoantibodies directed at the thyroid gland; the presence of an enlarged thyroid gland (goiter) is variable.

Approximately 10% of patients with DM have evidence of elevated TSH, indicating primary hy-

TABLE 14.21 Differential Diagnosis of Abnormal Thyroid Function Tests
Hypothyroidism
Congenital
Primary
Secondary
Tertiary
Acquired
Autoimmune thyroiditis
Endemic goiter
Postradiation (iatrogenic)
Hyperthyroidism
Focal
Thyroid carcinoma
Acute suppurative thyroiditis
Diffuse
Graves disease
Hashitoxicosis
Multinodular goiter

pothyroidism. This increase in TSH is strongly correlated with the presence of autoantibodies directed against the thyroid gland. For this reason, children with type 1 DM (insulin-dependent DM) are usually screened annually by obtaining T_4 and TSH levels.

Endemic goiter, a condition rarely seen in the United States, is primarily due to iodide deficiency. However, this condition is the most common cause of thyroid disease worldwide. The goiter results from low serum T_4 levels, which stimulate increased TSH secretion, causing an increase in iodide trapping and colloid formation.

As the survival rates of childhood brain tumors improve, **postirradiation (iatrogenic)** destruction of the thyroid gland, or of the pituitary production of TSH, or hypothalamic production of TRH is becoming more frequent. In this setting, the incidence of hypothyroidism is 35%–45%. Clearly, there is a relationship between the incidence of hypothyroidism, dose of radiation, age of the patient at the time of irradiation, and time elapsed since irradiation.

Hyperthyroidism caused by an overproduction of thyroid hormone may be due to a focal area within the thyroid gland or a process involving the entire gland. On physical examination, the detection of a discrete nodule or a diffusely enlarged gland would help to discriminate between the two entities.

Hashimoto thyroiditis, also known as lymphocytic infiltration of the thyroid gland, is more common in girls than in boys. A strong family history of thyroid disease is usually present. **Hashitoxicosis,** a term that describes the hyper-

thyroid phase of Hashimoto thyroiditis, results from either increased synthesis of thyroid hormone by the gland or destruction of the gland with subsequent release of thyroid hormone into the periphery. Ultimately, however, affected patients end up with a "burned-out" gland that underproduces thyroid hormone.

Management

Hypothyroidism

With the widespread availability of oral T_4 replacement, therapy of hypothyroidism is fairly straightforward. Treatment with T_4 is initiated in neonates at 10 μg/kg/day, tapered to 4 μg/kg/day between 1 and 10 years of age, and further tapered to approximately 2 μg/kg/day thereafter. All cases of hypothyroidism involve replacement therapy with T_4 regardless of cause. Careful monitoring of therapy, with checking of serum levels of T_4 and TSH every 3–4 months until stable, is essential because advancement in skeletal maturation may occur in overtreated patients.

Hyperthyroidism

Treatment for Graves disease is propylthiouracil at a dose of 6 mg/kg/day, divided three times daily, or methimazole at one-tenth of the propylthiouracil dose given once daily or divided two or three times daily. This agent, in the thioamide class of drugs, prevents the formation of T_4 and T_3 as well as the monodeiodination of T_4 to T_3 in the periphery.

Other options for therapy include thyroidectomy and radioactive iodine treatment. The recommended treatment of Graves disease involves propylthiouracil or methimazole for approximately 2 years, with an attempt to discontinue medication gradually. If remission does not occur, the subsequent recommendation is radioactive iodine treatment. If thyroid carcinoma is present, treatment involves thyroidectomy and dissection and removal of affected lymph nodes, followed by radiotherapy.

Leukopenia and skin rash occur in about 10% of patients treated with propylthiouracil; more serious problems, such as agranulocytosis, pericarditis, and systemic lupus erythematosus, have been reported. Propranolol, a β-adrenergic receptor blocker, at an initial dose of 2.5 mg/kg/day PO is useful to prevent some of the symptoms of sympathetic hyperactivity such as tachycardia and nervousness. Complications of propranolol therapy include bradycardia and exacerbation of reactive airway disease.

SUGGESTED READINGS

American Diabetes Association: Medical management of type I diabetes. Alexandria, VA, American Diabetes Association, 1994.

Bacon GE, Spencer ML, Hopwood NJ, et al: *A Practical Approach to Pediatric Endocrinology*, 3rd ed. Chicago, Year Book Medical Publishers, 1990.

Behrman RE, Keligman RM, Jenson HB (eds): *Nelson's Textbook of Pediatrics*, 16th ed. Philadelphia, WB Saunders, 2000

Biglieri EG, Kater CE: 17-Alpha hydroxylation deficiency. *Endocrinol Metab Clin North Am* 20:257–267, 1991.

Bonadio WA: Pediatric diabetic ketoacidosis: Pathophysiology and potential for outpatient management of selected children. *Pediatr Emerg Care* 8:287–290, 1992.

Chase HP, Garg SK, Jelley DH: Diabetic ketoacidosis in children and the role of outpatient management. *Pediatr Rev* 11:297–304, 1990.

Kaplan SA: *Clinical Pediatric Endocrinology*. Philadelphia, WB Saunders, 1990.

Kovacs L, Robertson GL: Syndrome of inappropriate antidiuresis. *Endocrinol Metab Clin North Am* 21:859–874, 1992.

McGillivray BC: Genetic aspects of ambiguous genitalia. *Pediatr Clin North Am* 39:307–317, 1992.

Miller WL: Congenital adrenal hyperplasias. *Endocrinol Metab Clin North Am* 20:721–749, 1991.

Siperstein MD: Diabetic ketoacidosis and hyperosmolar coma. *Endocrinol Metab Clin North Am* 21(2):415–431, 1992.

Vokes TJ, Robertson GL: Disorders of antidiuretic hormone. *Endocrinol Metab Clin North Am* 17:281–299, 1988.

Wilson JD, Foster DW: *Williams Textbook of Endocrinology*, 8th ed. Philadelphia, WB Saunders, 1992.

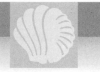

Chapter 15

Gastroenterology

Harvey W. Aiges

Gastrointestinal (GI) complaints are a significant part of ambulatory pediatrics. Abdominal pain, diarrhea, constipation, emesis, and GI bleeding are seen frequently. The pediatrician must determine whether a child's symptoms are caused by an abnormality of the GI tract or are related to a systemic disease. For example, otitis media or a urinary tract infection may manifest as diarrhea, whereas pharyngitis, pneumonia, or diabetes mellitus may manifest only as abdominal pain. The clinician must use a meticulous history and physical examination along with various clues such as the child's age and clinical appearance to determine the cause of the symptoms and to create a therapeutic plan.

Enormous advances have been achieved in caring for children on an ambulatory basis, greatly diminishing the need to hospitalize children for GI disorders. Some GI conditions obviously still necessitate the use of inpatient services. These include congenital GI anomalies and intestinal obstruction, GI hemorrhage, inflammatory diseases affecting the bowel, pediatric liver diseases, pancreatic disease, and peritonitis.

EVALUATION OF ABDOMINAL PAIN

Abdominal pain is the most frequent GI complaint that brings children and adolescents to the clinician. The child's complaints may be vague or quite specific.

Pathophysiology

The nature and site of the pain may aid in making a diagnosis. The pain may be **visceral** (from an abdominal viscera), **somatic** (parietal; from underlying peritoneal inflammation), or **referred** (from a more distal site). In general, visceral pain results from (1) a distention of the wall of a hollow organ or a stretching of the capsule of a solid organ, (2) inflammation, or (3) ischemia.

Clinical and Laboratory Evaluation

History
Most clinicians believe that the further away chronic or recurrent abdominal pain is from the umbilicus, the greater the likelihood that the

problem is organic. In addition, when a child complains of abdominal pain in different areas on different days without localization, an organic problem is less likely than when the pain is always in one area. Several helpful clinical pearls in the evaluation of abdominal pain are:

- Back pain associated with abdominal pain is infrequent and suggests involvement of a retroperitoneal organ or a process abutting the retroperitoneum (e.g., pancreatic disease, biliary disease, penetrating or perforating peptic ulcer).
- Acute organomegaly causes pain by the stretching of capsule of the organ. If an enlarged organ is nontender, it implies an adaptation of the capsule, which suggests chronicity.
- Rebound pain is rarely a helpful finding.
- Nocturnal GI symptoms are usually organic.
- Abdominal pain so severe that it causes children to writhe in agony is almost never organic in origin.

Physical Examination
Visceral pain tends to be poorly localized. The site of pain in hepatobiliary, pancreatic, and gastroduodenal disease tends to be the epigastrium, and small and large bowel disease tends to cause periumbilical symptoms. Abnormalities in the rectosigmoid colon, urinary tract, and pelvic organs generally result in suprapubic manifestations. Peritoneal pain is usually more sharp and constant and is localized to the area of the involved viscera. Signs are voluntary guarding and involuntary rigidity of the overlying abdominal musculature, with or without rebound pain.

Laboratory Evaluation
There are no specific laboratory studies for abdominal pain. However, pyuria, hematuria, glycosuria, or an abnormal chest radiograph (pneumonia) may direct the physician away from an intra-abdominal cause for the pain.

Differential Diagnosis

Acute abdominal pain in children is more frequently organic in nature, in contrast to chronic or recurrent abdominal pain, which is often functional. Although viral gastroenteritis is one of the most common causes of acute abdominal pain in children, it is most important for the clinician to work through the differential diagnosis carefully (Table 15.1). Several other GI problems cause acute abdominal pain. Nonintestinal causes (e.g., urinary tract disease, pharyngitis, diabetic ketoacidosis) may be extremely difficult to diagnose unless they are under specific consideration.

Chronic abdominal pain occurs in 10%–15% of children between 5 and 15 years of age. Three or more episodes of pain occurring over a period of 3 months is termed recurrent pain. The differential diagnosis list is long (Table 15.2).

Pediatric Pearl

Keep in mind that in about 90% of children with chronic and recurrent abdominal pain, the discomfort *does not* have an organic etiology.

TABLE 15.1 **Causes of Acute Abdominal Pain**

Common

Appendicitis
Bacterial enterocolitis
Dietary indiscretion
Food poisoning
Mesenteric lymphadenitis
Pharyngitis
Urinary tract infection
Viral gastroenteritis

Less Common

Incarcerated hernia
Gallbladder disease
Diabetes mellitus
Hepatitis
Intussusception
Meckel diverticulum
Pelvic inflammatory disease
Peritonitis
Pneumonia (especially lower lobes)
Trauma
Pregnancy (ectopic)
Henoch-Schönlein purpura
Obstruction (adhesions)
Acute rheumatic fever
Renal stones
Pancreatitis
Testicular torsion
Vasculitis
Obstructive nephropathy
Vascular insufficiency
Malignancy
Volvulus
Mittelschmerz
Sickle cell disease

TABLE 15.2 **Causes of Chronic or Recurrent Abdominal Pain**

Common

Irritable bowel syndrome (functional)
Psychogenic
Lactose intolerance
Constipation

Less Common

Food allergy
Acid-peptic disease
Mittelschmerz
Endometriosis
Sickle cell anemia
Collagen vascular disease
Recurrent pancreatitis
Parasitic infestation
Acute intermittent porphyria
Mesenteric cyst
Abdominal epilepsy
Inflammatory bowel disease
Helicobacter pylori infection
Dysmenorrhea
Hematocolpos
Urinary tract infection
Cystic fibrosis
Heavy metal poisoning
Enteric cyst (duplication)
Abdominal mass/malignancy
Familial Mediterranean fever
Abdominal migraine equivalent

The most common cause of chronic abdominal pain is irritable bowel syndrome (IBS). In children with acute abdominal pain, appendicitis must always be considered.

Appendicitis

Acute appendicitis is the most common childhood disease that requires emergency surgery. The diagnosis, which may be easy in a classic textbook case, is often unclear in children and may account for the significant number of cases that progress to perforation (see Chapter 25).

Irritable Bowel Syndrome

Irritable bowel syndrome (IBS), a poorly understood condition, affects a very large number of children and adults and is a major cause of school and work absences. A large number of endogenous and exogenous (e.g., infections, medications, teething, stress, diet) stimuli may precipitate GI dysmotility. Presumably, patients with IBS have a different electrophysiologic background in their gut, which allows the stimuli to cause alterations in intestinal motility, leading to symptoms. Research studies have demonstrated the variations in the electrophysiology, but routine GI evaluations (i.e., endoscopy, barium radiology studies, histology) are normal.

The clinical spectrum of IBS is diarrhea or constipation, with or without abdominal pain. Many affected children have a family history of IBS (formerly referred to as spastic colon). As infants, they frequently had colic and many, but not all, had chronic, nonspecific diarrhea until 3 years of age. At that time, a more constipatory phase, which lasts until adolescence, begins. By the teenage years, many patients present with recurrent or vague abdominal pain as the only symptom, although diarrhea at the time of examination is not unusual. At all stages, symptoms may increase with emotional or physical stress.

Diagnosis depends on a careful history and a normal physical examination. Routine blood studies [complete blood count (CBC), erythrocyte sedimentation rate (ESR), and SMA-20)] should be normal, as should stool and urine evaluations. A lactose breath hydrogen test after a lactose challenge may be helpful, but more invasive studies are not indicated if the history, physical examination, and routine studies are consistent with IBS.

Management

Management of acute and chronic abdominal pain depends on the underlying cause. The treatment for early acute appendicitis is emergency appendectomy. If the appendix has perforated prior to surgery, it is essential to correct fluid and electrolyte disturbances and begin aggressive antibiotic therapy.

Treatment of IBS involves education and reassurance. Medications are usually not useful, although an increase in fiber may help patients with alternating diarrhea and constipation. If patients cannot adapt to this functional problem and fail to participate in the normal "functions of daily living," psychologic intervention may be necessary.

ACUTE DIARRHEA

Diarrhea is most commonly defined as an increase in the number of stools or an increase in the fluid content of the fecal material. Almost everyone has diarrhea at some time during childhood.

Pathophysiology

Because there is considerable variation in stool number, volume, and consistency among individuals or even in the same child, the definition of diarrhea is imprecise. Stool volume in adults is nearly 100 g/day, with water being the primary constituent. Normal infants pass 5–10 g/kg/day, and stool volume in excess of 10 g/kg/day is often considered diarrhea. By 3 years of age, stool volume reaches adult levels. Stool volume greater than 200 g/day fits the generally accepted view of diarrhea in children and adults.

It is noteworthy that many infants and toddlers are said to have diarrhea by their parents but, in fact, do not. Infants may have as many as 10–12 bowel movements each day and not have diarrhea as long as there is no watery margin around the stool mass. Some toddlers, probably as a result of rapid intestinal transit time, have normal volume but unformed stools for many years. In such cases, reassurance of parents by the clinician can be extremely helpful to avoid dietary restrictions or medical workups.

In most cases, the cause of diarrhea is enteric infection. Most commonly, the infectious agents are usually viral. The cause of acute, self-limited, **bloody** diarrhea is usually bacterial.

Clinical and Laboratory Evaluation

History

The duration of acute diarrhea is short, usually less than 2 weeks. It is helpful to determine the frequency of bowel movements, as well as the consistency of the stool (a measure of the amount of water loss) and the presence of gross blood in the stool. The presence of mucus in the stool is not helpful. The color of the stool is more suggestive of transit time than any particular cause of diarrhea.

Physical Examination

The clinician must evaluate the patient's state of hydration by evaluating the anterior fontanelle (if opened), the mucous membranes, the turgor of the skin, the pulses, and the capillary refill. Evaluation of the stool for the presence of blood is most useful in determining whether antibiotic therapy is indicated.

Laboratory Evaluation

Stool analysis for blood, culture and sensitivity, and Wright stain is necessary. Serum electrolytes may be appropriate.

Differential Diagnosis (Table 15.3)

Acute diarrhea may result from infection with one or more of several agents.

TABLE 15.3 Causes of Acute Diarrhea

Infection
    Viral gastroenteritis
    Bacterial enterocolitis
    Others
Overfeeding (infant)
Food poisoning
Systemic infection
Antibiotic association
Hyperthyroidism

Rotavirus

Rotavirus, the most important cause of acute diarrheal disease during the winter months, may lead to particularly severe symptoms in younger infants. This virus accounts for as many as 80% of diarrheal episodes in children from 6 months to 2 years. Vomiting at the onset of disease is quite common and may last as long as 10 days. Dehydration is relatively common. The diagnosis may be confirmed on Rotazyme [enzyme-linked immunosorbent assay (ELISA)] testing of the stool. The Rotazyme test may stay positive for longer than 2 months and can therefore be misleading.

Norwalk-like Virus

The Norwalk-like virus is associated with both diarrhea epidemics and food poisoning. It usually affects children older than 5 years of age, lasts from 1–3 days, and frequently causes no fever. Enteric adenovirus, astrovirus, and mini-respiratory enteric orphan (REO) virus infections are also associated with childhood diarrhea. Viral agents do not produce blood or white blood cells (WBCs) in the stool [except in children who have human immunodeficiency virus (HIV) and are infected with cytomegalovirus or herpes simplex]. Therefore, stools that are positive for occult blood or have a positive Wright stain should prompt the clinician to consider a bacterial etiology in acute diarrhea and inflammatory bowel disease (IBD) in chronic diarrhea.

Escherichia coli

Enteroinvasive *Escherichia coli* may produce bloody diarrhea with fecal leukocytes. **Enterohemorrhagic** *E. coli* type 0157:H7 can cause a bloody diarrhea that produces hemolytic-uremic syndrome and thrombotic thrombocytopenic purpura. Hemolytic-uremic syndrome apparently occurs in about 10% of such infections. **Enterotoxigenic** *E. coli* is a leading cause of traveler's diarrhea.

Campylobacter jejuni

Campylobacter jejuni is the most common cause of bacterial enterocolitis in the United States. Children have a predilection for infection during the first decade of life. The illness, which lasts 3 days to 3 weeks, may mimic IBD. Abdominal pain, fever, nausea, and vomiting frequently accompany the diarrhea and occasionally precede it. The abdominal pain may persist for several weeks after the diarrhea subsides. Fecal blood and leukocytes are common.

Salmonella

Salmonella typhi infections are associated with typhoid fever (enteric fever). This serious infection, which is less common than the enterocolitis forms, arises from contaminated water or food. High, spiking fevers are the rule; if untreated, the fever may remain for 2–3 weeks. Nausea, vomiting, and splenomegaly are common. Diarrhea may occur, but constipation is often seen. Rose spots (a cutaneous vasculitis) are seen transiently over the abdomen, chest, and extensor surfaces. Intestinal perforation and hemorrhage, the most serious complications, occur in 1%–3% of patients, particularly in the second and third week of illness. Other complications include pneumonia, hepatitis, myocarditis, and meningoencephalitis.

Salmonella species other than *S. typhi* produce an enterocolitis that is usually associated with contaminated food and drink. The onset of symptoms is usually abrupt with headaches, chills, and abdominal pain followed by fever, vomiting, and diarrhea. The stools may be bloody. The course usually lasts 1–7 days but may be prolonged.

Shigella

Shigella sonnei and *S. flexneri* are the most frequent causes of **shigellosis** (bacillary dysentery). These organisms result in major damage to the distal colon and rectum. The clinical spectrum varies from mild, chronic diarrhea to an abrupt massive toxic process with a high mortality. The most common presentation involves abdominal cramps, fever, and vomiting. Diarrhea follows, often frequent with small volumes but mixed with blood and pus and associated with urgency and tenesmus. Meningismus and seizures often develop as a result of the presence of a neurotoxin. In rare cases, nephritis, arthritis, pneumonia, and the hemolytic-uremic syndrome have occurred. A high peripheral band count often accompanies this infection.

Yersinia enterocolitica

Yersinia enterocolitica causes diarrhea in infants and young children, whereas most older children develop a right lower quadrant mass or tenderness (acute ileitis or mesenteric lymphadenitis) that can mimic appendicitis or Crohn disease. Other organisms associated with enterocolitis in children include *Aeromonas hydrophila* and *Plesiomonas shigelloides*.

Clostridium difficile

Clostridium difficile (antibiotic-induced) colitis occurs when a patient's enteric flora is altered by antibiotics. Virtually all antibiotics are implicated, although the highest risk occurs with use of ampicillin, cephalosporins, and clindamycin. The colitis, which may be associated with the formation of a pseudomembrane, can be quite severe. Marked protein-losing enteropathy and grave toxicity (often with a very high WBC count) may be seen.

Management

The management of acute diarrhea should involve replacing fluid and electrolyte losses. Most cases resolve without complications, and the use of antispasmodic and antidiarrheal agents is contraindicated. The use of specific antibiotic treatments must be individualized. The major concerns with antibiotic treatment are (1) the emergence of resistant organisms that can worsen mild cases or (2) prolongation of the shedding state (a serious problem in nurseries and day-care centers).

    C. jejuni infection is self-limited, so in most cases, no treatment is necessary. In severely affected patients, oral erythromycin diminishes fecal excretion of the organisms with a decrease in symptoms. *Salmonella* enteritis is self-limited, and antibiotic therapy should be reserved for patients who are younger than 6 months of age, have bacteremia, or have salmonellosis while suffering from chronic illness or immunocompromise. However, all patients with *S. typhi* (typhoid fever) should receive appropriate antibiotics (usually chloramphenicol). Shigellosis is self-limited, but most clinicians treat this disease with ampicillin or trimethoprim–sulfamethoxazole. A minority suggest restricting antibiotics to only the most severe cases. Recent evidence suggests that antibiotic treatment of *Shigella* and enteroinvasive *E. coli* organisms that have a shiga toxin enhances the risk of the subsequent development of hemolytic-uremic syndrome. In antibiotic-induced colitis, therapy (as well as discontinuation of the offending agent) is usually necessary. Metronidazole (intravenous or oral) is the drug of choice. Oral vancomycin is very effective but quite expensive.

CHRONIC DIARRHEA AND MALABSORPTION

Chronic diarrhea is defined as diarrhea lasting longer than 2 weeks. The chronic nature of the diarrhea does not necessarily imply organic disease.

Pathophysiology

Chronic diarrhea may be the result of a dysmotility with normal absorption of nutrients (as in IBS), it may be secondary to a chronic infection (as in giardiasis), or it may be the result of severe intestinal mucosal damage from a variety of insults (especially in infants < 6 months of age). If the mucosa is compromised, nutrient malabsorption and diminished growth can be expected.

Clinical and Laboratory Evaluation

History

Again, it is important to determine the number and consistency of the stool. In addition, it is most critical to look at the child's growth curve. Chronic diarrhea that affects growth must be evaluated fully.

> ### ☀ Pediatric Pearl
>
> Chronic diarrhea associated with normal weight and length velocity is unlikely to have a serious organic cause.

Physical Examination

The physical examination is unlikely to help the clinician select a specific organic cause. A protuberant abdomen associated with loss of subcutaneous fat (in the buttocks and thighs) suggests malabsorption, as do clinical findings associated with various mineral and vitamin deficiencies. However, these markers only indicate what the growth curve already has; a workup is necessary.

Laboratory Evaluation

All children with chronic diarrhea and poor weight gain receive a workup to rule out a malabsorption syndrome. An acidic stool pH and the presence of reducing substances in the stool suggest carbohydrate malabsorption. A hydrogen breath test can measure lactose and sucrose malabsorption. A Sudan stain of the stool for fat and a 72-hour fecal fat study document fat malabsorption; abnormalities of fat-soluble vitamins A, D, E, and K also suggest this possibility. Ultimately, most workups end in a small bowel biopsy with duodenal fluid aspiration, which is of most help in diagnosing many opportunistic intestinal infections such as giardiasis, celiac disease, lymphangiectasia, and abetalipoproteinemia.

Differential Diagnosis (Table 15.4)

In small infants, a common cause of chronic diarrhea is a disorder commonly known as **intractable diarrhea of infancy**. The term signifies diarrhea in infants younger than 6 months of age that is associated with diffuse mucosal injury lasting longer than 2 weeks; the condition is often accompanied by malabsorption and malnutrition. Intractable diarrhea of infancy is most often the end result of many different disease entities, including cow's milk and soy protein intolerance; protracted infectious enteritis; Hirschsprung disease; and a host of rarer entities such as microvillus inclusion disease, autoimmune enteropathy, congenital transport defects (e.g., congenital chloridorrhea), and congenital carbohydrate malabsorption. Treatment of intractable diarrhea, regardless of the initial cause, is based on aggressive nutritional therapy, preferably via an enteral route.

A frequent cause of bloody diarrhea in infants as well as of intractable diarrhea is **cow's milk and soy protein intolerance**. These infants develop enterocolitis, which manifests itself during the first 3 months of life with vomiting, irritability, poor feeding, and diarrhea with blood-streaked stools. Symptoms usually resolve when the formula is removed. There is a large percentage of cross-reactivity between cow's milk and soy protein formula, so use of a casein hydrolysate formula is logical (see Chapter 4). When these infants are rechallenged with the offending formula, reactions occur in the first 24–48 hours. A small group of infants may experience life-threatening anaphylaxis.

The most common cause of chronic diarrhea in children between 6 months and 3 years of age is IBS (see INFLAMMATORY DISEASES OF THE BOWEl). Infection with the protozoan *Giardia lamblia* warrants consideration in young children. Transmission occurs through person-to-person contact or through ingestion of contaminated food and water. *Giardia* adheres to the microvilli of the proximal small bowel and may lead to a very variable clinical picture. Affected children may range from asymptomatic; to those with low-grade diarrhea and abdominal distention; to those with profound anorexia, weight loss, and malabsorption. Stool examination for ova and parasites may be normal in as many as 50% of patients, but a new test for detection of *Giardia* antigen in the stool is more sensitive. A small intestinal biopsy or aspiration of duodenal contents is the best way to make the diagnosis. Treatment is metronidazole or quinacrine.

Chronic diarrhea in toddlers may also represent the initial symptoms of primary malabsorption diseases. The overwhelming majority of children with malabsorptive disorders have cystic fibrosis, giardiasis, or gluten-induced enteropathy (celiac disease, sprue). Other causes of malabsorption are infrequent, except in patients with acquired immunodeficiency syndrome (AIDS) and other immunodeficiency syndromes. **Gluten-induced enteropathy** is an immune-mediated disease against gluten, a protein constituent of wheat, oats, barley, and rye. The α-gliadin fraction of gluten appears to induce a hypersensitivity reaction in the small intestine of genetically predisposed patients. This process results in a complete flattening of the villi and a deepening of the crypts. After gluten has been introduced into the diet

---

TABLE 15.4 **Causes of Chronic Diarrhea**

Common

Intractable diarrhea of infancy
Postinfection diarrhea
Carbohydrate malabsorption (lactose intolerance)
Dietary
    Overfeeding
    Allergic (cow's milk and soy protein intolerance)
Cystic fibrosis
Gluten-induced enteropathy (celiac disease)
Irritable bowel syndrome
Inflammatory bowel disease
Giardiasis
Constipation with encopresis

Uncommon

Immune deficiency states (HIV, primary)
Malnutrition
Secretary tumors (neuroblastoma)
Intestinal lymphangiectasia
Abetalipoproteinemia
Intestinal pseudo-obstruction
Intestinal tumors
Anatomical causes
    Blind loop
    Short bowel syndrome
    Hirschsprung disease
Pancreatic insufficiency
Eosinophilic gastroenteritis
Encopresis

HIV = human immunodeficiency virus.

(usually after 6 months), patients present with anorexia, irritability, weight loss, and failure to thrive. Diarrhea usually develops after significant failure to thrive. In some cases, diarrhea is not present, and children may manifest symptoms of constipation or protein-losing enteropathy.

A small bowel biopsy is absolutely necessary to establish the diagnosis. Clinical response to withdrawing gluten is often slow and frequently inconsistent and, therefore, inadequate. The anti-gliadin immunoglobulin A (IgA) and IgG and antireticulin and antiendomysial tests have made it much more easy to screen for the disease. These tests are useful in children with growth failure to determine whether a biopsy might be useful or to monitor compliance with a gluten-free diet. These tests can be abnormal in children with nonspecific mucosal injury; therefore, a positive test does not preclude the need for a biopsy.

Management

Management of the various causes of chronic diarrhea and malabsorption are disease specific. Where the cause is a food or food component, elimination is the first step in successful management. Treatment frequently leads to a cessation of the diarrhea and a marked improvement in weight gain and acceleration in linear growth.

VOMITING OR GASTROESOPHAGEAL REFLUX

All children have gastroesophageal reflux, and many experience vomiting during the first few years of life. It is essential to determine whether the vomiting is effortful or effortless, because the implications associated with the two conditions are so different.

Pathophysiology

Vomiting is the **forceful, effortful** ejection of gastric contents. It is important to remember that vomiting is controlled by the medullary emesis center in the floor of the fourth ventricle, which may be affected by gastrointestinal or nongastrointestinal stimuli. **Gastroesophageal reflux,** on the other hand, is the **effortless** regurgitation of gastric contents. However, it may be projectile. Transient relaxations of the lower esophageal sphincter, unrelated to swallowing, appear to cause gastroesophageal reflux. Other implicated factors are diminished lower esophageal tone, large hiatal hernias, and delayed gastric emptying. Virtually all infants have some degree

of gastroesophageal reflux, but only a small percentage have apparent complications (Table 15.5).

Clinical and Laboratory Evaluation

History
It is most critical to differentiate between vomiting (effortful) and gastroesophageal reflux (effortless) on the basis of history. The vast majority of infants with gastroesophageal reflux do well with time or conservative management. Vomiting, on the other hand, deserves serious evaluation if it is atypical, intractable, or chronic.

Physical Examination
The physical examination is helpful infrequently; however, abdominal distention suggests obstruction as a cause of vomiting, while palpation of a duodenal "olive" suggests hypertrophic pyloric stenosis. A good neurologic examination may be of help in guiding the physician to a central nervous system (CNS) cause for chronic vomiting.

Laboratory Evaluation
At all ages, vomiting (and the concomitant failure to eat) causes or results from a metabolic acidosis. If a child with vomiting has a metabolic alkalosis (often with hypochloremia), it is essential to consider gastric outlet obstruction (e.g., hypertrophic pyloric stenosis) or cystic fibrosis (failure to produce pancreatic bicarbonate). Electrolyte studies should be normal in gastroesophageal reflux.

Considerable controversy is associated with the use of the myriad studies available for diagnosis of gastroesophageal reflux. In patients with respiratory symptoms without clinical evidence of gastroesophageal reflux, barium upper GI se-

---

TABLE 15.5 **Complications of Gastroesophageal Reflux**

Apnea and bradycardia (SIDS)
Failure to thrive
Esophagitis
   Irritability
   Bleeding and anemia
   Strictures
   Barrett esophagus (premalignant)
Chest pain
Sandifer syndrome
Respiratory diseases
   Chronic cough
   Asthma
   Aspiration pneumonia
   Nocturnal cough

SIDS = sudden infant death syndrome.

ries and 24-hour pH probes can help establish gastroesophageal reflux as a cause of the respiratory disease. In patients with known gastroesophageal reflux, a technetium-99m (^{99m}Tc) scan of gastric emptying may be of help in establishing the cause of the gastroesophageal reflux. In cases of blood loss, anemia, chest pain, and dysphagia, endoscopy and esophageal biopsy may be useful. In general, esophageal testing must be well thought out and individualized to answer specific clinical questions.

Differential Diagnosis

In neonates, clinicians should view vomiting (especially if bile stained) with alarm; it suggests a congenital malformation causing obstruction or sepsis (see CONGENITAL GASTROINTESTINAL ANOMALIES AND INTESTINAL OBSTRUCTION). In infants, vomiting most frequently results from infectious gastroenteritis, but overfeeding, systemic infections, and pyloric stenosis (2–6 weeks of age) warrant consideration. In addition, vomiting may be the first manifestation of inborn errors of metabolism and the adrenogenital syndrome. In children and adolescents, gastroenteritis most commonly causes vomiting, but toxic ingestions and systemic infections are possible.

In individuals of all ages, vomiting, especially if chronic or recurrent, may be *nonintestinal* in etiology. It is critical to consider increased intracranial pressure as a cause of vomiting. Brain tumors, hydrocephalus, and CNS bleeding, as well as seizures and migraine headaches may manifest as vomiting. Metabolic derangements, especially metabolic acidosis, may cause vomiting, as in Reye syndrome, salicylate poisoning, and diabetic acidosis. Vomiting may also result from psychogenic causes, including bulimia. Of course, chronic vomiting may have a GI origin, such as achalasia, IBD, and late-onset intestinal obstructions (adhesions, webs, vascular insufficiency).

Management

Treatment of vomiting involves treatment of the underlying problem. In most cases of acute vomiting, no therapy is necessary beyond management of fluid and electrolyte imbalances.

Treatment of gastroesophageal reflux is controversial. Thickening of formula with dry cereal, long a mainstay of conservative therapy, has not proved to help. Most clinicians suggest the use of position therapy, consisting of a 30-degree prone upright stance immediately after feedings.

Medical therapy with prokinetic agents has limited efficacy. Bethanechol, a parasympathomimetic agent, may increase lower esophageal sphincter pressure, whereas metoclopramide, a dopamine agonist, can increase gastric emptying and increase lower esophageal tone. However, both agents have significant side effects. A newer prokinetic agent, domperidone, is under investigation. The use of antacids and histamine receptor type 2 (H_2) blockers may be beneficial in reducing acid reflux. Omeprazole, which completely blocks the hydrogen ion-secreting pump, holds significant promise for the future.

Surgery, via a Nissen fundoplication or other wrap procedure, is reserved for patients with gastroesophageal reflux and severe, intractable respiratory symptoms, failure to thrive, esophagitis with stricture formation, or Barrett esophagus. Patients with gastroesophageal reflux and severe neurologic disabilities and those with familial dysautonomia usually also require fundoplication.

CONSTIPATION AND ENCOPRESIS

Constipation is common in infants and children. No clear definition exists in pediatrics, but more people accept constipation as the infrequent passage of hard stools. **Encopresis**, a far less common condition, is a more confusing term, but it is a concept often used for fecal incontinence or soiling of formed or semiformed stool in the underwear (or elsewhere) by children older than 4 years of age. Fecal incontinence may occur with or without constipation.

Pathophysiology

Beyond the neonatal period, the vast majority of children with constipation have simple constipation as a result of a functional dysmotility or from voluntary withholding. Sometimes the withholding may become more severe; it may be as a result of problems with toilet training or fear of defecation secondary to a large or painful stool. If the stool retention remains untreated for a prolonged period, the rectal wall stretches, and the rectal vault enlarges.

Some children with this problem experience significant anorectal pain and repeatedly defecate small amount of stool to achieve relief. These children are classically dirty while awake and tend to have very little soiling when sleeping. Other children may have involuntary leakage of semiliquid stool around a hard stool mass. They usually claim that they have not experienced the urge to defecate. This stage is often termed **encopresis**. Encopresis may also occur in nonconstipated children who have severe psychogenic problems or in children with neuromuscular disorders.

Clinical and Laboratory Evaluation

History

Aggressive evaluation of children with constipation must take into account the fact that most children have simple constipation as an isolated problem. A good history, including a family history of constipation and IBS, aids in the diagnosis.

Physical Examination

A physical examination noting muscle tone, rectal tone, abdominal contents, and rectal contents is important. A large rectal vault suggests chronic constipation. A diastasis recti may enhance problems of constipation. A child may have some difficulty producing a good Valsalva maneuver, and an anterior displaced anus with a posterior rectal shelf may make defecation difficult.

Laboratory Evaluation

In routine cases of constipation, laboratory investigation is rarely necessary. In atypical cases or in those in which Hirschsprung disease is under consideration, however, a workup is necessary.

Differential Diagnosis (Table 15.6)

The exclusion of **Hirschsprung disease** in the differential diagnosis of chronic constipation is important. Hirschsprung disease, or congenital aganglionic megacolon, is due to a congenital absence in both the submucosal (Meissner) and myenteric (Auerbach) plexuses. It occurs in about 1 in 5000 live births and is often associated with Down syndrome and other congenital anomalies. There is a 4:1 male preponderance, but in long segment disease the ratio is diminished. The exact cause is unknown.

In Hirschsprung disease, the aganglionic segment is restricted to the rectum and sigmoid colon in the large majority (75%) of cases. Any length of bowel may be affected, however, ranging from the ultrashort segment (< 1% of cases) to that of the entire colon, with or without small bowel involvement (8% of cases). Functionally, there is sympathetic hyperactivity in the affected segment, leading to tonic contraction. The more proximal intestine is normally innervated and dilates in response to distal obstruction.

In 50%–75% of cases, diagnosis is made in newborns by the failure to pass meconium in the

TABLE 15.6	Differential Diagnosis of Constipation

Functional (simple) constipation
Stool withholding
Dietary
    Breastfeeding
    Low fiber
    Starvation
Psychogenic
Painful defecation
    (fissure, trauma)
Intestinal
    Hirschsprung disease
    Intestinal pseudo-obstruction
Anal atresia/stenosis
Drugs (narcotics, psychotropics)
Neuromuscular causes
    Hypotonia
    Spinal cord lesions
    Sacral malformation
    Myotonias
Metabolic causes
    Cystic fibrosis
    Hypothyroidism
    Hypokalemia
    Hypocalcemia/hypercalcemia
Typhoid fever

first 48 hours of life, followed by abdominal distention and bilious vomiting. This condition accounts for 25%–50% of all cases of neonatal intestinal obstruction. Dilation of the empty rectum by the first examiner results in explosive expulsion of retained fecal material and decompression of the proximal bowel. However, symptoms of obstruction return without repeated irrigation of the colon. Diarrhea secondary to enterocolitis develops in 25% of cases, if untreated. The mortality from enterocolitis is very high.

In 25%–50% of cases, early obstruction is not seen, and it is here where the differential diagnosis between functional constipation and Hirschsprung disease is problematic. Some of these cases involve nothing more than variable constipation punctuated by recurrent obstructive crises or fecal impaction. Still others may involve failure to thrive or anemia and hypoproteinemia (secondary to a protein-losing colopathy). Infrequently, children with this entity have nothing more than occasional constipation.

In the differentiation of simple constipation from Hirschsprung disease, it is wise to remember that the urge to defecate or straining rarely occurs in Hirschsprung disease because stools are retained proximal to the anorectum. Children with Hirschsprung disease rarely soil, and they pass small, ribbon-like stools (because they must pass the hypertonic, constricted aganglionic zone) unlike the very large stools often found in children with functional constipation. In addition, the rectum is tight and narrow and almost always free of stool in children with Hirschsprung disease. In contrast, children with constipation or retention have a large rectal vault full of stool.

The diagnosis of Hirschsprung disease is based on rectal suction biopsy that demonstrates both an absence of ganglion cells in the plexus and hyperplastic sympathetic nerve fibers. An increase in acetylcholinesterase activity by histochemical staining helps confirm the diagnosis. Anorectal manometry (failure of internal sphincter relaxation with rectal distention) and barium enema (evidence of a transition zone, delayed emptying) aid in the diagnosis of difficult cases.

Management

Treatment is indicated in constipation and stool withholding in cases in which it has been possible to rule out other causes such as Hirschsprung disease, hypothyroidism, and neurofibromatosis. Failure to treat may lead to an increase in problems and may eventually result in further stool withholding and encopresis. In infants, a malt extract or lactulose added to the formula may be effective in the management of functional constipation. In older children, diet manipulation with added fiber, or, if necessary, stool softeners or cathartics such as senna (Senokot) may be appropriate. In some cases, when there is a large amount of retained stool in the rectal vault, enemas and rectal cathartics may be necessary before oral preparations are used. In very difficult cases, large doses of oral (or nasogastric) electrolyte preparations may be indicated.

Treatment of Hirschsprung disease involves surgery directed at pulling innervated bowel through the distal rectal segment. The specific choice of endorectal pull-through is determined by the length of aganglionic bowel present.

ACID-PEPTIC DISEASE AND *HELICOBACTER PYLORI* INFECTION

The topic of acid-peptic disease in children, always vague in comparison to the more substantial literature and experience in adult gastroenterology, is now in enormous flux, given the emergence of *Helicobacter pylori* as an important agent in gastroduodenal disease. Historically, acid-peptic disease referred to a variety of entities, including dyspepsia, gastritis, duodenitis, and ulcers of the proximal GI tract related to excess acid secretions.

Pathophysiology

The etiology and pathophysiology of acid-peptic disease has now come into question, but the clinical picture remains the same. It is important to attempt to determine the underlying cause, so that appropriate, curative treatment can be given.

Clinical and Laboratory Evaluation

History
Upper intestinal inflammatory disease may be asymptomatic in children or manifest as epigastric discomfort and nausea. For example, children younger than 10 years of age with peptic ulcers may have no symptoms. Abdominal pain, when present, may be appreciated as burning. It can be nocturnal. Bleeding, whether via hematemesis or blood in the stool, may be a concomitant finding or the only sign of upper tract disease. Although bleeding from peptic ulcers can occur in the absence of a precipitating event, there is often a history of upper respiratory infection, stress, or salicylate ingestion. More than 30% of children with peptic ulcers have a positive family history.

Physical Examination
Physical examination may reveal tenderness in the epigastric region or may be normal.

Laboratory Evaluation
Currently, the best way to evaluate upper intestinal inflammation is via upper endoscopy with biopsies. This examination is simple and safe. In most centers, the optimal method for diagnosing *H. pylori* is by gastric biopsy. A C-13 breath test will soon be available. It is important to test the stool for occult or frank blood.

Differential Diagnosis

Acid-peptic disease may take the form of several conditions. **Gastritis** may be localized or diffuse. Acute gastritis is often the sequelae of viral infections, use of nonsteroidal anti-inflammatory drugs (NSAIDs), and various toxins. Gastritis is also associated with toxic conditions and severe sepsis. Although abdominal or epigastric pain with nausea may be present, the hallmark of erosive gastritis is hematemesis, which can be significant.

Ulcers in the stomach or duodenum of children are not uncommon. However, the frequency of ulcers is unknown, in part because many ulcers in children may be asymptomatic. The most prevalent symptom is epigastric pain, but many children with ulcers have no pain. Bleeding is thought to occur in 10%–20% of children with ulcers. Most gastric ulcers are found in the prepyloric area, while most duodenal ulcers are found in the bulb. Ulcers in preschoolers tend to be gastric in location, whereas in older children they are more likely to be duodenal.

Zollinger-Ellison syndrome is an entity characterized by severe peptic ulcer disease, gastric hypersecretion, and non–beta islet cell tumors of the pancreas. These tumors, referred to as gastrinomas, contain and release large amounts of gastrin into the circulation. Although most gastrinomas arise within the pancreas, they may originate as solitary or multiple tumors in other areas such as the wall of the duodenum, the hilus of the spleen, or the lymph nodes of the peritoneal cavity. One-fourth of gastrinomas occur in patients with multiple endocrine neoplasia type 1, an entity of parathyroid, pituitary, and islet cell tumors. Zollinger-Ellison syndrome warrants consideration in patients with peptic ulcers that are not responsive to routine therapy, multiple ulcers that occur in atypical areas, or ulcers associated with chronic diarrhea. Diagnosis is made by the marked increase in gastrin levels seen after administration of secretin. If gastrin levels are high, an attempt to localize and identify the tumor should be undertaken.

***H. pylori* infection** probably plays an important role in the development of inflammation and ulcers in the proximal bowel in children. It is also possible that *H. pylori* may contribute to the development of recurrent abdominal pain in children. Data in adults are striking. *H. pylori* is seen in 100% of adults with antral gastritis, 100% of patients with duodenal ulcers, and about 80% of patients with gastric ulcers that are unrelated to the use of NSAIDs. *H. pylori* is also seen in 60% of adults who have no upper GI symptoms. In addition, there is growing evidence that longstanding *H. pylori* infection, even in asymptomatic patients, may be a risk factor for the development of gastric carcinoma.

Management

Upper GI diseases related to gastric acid respond well to antacids or H_2 blockade. The duration of therapy is controversial. The most appropriate approaches to treating and eradicating *H. pylori* in children are still under investigation. Treatment of Zollinger-Ellison syndrome includes removal of the tumor and its metastasis, if possible, along with aggressive medical therapy with omeprazole or an H_2 blocker, often in conjunction with anticholinergic agents.

CONGENITAL GASTROINTESTINAL ANOMALIES AND INTESTINAL OBSTRUCTION

Neonates with GI anomalies often manifest signs and symptoms within hours or days of birth. Intestinal obstruction is the most frequent and the earliest clinical presentation of many of these entities. Accurate and early diagnosis is critical to avoid many of the long-term complications of these problems.

Pathophysiology

Congenital anomalies of the GI tract and the abdominal wall are the result of developmental abnormalities or intrauterine insults. The physician should be aware of possible GI congenital anomalies and their relationship to other congenital problems.

Clinical and Laboratory Evaluation

History
Immediately after birth, clinical clues about congenital anomalies resulting in intestinal obstruction can be gained by a history of polyhydramnios, a single umbilical artery, or meconium staining. Although intestinal obstruction is most frequently seen in association with congenital anomalies in the first few hours or days of life, it may occasionally present later in childhood.

Pediatric Pearl

There is a great urgency to investigate any possibility of intestinal obstruction (bilious vomiting, abdominal distention) **in neonates,** because obstruction may be associated with impaired blood flow to the affected segment of gut.

The resulting ischemic changes may lead to catastrophic problems, with loss of large areas of bowel and overwhelming sepsis.

Physical Examination
In the delivery room, several congenital problems such as omphalocele, gastroschisis, and imperforate anus are apparent on simple inspec-

tion. In addition, intestinal obstruction may be one of a collection of anomalies associated with a diverse list of autosomal abnormalities such as cleft palate, skeletal deformities, and craniofacial dysplasia.

Laboratory Evaluation

Fetal sonography may ascertain congenital anomalies in neonates. Usually, other studies are not helpful.

Differential Diagnosis>

Intestinal obstruction may result from one or more conditions.

Omphalocele and Gastroschisis

An **omphalocele** is a congenital hernia involving the umbilicus, which is usually covered by a sac composed of the fused layers of amnion and peritoneum. Although there is a central defect in the skin and linea alba, the remainder of the abdominal wall is intact, including the surrounding musculature. A variable amount of viscera may herniate into this sac. Of affected patients, 35% have other GI defects, including malrotations; 20% have congenital heart disease; and 10% have Beckwith-Wiedemann syndrome (gigantism, visceromegaly, macroglossia, hypoglycemia, omphalocele). In addition, extrophy of the bladder, vesicoenteric fistulae, or other renal abnormalities may be present. It is possible to miss a small occult omphalocele; therefore, the cord tie on the umbilicus should be at least 5 cm from the abdominal wall to avoid damage to the viscera.

A **gastroschisis** is a full-thickness, complete abdominal wall defect, usually to the right of a normal umbilicus, and a sac never covers the extruded viscera. An omphalocele with a ruptured sac may be difficult to distinguish from a gastroschisis. Of affected infants, 14% have an associated jejunoileal malformation (often a atresia), often with an abnormally short nonrotated midgut, but only 4% have an extraintestinal anomaly. Between 50% and 60% are premature.

The surgical management of an omphalocele and a gastroschisis and the associated prognosis depends on the size of the hernia, the presence or absence of a covering sac, and the severity of any associated anomalies. It is easy to repair a small omphalocele in the base of the umbilical cord with an intact membrane in a single-stage procedure. In cases in which the defect is large or there is no intact membrane, the surgeon must use many creative techniques to achieve reduction of

the extruded abdominal contents into the peritoneal cavity without compromising the viscera.

Umbilical Hernia

An **umbilical hernia** results from the incomplete closure of the fascia of the umbilical ring. This type of hernia, which is much more common in premature infants and blacks, is found in about 40% of black children younger than 1 year of age. If the defect is less than 0.5 cm, it is predicted that healing will occur spontaneously by 2 years of age. If the ring is between 0.5 and 1.5 cm, healing is usually complete by 4 years of age. Surgical correction warrants consideration if the defect is larger than 1.5 cm at 2 years of age or if incarceration of viscera has occurred. Reducing the hernia by strapping a device (such as a coin) over the ring does not help the healing process.

Meckel Diverticulum

The most common anomaly of the GI tract, **Meckel diverticulum** is a blind omphalomesenteric duct that results from persistence of the duct communication between the bowel and the yolk sac. It is described as an antimesenteric outpouching of the ileum, about 2 feet (60 cm) from the ileocecal valve, and is present in about 2% of the population with a male predominance at 2:1. Ectopic GI and pancreatic tissue is seen in nearly 50% of cases, with 85% of the tissue being gastric.

In the vast majority of cases, Meckel diverticulum causes no symptoms, but about 2% of cases are associated with complications, most occurring in children younger than 2 years of age. Painless rectal bleeding (85%), intestinal obstruction (intussusception or volvulus, 10%) and pain mimicking appendicitis (5%) are the most common problems encountered. The rectal bleeding is secondary to ulceration of the ileal mucosa adjacent to the ectopic gastric mucosa of the diverticulum. The bleeding can manifest as recurrent occult blood to sudden, massive, wine-colored hemorrhage with shock.

The diagnosis of Meckel diverticulum is often made clinically by excluding other causes of painless rectal bleeding. Radionuclide imaging with ^{99m}Tc pertechnetate after enhancement with cimetidine may be helpful in identifying gastric mucosa in the diverticulum in as many as 80% of cases. A surgical wedge resection of the diverticulum is curative.

Diaphragmatic Hernia

A **diaphragmatic hernia** results from incomplete closure of the membranous pleuroperitoneal folds that normally form the lateral and posterior aspects of the diaphragm. The last portions of the diaphragm to close are the posterolateral triangular canals, the foramen of Bochdalek, through which the great majority of hernias occur. Between 80% and 90% of these are left-sided hernias, and 2% are bilateral. When the diaphragm is forming, the midgut is rapidly elongating and returning from its extracoelomic position in the yolk sac. Therefore, if there is a defect in the diaphragm, the gut takes the path of least resistance and enters the thorax. About 2% of diaphragmatic hernias are associated with a retrosternal defect, the foramen of Morgagni. These hernias are usually less severe because the retrosternal space is smaller, so less abdominal viscera can enter.

The majority of infants with diaphragmatic hernia manifest symptoms of respiratory distress in the delivery room or shortly after birth as the herniated bowel fills up with air. However, some patients may present later in life with symptoms of chronic cough or congestion. Survival correlates with the time respiratory distress appears (the earlier the symptoms, the lower the survival rate) and the existence of pulmonary hypoplasia.

Esophageal Atresia and Tracheoesophageal Fistula
In the embryonic process, **esophageal atresia** and **tracheoesophageal fistula** occur when the septation between the ventral tube of the foregut the dorsal esophagus develops abnormally. The clinical clues to the diagnosis are polyhydramnios and excessive oral secretions. If these are present, a radiograph with a radiopaque nasogastric tube inserted may be very helpful by showing the coiling of the tube in the air-filled proximal esophageal pouch, heart size, the presence of air in the GI tract, any abnormal gas pattern, and the skeletal structures.

Between 35% and 40% of patients with tracheoesophageal fistula have significant associated anomalies, and in more than 50% of cases, there are more than two malformations. The most common associated anomalies are cardiovascular [patent ductus arteriosus (PDA), vascular rings, or coarctation]; GI (imperforate anus, malrotation, and duodenal atresia); and finally, the syndrome of vertebral, vascular, anal atresia, tracheoesophageal fistula, renal, and radial limb dysplasia (VATERL syndrome). Most deaths in patients with tracheoesophageal fistula appear to be more related to other severe abnormalities than to the tracheoesophageal fistula.

In all, at least 95 subtypes of esophageal atresia and tracheoesophageal fistula have been described. The most common variety of esophageal atresia (85%–90%) is a blind proximal esophageal pouch with a distal tracheoesophageal fistula. The next most common form (8%) is a proximal esophageal pouch without a tracheoesophageal fistula. In both of these forms, coiling of the nasogastric tube occurs. Infants with tracheoesophageal fistula without an esophageal atresia, the so-called H-type tracheoesophageal fistula (4%), often present with chronic cough or choking while feeding.

Treatment of esophageal atresia and tracheoesophageal fistula is surgical division of the fistula and primary anastomosis of the esophagus. Many patients, especially if premature or sick, require staged treatments. If the gap between the two ends of the esophagus is too great, a colonic interposition may be necessary. The survival rate in term infants without other abnormalities is greater than 90%. However, complications are common. Postoperative leaks occur in as many as 10% of all cases. Most patients with these entities have abnormal esophageal motility and lower esophageal sphincter dysfunction. These result in significant gastroesophageal reflux with complications of chronic esophagitis, stricture formation, and recurrent pneumonia.

Hypertrophic Pyloric Stenosis
The obstruction of the pylorus is the result of marked hypertrophy of the circular musculature of the pylorus. Hypertrophic pyloric stenosis occurs once in every 500 births with a 4:1 ratio in favor of males. Familial cases occur in 5% of siblings and as many as 25% of children if the mother was affected. The relationship to being firstborn, being breastfed, or other feeding practices is unclear. It has been postulated that the condition may be an early manifestation of gilbert syndrome precipitated by starvation.

The clinical manifestations of hypertrophic pyloric stenosis are projectile, nonbilious vomiting beginning at 2–6 weeks of life. (Ten percent of cases begin within the first 2 weeks of life, and rare cases have been reported at 6 months or beyond.) The frequency of the vomiting is variable at first and may be lessened by frequent feeding, especially of clear liquids. The vomiting becomes more severe and projectile as the gastric outlet becomes more obstructed. Palpation of the pyloric tumor or "olive" is diagnostic. The mass is palpable to the right of the umbilicus; it is best felt during a feeding or just after vomiting. A visible upper abdominal peristaltic wave is often apparent.

Laboratory results are often normal early in the course of disease, but in severe or protracted cases, a hypokalemic, hypochloremic metabolic alkalosis occurs, associated with malnutrition and dehydration. If clinical or laboratory results are inconclusive, abdominal ultrasound or an upper GI series are helpful.

Pediatric Pearl

Hypertrophic pyloric stenosis is occasionally associated with mild, unconjugated hyperbilirubinemia.

Treatment of hypertrophic pyloric stenosis consists of nasogastric decompression and correction of fluid and electrolyte abnormalities. The Fredet-Ramstedt pyloromyotomy is curative and associated with a very low mortality. Complications such as duodenal hematoma are treated expectantly.

Anomalies of the Small Intestine

DUODENAL ANOMALIES. Duodenal obstruction, which results from atresia (40%–60%), stenosis (35%–40%), or a web (5%–15%), manifests as a high intestinal blockage. The vast majority of atresias and webs are near or just distal to the ampulla of Vater. Atresia and web anomalies result from failure of the lumen to recanalize during the 8th to 10th week of gestation. **Duodenal atresia** is associated with trisomy 21 (30% of cases), prematurity (25%), and other anomalies (30%). **Duodenal stenosis** is most often due to extrinsic duodenal obstruction such as annular pancreas, peritoneal bands, or ectopic pancreatic tissue.

Clinically, affected infants present with bilious vomiting on the first day of life, without abdominal distention. High-grade duodenal obstruction is very clearly seen on an abdominal radiograph as a typical "double bubble" sign, which is actually distention of the stomach and duodenum. Treatment is a surgical bypass of the obstruction except for webs (the "wind sock" deformity), which involves surgical resection.

JEJUNOILEAL ANOMALIES. Jejunoileal atresia, which is more common than duodenal atresia (2:1), most often results from an impaired vascular supply. Ileal atresia occurs much more often than jejunal atresia. Atresias are 15 times more common than stenoses. About 50% of cases have an associated major malformation, including malrotation, Down syndrome, or cystic fibrosis.

Infants with small bowel atresia distal to the duodenum have bilious or fecal vomiting and abdominal distention. An abdominal radiograph shows dilated loops of bowel, often with air-fluid levels. A barium enema may reveal an unused, small colon (microcolon), particularly with very distal small bowel obstructions. An oral contrast small bowel study is contraindicated in the presence of a complete obstruction.

Meconium ileus is a common cause of neonatal intestinal obstruction. This defect is the earliest manifestation of cystic fibrosis, occurring in 10%–15% of patients with the disease. Patients with the defect almost certainly have cystic fibrosis, although there have been reports of meconium ileus without cystic fibrosis. Meconium ileus should not be confused with **meconium plug syndrome,** a relatively mild condition associated with inspissated rubbery meconium that plugs the distal colon and rectum. Most patients have no further problems, but it is necessary to rule out Hirschsprung disease, cystic fibrosis, and hypothyroidism.

MALROTATION AND MIDGUT VOLVULUS. Malrotation and other disorders of intestinal fixation ranks as the second most common cause of neonatal intestinal obstructions, just behind intestinal atresias. **Malrotation of the small bowel** is due to abnormal movement or rotational arrest of the intestine around the superior mesenteric artery when the midgut returns to the coelomic cavity via a 270-degree counterclockwise rotation. The result is an abnormal mesenteric fixation of the small intestine and cecum, with obstructive bands.

Nonrotation of the midgut is often a finding in omphalocele, gastroschisis, and diaphragmatic hernias. Malrotation or incomplete rotation may produce duodenal obstruction, volvulus, and internal hernias. Less acute presentations usually occur after 1 month of age and may manifest as chronic intermittent obstruction, malabsorption, protein-losing enteropathy, or recurrent pain and vomiting. However, more than 50% of cases present as high intestinal obstruction (a midgut volvulus) in the first week of life, with bilious vomiting, distention, and some bleeding.

It is possible to make the diagnosis by a barium enema that shows the cecum in the right upper quadrant or by an upper GI series that reveals an abnormal duodenal sweep with the ligament of Treitz absent or in an abnormal position.

Pediatric Pearl

Neonatal midgut volvulus is an **absolute surgical emergency,** and all haste should be extended to make the diagnosis in order to avoid bowel ischemia and intestinal perforation. Any undue delay in making the diagnosis frequently results in massive bowel resection and a "short gut" syndrome.

ENTERIC DUPLICATIONS. Enteric duplications occur throughout the GI tract. Their etiology is unclear. Ileal duplications are the most common, and gastric duplications are the most rare. Small bowel duplications often contain gastric mucosa, and a technetium radio imaging study may be useful in making the diagnosis. The lesions may be asymptomatic, but most seem to cause problems eventually. Complications can be bleeding from the ectopic gastric mucosa, bacterial overgrowth and malabsorption from a communicating duplication (a blind loop), and obstruction from the cyst. Treatment is surgical resection of the duplication.

INTUSSUSCEPTION. Intussusception is the invagination or telescoping of one portion of the intestine into itself. The majority of cases occur in children younger than 1 year of age, including, infrequently, neonates. Clinically, intussusception produces intermittent, colicky abdominal pain interspersed with intervals in which the patient appears perfectly well. After several episodes of such pain, vomiting (80%) and blood per rectum (95% of infants; 65% of older children) becomes evident. It is important to note that intussusception may present in a nontypical fashion. Apathy and altered states of consciousness may be the only signs. This presentation makes diagnosis difficult unless the clinician has a high index of suspicion.

Pathologically, the mesentery of the invaginated bowel becomes entrapped, causing venous compression and edema. This process continues until the tissue pressure exceeds arterial inflow pressure, with resultant cessation of arterial circulation and ischemia.

Early in the progression of the intussusception, there may be few significant findings. Later, a mass, which is often sausage-shaped, may be palpable in 85% of patients. As the intussusception passes further along the colon, it may be situated behind the right costal margin and be impossible to palpate.

The majority of intussusceptions involve the ileocecal junction (95%). Clearly defined pathology at the lead point occurs in 2%–8% of cases and includes Meckel diverticulum, polyps, enteric duplications, Henoch-Schönlein purpura, cystic fibrosis, and tumors. In the remainder of cases (> 90%), no identifiable lead point pathology is apparent, but a variety of viral infections causing enlarged Peyer patches have been implicated.

The barium enema is the hallmark of diagnosis and treatment. First-line treatment for intussusceptions is usually hydrostatic reduction by barium enema at a height of 3.0–3.5 feet above the table. It is not successful unless there is free flow of barium into multiple loops of small intestine. Hydrostatic reduction is successful in about 85% of cases. Failures or nonattempts occur when high-grade obstruction is evident. In these cases, surgical reduction is necessary. Most recently, the success of air-mediated enemas has been documented, with increasingly good results.

Most intussusceptions with a pathologic lead point do not reduce as a result of barium pressure. The older the child, especially after the age of 6 years, the more likely it is that the lead point is pathologic, especially a lymphoma. In these cases, it is recommended that a search be made for a lead point even if hydrostatic reduction is successful.

Recurrent intussusception following barium reduction occurs in about 5% of patients. Multiple recurrences can occur in the same patients, and in each occurrence the appropriate therapy is still enema reduction. There is a 3% recurrence rate even with surgical reduction.

ANORECTAL ANOMALIES/IMPERFORATE ANUS. Anorectal anomalies arise from incomplete division of the cloaca by the urorectal septum or incomplete convergence of the anal tubercles around the end of the hindgut. These malformations, which occur in 1:4000 to 1:5000 births, mostly affect full-term, appropriate-for-gestational age infants; there is a slight male preponderance. In two-thirds of the cases, these malformations are associated with other anomalies. The other systems most commonly affected are the vertebral column, the CNS, and the genitourinary system.

Inspection of the perineum is helpful in most cases. The **imperforate anus** should be obvious to the naked eye. Meconium may be seen emerging from the vagina, urethra or from a pinpoint anal opening. In infants with an anal membrane, no meconium is passed, but a greenish bulging membrane may be seen.

There are approximately 30 subtypes of anorectal anomalies, in essentially two major groups: the **supralevator (high) imperforate anus** and the **translevator (low) imperforate anus**. This classification is based on the location of the blind pouch. That is, high pouches, which are more common (75%), are at or above the puborectalis sling (supralevator), and low pouches are below the sling (translevator). In both groups, the rectal pouch may end blindly or communicate by a fistula with a nearby viscus or the perineal skin. The vast majority of fistulas are present only in cases of high imperforate anus and involve the urinary tract in males and the genital tract in females. Infants with a low pouch may exhibit a perineal bulge when crying or have a perineal fistulous aperture.

Contrast radiographs of the fistula or instillation of contrast into the rectum should allow delineation of the defect. Sonography and CT may also help define the blind pouch. Treatment is surgical except in anal stenosis, in which simple dilation is adequate. Fecal continence is achieved in more than 90% of children with low pouches, but in only 30%–70% of those with high pouches.

INGUINAL HERNIA. The incidence of inguinal hernia is highest in the first year of life with a peak in the first month of life. Boys are affected six times more than girls, but in both, 60% of hernias occur on the right side, 30% on the left, and 10% bilaterally.

Inguinal hernia occurs when a patent processus vaginalis contains some portion of the abdominal viscera. During development, a peritoneal sac precedes the testicle as it descends from the genital ridge into the scrotum. The lower portion of this sac (processus vaginalis) eventually envelopes the testes and forms the tunica vaginalis and the rest of the sac regresses. In almost 50% of children, the processus vaginalis remains patent, and in some, abdominal contents become trapped.

The symptoms of an incarcerated hernia are abdominal pain, irritability, and vomiting. If there are ischemic changes, pain increases and the vomiting may become bilious, which indicates that there is intestinal obstruction. Inguinal hernia presents as a bulge in the groin that often extends into the scrotum. If a child is relaxed and not crying, usually the hernia reduces either on its own or with manual manipulation by the clinician.

Initially, nonoperative management of an incarcerated inguinal hernia without strangulation is appropriate. After hernia reduction, which occurs in 81% of children, elective surgical repair should take place within 48 hours. However, if an inguinal hernia does not reduce spontaneously, repair is essential because of the high risk of irreducible incarceration and strangulation, especially in the first few months of life. If strangulation occurs, infarction of the contents of the sac results, and an abdominal catastrophe ensues.

GASTROINTESTINAL BLEEDING

Bleeding can occur at any location in the GI tract, and the diagnosis depends to a large extent on the patient's age, the site of the bleeding, and the color of the blood. Because GI hemorrhage can be so frightening to the child and the family, a calm and logical approach to the diagnosis and treatment of the bleed is warranted. In the great majority of cases, bleeding in children is easy to control or stops spontaneously, and a cause determined.

Pathophysiology

Hematemesis is the vomiting of blood. The blood is either bright red or "coffee ground" in appearance if it has been altered by gastric acid. Hematemesis implies that the site of bleeding is proximal to the ligament of Treitz. Blood from the upper GI tract, if vigorous, appears per rectum as black or "tarry" stool (i.e., **melena**). The melenotic stool is coal-black, shiny, sticky, and frequently foul smelling. Bleeding from distal small bowel or colon is usually bright or dark red, but may be black, especially if intestinal transit time is prolonged. **Hematochezia** is the passage of bright red or maroon colored blood in or on the stool. The site of this bleeding is usually in the left colon or anorectal. Occult GI bleeding suggests significant, continuing blood loss in the absence of a visible change in the color or consistency of the stools.

Clinical and Laboratory Evaluation

The physician approaching a child with a presumed GI bleed must first be sure that blood is actually present. Drinks such as Kool-Aid and Hawaiian Punch, gelatins, beets, and tomato sauces mimic hematochezia, and bismuth compounds, iron supplements, charcoal, and spinach simulate melena.

History

Parents tend to overestimate the severity of the blood loss for two reasons: (1) they are anxious and (2) small amounts of blood mixed with toilet water may appear copious. The character of blood loss is important. Because hematemesis implies that the bleeding is proximal to the ligament of Treitz, a history of epistaxis, hemoptysis, or oropharyngeal trauma may preclude the need for a GI workup. Bright red blood, which appears only on the toilet paper, or in the toilet water, or on the surface of the stool, suggests anorectal pathology (e.g., anal fissure, distal polyp, proctitis). If the parents describe black stools with a normal fecal odor, one should be skeptical, because melena is associated with a strong, foul odor.

Past medical history may also be helpful. Evidence of fever (enterocolitis); family pathology (polyps, bleeding diathesis, family cancer syndromes); ingestions of drugs, dyes, or foreign bodies; systemic illnesses (liver disease, collagen vascular disease, IBD, gastroesophageal reflux); or prior symptoms (trauma, colicky pain, constipation with defecation) can be extremely helpful.

Physical Examination

Evaluation of the skin and mucous membranes for signs of Peutz-Jeghers syndrome, angiomata, jaundice, or evidence of bleeding disorders is warranted. Careful examination of the abdomen is important. Hepatosplenomegaly may indicate portal hypertension (and variceal bleeding) or sepsis, while an abdominal mass may suggest intestinal duplication or intussusception.

Laboratory Evaluation

A Hemoccult test is essential, and if positive, it is appropriate to eliminate extraintestinal sources of bleeding such as nose, mouth, pharynx, and vagina. If significant GI bleeding is actually present, it is necessary to insert a nasogastric tube and aspirate fluid unless a distal source is obvious (anal fissure, distal polyp, or IBD). If the nasogastric tube aspirate is positive for blood, the bleeding is almost surely proximal to the ligament of Treitz.

POSITIVE NASOGASTRIC ASPIRATE. If the nasogastric aspirate is positive for blood, an upper endoscopy within the first 24 hours is the procedure of choice to ascertain the etiology of the bleeding; this establishes the source in more than 90% of cases. The most common causes of upper GI bleeding in children (in order of frequency) are gastritis, esophagitis, duodenal ulcers, and esophageal varices. Endoscopy is necessary in children with active bleeding and known esophageal varices, because lesions other than varices are the source of the bleeding in as many as 50% of cases.

In unusual cases, in which endoscopy and barium studies fail to elucidate the source of bleeding, or in which bleeding is brisk (> 0.5 ml/min), arteriography may be appropriate. This examination, via the superior and inferior mesenteric arteries and the celiac axis, may reveal the more common causes of bleeding as well as unusual causes such as hematobilia from trauma, hepatic artery aneurysms, gastropancreatic duplication cysts, or arteriovenous malformations and hemangiomas.

If arteriography has not been helpful or cannot be performed, it is possible to label red blood cells (RBCs) with a radioactive marker and then scan the abdomen to detect the site of active bleeding. Both arteriography and tagged RBC

studies are technically unfeasible if barium studies have recently taken place.

NEGATIVE NASOGASTRIC ASPIRATE. The approach to a child with rectal bleeding and a negative nasogastric aspirate is predicated on the color and amount of blood and the child's symptoms. If bright red blood is in the toilet water or coating the stool, an **anal fissure** is by far the most likely diagnosis. Therefore, a careful perianal examination is indicated. The clinician should exert constant thumb pressure on both sides of the anus to evert the area. If an anal fissure is not apparent, the pediatrician should suspect distal polyps or proctitis. A digital rectal examination and a proctosigmoidoscopy are necessary.

If the blood is darker in color, admixed with the stool, and usually unassociated with abdominal pain and diarrhea, a Meckel diverticulum, enteric duplication, or proximal polyp are suspected. A Meckel scan is necessary initially, followed by colonoscopy and air contrast barium enema.

If the blood is admixed with the stool and associated with abdominal pain or diarrhea, consideration of IBD, infectious or allergic colitis, or vasculitis is warranted. Appropriate blood and stool studies are necessary prior to endoscopy and barium studies.

In a totally asymptomatic child who presents with occult blood in the stool and anemia, a thorough workup may be indicated. A Meckel scan is necessary initially, followed by upper and lower endoscopy, an air contrast barium enema, and finally an upper GI barium study.

If the entire workup is negative and significant rectal bleeding persists or recurs, an exploratory laparotomy may be indicated. A laparotomy most often reveals a Meckel diverticulum in the face of a completely negative workup. Other possible diagnoses include intussusception, small bowel tumors, duplications, and vascular lesions of the bowel.

Differential Diagnosis: Etiology by Age
(Table 15.7)

Newborns (birth to 1 month)

GI bleeding in neonates differs from that in older children. Several causes are very specific to this age group, and the mortality associated with bleeding is much higher than at any other time in childhood. However, the cause of the bleeding is often not determined because the bleeding often stops in less than 24 hours, and no evaluation is performed. Undiagnosed bleeding is usually the

TABLE 15.7 Differential Diagnosis of Gastrointestinal Bleeding

Upper Gastrointestinal Tract Bleeding

Conditions specific to neonates
   Swallowed maternal blood
   Hemorrhagic disease of the newborn
   Hemorrhagic gastritic/stress ulcer
Acid/alkali disease
   Esophagitis
   Gastritis/duodenitis
   Peptic ulcers
Esophageal/gastric varices
Mallory-Weiss tear
Hematobilia
Swallowed blood (oropharyngeal)

Lower Gastrointestinal Tract Bleeding

Anal fissure
Enterocolitis
   Neonatal ischemia
   Infection
      Bacterial
      Parasitic
      Viral (immunocompromised)
   Allergic
      Cow's milk protein/soy protein intolerance
      Eosinophilic gastroenteropathy
   Inflammatory bowel disease
   Antibiotic-induced colitis (*Clostridium difficile*)
Midgut volvulus
Juvenile polyps and tumors
Vascular malformations
Meckel diverticulum
Duplication (enteric cysts)
Intussusception
Nodular lymphoid hyperplasia
Vascular abnormalities
   Henoch-Schönlein purpura
   Hemolytic-uremic syndrome
   Autoimmune vasculitis
   Infectious vasculitis
   Ischemia
Foreign body
Trauma

result of **hemorrhagic gastritis or stress ulcers** caused by a perinatal insult such as hypoxia, sepsis, or a CNS lesion that renders the gastric mucosa vulnerable to the effects of the relatively high gastric acidity in newborns. Other frequently recognized causes of neonatal bleeding are **hemorrhagic disease of the newborn** and **anal fissures.** Another source of GI bleeding in neonates is **swallowed maternal blood,** which may appear as hematemesis or even massive dark rectal bleeding. The **Apt test** readily provides a diagnosis. This test differentiates fetal from maternal blood by adding sodium hydroxide to a supernatant of the blood.

Fetal blood remains pink due to the alkaline resistance of fetal hemoglobin, while adult hemoglobin changes to a brown color.

Necrotizing enterocolitis in preterm or stressed infants and enterocolitis secondary to **Hirschsprung disease** may result in occult to moderate rectal bleeding (see CONGENITAL GASTROINTESTINAL ANOMALIES AND INTESTINAL OBSTRUCTION, DIFFERENTIAL DIAGNOSIS). **Midgut volvulus** associated with malrotation of the bowel is a grave emergency that can produce melena or hematochezia. All three of these entities are life threatening and require rapid diagnosis and aggressive intervention with fluid replacement, antibiotics, bowel decompression, or surgery.

Cow's milk protein allergy may also manifest as occult or significant rectal bleeding (see GASTROINTESTINAL BLEEDING). Affected infants may also have diarrhea, wheezing, atopic dermatitis, or rhinitis. Symptoms usually resolve with cessation of the cow's milk feedings. If refeedings begin, symptoms may recur within hours, and are associated with a peripheral leukocytosis with or without an eosinophilia. It is possible to diagnose cow's milk–induced colitis by obtaining a rectal biopsy with an inflammatory reaction with a predominance of eosinophils while the infant is on the offending agent. Treatment involves changing to a casein hydrolysate formula (soy-based formulas often cross-react with cow's milk protein).

Children

ANAL FISSURES. Perianal fissures are the most common cause of nonmassive, bright red anal bleeding in children. Blood tends to streak the stool and may be mixed with flecks of mucus. Fissures usually result from the trauma of passing a large, hard stool, but they may occur in children who pass softer stools, but who frequently strain. These fissures, or stercoral ulcers, are usually present in the midline, along the median raphe. Rectal prolapse (incomplete) or procidentia (complete) may also cause bright red rectal bleeding. These lesions are most often the result of constipation and straining, but it is necessary to rule out cystic fibrosis and parasitic infestation.

MALLORY-WEISS TEARS. Mallory-Weiss tears consist of a laceration of the posterior wall of the gastroesophageal junction that may extend through the muscularis mucosae. The tears, which are more often on the gastric side, follow forceful emesis or repeated retching. They may cause massive upper GI bleeding and are often difficult to diagnose without careful upper endoscopy. Selective celiac arteriography also demonstrates the lesions. Clinicians have reported the existence of Mallory-Weiss tears in children as young as 16 weeks of age. Bleeding usually stops spontaneously, and surgery is rarely indicated.

GASTRITIS/STRESS LESIONS. Erosions of the intestinal mucosa may occur acutely following major trauma, burns, shock, or severe sepsis. These lesions are superficial, multiple, and occur mostly in the fundus of the stomach. **Cushing ulcers,** which occur with intracranial surgery and head injury, tend to be single and deep, and may involve the esophagus, stomach, and duodenum. The pathogenesis of these lesions are unclear, but it appears that gastric mucosal ischemia interferes with the normal buffering ability. Duodenal reflux of bile salts due to ileus may add to the ulceration.

ACID-PEPTIC DISEASE (SEE ACID-PEPTIC DISEASE AND *HELICOBACTER PYLORI* INFECTION). Peptic ulcers may present as hematemesis, melena, or both. About 25% of children with peptic ulcers present with GI bleeding.

PORTAL HYPERTENSION AND VARICES. Obstruction to portal venous flow leads to **portal hypertension** with subsequent **esophageal or gastric varices** and splenomegaly with hypersplenism. Prehepatic portal vein obstruction usually follows neonatal events such as omphalitis or catheterization of the umbilical vein with thrombus formation. Intrahepatic causes are usually secondary to cirrhosis. Variceal bleeding may be the first evidence of cirrhosis (e.g., with cystic fibrosis) or may be related to noncirrhotic causes of intrahepatic venous stasis such as congenital hepatic fibrosis or nodular regenerative hyperplasia. Hemorrhage from varices is infrequent in the first year of life, but 67% of patients bleed with varices before 5 years of age and 85% by 10 years of age.

There is little evidence that varices bleed because of erosive mucosal damage. The risks of bleeding are more likely related to increased portal vein pressure and the diameter of the varices. Most variceal bleeding stops spontaneously in children, because of their ability to respond to a "preshock" state with excellent vasoconstriction. If bleeding fails to cease, intravenous agents such as somatostatin or vasopressin may be necessary. Injection sclerotherapy has become extremely effective in controlling variceal bleeding, but it is preferable to use these injections of a sclerosing agent such as sodium morrhuate on an elective, rather than on an emergent basis. Emergency surgical interventions for acute bleeding such as portal-systemic shunting or esophageal transection with devascularization are associated with a high morbidity; it is essential to avoid them, if at all possible.

OTHER CAUSES OF BLEEDING. Important causes of GI bleeding such as intussusception, Meckel diverticulum, and enteric duplications are described previously (see INTUSSUSCEPTION, MECKEL DIVERTICULUM, and ENTERIC DUPLICATION). In addition, many systemic diseases associated with vasculitis and microangiopathy may have GI bleeding as one of their manifestations. **Henoch-Schönlein purpura,** the most common vasculitis of childhood, may have rectal bleeding as part of its clinical picture in addition to the classic features of abdominal pain, nephritis, lower extremity and buttock purpura, and arthralgia. It is believed that the GI pain and bleeding are related to the anaphylactoid vasculitis that can lead to submucosal hemorrhage. Accumulation of submucosal hemorrhage may become the lead point for an intussusception.

Bloody diarrhea may often be the presenting symptom of **hemolytic-uremic syndrome**. A verotoxin produced by *E. coli* 0157:H7, or the cytotoxin such as shiga, which is produced by *Shigella dysenteriae,* may induce this microangiopathy. The GI symptoms of severe abdominal pain and bloody diarrhea may be secondary to the infection or may be related to thrombosis of intestinal blood vessels. The GI symptoms usually precede the platelet consumption, hemolysis, and acute renal insufficiency by several days. Other vasculitic disorders such as Rocky Mountain spotted fever and collagen vascular diseases can cause lower GI bleeding. In addition, hemangiomas of the GI tract that are usually cavernous in nature, involving the rectosigmoid, can cause bleeding.

Management

Treatment is disease specific (see DIFFERENTIAL DIAGNOSIS). Most often, physicians in GI and pediatric surgical subspecialties are involved in diagnosing the etiology and guiding the management of individual children.

INFLAMMATORY DISEASES OF THE BOWEL

Inflammatory bowel disease (IBD), including ulcerative colitis and Crohn disease, is a major cause of chronic disease. Epidemiologic studies of IBD in children are limited. The incidence of

IBD, which is highest in northwestern Europe and North America, is more common among whites than nonwhites. Males and females are equally affected. Susceptibility appears to be increased for Jews, especially those of a middle European background. Researchers have clearly shown the family aggregation of IBD. At the time of diagnosis of either ulcerative colitis or Crohn disease, the chances of finding IBD in a first-degree relative of the proband are 5%–25%.

Pathophysiology

Despite great efforts from many research groups, the etiology and pathophysiology of IBD are still unclear. To date, no convincing evidence implicates a viral, chlamydial, bacterial, or mycobacterial pathogen as the causative agent. However, it is possible that any, or all of these agents may trigger the disease in predisposed patients. Recent, exciting work suggests that defects in immunoregulation involving the gut-associated lymphoid tissue and the complex mixture of antigens and pathogens in the bowel lumen may play a major role in the development and progression of the diseases, but more clarification is needed.

Chronic **ulcerative colitis** and **Crohn disease** are the major inflammatory diseases of the intestine. Affected adolescents frequently present with these conditions. Increasing numbers of children younger than 12 years of age have received these diagnoses; however, this may represent improved recognition by clinicians rather than a true increase in the incidence among very young patients.

Ulcerative colitis and Crohn disease are distinct pathologic entities but share many signs and symptoms. Ulcerative colitis is defined as a chronic inflammatory process limited to only the **mucosal** layer of the large intestine. Crohn disease, on the other hand, is a chronic **transmural** inflammatory process, involving noncaseating granuloma formation, which may involve any portion of the GI system from the mouth to the anus, including the ileum in about 85% of cases (Table 15.8).

Clinical and Laboratory Evaluation

History

Abdominal pain and **diarrhea** are the most common complaints of children with IBD, both at initial diagnosis and at relapse. Many patients with IBD who have abdominal pain and diarrhea of an urgent nature may choose not to eat at certain times, so as to avoid embarrassing accidents. Abdominal pain and diarrhea may be nocturnal and awaken the patient.

Pediatric Pearl

The occurrence of nocturnal pain and diarrhea that awakens the patient helps distinguish IBD from IBS, in which symptoms tend to occur only when the patient is awake.

TABLE 15.8 **Clinical Features of Inflammatory Bowel Disease (Colonic): Ulcerative Colitis versus Crohn Colitis**

Feature*	Ulcerative Colitis	Crohn Colitis
Macroscopic		
Distribution	Continuous with rectum	Segmental
Rectal involvement	Usual (98%)	Usual (80%–85%)
Terminal ileum	Usually normal	Involved (85%)
Mucosa	Diffusely involved	Discrete ulcers, fissures, cobblestoning
Serosa	Usually normal	Congestion, thickening
Fistulas	Absent	Present
Pseudopolyps	Common	Common
Strictures	Uncommon	Common
Microscopic		
Inflammation	Diffuse, mucosal, submucosal	Patchy, transmural
Ulceration	Mucosal, submucosal	Deep
Crypt abscesses	Common	Common
Granulomata	Absent	Common (60%–75%)
Fibrosis (serosal)	Absent	Present

*Subtotal colectomy specimen.

Physical Examination

Children and adolescents with IBD may have a normal examination or a myriad of clinical manifestations such as poor growth, cachexia, and sexual delay. findings that should alert the physician include perianal lesions, clubbing, and rashes such as erythema nodosum.

GASTROINTESTINAL MANIFESTATIONS. The **abdominal pain** of IBD tends to be crampy, usually localized to the lower abdomen and tends not to be significantly improved by the passage of flatus or a bowel movement. The **diarrhea** may be of variable volume with small volume stools often being accompanied by tenesmus or urgency. These symptoms suggest active inflammation in the distal rectosigmoid. Visible **blood per rectum** is suggestive of active colonic inflammation in IBD, while Crohn disease of the small bowel is more frequently associated with occult blood or no blood at all. In a subgroup of patients with IBD, blood loss may be brisk, causing severe anemia, hemodynamic abnormalities with orthostatic changes, and requiring aggressive intervention.

EXTRAINTESTINAL MANIFESTATIONS. An important part of the clinical picture of IBD is the wide range of extraintestinal manifestations that can be seen in children with ulcerative colitis and Crohn disease (Table 15.9). The extraintestinal problems may present before the onset of intestinal symptoms, or at any time after the diagnosis has been made.

It is important to remember that many patients with IBD, especially with small bowel Crohn disease, may present with more subtle findings and have little or no intestinal findings. The presentation may be one of poor growth and sexual retar-

dation, fever of unknown origin, arthritis, perianal disease or a seeming feeding disorder. **Anorexia** is common and is frequently associated with inadequate intake of micro- and macronutrients. In Crohn disease there may be early satiety with solid foods, reflecting upper GI involvement. In patients without evidence of Crohn disease of the stomach and duodenum, there has been speculation that the anorexia may be related to a chronic *H. pylori*–negative gastritis or to a proximal bowel motility disturbance.

Perianal lesions, which are by far the most common of the extraintestinal problems, are also the most difficult to treat. In one study of 149 children and adolescents with Crohn disease, researchers found a 49% prevalence of perianal disease. Of these 71 patients, 51 had fissures and large anal tags (sentinel tags), 10 had fistulae, and 12 had abscesses. Because these lesions may precede the classic signs and symptoms of IBD, it reinforces the importance of the clinician's doing an adequate perianal evaluation in all children with unexplained illness.

Delayed growth and sexual maturation, which is common in Crohn disease, may be the most devastating part of IBD for adolescents. In contrast, growth retardation infrequently affects patients with ulcerative colitis. Severe linear growth retardation occurs in about 30% of children with Crohn disease and the growth impairment frequently antedates the diagnosis, may precede weight loss, and can be the earliest indicator of the disease. In addition, growth curves reveal that as many as 60% of children with Crohn disease drop two standard deviations or more from their best height percentile for age during adolescence. Nineteen percent remain two standard deviations below their best height percentile at maturity.

Experts have attributed this marked growth delay to a combination of factors, including inadequate caloric intake, chronic inflammation and hypermetabolism, excessive enteric protein loss, and some degree of malabsorption. Recent data show that young adults with Crohn disease who received treatment with aggressive nutritional support still do not reach their ultimate predicted height. This suggests that other, still not elucidated, factors may be involved. There is growing evidence that indicate that the cytokines responsible for mediating inflammation in the bowel also have a direct growth-inhibiting effect.

Fever, which occurs in 25%–50% of children with IBD, often without a discernible focus of infection, may be a frequent diagnostic and therapeutic dilemma. **Anemia** is common and usually

---

TABLE 15.9 **Extraintestinal Manifestations of Inflammatory Bowel Disease**

Perianal disease
Hepatobiliary disease
Mouth lesions
Cutaneous lesions
Vasculitis
Vascular thrombosis
Anemia, thrombocytosis
Arthritis, arthralgias
Ocular disorders
Myocarditis, pericarditis
Nephrolithiasis
Pulmonary fibrosis

results from either blood loss or lack of incorporation of iron into erythrocytes in the bone marrow. In the anemia of chronic IBD, the erythrocytes are hypochromic and microcytic. However, iron is present in the bone marrow and normal serum ferritin concentrations reflect normal total body iron stores. Laboratory studies reveal a low serum iron with a normal to high total iron binding capacity. The low serum iron probably relates to the deposition of available iron in the reticuloendothelium system.

Although **arthralgias** are common, frank arthritis occurs infrequently in children and adolescents with IBD. Joint deformities, resulting from chronic inflammation, are very rare in IBD and should suggest the possibility of another autoimmune disease such as rheumatoid arthritis or systemic lupus erythematosus. Aseptic necrosis of the hip is quite rare, even if the particular child or adolescent is undergoing chronic steroid therapy. Adolescents with IBD often complain of chronic lower back pain and tenderness. A few have sacroiliitis, but in most, diagnostic studies reveal no specific skeletal or joint abnormality, but signs and symptoms often remit with NSAIDs.

Hypoalbuminemia, which is almost always seen with active IBD, results from protein loss due to bowel inflammation. This can be confirmed by looking for increased amounts of α_1-antitrypsin in the stool. Protein malabsorption in IBD is usually not clinically significant. In addition, protein intake is usually adequate despite poor caloric intake.

Colorectal cancer is a formidable problem for patients with long-standing IBD. The two most important risk factors for developing colorectal cancer are disease duration and anatomic extent of disease. Therefore, it is suggested that all patients with colonic involvement, including those patients with Crohn colitis, should have colonoscopy surveillance after 8 years of disease. This suggestion most definitely pertains to children and adolescents with IBD.

Laboratory Evaluation

In IBD, the ESR is often elevated, but normal values may be seen even in acute fulminant colitis. If the ESR is elevated, it is more likely to be indicative of IBD than IBS, in which laboratory data should be normal. Evaluation of stool cultures and analysis of stools for ova and parasites and fecal Wright stain is necessary. A low serum albumin indicates protein loss from inflamed bowel mucosa, whereas a low serum cholesterol often reflects loss of bile salts in the feces due to the presence of significant ileal disease. The serum

immune markers antineutrophil cytoplasmic antibody (ANCA) and anti–*Saccharomyces cerevisiae* antibody (ASCA) are being used increasingly to help in differentiating IBD from other entities. ANCAs are present in the sera of 60%–80% of patients with ulcerative colitis, in < 20% of patients with Crohn disease, and in about 6% of the general population. ASCAs are present in 60%–70% of patients with Crohn disease and very infrequently in patients with ulcerative colitis or in children without IBD.

Currently, it is usual to obtain an upper GI with small bowel series and to perform a colonoscopy with multiple biopsies. During this procedure, it is necessary to take biopsies from even normal looking mucosa, because histologic inflammation may be present in tissue that appears normal endoscopically.

It is very useful to determine growth velocity curves, Tanner staging for sexual maturation, and bone ages as a way of assessing a child's growth and development and potential for future maturation. A lactose breath hydrogen test may be helpful in determining whether milk can or cannot be used in the diet. It is also a good idea to perform a Mantoux skin test for tuberculosis at the time of diagnosis, in case steroid therapy becomes necessary. Radiographs and bone scans are necessary in the child with chronic joint discomfort to determine whether the problem is related to osteonecrosis.

Differential Diagnosis

Despite these seemingly clear differences between ulcerative colitis and Crohn disease, it is often very difficult to distinguish between the two conditions when the disease is strictly limited to the colon. In a child with Crohn disease and only colonic involvement without perianal disease or granuloma detected through biopsy, it may be necessary to defer a precise diagnosis. Involvement of the rectum, once considered exclusive to ulcerative colitis, occurs in 80%–85% of children with Crohn disease. Moreover, the finding of a normal rectum through endoscopy, once thought of as inconsistent with ulcerative colitis, actually can occur with this disease. Biopsy specimens of mucosa that appears to be normal may show varying degrees of inflammation and granulomata (see Table 15.8).

Certain radiographic features may help distinguish ulcerative colitis from Crohn disease (Table 15.10). However, the distribution of the disease as shown by radiographic examination (continuous versus segmental) is nonspecific; often, it does not reflect the extent of the inflam-

TABLE 15.10 Inflammatory Bowel Disease (Colonic): Radiographic Differentiation in Ulcerative Colitis versus Crohn Colitis		
Radiographic Feature	Ulcerative Colitis	Crohn Colitis
Terminal ileum	Usually normal	Often involved (65%), stenotic, irregular
Symmetry	Usually symmetric	Often asymmetric
Foreshortening	Common	Common
Mucosa	Shallow ulceration, pseudopolyps	Longitudinal fissures, cobblestone appearance; pseudopolyps
Fistulas	Absent	Present
Sinus tract	Absent	Present
Strictures	Uncommon (suggests carcinoma)	Frequent

mation. In fact, barium enema studies may be normal in as many as 25% of children with inflammatory colitis that has been documented endoscopically and histologically.

The differential diagnosis of IBD is broad and causes of chronic diarrhea, such as amebiasis, giardiasis, *Yersinia enterocolitica,* and *Campylobacter jejuni* must be entertained. In the appropriate setting, the diagnosis of tuberculosis, allergic enteropathies (including gluten-induced enteropathy), vasculitis, and neoplasms (especially intestinal lymphoma) must be considered.

Management

It is necessary to gear all therapeutic approaches to children and adolescents with IBD toward having the patient perform the functions of daily living as normally as possible. This means the suppression of incapacitating symptoms, promotion of normal growth and development, and control of complications. The clinician should take care to avoid excessive or inappropriate therapy. Treatment requires a careful balance between sufficient intervention to improve the patient's quality of life and avoidance of the deleterious side effects of overtreatment.

Nutritional Support

Although the growth failure and sexual retardation in IBD is multifactorial, inadequate caloric intake seems to play a major role. It is necessary to provide nutritional support to provide adequate calories and the proper macro- and micronutrients either orally, enterally, or parenterally.

Adolescents with IBD often require 80–90 kcal and 3.00 g protein/kg ideal body weight/day to achieve their height potential (healthy adolescents need 60 kcal and 2.25 g/kg/day). For children with asymptomatic or mildly symptomatic ulcerative colitis and Crohn disease but who have inadequate weight and height gain and delayed sexual maturation, the use of oral liquid supple-

mentation is encouraged. Supplementing the usual diet with these drinks can result in adequate caloric intake and improved growth. However, many patients cannot or will not accept this approach because of the volume needed, the taste of the liquid, or their own gastric dysmotility.

Nasogastric infusions of formula also result in improved growth. The use of nocturnal nasogastric infusions after insertion of the tube by the patient at home allows for significant increases in weight and height and normal attainment of puberty. The approach, with the tube being removed in the morning, allows the patient to pursue normal activities. It permits flexibility because the feedings can be discontinued on weekends and vacations, if necessary.

High-calorie intravenous infusions through a central venous line during sleep also provide a possible source of increased calories. The line is capped during the day, making normal activity possible. However, this approach is riskier than tube feedings because it can occasionally cause line sepsis or hepatobiliary dysfunction.

Medical Therapy

As previously mentioned, new evidence suggests that IBD may be a result of defects in gut immunoregulation with perturbations in T-cell regulation as a key (see INFLAMMATORY DISEASES OF THE BOWEL, PATHOPHYSIOLOGY). New therapeutic modalities such as cytokine manipulation (including infliximab, an anti–tumor necrosis factor alpha monoclonal antibody) are in their infancy and herald an exciting new era in treatment of IBD. At present, the major modes of therapy are aminosalicylates, corticosteroids, immunosuppressive agents such as 6-mercaptopurine, and antibiotics.

5-AMINOSALICYLATES. The mechanisms of action of the 5-aminosalicylate compounds are unclear but probably involve inhibition of cyclo-oxygenase, and, especially, lipoxygenase pathways as well as scavenging of oxygen radicals. Several oral and rectal preparations are now available. Some of the oral medications are effective in small bowel disease as well as the previously recognized colonic efficacy. In ulcerative colitis, preparations of 5-aminosalicylates are effective in newly diagnosed mild disease, active disease at relapse, and maintenance of remissions. In Crohn disease, 5-aminosalicylate preparations play an effective role in treatment of active colonic disease and may contribute to the treatment of active small bowel disease. In addition, in Crohn disease, 5-aminosalicylates may prevent relapses, especially if patients have ileal disease or a history of resection.

CORTICOSTEROIDS. Corticosteroids have long been the gold standard for treatment of moderate-to-severe ulcerative colitis and Crohn disease. As clinicians gain more experience and success with new methods of immunomodulation, steroid use is diminishing. Rectal corticosteroids, in foam or enema form, are often effective in children with mild active ulcerative colitis of Crohn colitis who have predominant symptoms of distal left-sided colitis such as tenesmus and urgency. Pediatricians often prescribe them in conjunction with oral 5-aminosalicylate preparations. Although mucosal absorption of the rectal corticosteroids is small, some clinicians who are wary of any steroid effect are more frequently using 5-aminosalicylate enemas [mesalamine (Rowasa)] in these circumstances with little loss of symptom control.

Oral corticosteroids (prednisone) at doses of 0.5–1.0 mg/kg/day and intravenous hydrocortisone at 0.5–1.0 mg/kg/dose given every 6 hours is usually effective in moderate-to-severe disease. After a remission is achieved, patients are slowly weaned and begin taking a 5-aminosalicylate preparation. Some patients have symptom breakthrough with reduced dosages of steroids and need continuous treatment. A subgroup of these may be successful with steroids on an alternate-day basis, thus avoiding the linear growth–retarding effect. When long-term daily steroids are necessary, alternate treatment plans may become necessary because of the significant long-term complications of corticosteroid use such as growth suppression, osteoporosis, cataract formation, and aseptic necrosis of the bones. In addition, and most importantly in adolescents, the many disturbing cosmetic side effects from steroid use (cushingoid facies, hirsutism, striae, acne) lead to poor compliance.

IMMUNOSUPPRESSIVE DRUGS. 6-mercaptopurine is the most commonly prescribed immunosuppressive for adolescents with intractable Crohn disease.

Studies have found that the drug is an effective long-term therapy. In addition, it has the important advantage of having a significant steroid-sparing effect, which is of particular benefit to adolescents. When used at a daily dose of 1.0–1.5 mg/kg/day to a maximum of 75 mg/day, no evidence of neutropenia, serious infection, or other untoward reactions is apparent.

It is unclear whether 6-mercaptopurine has efficacy in ulcerative colitis. Cyclosporine and intravenous gamma globulin are also being evaluated in children and adolescents with IBD.

ANTIBIOTICS. Metronidazole (Flagyl) has been found to have a steroid-sparing effect on adolescents with active or steroid-dependent Crohn disease. The dosage used has been 15–20 mg/kg/day. The mechanism of action is unclear. A large number of adolescents on chronic metronidazole therapy develop paresthesias and dysesthesias, which are reversible with discontinuation of the drug. However, the frequency and severity of symptoms have limited the acceptance of this effective therapy. Other oral antibiotics such as tetracycline and ciprofloxacin (in older children) may suppress symptoms of bacterial overgrowth in some patients with Crohn disease.

Surgery

ULCERATIVE COLITIS. Emergency surgical intervention may be necessary because of acute fulminant colitis, massive intestinal bleeding, free perforation, or toxic megacolon. Elective surgery is appropriate for dependence on growth-suppressive steroids, continuous debilitating symptoms despite medical therapy, and the presence of colonic dysplasia in noninflamed tissue or evidence of malignancy on surveillance colonoscopy. This surveillance is suggested for patients with ulcerative colitis and Crohn colitis for longer than 8 years.

Surgery in ulcerative colitis is curative and eliminates the risk of malignancy. The initial surgical approach in adolescents with presumed ulcerative colitis consists of a subtotal colectomy and ileostomy. The distal sigmoid and rectum are left intact. The subtotal colectomy specimen should be closely evaluated to confirm the clinical impression of ulcerative colitis. If so, patients may opt to have their traditional ileostomy converted to an endorectal pull-through or ileoanal anastomosis within the next 6–12 months.

CROHN DISEASE. Surgical intervention is recommended to deal with complications that are unresponsive to medical therapy such as intestinal obstruction, perianal disease, and fistulae. Resection of a localized diseased segment may be preferable to chronic medications. Recurrence after surgical resection in Crohn disease is greater than 90%, so surgery should be considered after careful deliberation. Multiple intestinal resections may lead to a "short gut" problem. Patients with intestinal strictures leading to recurrent partial obstruction may undergo stricturoplasty, a bowel-sparing technique that creates a patent lumen.

LIVER DISEASE IN CHILDREN AND ADOLESCENTS

The understanding of the embryology and development of the fetal liver and the pathophysiology of pediatric liver disease has increased dramatically in the last two decades. Despite this increased knowledge, medical treatment of many of the hepatobiliary disorders of childhood has continued to be frustrating. However, optimism has arisen in view of the advances in gene therapy and the increased availability and improved techniques in liver transplantation.

NEONATAL CHOLESTASIS

Neonatal cholestasis is far less common than unconjugated hyperbilirubinemia. Despite its relative infrequency, neonatal cholestasis is always pathologic. Therefore, the clinician should consider the possibility of cholestasis in a jaundiced infant.

Pathophysiology

The terms neonatal cholestasis and neonatal conjugated hyperbilirubinemia are often used interchangeably, although it is technically incorrect and occasionally clinically confusing. **Cholestasis** refers to an impedance to bile acid flow, which may have significant pathophysiologic implications, while **conjugated (direct) hyperbilirubinemia,** which frequently but not invariably accompanies the cholestasis, is more of a clinical marker rather than a cause of disease. Although there is some controversy over the exact definition of conjugated hyperbilirubinemia, most would accept as abnormal a direct bilirubin level of more than 2 mg/dl, or more than 50% of the total bilirubin level. Unlike neonatal unconjugated (indirect) hyperbilirubinemia, which is more frequently physiologic rather than pathologic, **conjugated hyperbilirubinemia should always be viewed as abnormal** and should not be ignored. Early recog-

nition of cholestasis in infants and prompt diagnosis of the underlying disorder are imperative to identify those disorders that respond to specific treatment. Several conditions may cause neonatal cholestasis (Table 15.11).

Clinical and Laboratory Evaluation

The key to the evaluation of infants with cholestasis is to determine which of them have conditions that are surgically correctable (extrahepatic biliary atresia, choledochal cyst) or amenable to treatment with diet and medication (tyrosinemia, galactosemia, fructosemia). Promptness of diagnosis and therapy may have tremendous implications for prognosis.

History and Physical Examination
Most infants with neonatal cholestasis present with jaundice, dark urine, acholic stools, and varying degrees of hepatomegaly. It is necessary to evaluate infants for evidence of congenital anomalies, splenomegaly, skin rash, and neurologic signs.

> **Pediatric Pearl**
>
> Note that patients with extrahepatic biliary atresia, choledochal cyst, and many of the intrahepatic causes of neonatal cholestasis look remarkably well despite the jaundice. On the other hand, infants with cholestasis who appear toxic should point the clinician toward an infectious or metabolic etiology.

Laboratory Evaluation
Laboratory tests that evaluate liver function are not particularly helpful in distinguishing the various causes of infantile cholestasis. Blood tests that may be useful include titers for toxoplasmosis, congenital syphilis and viruses, rubella, cytomegalovirus, herpes simplex virus (TORCH); hepatitis A, B, and C markers; α_1-antitrypsin levels and phenotypes; thyroid function; as well as iron and ferritin levels. Viral and bacterial cultures as well as urine for metabolic studies (e.g., reducing substances, amino acids) are necessary when clinically indicated.

Helpful studies are **hepatobiliary ultrasonography,** which can make or exclude the diagnosis of choledochal cyst as well as suggest biliary atresia, and **hepatobiliary scintigraphy** (e.g., HIDA scan) after premedication with phenobarbital, which can exclude biliary atresia if the isotope

TABLE 15.11 Causes of Neonatal Cholestasis

Extrahepatic Causes

Biliary atresia
    Polysplenia syndrome
    Immotile cilia syndrome
Choledochal cyst
Spontaneous bile duct perforation
Obstruction (tumors, stones, sludge, anomalies)

Intrahepatic Causes

Infectious
    Bacterial sepsis (*Escherichia coli, Listeria*)
    Urinary tract infection, endotoxemia
    TORCH syndrome
    Syphilis
    Other viral infections
        Hepatitis B
        Hepatitis C
Metabolic
    α_1-Antitrypsin deficiency
    Cystic fibrosis
    Hypothyroidism, hypopituitarism
    Tyrosinemia
    Galactosemia, fructosemia, glycogen storage disease IV
    Disorders of lipid metabolism (Gaucher, Niemann-Pick, Wolman)
    Neonatal iron storage disease
Toxic
    Total parenteral nutrition–related conditions
Anatomic
    Inspissated bile syndrome
    Congenital hepatic fibrosis
    Caroli disease (cystic dilation of intrahepatic ducts)
Idiopathic
    Familial
        Alagille syndrome (syndromic paucity of intrahepatic ducts)
        Byler disease
        Agneas syndrome (hereditary cholestasis with lymphedema)
        Benign recurrent cholestasis
        Zellweger syndrome (cerebrohepatorenal syndrome)
        Other defects in bile acid metabolism
    Sporadic
        "Idiopathic" neonatal hepatitis
        Nonsyndromic paucity of intrahepatic bile ducts

TORCH = toxoplasmosis, rubella, cytomegalovirus, herpes simplex.

passes from the liver into the intestine. Ultimately, a **liver biopsy** may be necessary to ascertain the diagnosis.

Differential Diagnosis

Although the differential diagnosis of neonatal cholestasis is varied, the clinical presentation in many of these disorders is similar, reflecting a similar response to the underlying decrease in bile flow. The most common disorders causing neonatal cholestasis in full-term infants are extrahepatic biliary atresia and some of the idio-

pathic causes (paucity of intrahepatic bile ducts and idiopathic neonatal hepatitis). **Extrahepatic biliary atresia** appears to be related to a perinatal inflammatory process that continues postnatally, finally obliterating part of the extrahepatic tree. The process appears to involve the intrahepatic structures as well but to a lesser degree. The etiology is unknown, but REOvirus has been causally associated in some patients. Infants are usually healthy but acquire jaundice in the 2nd or 3rd week of life. Their stools eventually become acholic but develop a greenish coloration related to the shedding of bilirubin-filled intestinal mucosal cells, which may fool parents and physicians. Trisomy 13 and 18, polysplenia, and immotile cilia syndromes may be associated with biliary atresia.

Paucity of intrahepatic bile ducts is being recognized more frequently as a cause of neonatal cholestasis. The syndromic form, **Alagille syndrome** (arteriohepatic dysplasia) consists of paucity of the ducts and cardiac lesions (valvular or peripheral pulmonic stenosis), along with classic facies, butterfly vertebra, posterior embryotoxon in the eye and renal dysplasia. Growth failure and mild mental retardation is also seen. The nonsyndromic form of paucity of intrahepatic ducts is probably a morphologic endpoint to multiple different insults to the neonatal liver. It may occur frequently in sick neonates and prematures who have hypoxia, hypoperfusion, and sepsis. The prognosis for the syndromic form is usually better. Liver biopsy may be used to diagnose both forms.

Management

If a percutaneous liver biopsy shows bile duct proliferation (a manifestation of extrahepatic obstruction), exploratory laparotomy is warranted. If the procedure confirms biliary atresia, a Kasai procedure (portoenterostomy) to connect the bowel lumen with the porta hepatis is appropriate. If the surgery is successful, bile drainage occurs. Success is often related to early operation. The Kasai procedure is palliative, not curative, and a liver transplant may eventually be necessary.

ACUTE HEPATITIS

In the last few years, clinicians have learned a great deal about the viruses that cause hepatitis. There are at least five such viruses, causing hepatitis A, B, C, D, and E. These viruses are different from other viruses that cause hepatic inflammation (e.g., Epstein-Barr virus, herpes virus, cytomegalovirus) because in general they cause hepatitis itself rather than a wider clinical illness that may include hepatitis. Hepatitis D infection, which occurs only in conjunction with hepatitis B infection, is very infrequent in the United States, and hepatitis E has been found only in Americans who have traveled to endemic areas.

Hepatitis A

The incidence of infection with hepatitis A (HAV), a RNA picornavirus, has been declining steadily in the last 25 years as sanitary conditions have im-

proved. However, the exact incidence is difficult to ascertain, because so many cases are subclinical or anicteric and therefore are not reported. The transmission of HAV is almost always by the fecal–oral route, although percutaneous transmission may occur. The incubation period is 25 days. The diagnosis is made on serologic grounds based on an IgM antibody that is first seen at the onset of clinical symptoms (about 5 weeks after exposure); it is evidence of acute infection. The antibody remains positive for 4–12 months. The IgG anti-HAV antibody, which develops at the end of the infection and remains positive for many years, is evidence of previous HAV infection.

Symptoms of HAV are increasingly apparent in accordance with increasing age. Eighty-five percent of children younger than 2 years of age who are infected are asymptomatic, as are 50% of those 2–4 years of age. Adolescents are usually symptomatic; 75%–97% are ill, and 40%–70% are icteric. Nausea, vomiting, malaise, anorexia, and cholestatic jaundice with pruritus (bilirubin > 10 mg/dl) may be severe, but almost all patients recover without evidence of fulminant hepatitis or chronic liver disease.

No therapy is indicated, but immunoglobulin given prior to exposure or during the incubation period of HAV is protective against clinical illness. Close personal contacts and household members of patients with HAV should receive immunoglobulin within 2–4 weeks of exposure, but treatment of casual contacts such as schoolmates is not necessary. A safe and effective inactivated hepatitis A vaccine is available.

Hepatitis B

Hepatitis B virus (HBV), a DNA hepadnavirus, is most often transmitted parenterally and has an incubation period of 45–75 days. The presence of surface antigen to the virus (HBsAg) signifies infection with HBV. Antigenemia may appear early in the illness and may diminish before the symptoms have disappeared. Therefore, a second marker such as hepatitis B core antibody (anti-HBc) is usually needed to confirm the diagnosis of acute infection. Although the hepatitis B e antigen (HBeAg) is not necessary for diagnosis, it is an important marker, indicating viral infectivity.

More patients with HBV infection are symptomatic than those with HAV infection. Infants and children tend to be asymptomatic, whereas adolescents commonly have clinical evidence of fever, malaise, anorexia, nausea, and vomiting. Twenty-five percent of adolescents are icteric. In as many as 10% of cases, extrahepatic (immune complex) symptoms predominate. A common presentation is a "serum sickness-like" illness with urticaria, arthritis, angioedema, and a maculopapular rash. Other presentations include nephritis, nephrosis, myocarditis, and pancreatitis.

Fulminant, life-threatening hepatitis, although rare, can occur with HBV. An asymptomatic carrier state [HBsAg(+), anti-HBs(−) for > 6 months] occurs in < 0.1% of American Caucasians but in 10% of patients from the Pacific Rim. Carriers are at risk for cirrhosis and hepatocarcinoma. More than 90% of infants who acquire the infection perinatally become chronic carriers. The hepatitis B vaccine leads to prevention. In addition, all neonates of HBsAg(+) mothers, intimate contacts of patients with acute or chronic HBV, and individuals with needlestick exposure to HBsAg(+) blood should receive the vaccine along with hepatitis B immunoglobulin for its synergistic effect.

There is no specific treatment for acute HBV infection, but interferon alfa and lamivudine may be effective in adults with chronic hepatitis B infection. Evaluation of the safety and efficacy of these drugs in children is currently underway.

Hepatitis C

In the United States, hepatitis C (HCV), a RNA flavivirus, causes the vast majority of cases of non-A, non-B hepatitis. Transmission is predominately parenteral. Sexual and perinatal transmission may occur (at a low frequency), and household contacts may be at risk. Antibody against HCV (anti-HCV) signals infection and probably infectivity, but not immunity. The antibody is not protective. Because there is a high false-positive anti-HCV rate with the ELISA method, all positive results should be confirmed with a recombinant immunoblot assay or polymerase chain reaction assay.

Mortality from acute infection is less than 1%, but chronic disease occurs in more than 50% of infected cases. This is usually manifested by a fluctuating pattern of aminotransferase elevation, which occurs in about 80% of chronic cases. Many patients with chronic disease develop chronic active hepatitis, which may lead to cirrhosis and hepatocarcinoma. Again, the use of interferon alfa and ribavirin in adults with chronic active HCV has been promising, and use in children is under evaluation.

CHRONIC HEPATITIS

Chronic hepatitis is defined as an inflammatory reaction of the liver that continues for at least 6 months. The cause of many of the cases is un-

known. Infections with HBV and HCV are the most frequently identifiable causes. Other causes are drugs such as α-methyldopa, isoniazid, and nitrofurantoin; Wilson disease; $α_1$-antitrypsin deficiency; and IBD. The two types of chronic hepatitis seen in children are chronic persistent hepatitis and chronic active hepatitis.

Chronic persistent hepatitis, a benign form of chronic hepatitis, is most often associated with a bout of acute viral hepatitis that does not resolve for unclear reasons that probably relate to the interaction of host immunity factors and the causal agent. It is the most common form of chronic hepatitis. Patients may be totally asymptomatic or may complain of fatigue or mild pain in the right upper quadrant. Serum aminotransferase levels are elevated and may remain so for many years. The diagnosis is confirmed by a needle biopsy of the liver, which should be performed after abnormal liver function tests have persisted for at least 6 months. On biopsy, chronic persistent hepatitis is apparent as normal liver architecture with expansion of the portal areas by a mononuclear infiltrate. The limiting plate between the portal area and the lobule is intact and piecemeal (individual) necrosis of hepatocytes is not seen. A self-limited condition, chronic persistent hepatitis requires no therapy.

Chronic active hepatitis refers to a continuing inflammatory process of the liver that often progresses to severe, irreversible destruction (cirrhosis) and death. The mechanism(s) involved in the evolution and continuation of this disease are not completely clear, but abnormal immune reactivity appear to play a role. Both autoimmune chronic active hepatitis and HBsAg(+) chronic active hepatitis are seen with some frequency in adolescents. Hepatitis C and D also may evolve into chronic active hepatitis. In children with HIV infection, other viral agents such as cytomegalovirus, rubella, and Epstein-Barr virus are implicated in chronic active hepatitis.

Autoimmune chronic active hepatitis, which most frequently affects adolescent and young women, has also been called lupoid hepatitis, plasma cell hepatitis, and HBsAg(−) chronic active hepatitis. The clinical picture is variable. Affected patients may presents with (1) a prolonged typical attack of presumed viral hepatitis, (2) malaise with or without jaundice, or (3) hepatosplenomegaly found on a routine examination. In addition, these young women may have amenorrhea (primary or secondary), acne, erythema nodosum, arthritis, or arthralgia. Extrahepatic disorders such as thyroiditis, IBD, or nephritis may be present in many cases.

Patients with autoimmune chronic active hepatitis have elevated classical liver function tests. In addition, they have markedly elevated serum IgG levels (often 2500–5000 mg/dl), anti–smooth muscle antibody (70%), and other autoimmune markers such as antimitochondrial and antinuclear antibodies.

It is possible to diagnose autoimmune chronic active hepatitis by liver biopsy; an inflammatory reaction of plasma cells and lymphocytes extends beyond the portal area, eroding the limiting plate of the hepatocytes, causing individual, or piecemeal, hepatocellular necrosis. If the cellular necrosis is more advanced, as it often is at diagnosis, areas of necrosis are replaced by fibrosis. Treatment with oral corticosteroids and 6-mercaptopurine (as a prednisone-sparing agent) are effective in many cases. Progression to cirrhosis may occur despite a good biochemical response to treatment.

OTHER LIVER DISORDERS

Gilbert Syndrome

Gilbert syndrome is a common form of mild unconjugated hyperbilirubinemia. It is often first noticed in adolescents; the jaundice is noted with stress, fasting, or menstrual periods. The serum bilirubin levels are usually less than 3 mg/dl but may be as high as 7–8 mg/dl. The diagnosis is predicated on a mild fluctuating indirect hyperbilirubinemia in the presence of normal liver function tests and the absence of hemolysis. Hepatic glucuronosyltransferase activity is diminished. The benign nature of this syndrome makes therapy superfluous.

Wilson Disease

Wilson disease (hepatolenticular degeneration), an autosomal recessive disorder, results from excessive accumulation of copper in the liver, brain, eyes, kidneys, and bone. The abnormal gene that causes this condition is located on chromosome 13. The precise biochemical defect is unknown, but it is clear that biliary excretion of absorbed copper is inadequate. Although the accumulation of copper in tissues begins in infancy, clinical disease before age 6 years is rare. However, about 50% of patients develop symptoms by 15 years of age. Clinical manifestations include hepatosplenomegaly and jaundice that resemble chronic active hepatitis (more common in children), a Coombs-negative hemolytic anemia, deterioration of neuropsychiatric behavior, and renal tubular acidosis. Kayser-Fleischer rings (golden discoloration in the limbic region of the cornea) is common and can be diagnosed by slit lamp examination.

No single test is diagnostic of Wilson disease, and the workup can be frustrating. However, it is necessary to explore all avenues if the disease is suspected, because therapy is so effective. Low serum copper and low serum ceruloplasmin levels suggest the diagnosis, but both may be normal. Quantitation of the urinary copper level, which is usually extremely high in this disorder, is the best screening test in association with a slit lamp examination. Once the diagnosis is established, treatment with d-penicillamine (a copper chelator) should begin. Prognosis depends on early diagnosis and effective chelation.

α_1-Antitrypsin Deficiency

Homozygous α_1-antitrypsin deficiency, an autosomal recessive disorder, is associated with neonatal cholestasis and childhood liver disease resembling chronic active hepatitis or early adult-onset emphysema. α_1-Antitrypsin, a glycoprotein produced by hepatocytes, inhibits trypsin, pancreatic elastase, and acid proteases of alveolar macrophages. Uninhibited proteolytic activity of these enzymes in the face of the disorder can cause liver, pulmonary, or pancreatic injury. The diagnosis is made by measuring levels of α_1-antitrypsin or by doing a phenotype of the protease-inhibitor (Pi) system. There is no treatment at present, but liver transplantation has been performed in cases with severe hepatic involvement.

Pancreatic Disease

Diseases of the exocrine pancreas are relatively uncommon in children. Many of the pediatric diseases that affect the pancreas are the result of inborn errors of metabolism such as cystic fibrosis and Schwachman-Diamond syndrome (pancreatic insufficiency, cyclical neutropenia, dysostosis, and growth retardation).

Pancreatitis may be secondary to duct obstruction or perichymal inflammation, which causes release of proteases that cause more inflammation and edema. Causes include infectious agents (mumps, Epstein-Barr virus, coxsackie B4), drugs (corticosteroids, alcohol), trauma, stones, or diseases (cystic fibrosis), and α_1-antitrypsin deficiency. Recurrent pancreatitis suggests abnormalities of cholesterol and triglyceride metabolism or an anatomic defect such as pancreas divisum (a failure of fusion of the dorsal and ventral embryonic pancreas).

Patients with pancreatitis are often very toxic-appearing, with severe epigastric pain radiating to the back and nausea and vomiting. Laboratory findings include elevated amylase and lipase levels. Abdominal ultrasonography may be helpful. Treatment is directed at massive fluid replacement, bowel rest, and nasogastric decompression. Pseudocysts may form and may require surgery if they do not resolve.

Peritonitis

Peritonitis is defined as a chemical or infectious inflammation of the peritoneal lining of the abdominal cavity. Infectious peritonitis may be either primary or secondary. The clinical presentation includes fever, severe abdominal pain, and vomiting. However, corticosteroids may suppress the manifestations. Diagnosis is made by abdominal paracentesis that reveals organisms and many leukocytes.

Primary peritonitis, also called spontaneous or idiopathic peritonitis, is an infection of the peritoneal cavity in which the source of the infection arises outside of the abdomen and reaches it by either hematogenous or lymphatic spread. Most cases of primary peritonitis in children occur in patients with nephrotic syndrome or cirrhosis. The usual responsible bacteria in primary peritonitis are *Streptococcus pneumoniae* and gram-negative enteric organism such as *E. coli* and *Klebsiella pneumoniae*.

Secondary peritonitis is an inflammatory response to the rupture of an abdominal viscus, spillage of an abdominal abscess, trauma, or a vascular accident. Enteric gram-negative organisms such as *E. coli* and anaerobic organisms such as *Bacteroides fragilis* are the most frequently found pathogens. Treatment is appropriate antibiotics.

SUGGESTED READINGS

Camilleri M: Management of the irritable bowel syndrome. *Gastroenterology* 120:652–668, 2001.

Markowitz J: A primer on pediatric inflammatory bowel disease. *Contemp Pediatr* 13:25–46, 1996.

Mieli-Vergan G, Vergan D: Progress in pediatric autoimmune hepatitis. *Semin Liver Dis* 14:282–288, 1994.

Motil KJ, Grand RJ, Davis-Kraft L, et al: Growth failure in children with inflammatory bowel disease. A prospective study. *Gastroenterology* 105:681–691, 1993.

Orentstein SR, Izadnia F, Khan S: Gastroesophageal reflux disease in children. *Gastroenterol Clin North Am* 28:947–969, 1999.

Ramirez RO, Sokol RJ: Medical management of cholestasis. In *Liver Disease in Children*. Edited by Suchy FJ. St. Louis, Mosby, 1994, pp 356–388.

Rasquin-Weber A, Hyman PE, Cucchiara S, et al: Childhood functional gastrointestinal disorders. *Gut* 45:60–68, 1999.

Romero R, Lavine JF: Viral hepatitis in children. *Semin Liver Dis* 14:289–302, 1994.

Sakorafas GH, Tsiotou AG: Etiology and pathogenesis of acute pancreatitis: Current concepts. *J Clin Gastroenterol* 30:343–356, 2000.

Shuppan D: Current concepts of celiac disease pathogenesis. *Gastroenterology* 119:234–242, 2000.

Treem WR: Gastrointestinal bleeding in children. *Gastrointest Endosc Clin North Am* 4:75–97, 1994.

Chapter 16

Hematology and Oncology

Gary V. Dahl and Kaveri Suryanarayan

 Hematology

Hematologic disorders may be categorized on the basis of the blood constituents involved in the disease process: cellular components (red blood cells [RBCs], white blood cells [WBCs], and platelets) and plasma components (coagulation factors). The fundamental pathophysiology underlying most hematologic disorders is based on the limited life span of marrow-derived blood cells. RBCs survive in the circulation for 120 days, platelets for approximately 5–10 days, and neutrophils for only 2 days. Either the senescent cells die or the reticuloendothelial system removes them from the circulation. The end-stage cells cannot replace themselves. (In contrast, the lymphocytes, which are generally long-lived, travel among the blood, lymphatics, and tissues.) Because of the limited life span of RBCs, platelets, and neutrophils, the bone marrow must constantly produce new cells. Abnormalities that occur at any stage of this process result in various clinical presentations.

Hematopoiesis takes place in the bone marrow as a series of orderly, programmed steps in which mature blood cells are produced from immature progenitors. The majority of cells in the bone marrow are **committed** to one hematopoietic lineage; they have acquired characteristics of the appropriate lineage (e.g., hemoglobin for the RBCs, primary and secondary granules for the neutrophils). These **precursors,** which are recognizably differentiating into mature blood cells, progressively lose their ability to proliferate as they mature. Less mature cells in the bone marrow, the progenitors, are committed to one or more hematopoietic lineages but have not morphologically differentiated. The least mature progenitors are capable of differentiating into all hematopoietic lineages (**pluripotentiality**) and can replace themselves (self-renewal).

Progenitors, which are extremely rare, represent less than 1/10,000 nucleated marrow cells.

They are called **hematopoietic stem cells**. A single hematopoietic stem cell can give rise to over 1,000,000 mature blood cells.

Any sort of interference with the survival of the mature blood cells or the production of new blood cells may result in disease. (A common abnormality of RBC production is iron deficiency anemia.) Blood cell function is abnormal in some inherited diseases. These genetic conditions are a result of mutations that affect the ability of the RBCs to perform gas exchange, the ability of the neutrophils to kill microorganisms, or the ability of the platelets to form primary blood clots.

The liquid component of blood contains many essential proteins in addition to blood cells: the clotting factors required for blood coagulation, the immunoglobulins that serve as antibodies, and the complement proteins used for lysis of organisms that have been bound to antibodies. Much of pediatric hematology and immunology concerns inborn errors that result in nonfunction of these important proteins. Acquired illnesses that result in consumption of these proteins also occur.

BLOOD CELL DISORDERS

Disorders of blood cells can be classified as quantitative, qualitative, or both.

- **Quantitative disorders** are due to problems with bone marrow production of cells or loss of blood from the circulation (Figure 16.1). In children, abnormally low blood counts are more common than abnormally high counts (i.e., anemia and thrombocytopenia are more common than polycythemia and thrombocytosis).
- **Qualitative disorders** are due to inherent abnormalities in the blood cells themselves. However, they often lead to quantitative problems as well (i.e., hemolytic anemia due to a qualitative abnormality in hemoglobin such as sickle cell anemia).

A Quantitative Approach to hematologic abnormalities

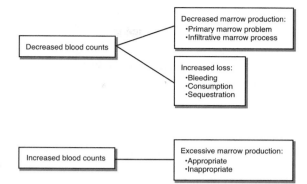

FIGURE 16.1. Significance of quantitative abnormalities in blood counts.

ANEMIA

Anemia is an abnormally low hemoglobin, hematocrit, or **RBC count**. It can be classified using either the previously discussed production–destruction approach or a morphologic approach based on the appearance of the RBCs on a peripheral blood smear and RBC parameters such as **mean corpuscular volume (MCV)** and **mean corpuscular hemoglobin concentration (MCHC)**. Because the values of RBC parameters vary with age, the pediatrician must be aware of the normal age ranges before determining that a child has a microcytic, normocytic, or macrocytic anemia.

Clinical and Laboratory Evaluation

History
In evaluating children with anemia, a careful history is essential. It is necessary to ask about a family history of anemia, transfusion requirements of relatives, or histories suggestive of chronic hemolysis (e.g., splenectomy or gallbladder disease). A dietary history is essential for determining whether the intake of iron, folate, and vitamin B_{12} is adequate. For example, vegans (vegetarians who consume no animal food or dairy products) may develop folate deficiency. In addition, the onset of hemolysis in children with **glucose-6-phosphate dehydrogenase (G6PD) deficiency** is sometimes associated with intake of certain foods (e.g., fava beans). It is necessary to obtain a history of pica or other possible exposure to **lead poisoning**. Questions regarding melena, hematochezia, hematemesis, or abdominal pain are appropriate; these may indicate chronic blood loss from the gastrointestinal (GI) tract. In adolescent girls, excessively heavy menstrual bleeding is notewor-

thy. Patients with hemolytic anemias may relate a history of dark-colored urine.

Physical Examination
Physical signs of anemia include pallor of the skin, oral mucosa, and nail beds. Infants with iron deficiency anemia secondary to excessive milk consumption are frequently obese. Tachycardia may occur as a physiologic response to anemia, and patients may also develop a systolic flow murmur. In long-standing moderate-to-severe anemia, signs of congestive heart failure such as edema, hepatomegaly, and splenomegaly may be present. The presence of jaundice is a sign of hemolysis. The facial appearance of children with untreated thalassemia are altered by increased bone marrow production (medullary expansion). Children with Fanconi anemia have microcephaly and an unusual bird-like facies. Adenopathy should be carefully noted; it may indicate either infection or malignancy. Abdominal examination should focus on determining the presence of hepatosplenomegaly, adenopathy, mass, or tenderness. The extremity examination is important for diagnosing several underlying causes of anemia. Children with arthritis and a secondary anemia may have a systemic rheumatologic, oncologic, or infectious disease. Children with Fanconi anemia usually have absent or hypoplastic thumbs. Children with sickle cell disease have extremities that may show signs of acute swelling and tenderness due to sickling or osteomyelitis.

It is important to note that the signs and symptoms of anemia vary with the degree of anemia and the rapidity with which it has developed. When anemia has developed over a period of time, pallor, fatigue, headache, and lightheadedness are more likely. When the onset of anemia is fairly acute, cardiovascular symptoms related to reduced oxygen-carrying capacity and resultant tissue hypoxia are more common.

Laboratory Evaluation

A **complete blood count** (CBC) with RBC parameters, peripheral blood smear, and reticulocyte count are part of the initial evaluation. Other tests that may be helpful include serum bilirubin and lactate dehydrogenase (LDH), which may be elevated with hemolysis, and a Coombs test, which may identify antibodies to the RBCs causing he-

molysis. Once a differential diagnosis has been generated from the clinical evaluation, CBC, and peripheral smear, other tests should be ordered judiciously. The laboratory evaluation of anemia can be expressed as an algorithm (Figure 16.2).

Differential Diagnosis

Anemias in children may be classified in terms of RBC production, RBC destruction, or blood loss (Table 16.1). In addition, this group of disorders may be organized somewhat differently with the same primary categories (Table 16.2).

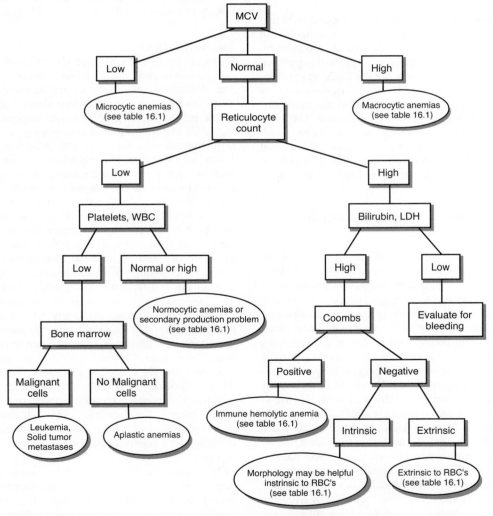

Diagnostic Approach to anemia
(Boxes represent diagnostic tests and results. Oval boxes represent diagnosis.)

FIGURE 16.2. Diagnostic approach to anemia. Boxes represent diagnostic tests and results. Oval boxes represent diagnoses. LDH = lactate dehydrogenase; MCV = mean corpuscular volume; RBC = red blood cell; WBC = white blood cell.

TABLE 16.1 Classification of Anemia

Production

Primary production
    Microcytic
        Fe deficiency
        Lead poisoning
        Thalassemia*
        5′ nucleotidase deficiency
    Macrocytic
        Folate, vitamin B_{12} deficiency
        Diamond-Blackfan anemia[†]
        Myelodysplastic syndrome
    Normocytic
        Viral suppression
        Transient erythroblastopenia of childhood
        Diamond-Blackfan anemia[†]
        Aplastic anemia
        Renal failure
Secondary production
    Infiltrative disease (leukemia, solid tumor metastases)

Destruction (hemolysis)

Intrinsic to red blood cells
    Hemoglobinopathy
        Sickle cell syndromes
        Thalassemia*
        Other unstable hemoglobins
    Membrane
        Hereditary spherocytosis
        Hereditary elliptocytosis
    Enzyme
        Glucose-6-phosphate dehydrogenase (G6PD) deficiency
        Pyruvate kinase deficiency
        Glutathione reductase deficiency
Extrinsic to red blood cells
    Immune
        Autoimmune
            Idiopathic
            Secondary
                Infection-associated
                Drug-induced
                Associated with other autoimmune diseases (e.g. systemic lupus erythematosus)
        ABO/Rh incompatibility
    Nonimmune
        Microangiopathic
            Sepsis
            Disseminated intravascular coagulation
            Hemolytic-uremic syndrome, thrombotic thrombocytopenic purpura
            Prosthetic heart valve
        Hypersplenism

Blood loss

---

*Thalassemia is included in both production and destruction categories.
[†]Diamond-Blackfan anemia may be macrocytic or normocytic.

TABLE 16.2 **Alternative Classification of Anemias Due to Abnormalities of Production**

Anemia due to deficiencies of substrate
Iron deficiency anemia
Vitamin B_{12} or folate deficiency

Anemia due to suppression of production
Transient or acquired
Transient erythroblastopenia of childhood
Aplastic crisis due to parvovirus B19
Congenital
Diamond-Blackfan anemia
Sideroblastic anemia
5'-nucleotidase deficiency
Other conditions
Bone marrow infiltrative process
Anemia of chronic disease

Management

The treatment of anemia is based on the underlying cause, the degree of anemia and the clinical status of the patient. The approach to the management of anemia is twofold. One, the severity of the situation must be assessed for the necessity of immediate interventions such as blood transfusions or other supportive care. Two, the cause of the anemia must be determined. Most children with anemia that general pediatricians most frequently encounter are not acutely ill, and a careful determination of the etiology is the first step.

Abnormalities of Erythrocyte Production

Anemias due to decreased RBC production are due to deficiencies of substances needed for the synthesis of erythrocytes (iron, B_{12}, or folate), exposure to toxins such as lead, suppression of production (such as that associated with viruses, which may be the mechanism for **transient erythroblastopenia of childhood)**, or a primary failure of erythropoiesis (**Diamond-Blackfan anemia or aplastic anemia**).

IRON DEFICIENCY ANEMIA. Classically, the cause of iron deficiency anemia in children is inadequate dietary intake of iron. The clinical scenario may be that of a toddler who is drinking large quantities of cow's milk from the bottle and eating little in the way of solid food. The lack of iron in cow's milk, combined with the exclusion of iron-rich food and chronic microscopic blood loss in the GI tract (thought to be due to inflammation associated with milk-protein allergy) leads to a **hypochromic, microcytic anemia**. The child can be quite anemic, with hemoglobin concentrations as low as 2 g/dl, and still be hemodynamically stable because of the gradual onset and the body's ability to compensate for a chronically decreased oxygen-carrying capacity.

Laboratory studies to assess iron status are serum iron, ferritin (a measure of iron stores), and total iron-binding capacity (Table 16.3). Depending on the child's clinical state, if iron deficiency is the cause, the initiation of oral iron supplements results in a **reticulocytosis** in several days and a rise in hemoglobin soon after. Consideration must also be given to the possibility of **lead poisoning**, because iron deficiency is often seen in children who also have lead toxicity.

It is sometimes difficult to distinguish between iron deficiency and **thalassemia trait**. The **Mentzer index** can assist in the diagnosis of thalassemia trait during the assessment of microcytic anemia.

Pediatric Pearl

The Mentzer index, which is the ratio of the MCV to the RBC number, is useful as a screening test to differentiate between iron deficiency and thalassemia. If the MCV/RBC is less than 13, thalassemia is more likely; if it is greater than 13, iron deficiency is more likely.

TABLE 16.3 **Laboratory Evaluation of Iron Deficiency Anemia and β Thalassemia Trait**

Feature	Iron Deficiency Anemia	β Thalassemia Trait
MCV/RBC (Mentzer index)	> 13	< 13
RBC morphology	Hypochromia	Target cells/hypochromia
Serum iron	Decreased	Normal
Iron-binding capacity	Increased	Normal
% Saturation	Decreased	Normal
Serum ferritin	Low	Normal
Hemoglobin A_2	Decreased	Increased
Hemoglobin F	Normal	Normal or increased

MCV = mean corpuscular volume; RBC = red blood cell.

Coexisting diseases (e.g., hemolysis), which alter the RBC, invalidate the Mentzer index as a diagnostic tool. Other tests that may be helpful are serum tests for iron stores and quantitation of subtypes of hemoglobin by hemoglobin electrophoresis (see Table 16.2). Once iron deficiency is excluded, the diagnosis of either α or β thalassemia depends on measurement of HgA_2 and HgbF levels.

VITAMIN B$_{12}$ OR FOLATE DEFICIENCY ANEMIA. Deficiencies of vitamin B_{12} or folate, which are associated with **macrocytic (megaloblastic) anemia,** are seen less commonly than iron deficiency in pediatrics. Vitamin B_{12} deficiency may result from inadequate dietary intake (e.g., vegan diet) or inadequate intestinal absorption of vitamin B_{12} (e.g., inflammatory bowel disease, surgical resection of the terminal ileum, genetic defect in intrinsic factor, or rare parasitic infections). Folate deficiency may also result from inadequate dietary intake (intake of goat's milk instead of cow's milk) or inadequate intestinal absorption (inflammatory bowel disease). Treatment consists of administration of vitamin B_{12} or folate orally or intramuscularly.

TRANSIENT OR ACQUIRED SUPPRESSION OF ERYTHROCYTE PRODUCTION. Transient suppression of RBC production as an abnormal response to a viral infection is the suspected cause of **transient erythroblastopenia of childhood.** Several viruses have been associated with this condition (e.g., human herpes virus 6). Children with transient erythroblastopenia of childhood may require transfusion if they present with very low hemoglobin values without evidence of reticulocytosis. If reticulocytosis does not occur after several weeks, evaluation for other causes of hypoplastic anemia should proceed.

Pediatric Pearl

Children with chronic hemolytic anemia (e.g., sickle cell anemia, hereditary spherocytosis) who are dependent on a high reticulocyte count to maintain their hemoglobin are at risk of more severe anemia, or aplastic crisis, when reticulocytosis ceases as a result of viral infection. Classically, this is due to infection with **parvovirus B19**.

CONGENITAL SUPPRESSION OF ERYTHROCYTE PRODUCTION. Congenital anemias are rare entities such as sideroblastic anemia and 5′ nucleotidase deficiency. A more common congenital anemia, although still quite rare, is **congenital red cell aplasia,** also known as **Diamond-Blackfan anemia,** which manifests as either a normocytic or macrocytic anemia in the first year of life. Associated physical abnormalities occur in approximately 25% of cases (most commonly, radial and thumb abnormalities; sometimes abnormalities of the face and head). These physical abnormalities themselves have no prognostic significance. Recent studies have shown an abnormality in a ribosomal protein encoded on chromosome 19 in a subset of patients with Diamond-Blackfan anemia while other studies have shown linkage to chromosome 8. Bone marrow aspiration or biopsy, which is warranted if Diamond-Blackfan anemia is suspected, shows marked reduction of RBC precursors. Treatment for patients with this condition include corticosteroid therapy, chronic transfusion, and allogeneic bone marrow transplantation (BMT).

SECONDARY CAUSES OF SUPPRESSION OF ERYTHROCYTE PRODUCTION. Infiltration of the bone marrow space can interfere with RBC production. Usually, this is also associated with leukopenia and thrombocytopenia. Diseases such as leukemia, solid tumor metastases, or rare stromal bone marrow disease (e.g., osteopetrosis) can be diagnosed with bone marrow studies.

Anemia of chronic disease, which is usually normocytic, should only be a diagnosis of exclusion in chronically ill patients when there is no other explanation for anemia. Although iron stores are normal, serum ferritin is often increased because inflammation caused by the underlying condition.

Abnormalities Due to Increased Erythrocyte Destruction

Hemolysis, or erythrocyte destruction, may result from a variety of causes. The hemolytic anemias are marked by RBCs with a shortened life span. Normally, RBCs survive in the circulation for 120 days. When the senescent cells are removed by the reticuloendothelial system, the iron contained in the hemoglobin is recycled. The normal **reticulocyte count** of 0.8%–1% reflects the need to replace approximately 1/120 of the RBC volume each day. If the production capacity of the bone marrow is normal, hemolytic anemias result in increased reticulocyte levels. Diseases that shorten the RBC lifespan can be **intrinsic** to the RBC, or due to **extrinsic** factors.

THALASSEMIAS. The thalassemias are the most common single gene disease in humans. A heterogeneous group of disorders of hemoglobin synthesis, all thalassemias are characterized by the absence or reduced output of either the α or β globin chains. If production of the α and β proteins is not precisely balanced, then an abnormal hemoglobin resulting from aggregation of excess chains is produced in the developing RBCs, which usually die prematurely in the bone marrow. The resultant anemia leads to increased stimulus for RBC production and increased RBC precursors in the bone marrow, spleen, and liver. The dying RBCs also result in chronic hemolysis as evidenced by the appearance of jaundice.

Thalassemias are classified on the basis of whether production of the α or β globin chains is defective. The degree of clinical disease depends on the number of normal genes present. Humans normally have two β globin genes and four α globin genes. In **α thalassemia,** patients have a deletion of one or more of the four α globin genes. Patients with one or two gene deletions have **α thalassemia trait**. Patients with one gene deletion are silent carriers, those with two deletions have a mild anemia, and those with three deletions have a more severe anemia. In these latter patients, levels of hemoglobin H, consisting of four β globin chains, increase. Deletion of all four genes usually results in fetal demise due to hydrops fetalis (**hemoglobin Bart hydrops fetalis syndrome**). Hemoglobin Bart is a homotetramer consisting of four γ chains, because no α chains are produced.

At birth the major hemoglobin is fetal hemoglobin, which is composed of two α and two γ globin chains. In contrast to the α globin gene, β globin is not expressed until after birth, when production of γ globin decreases. Levels of adult hemoglobin, composed of two α and two β globin chains, are low at birth and increase gradually over the first few months of life. Thus, symptoms of **β thalassemia** are usually not evident until 4–6 months of age. Similar to α thalassemia, the severity is related to the number of genes deleted; however, there are only two β globin genes. To complicate matters further, some defective β globin genes produce no β globin at all (β^0 thalassemia), whereas others produce intermediate levels of β globin (β^+ thalassemia). Patients who are heterozygous for a β-globin deletion have **β thalassemia minor** with a mild or moderate anemia that usually does not require transfusion. Patients who are homozygotes have **β thalassemia major (Cooley anemia)** and suffer from severe anemia and hepatosplenomegaly that develops within the first year of life. If patients are not treated, then expansion of the bone marrow space (**extramedullary hematopoiesis**) results in characteristic abnormal facies and pathologic fractures of long bones.

The form of thalassemia most often encountered by general pediatricians is that of **thalassemia trait,** either α or β. Because of genetic differences in populations, the more severe thalassemia syndromes are seem more commonly outside of the United States. β thalassemia major is encountered in the Mediterranean, Asian, and African populations and the α thalassemia syndromes in the Asian and African populations. Typically, severe α thalassemia is not seen in Africans, because they tend not to have two gene deletions on the same chromosome.

Asymptomatic children with thalassemia trait usually present with **microcytic anemia** on routine screening for anemia. The primary considerations for initial management consist of excluding iron deficiency anemia or lead toxicity. Mild thalassemia syndromes usually require no specific treatment. Patients with β thalassemia are treated with hypertransfusion regimens designed to maintain a hemoglobin level above 12 g/dl. These patients also receive iron chelation therapy with subcutaneous deferoxamine to prevent the deleterious consequences of chronic iron overload due to repeated transfusions. BMT with a compatible sibling donor has now become a major therapeutic option for patients with β thalassemia major.

Genetic counseling at an appropriate age should be provided because individuals with thalassemia trait can pass on the affected gene to their children, potentially resulting in one of the more severe thalassemia syndromes. Parents of newly identified patients should receive counseling regarding future pregnancies.

SICKLE CELL DISEASE. Sickle cell disease is a chronic hemolytic anemia caused by a point mutation in the β globin gene, which results in the substitution of valine for glutamic acid in the sixth amino acid position of the β globin chain. This abnormal hemoglobin polymerizes and condenses when it is in the deoxygenated state, leading to distortion of the RBC membrane and the characteristic sickle morphology. Sickle cells cause occlusion of vessels through their interactions with the vascular endothelium as well as cytokine release by activated WBCs and adhesive plasma proteins. The abnormal behavior of the sickle RBCs in the capillaries results in the characteristic painful crises and end-organ damage of sickle cell disease. Cells that leave the capillary bed become reoxygenated on entering the arterial circulation, reform to normal shape, but then enter the capillaries again. The chronically damaged RBCs have a shortened half-life, leading to hemolysis and anemia.

A CBC indicates anemia with a hemoglobin level usually around 7 g/dl, an elevated WBC count, and a reticulocyte count of 10%–25%. Characteristic sickle morphology is evident as well as target cells and poikilocytes. Hemoglobin electrophoresis shows the presence of hemoglobins S and F.

Homozygous hemoglobin S (sickle hemoglobin) is the most common sickling syndrome. Other sickling syndromes, which may be clinically indistinguishable from homozygous hemoglobin S are the double heterozygote conditions of hemoglobin SC (hemoglobin C is another mutation in the β chain) and hemoglobin S-β thalassemia.

The clinical complications of sickle cell disease become apparent when affected children are about 6 months old. Before that time, most of the hemoglobin is fetal hemoglobin, or hemoglobin F, which consists of two α chains and two γ chains. However, by 6 months of age, most of the hemoglobin is hemoglobin S, consisting of two α chains and two β^S chains (superscript S denotes the sickle mutation in the β chain).

The clinical result of having hemoglobin S is vaso-occlusion and resultant tissue infarction. Acutely, the infarction produces pain that is often termed **pain crisis** or **vaso-occlusive crisis** due to small vessel occlusion and infarction of bone and bone marrow. In infants, vaso-occlusion usually presents in the hands and feet with soft tissue swelling and pain, which is usually symmetrical (**dactylitis**). It is sometimes difficult to distinguish the bony pain and swelling of vaso-occlusive crises from osteomyelitis. In older children and adults, vaso-occlusive crises usually occur in the larger long bones, the back, and abdomen. The latter condition is easily confused with an acute abdomen due to infection. Sickling may also occur in the central nervous system (CNS) vasculature, resulting in strokes and infarction. Penile vaso-occlusion can produce painful priapism. Repeated vaso-occlusion over many years, whether symptomatic or asymptomatic, leads to chronic organ damage. Virtually every organ can be affected (Table 16.4). Of particular importance are the risk of complications due to chronic hemolysis (chronic anemia, increased bilirubin, increased incidence of gallstones and aplastic crisis).

The management of sickle cell disease begins at birth, with affected children most commonly identified by the nationwide newborn screening program. In addition to the well-child evaluations and anticipatory guidance that all children receive, children with sickle cell disease should be followed in a parallel manner by a pediatric hematologist (Table 16.5).

The management of the complications of sickle cell disease depends on their severity. Pain crises are treated with hydration and analgesia [nonsteroidal anti-inflammatory drugs (NSAIDs) such as ibuprofen or ketorolac or narcotics such as morphine]. Infectious complications are treated with appropriate antibiotics. The management of other complications can be found in Table 16.4.

The only currently available definitive treatment for sickle cell disease is BMT. Because of the potential morbidity and mortality of BMT, this therapy is considered only if such severe complications as stroke have occurred. Several ongoing clinical studies are evaluating hydroxyurea to increase hemoglobin F production and prevent clinical complications. Hydroxyurea is effective at increasing fetal hemoglobin concentration, and it appears to be well tolerated with mild, reversible myelosuppression. Patients who receive hydroxyurea have fewer painful and other acute vaso-occlusive events.

OTHER HEMOLYTIC ANEMIAS. In children with hemolytic anemia, the history is frequently helpful in narrowing the diagnostic workup. However, laboratory tests are usually required for definitive diagnosis.

A family history of hemolytic anemia suggests a genetic cause. Patients with hereditary spherocytosis are frequently treated with splenectomy; a family history of splenectomy is suggestive. Similarly, relatives may have a history of gallstones; they are common in chronic hemolytic anemias. Using the history to establish a pattern of hemolysis is sometimes helpful. Patients with chronic hemolysis from energy production defects such as pyruvate kinase deficiency or membrane defects may have long-standing histories of hemolysis, iron-unresponsive anemia, and jaundice going back to the neonatal period. Patients with G6PD deficiency or autoimmune hemolytic anemia are more likely to have a sudden onset of pallor, jaundice, and dark urine. G6PD deficiency is X-linked and thus affects primarily males. Patients with G6PD deficiency may also have a history of drug ingestion, especially sulfa drugs, quinines, or nitrofurans, or eating of foods such as fava beans. Patients with autoimmune hemolytic anemia frequently have a history of antecedent infection.

TABLE 16.4 **Clinical Complications of Sickle Cell Disease**

Organ/System	Complication	Symptoms	Management	Other
Bone	Infarction	Pain, tenderness, swelling	Hydration, analgesia	Dactylitis in infants
	Osteomyelitis	Fever, pain, tenderness, swelling	Antibiotics	Risk for encapsulated organisms such as *Streptococcus pneumoniae* and *Salmonella*
	Avascular necrosis of the femoral or humeral head	Hip or shoulder pain	Orthopedic interventions such as hip replacement	
Lungs	Acute chest syndrome	Chest pain, hypoxia, infiltrate on chest x-ray	Exchange transfusion	
	Chronic lung disease	Symptoms of pulmonary hypertension		
Central nervous system	Stroke	Paresis	Exchange transfusion, chronic transfusion therapy, BMT if sibling is an HLA-match	Transcranial Doppler studies to identify patients with high risk of stroke
Spleen	Sequestration	Splenomegaly, anemia, thrombocytopenia	Transfusion (simple or exchange)	Splenectomy after second sequestration
Immune system	Sepsis, infection Functional asplenia	Fever and other symptoms, depending on site	Antibiotics, immunization,* penicillin prophylaxis	Risk for encapsulated organisms
Hematopoietic system	Accelerated hemolytic crisis	Symptoms of anemia, jaundice	Transfusion if needed, hydration	
	Aplastic crisis	Symptoms of anemia	Transfusion	Due to parvovirus B19
Skin	Ulceration of lower extremities			
Genitourinary system	Priapism		Hydration, transfusion (simple or exchange)	
	Hyposthenuria			
Gastrointestinal system	Cholecystitis	Abdominal pain	Cholecystectomy	
Eyes	Retinopathy			
Cardiac system	Cardiomyopathy			
Endocrine system	Growth and pubertal delay			

BMT = bone marrow transplantation, HLA = human leukocyte antigen.
*Particularly against encapsulated organisms such as *Streptococcus pneumoniae* and *Haemophilus influenzae*.

The physical examination should focus on looking for signs of hemolysis and assessing the severity of anemia. Patients with severe hemolysis, especially of sudden onset, may have signs of high-output congestive heart failure. Jaundice is always present in patients with severe hemolysis. Splenomegaly is common in older children with RBC membrane defects.

TABLE 16.5	Routine Hematologic Care of the Child with Sickle Cell Disease
Time of Visit	**Intervention**
Initial visit	Review electrophoresis result
	Initiate penicillin prophylaxis
	Initiate parent education regarding potential complications (continue at every visit)
	Ensure patient receives pneumococcal vaccines along with routine immunizations of childhood
	Refer to hematologist when hemoglobin electrophoresis results are obtained, usually at 2–3 months of age
6 months	Reinforce parent education
12 months	Start folic acid if reticulocyte count > 3%
18 months	Reinforce parent education
2 years	Initiate transcranial Doppler studies and repeat every 6 months-1 year until 10 years of age to identify children at risk of stroke
Annual visits	Provide ongoing education regarding potential complications
	Perform regular eye examinations and renal function tests

Except in patients with an aplastic crisis caused by viral infection, the **reticulocyte count** is elevated in all hemolytic anemias. Supportive evidence for the presence of hemolysis includes measurement of the serum bilirubin level and the presence of urinary urobilinogen. The peripheral blood smear frequently indicates the diagnosis in patients with hereditary spherocytosis, elliptocytosis, or stomatocytosis, who have changes in RBC morphology typical of each disease. Additional laboratory tests required for specific diagnoses are described for each individual condition.

HEMOLYSIS DUE TO MEMBRANE ABNORMALITIES. Inherited disorders of the RBC membrane are due to abnormal proteins or abnormal protein interactions in the lipid bilayer. The result is decreased deformability and increased fragility of the RBC, which hemolyzes in the splenic microcirculation.

Hereditary spherocytosis, which has both autosomal dominant and autosomal recessive forms, is due to defects in the cell surface associated proteins spectrin, ankyrin, or band 3. On peripheral blood smear, the cells appear to be spheres rather than the characteristic biconcave disk (i.e., absent normal central pallor). The diagnosis is confirmed by incubating the RBCs in a progressively hypotonic solution and measuring the percent that undergo hemolysis at decreasing concentrations of NaCl (**osmotic fragility test**). An MCHC at or above the upper limit of normal on an automated CBC should prompt suspicion of hereditary spherocytosis.

Hereditary elliptocytosis is inherited in an autosomal dominant fashion. The pathophysiology involves several potential sites of defects in

cell surface–associated proteins. Penetrance may vary; most individuals have greater than 60% elliptocytes on peripheral blood smear, but some may have less than 10%. Hemolysis may be mild, but patients with homozygous elliptocytosis may have pyropoikilocytosis due to a compound heterozygosity for elliptocytosis and a separate "silent carrier" protein defect. Pyropoikilocytosis is characterized by very abnormal RBCs of aberrant shapes and a high degree of hemolysis. Both hereditary spherocytosis and hereditary elliptocytosis can be treated with splenectomy to remove the site of hemolysis. However, the RBC defect remains and is visible on the blood smear.

HEMOLYSIS DUE TO ENZYME DEFECTS. **G6PD deficiency,** the most common RBC enzymopathy, is an X-linked defect in which both males and females may be symptomatic. Frequency is highest in Mediterranean, African, and Asian countries. The dehydrogenase enzyme is part of the hexose monophosphate shunt that replenishes the supply of reduced glutathione in RBCs to reduce oxidants produced during stress. Without an adequate supply of reduced glutathione, the unbuffered oxidants damage the RBC membrane, resulting in hemolysis. There are different variants of G6PD deficiency, which can be grouped according to the ethnic background of the individual.

To make the diagnosis of G6PD deficiency, RBC enzyme levels are measured. However, this measurement may be inaccurate immediately following an acute episode of hemolysis because the deficient cells have hemolyzed, leaving only new reticulocytes with increased levels of enzyme. The oxidant stresses that precipitate acute hemolysis in individuals with G6PD are infection, drugs, chemicals (e.g., naphthalene) and, in the Mediterranean variant, fava beans. Avoidance of known precipitants and supportive care are important aspects of the management of the disease.

Pyruvate kinase deficiency, a rare deficiency, is inherited in an autosomal recessive pattern. It is the most common enzyme deficiency in the glycolytic pathway. The decreased ATP production in the cell caused by the deficiency is thought to result in accelerated aging and subsequent hemolysis of RBCs.

EXTRINSIC CAUSES OF HEMOLYSIS. In immune-mediated hemolysis, alloimmune antibodies to antigens on RBCs can cause hemolysis as the antibody-coated cells are destroyed by the spleen. Alloimmune hemolysis is most classically seen in the neonatal period with ABO or Rh incompatibility where the mother is antigen (A, B or Rh)-negative and the fetus is antigen-positive. The mother makes antibodies to the RBC antigens on the fetal RBCs, which are then destroyed. Transfusion of incompatible blood products can also result in an alloimmune-mediated hemolysis that can be life-threatening.

Pediatric Pearl

A Coombs test is used to identify antibodies that bind antigens on RBCs and indicates an immune-mediated hemolytic anemia.

Autoimmune hemolysis can be idiopathic or secondary to infection, exposure to certain drugs, or associated with a systemic process such as systemic lupus erythematosus (SLE).

In **nonimmune hemolysis,** hemolysis can occur in the spleen as a result of hypersplenism or inappropriate removal of normal RBCs from the circulation. **Microangiopathic hemolysis** can occur outside the spleen in diseases such as disseminated intravascular coagulation (DIC), hemolytic uremic syndrome, and thrombotic thrombocytopenia purpura, as well as secondary to mechanical shearing forces such as with prosthetic heart valves.

WHITE BLOOD CELL DISORDERS

WBCs consist of two major cell types: myeloid cells (neutrophils, monocytes, basophils, eosinophils) and lymphocytes. **Myeloid cell disorders,** which are presented below, can be grouped into quantitative and qualitative abnormalities. For

lymphoid cell disorders, see the discussion of the evaluation of lymphadenopathy in the oncology section of this chapter as well as Chapter 17.

Pathophysiology

Defects of neutrophil number or function can result in susceptibility to infections. Because neutrophils are important for killing bacteria and fungi, infection with these organisms are most commonly observed in neutropenic patients. Infection with viruses is generally not problematic in patients with neutrophil disorders. Patients frequently develop cutaneous infections or infections at mucosal surfaces such as the mouth, lungs, or GI tract. In patients with severe neutropenia, occult infection may occur with minimal signs on physical examination.

Developmental changes in neutrophil number occur, just as they do for RBC. Newborns normally have neutrophils representing 60% of the total WBC count. This number declines with age, and lymphocytes become predominant until the age of 4–5 years, when neutrophil predominance recurs. The number of neutrophils is best quantified as the **absolute neutrophil count (ANC),** which is calculated as the percent of neutrophils and bands $\times$ 100 $\times$ WBC/mm^3. Normally, the ANC of infants older than 2 weeks of age to 1 year of age is over 1000/mm^3, and the ANC of older infants and children is greater than 1500/mm^3. In general, the risk of infection rises with the degree of neutropenia.

Pediatric Pearl

Children with **ANCs** less than 500/mm^3 are at highest risk of developing overwhelming infection.

Clinical and Laboratory Evaluation

History

Evaluation of the medical history of children with suspected disorders of neutrophil function or number should primarily focus on infectious diseases. It is necessary to search for a family history of severe, recurrent, or fatal bacterial infections. The history of the particular child, especially with regard to growth, infections of the skin, periodontal tissues, sinuses, and lower respiratory tract, is important. Unusual findings are delayed separation of the umbilical cord [leukocyte adhesion deficiency (LAD)] and widespread granuloma formation [chronic granulomatous disease (CGD)].

Physical Examination

The level of acuity should be assessed first. Children in shock are probably septic and require prompt attention to potential bacterial or fungal infections. Neutropenic children who are febrile, even though they are not in shock, also require immediate diagnosis and treatment for presumed infection. Many children with neutrophil disorders appear to be chronically ill with abnormal weight and height, diminished muscle mass, and listlessness. The examination of neutropenic children must take into account the fact that most of the physical findings of infection (e.g., redness, swelling) require neutrophilic infiltration to become manifest and thus may be absent in these patients. Thus, only local tenderness may mark an area of infection. Careful palpation of potentially infected areas is therefore essential to determine whether infection is present. A perianal exam is particularly important. The condition of the teeth and mouth is noteworthy; neutrophilic disorders frequently result in chronic oral infections. Children with Chédiak-Higashi syndrome have abnormal pigmentation with very pale skin and silver hair.

Laboratory Evaluation

The laboratory examination begins with a CBC to determine whether neutropenia is present. The morphology of the neutrophils may also provide a clue. In LAD, the WBC count becomes very elevated ($> 30,000/mm^3$). In suspected CGD, the nitroblue tetrazolium test, which is based on the ability of the neutrophil respiratory burst to alter the color of an oxidized compound, is warranted. Specialized tests of neutrophil function are necessary to diagnose other disorders such as LAD, actin deficiency, or Chédiak-Higashi syndrome.

Differential Diagnosis

Quantitative Myeloid Cell Disorders

Neutropenia is used to describe a decreased number of neutrophils. Neutropenia can be congenital or acquired, and etiologies are listed in Table 16.6.

CONGENITAL NEUTROPENIAS. **Kostmann syndrome,** or **congenital agranulocytosis,** results from maturational arrest of myeloid precursors in the bone marrow. Life-threatening bacterial infections develop soon after birth. Affected patients have an increased incidence of leukemia and myelodysplastic syndrome. Treatment may involve granulocyte colony-stimulating factor (G-CSF).

Shwachman-Diamond syndrome is a syndrome of short stature, exocrine pancreatic dys-

TABLE 16.6 Causes of Neutropenia in Childhood

Congenital
Kostmann syndrome
Shwachman-Diamond syndrome
Congenital benign neutropenia
Cyclic neutropenia

Acquired
Drug induced
Toxins
Infection (suppression and destruction)
Immune-mediated
Alloimmune
Autoimmune
Hypersplenism

function, and neutropenia. Aplastic anemia develops in as many as 25% of patients, and leukemia in at least 5%. Inheritance is autosomal recessive.

Congenital benign neutropenia, as the name implies, is not associated with increased risk of infection. The condition may be familial.

Cyclic neutropenia leads to periods of normal WBC counts that alternate with periods of neutropenia (mean oscillatory period, about 21 days). The disease, which may also be familial, is autosomal dominant in 10% of cases. Recurrent fever, gingivitis, mouth ulcers, and lymphadenopathy may develop during periods of neutropenia.

ACQUIRED NEUTROPENIAS. **Decreased marrow production** leading to neutropenia may be associated with drugs such as chemotherapeutic agents, anticonvulsants, immunosuppressive agents, and other medications. Toxins such as benzene may also have a similar effect. Viral or bacterial infections and leukemia or metastatic solid tumors in which malignant cells infiltrate the bone marrow may also suppress bone marrow function and cause neutropenia.

Increased peripheral destruction or consumption may be a result of overwhelming infection if the rate of consumption of neutrophils at the site of infection exceeds the rate of production in the bone marrow. Immune-mediated neutropenia can be alloimmune, which is seen in neonates with maternally-generated antibodies, or autoimmune, such as with lupus. In **hypersplenism,** WBC trapping in the spleen can lead to neutropenia.

NEUTROPHILIA. An increased neutrophil count is most often seen with infection. A **leukemoid reaction** is a markedly increased WBC count in which the differential consists of immature myeloid precursors not usually seen in the periphery. Leukemoid reactions are common in infants with infection and, in particular, those with Down syndrome.

Acute myeloid leukemia (AML) may be associated with a high WBC count, but most often the cells seen on the peripheral blood smear are very immature myeloid cells known as **blasts,** as opposed to the mature neutrophils, band forms, and myelocytes seen with a leukemoid reaction (see ACUTE MYELOID LEUKEMIA). Often a bone marrow aspirate is needed to differentiate leukemia from a leukemoid reaction.

Qualitative Myeloid Cell Disorders

Neutrophil dysfunction may be due to rare genetic mutations that can occur at various sites in the pathway of normal neutrophil function. Inheritance may be X-linked or autosomal recessive.

Chronic granulomatous disease (CGD) results from the inability of WBCs to form the bactericidal product hydrogen peroxide due to mutations in the neutrophil oxidase system. Children with CGD have lymphadenopathy and recurrent abscesses that require drainage.

Leukocyte adhesion deficiency (LAD) is due to an inherited deficiency of adherence glycoproteins (CD11, CD18) that normally allow the WBCs to adhere to endothelium and migrate to sites of infection. Affected children have poor wound healing, with recurrent infections of the skin and mucosal surfaces.

Defects in opsonization include deficiencies in the complement system. Patients with absent or dysfunctional spleens, such as patients with sickle cell disease, can also have defective opsonization.

Chédiak-Higashi disease is an autosomal recessive disorder in which there is abnormal fusion of the neutrophil granules resulting in the formation of giant granules that interfere with bacterial killing. The disorder is associated with partial oculocutaneous albinism, photophobia, and rotary nystagmus.

Management

The treatment of neutropenia includes the immediate management of infection as well as long-term efforts to either minimize infection or treat the underlying disorder. It is assumed that children with neutropenia and fever are infected, and they usually receive broad-spectrum antibiotics. The precise combination of antibiotics largely depends on institutional experience and patterns of antibiotic resistance in the community. Patients with localizing signs of infection (e.g., staphylococcal skin abscess) can be treated with a more specific antibiotic regimen.

Treatment of the underlying cause of the neutropenia is dependent on the precise etiology. Congenital agranulocytosis has been cured by histocompatible BMT. Patients have also been successfully treated with chronic administration of recombinant G-CSF, a hormone that regulates the differentiation of myeloid cells. Autoimmune neutropenia is treated with immunosuppressive therapy. If a drug is suspected of causing neutropenia as an idiosyncratic reaction, every effort must be made to withdraw the offending drug. Neutropenia from chemotherapeutic drugs may require modification of subsequent doses. Patients with benign congenital neutropenia and cyclic neutropenia benefit from careful oral and skin hygiene and cautious use of antibiotics.

The management of defects of neutrophil function must focus both on the immediate treatment of existing infections and on long-term management. The presenting infections for children with either LAD or CGD are frequently serious, requiring intensive antibiotic therapy. Leukocyte transfusions have been used as an adjunct to the treatment of LAD-associated infections. The optimal treatment for LAD is histocompatible BMT from a sibling donor, which can be curative. Unfortunately, most patients do not have access to a donor and receive only supportive therapy with antibiotics. CGD is also responsive to BMT but because of the infrequency of matched donors and the relatively high risk associated with BMT, most patients are currently receiving alternative treatment. Treatment with interferon-gamma decreases the risk of infections in patients with CGD, although the beneficial effect is probably not due to enhanced activity of the oxidative burst. Supportive care also includes use of prophylactic antibiotics, especially trimethoprim-sulfamethoxazole.

PLATELET DISORDERS (SEE DISORDERS OF HEMOSTASIS AND THROMBOSIS)

SYNDROMES OF BONE MARROW FAILURE

When bone marrow fails to function, a loss of effective production of mature RBCs, myeloid cells, and platelets occurs. This loss of production is due either to a decreased number of hematopoietic precursors or to reduced function of the precursors. Only one or two cell lines may be affected. The **congenital bone marrow failure syndromes,** which are characterized by cytopenias often accompanied by congenital anomalies, include **Fanconi anemia, thrombocytopenia absent radii,** and **dyskeratosis congenita.** Acquired bone marrow failure syndromes include **aplastic anemia** and **paroxysmal nocturnal hemoglobinuria.** Except for thrombocytopenia absent radii, in which the hematologic abnormality usually resolves after the first year of life, BMT may be required and can be curative; however, the potential morbidity associated with the procedure may be significant. Patients with Fanconi anemia and dyskeratosis congenita are at increased risk for the development of AML and require frequent and careful monitoring.

DISORDERS OF HEMOSTASIS AND THROMBOSIS

Trauma to blood vessels constantly occurs in day-to-day activities, and a complex system for the regulation of blood clotting has evolved to protect the body from serious bleeding. Bleeding disorders may involve defects of the **platelet system,** which forms the initial platelet plug at the site of vessel injury, or the **coagulation system,** which forms the clot that stabilizes the vessel until tissue repair occurs. These two components also interact in complex ways. Platelets are fragments of megakaryocytes, precursor cells that reside in the bone marrow. Production of megakaryocytes is under the control of a secreted protein called thrombopoietin, much as RBC production is controlled by erythropoietin.

Pathophysiology

The first step in blood clotting occurs when endothelial cells are damaged (e.g., by trauma). Platelets do not normally stick to the endothelium, but after injury, they attach to the endothelial cells through several mechanisms. Damaged endothelial cells bind a circulating protein, **von Willebrand factor (vWF),** which in turn binds to the platelets and mediates the association of platelets with the endothelium. Exposed collagen also leads to the binding of platelets to damaged tissue. After one platelet adheres to the endothelium or tissue, it becomes activated, releases mediators of clotting and inflammation, and aggregates with other platelets. The aggregated platelets congeal to form a platelet plug,

which usually stops bleeding from the damaged blood vessel within minutes.

In addition to the platelet plug, blood clotting involves a series of enzymatic reactions that result in the transformation of a plasma protein, fibrinogen, into polymerized fibrin strands. The fibrin acts as a cement that stabilizes the platelet plug. The generation of fibrin is the culmination of two different pathways, one initiated by proteins extrinsic to the plasma, and the other started by proteins present in the plasma (Figure 16.3). The clotting cascade contains proteins with protease activity, which results in partial cleavage and activation of the next protein in the pathway.

Clinical and Laboratory Evaluation

History
Evaluation of children for bleeding disorders usually occurs for two reasons: (1) history of unusual bleeding or (2) an abnormal result on a routine screening test, often obtained prior to an elective surgical procedure. If bleeding is present, a careful description of the bleeding episode is helpful in determining the cause.

Pediatric Pearl

Mucocutaneous bleeding is more typical of platelet or collagen vascular disorders, whereas joint or soft tissue bleeding is more characteristic of clotting factor deficiencies.

Serious bleeding episodes may be seen in children with preexisting bleeding disorders who are suffering from an acute exacerbation or undergoing surgery as well as in patients with bleeding diatheses acquired as the result of other illness. Patients with severe bleeding usually carry the diagnosis of a bleeding disorder and have a preexisting history, but they may have a newly acquired disorder with no previous history. Occasionally, detection of inherited bleeding disorders occurs after the onset of severe bleeding that requires hospitalization.

The history should focus on sites of previous bleeding. Petechiae (nonblanching lesions < 2 mm in size) usually indicate a platelet disorder, rather than a clotting protein disorder. Bleeding from the nose, purpuric bleeding in the skin, intracranial hemorrhage, GI tract bleeding, or genitourinary tract bleeding can occur with either condition. Children with a history of fat malabsorption are susceptible to vitamin K deficiency. Children with liver disease may develop a coagulopathy due to lack of production of a number of clotting proteins. Children with known platelet or coagulation disorders who complain of headache must be carefully evaluated and presumptively treated for CNS hemorrhage. When evaluating children with suspected coagulation disorders, a careful family history is warranted. Factor VIII and factor IX deficiencies, the most common forms, are both X-linked and affect only males.

Physical Examination

The physical examination should include a thorough evaluation for sites of bleeding. In children with suspected platelet disorders, it is necessary to search for petechiae. In addition, a careful examination for signs of systemic lupus erythematosus (SLE) is useful; **immune thrombocytopenia purpura** (ITP) may be associated with SLE, especially in older children. Children with suspected thrombocytopenia with significant adenopathy, organomegaly, or bone pain are more likely to have leukemia or a malignancy other than ITP. Signs of chronic hepatic disease such as varices may be present. Deep hematomas are usually the result of a clotting protein abnormality. Patients with iliopsoas hemorrhages may present with abdominal pain that mimics appendicitis as well as neurologic signs due to compression of the lumbar plexus. Patients with known clotting abnormalities who have major trauma warrant careful examination for sites of bleeding in soft tissues, the mouth, abdomen, and brain.

Laboratory Evaluation

The major coagulopathies encountered in children are characterized by certain laboratory abnormalities (Table 16.7). Initially, the pediatrician should be able to distinguish platelet from coagulation protein disorders. The combination of the platelet count and the bleeding time detects numerical and functional defects of platelets. The bleeding time is abnormal (> 10 minutes) in both numerical and qualitative disorders of the platelets. The prothrombin time (PT) detects defects of the extrinsic and common pathways, whereas the partial thromboplastin time (PTT) evaluates the intrinsic and common pathways. Special platelet coagulation studies are now available to evaluate platelet function; these tests should be considered instead of bleeding time.

The bleeding time is performed by using a special template to create a 1-cm long, 1-mm deep incision, repeatedly blotting the wound, and measuring the time required for bleeding to stop. [Because the results of a bleeding time can be influenced by the technique of the person performing the test (e.g., site of incision, amount of pressure with which the template is held against the skin to make the incision), the results have the potential to be misleading.]

In children with abnormal screening tests but with no significant bleeding history, the laboratory evaluation can be more focused (Figure 16.4). Specific tests of factor levels are necessary to further define inherited deficiencies.

PLATELET DISORDERS

Quantitative Disorders of Platelets

Platelets arise from megakaryocytes in the bone marrow. As the platelet count decreases, the risk of bleeding increases. A platelet count below

---

TABLE 16.7 Laboratory Abnormalities in Coagulopathies

Type of Coagulopathy	PT	PTT	Platelets	Factor Levels
Factor VIII deficiency (hemophilia A)	Normal	Prolonged	Normal	VIII decreased
Factor IX deficiency (hemophilia B)	Normal	Prolonged	Normal	IX decreased
Factor VII deficiency	Prolonged	Normal	Normal	VII decreased
Vitamin K deficiency	Prolonged	Prolonged	Normal	Normal
Liver disease	Prolonged	Prolonged	Normal	Decreased*
Disseminated intravascular coagulation	Prolonged	Prolonged	Decreased	Decreased
vWD	Normal	Normal or prolonged	Normal, decreased in type IIB vWD	VIII decreased in type III vWD
Thrombocytopenia	Normal	Normal	Decreased	Normal

PT = prothrombin time; PTT = partial thromboplastin time, vWD = von Willebrand disease.
*Factor VIII is made in endothelial cells and levels are not decreased in liver disease.

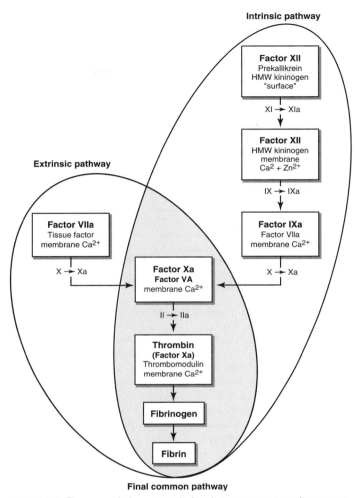

FIGURE 16.3. The coagulation cascade involves enzyme complexes comprised of serine proteases, cofactors, divalent cations, and a tissue surface. The intrinsic and extrinsic pathways converge to a shared final common pathway. The prothrombin time measures the intrinsic pathway; the activated partial thromboplastin time measures the extrinsic pathway. *HMW* = high molecular weight.

normal (150,000/mm^3) is termed **thrombocytopenia,** which may be due to decreased production in the bone marrow or increased destruction peripherally.

Causes of decreased bone marrow production of platelets include infection; an infiltrative bone marrow process such as leukemia; and congenital abnormalities in platelet production such as **congenital megakaryocytic hypoplasia, thrombocytopenia absent radii, aplastic anemia,** or **Wiskott-Aldrich syndrome**. An X-linked disease, Wiskott-Aldrich syndrome causes variable degrees of thrombocytopenia and both cell-mediated and humoral immune deficiency. Af-

fected boys, who have frequent infections with encapsulated organisms, may have eczema. The disease is allelic with isolated X-linked thrombocytopenia, both being due to mutations of a gene called *WASP*.

Increased destruction of platelets in children is most commonly due to **ITP**. Children usually have a history of antecedent viral infection. Patients most often present with extensive bruising, and platelet counts can be quite low (< 10,000/mm^3). Associated bleeding may occur, and intracranial hemorrhage occurs in less than 1% of patients. Treatment includes intravenous immunoglobulin, anti-D antibody in Rh+ pa-

Approach to Prolonged Partial Thromboplastin Time

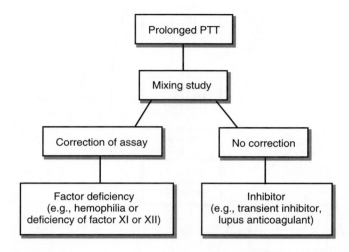

FIGURE 16.4. Approach to the evaluation of prolonged partial thromboplastin time (PTT).

tients only, and steroids. Rarely, platelet transfusions are used in emergent situations. For patients with chronic ITP (lasting > 6–12 months), splenectomy may be considered.

Immune-mediated platelet destruction can also be encountered in autoimmune disorders such as SLE. Thrombocytopenia due to peripheral destruction or consumption can be due to **disseminated intravascular coagulation (DIC)** associated with infection, or the **Kasabach-Merritt syndrome,** which is the occurrence in infants of localized DIC within a giant congenital hemangioma.

Thrombocytosis is an abnormally high platelet count, defined as greater than $450,000/mm^3$. Because platelets are an acute phase reactant, thrombocytosis may be seen in the setting of infection or other stress; this condition is a common finding in patients with **Kawasaki disease** (see Chapter 13). Thrombocytosis can also be seen in iron deficiency or in states of increased production of another cell line such as in patients with chronic hemolytic anemia (e.g., patients with sickle cell disease often have elevated platelet counts). Thrombocytosis is also associated with neuroblastoma. Although thrombocytosis may also be seen with certain types of myelodysplastic syndrome. this condition is much more common in adults.

Qualitative Disorders of Platelets

The most common inherited bleeding disorder is **von Willebrand disease,** due to decreased, absent, or abnormal vWF, which is necessary for platelet adhesion to the vascular endothelium as well as for stabilization of clotting factor VIII. Affected children may have mucosal bleeding (epistaxis, bleeding with tooth eruption, heavy menstrual bleeding); the extent varies depending on the type of disorder. Type I disease (all multimers present) is due to a mild quantitative decrease in vWF, type II disease (large multimers absent) is due to qualitative abnormalities of vWF, and type III disease (all multimers absent) is the most severe with essentially no detectable vWF. Laboratory evaluation includes vWF levels; vWF multimeric analysis; factor VIII levels; and ristocetin cofactor assay, which is an indirect measure of platelet aggregation. Formal platelet aggregation studies are usually not necessary.

Treatment for patients with mild disease consists of desmopressin (1-desamino-8-D-arginine vasopressin), which promotes endothelial release of vWF. Many subtypes of type II disease do not respond to desmopressin, which is contraindicated in some (patients with the IIB subtype) because it causes thrombocytopenia. In patients who are not candidates for desmopressin, concentrates of plasma-derived vWF and factor VIII such as antihemolytic factor/vWF complex (human), marketed as Humate P, are available. Antifibrinolytic agents such as ε-aminocaproic acid are used to stabilize clots in patients with mucosal bleeding.

CONGENITAL COAGULATION DISORDERS (HEMOPHILIAS)

The two most common inherited deficiencies of coagulation proteins are due to mutations in the genes for factor VIII (**hemophilia A**) and factor

IX (**hemophilia B or Christmas Disease**). Factor VIII deficiency accounts for approximately 80% of cases. Both diseases are X-linked. The family history is usually positive. The clinical severity depends on the level of coagulation protein activity in the plasma, which can vary considerably; however, severity tends to be similar among affected family members. Affected boys may present in infancy with excessive bleeding after circumcision or hematoma formation after intramuscular injection. As they become older, easy bruising and severe bleeding into soft tissues or joints after minimal trauma occurs. Most patients have experienced severe bleeding by the end of the first year of life. Diagnosis is confirmed by abnormalities of the PTT and by specific assays for factors VIII or IX. Treatment consists of infusion of appropriate recombinant factor concentrates.

Other less common factor deficiencies include those of factors VII, XI, and XII. Factor XII deficiencies are not associated with clinical bleeding, although the PTT is prolonged. Deficiencies of factors V, X, prothrombin, and factor XIII are not detected by PT or PTT.

ACQUIRED COAGULATION DISORDERS

Vitamin K Deficiency

Deficiency of vitamin K, a fat-soluble vitamin, results in the inability to carboxylate the vitamin K–dependent clotting factors (II, VII, IX, and X). Carboxylation is necessary for the formation of coagulation complexes between the clotting factors and the phospholipid membranes of platelets and endothelium. PT and PTT are both prolonged.

In neonates, **hemorrhagic disease of the newborn** occurs as a result of poor transfer of vitamin K across the placenta, relative deficiency of clotting factors in the neonate, and the low concentration of vitamin K in breast milk. An early form of this disease occurs in mothers treated with certain medications (e.g., anticonvulsants, warfarin) while pregnant. A routine intramuscular injection of vitamin K at birth prevents classic hemorrhagic disease of the newborn, which occurs at 2–7 days of age.

In older children, vitamin K deficiency is seen in the setting of malabsorption, prolonged antibiotic therapy, or warfarin (rat poison) ingestion. Treatment with vitamin K intramuscularly corrects the PT in 4–8 hours. If immediate correction is indicated, fresh frozen plasma or pro-

thrombin complex concentrates can be administered to supply carboxylated clotting factors.

Other Acquired Coagulation Disorders

DIC or consumption coagulopathy may occur in the presence of diseases, particularly sepsis, which cause hypoxia, acidosis, shock, or tissue necrosis. Widespread intravascular deposition of fibrin leads to further tissue ischemia, generalized hemorrhage, and a hemolytic anemia. Bleeding may begin around the sites of intravenous lines or surgical incisions. Infarcts may occur of both internal organs and areas of the skin.

The vast majority of patients with **liver disease** have some form of coagulation defect as determined by laboratory testing, although clinically significant bleeding develops in a much smaller group of patients. The abnormality results from a decrease in the synthesis of all the clotting factors except factor VIII. The severity is related to the degree of hepatic damage.

THROMBOPHILIA (HYPERCOAGULABILITY)

Just as coagulation factors are needed to form a clot, factors are needed to prevent extension of the clot beyond what is necessary. Clinically, venous or arterial thromboses and pulmonary emboli are potential signs of hereditary hypercoagulable states. The evaluation of children with thromboembolism should be directed toward identifying whether there is an underlying hereditary or acquired abnormality leading to thromboses involving veins, arteries, or the microvasculature. The list of factors that play a role in regulating the extent of thrombus formation is growing as research in the field identifies new factors and new genetic mutations.

Several environmental factors can increase the risk of thrombosis, including postoperative immobility, infection, smoking, dehydration, an indwelling venous catheter, and certain medications (e.g., oral contraceptives, L-asparaginase). Evaluation for inherited predisposition is indicated to determine if long-term anticoagulation is necessary. In many situations, once the environmental factor is removed, there is no need for long-term anticoagulation.

Evaluation of patients with a suspected inherited predisposition to thrombophilia includes assays for deficiencies of **protein C, protein S,** and **antithrombin III** (measured by levels of protein activity); genetic analyses for the **factor V Leiden** mutation, which confers resistance to activated protein C, **prothrombin mutation,** and **methylene tetrahydrofolate reductase mutation;** and serum tests for **lupus anticoagulant** and **anticardiolipin antibody** (associated with the **antiphospholipid syndrome**).

EXCESSIVE BLEEDING IN SURGICAL PATIENTS

Pediatricians are often asked to evaluate surgical patients for hematologic problems both pre- and postoperatively. The usual reasons for consultation are concern about either anemia or bleeding. Accordingly, clinicians should seek a past medical history of anemia or bleeding. The reason for surgery should be considered in determining whether a hematologic problem exists. For example, a child undergoing abdominal surgery for GI bleeding (e.g., Meckel diverticulum) might have iron deficiency anemia. The physical examination should also focus on signs of either anemia or bleeding.

Preoperative Evaluation

Screening laboratory tests are frequently useful. In general, for moderate- to high-risk surgery (e.g., orthopedic, intra-abdominal, cardiac, neurologic), a CBC with platelet count, PT, and PTT is warranted. For low-risk surgery (e.g., herniorrhaphy), a hematocrit is usually adequate if the history and physical examination are normal. Elective surgery can usually be performed when the hemoglobin level is 10 g/dl, the platelet count is normal, and the PT/PTT are normal. If the hematologic tests are abnormal in a child scheduled for elective surgery, it is better to postpone the surgery until the cause of the abnormality is determined. If surgery is urgent, then correction of the abnormality may be necessary. Management of the anemic child might include packed RBCs to achieve a hemoglobin of 10 g/dl. In patients with thrombocytopenia, transfusion to a platelet count of greater than 50,000/mm³ is adequate, but additional intra-operative platelet transfusions may be necessary. Correction of clotting abnormalities might include infusions of fresh frozen plasma or cryoprecipitate, with administration of vitamin K to correct the defect.

Postoperative Bleeding

A careful examination of the patient is essential. Children with bleeding only at the site of surgery are likely to have a surgical problem, rather than a bleeding diathesis, especially if the preoperative history, physical examination, and screening tests are normal. The pediatrician should look for other sites of bleeding (e.g., endotracheal tube, mucous membranes, skin, sites of intravenous or intra-arterial line).

Diffuse bleeding may be due to **DIC** or a previously undiagnosed bleeding diathesis. Surgical patients who have undergone open heart surgery, neurosurgery, trauma, or sepsis are at particular risk for DIC. Laboratory tests for the patient with excessive postoperative bleeding should include a CBC with platelet count, PT, PTT, **fibrin split products,** and **fibrinogen** levels. Patients with DIC have a low platelet count, prolonged PT and PTT, elevated fibrin split products, and decreased fibrinogen levels. The blood smear may also show microangiopathic changes in RBC morphology.

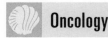 Oncology

LYMPHADENOPATHY

Hematologists–oncologists and infectious disease specialists are frequently asked to examine children with lymphadenopathy, which usually occurs as a result of infection or infiltration with inflammatory or malignant cells. Lymphoid tissue grows at a very rapid rate during childhood. Because children are constantly being exposed to new infectious agents, lymphadenopathy is a frequent occurrence, and palpable lymph nodes in the cervical, axillary, and inguinal areas are common. Lymph nodes more than 2.5 cm in diameter or located in other areas are more likely to indicate the presence of a disease process.

Localized lymphadenopathy is more frequently associated with a bacterial or fungal infection in the region drained by that particular group of lymph nodes. Thus, a basic knowledge of patterns of regional lymph node drainage is useful in the assessment of lymphadenopathy. For example, a child with isolated submental or submandibular lymphadenopathy may have a dental or gingival infection but is unlikely to have a scalp infection. Diffuse adenopathy is more suggestive of viral infection, storage disease, leukemia, or chronic autoimmune disease. Popliteal and inguinal lymphadenopathy may be due to a lower extremity infection. When a lymph node is enlarged as a result of infection, resolution of the infection is associated with shrinkage of the lymph node back to normal size.

When a lymph node has been enlarged for a prolonged period, usually more than 1 month, the lymphadenopathy is considered chronic. Administration of appropriate antibiotic treatment leads to the resolution of most infection-related adenopathy within 2 weeks.

Clinical and Laboratory Evaluation

History

The history should focus on the duration of lymphadenopathy and antecedent history. A history of trauma or infection to distal areas drained by the node is particularly important. Exposure to bacteria via a cat scratch, tick bite, rodent or other animal bite, or distal wound warrants careful exploration. Generalized symptoms such as fever, anorexia, weight loss, joint or bone pains, and diarrhea may indicate a systemic illness.

Physical Examination

Experience with palpation of lymph nodes is invaluable in the assessment of lymphadenopathy. Lymph nodes should be characterized by location, number, size, consistency, mobility, and attachment to skin and soft tissues. Infected lymph nodes may be fluctuant, tender, and matted together and have overlying superficial erythema. A sinus tract, with or without drainage, is relatively common in **tuberculosis** but can also be seen in **aspergillosis** or **actinomycosis.** Lymph nodes that are enlarged as part of the systemic response to infection tend to be diffuse and not fluctuant, but may be tender. Lymph nodes that are enlarged because of malignancy tend to be rubbery and firm and can be matted down, especially if the malignancy is a solid tumor. Supraclavicular lymph nodes on the left side may be derived from an intra-abdominal malignancy spreading through the thoracic duct, such as Hodgkin or non-Hodgkin lymphoma. Right-sided supraclavicular lymphadenopathy is more often associated with intrathoracic or pulmonary diseases.

Other noteworthy physical features include hepatosplenomegaly, jaundice, wasting, bruising, petechiae, or pallor. A detailed examination to look for evidence of local infection in the areas drained by regional lymph nodes is necessary (e.g., throat in the presence of cervical lymphadenopathy).

Laboratory Evaluation

Children with lymphadenopathy should have a CBC, a tuberculin skin test, and culture of relevant primary sites of infection (e.g., throat with cervical adenitis). A chest radiograph is necessary if no localized site of infection can be identified to account for the lymphadenopathy. In children with diffuse adenopathy, appropriate serologic tests include those for Epstein-Barr virus, cytomegalovirus, and *Toxoplasma gondii*. If localized adenopathy persists despite an appropriate course of antibiotics, usually of 2 weeks' duration, an excisional lymph node biopsy may be indicated.

If leukemia is suspected, a bone marrow aspirate should be obtained prior to referral to a surgeon, because a leukemic marrow would make a surgical node biopsy unnecessary. The biopsy material should be stained for histopathology and for evidence of infection, including Gram stain, acid-fast bacteria, and fungal stains. It should be sent for culture for these organisms. In the event that the lymph node demonstrates malignancy, the pathology laboratory should be prepared to perform a careful analysis for lymphoma or leukemia with monoclonal antibody staining and cytogenetics. It is essential that the pediatrician, surgeon, and pathologist coordinate the tests to be done in advance of the biopsy.

Differential Diagnosis

The differential diagnosis of lymphadenopathy is quite extensive, including infections, noninfectious inflammatory diseases, malignancies, and storage diseases. It may help to distinguish localized from generalized lymphadenopathy according to its common causes (Table 16.8). Not all swellings are due to lymphadenopathy. Congenital malformations such as thyroglossal duct cysts, branchial cleft cysts, cystic hygromas, or tumors such as neuroblastoma and rhabdomyosarcoma can cause neck masses that may be mistaken for lymphadenopathy.

Management

The management of children with localized lymphadenopathy depends on the suspected etiology. In children with infections of the oropharynx such as streptococcal pharyngitis, treatment with a β-lactam antibiotic (e.g., amoxicillin, amoxicillin–clavulanic acid, cefuroxime) is adequate. When *Staphylococcus aureus* is suspected, a β-lactamase-resistant antibiotic is required. Parenteral administration may be necessary if swallowing difficulties or severe emesis is present.

For children with infections of the extremities causing regional lymphadenopathy, coverage for both streptococcus and staphylococcus is recom-

TABLE 16.8	Common Causes of Lymphadenopathy

Generalized Lymphadenopathy	Localized Lymphadenopathy
Bacterial infections	Occipital/posterior auricular region
Pyogenic bacterial infection	Local scalp infection (e.g., impetigo)
Tuberculosis	Ringworm
Brucellosis	Pediculosis
Typhoid fever	Roseola (HHV-6 infection)
Syphilis	Preauricular
Fungal infections	Chlamydia
Histoplasmosis	Catscratch disease
Coccidioidomycosis	Trachoma
Viral infections	Tularemia
Epstein-Barr virus (infectious mononucleosis)	Sarcoidosis
Cytomegalovirus	Submaxillary/submental region
Human immunodeficiency virus (HIV)	Dental caries and abscesses
Measles	Bacterial gingivitis
Rubella	Herpes simplex stomatitis
Parasitic infections	Cervical region
Toxoplasmosis	Viral infections
Malaria	Respiratory viruses
Inflammatory diseases (noninfectious)	Epstein-Barr virus
Systemic lupus erythematosus	Cytomegalovirus
Juvenile rheumatoid arthritis	Bacterial
Serum sickness	Upper respiratory tract infection (e.g., group A hemolytic streptococcus)
Sarcoidosis	*Staphylococcus aureus* infection
Neutrophil disorders	Head and neck impetigo
Chronic granulomatous disease	Tuberculosis and atypical *Mycobacterium*
Leukocyte adhesion deficiency	Parasitic: *Toxoplasma gondii*
Storage disease	Other
Gaucher disease	Kawasaki disease
Niemann-Pick disease	Sarcoidosis
Malignancies	Malignancy
ALL	Hodgkin disease
Acute myeloid leukemia	Non-Hodgkin lymphoma
Hodgkin lymphoma	ALL
Non-Hodgkin lymphoma	Histiocytosis X
Neuroblastoma	Supraclavicular region
Rhabdomyosarcoma	Hodgkin disease
	Non-Hodgkin lymphoma
	Metastatic solid tumors (e.g., rhabdomyosarcoma, carcinomas)
	Axillary region
	Infection of the arm (e.g., cellulitis, impetigo)
	Catscratch disease
	Rat-bite fever
	Rheumatoid fever
	Epitrochlear region
	Infection of the forearm or hand (e.g., cellulitis)
	Impetigo
	Sporotrichosis
	Tularemia
	Mediastinal region (examined radiographically)
	Tuberculosis
	Sarcoidosis
	Histoplasmosis
	Coccidioidomycosis
	Hodgkin disease
	Non-Hodgkin lymphoma
	ALL

TABLE 16.8 Common Causes of Lymphadenopathy	
Generalized Lymphadenopathy	**Localized Lymphadenopathy**
	Neuroblastoma
	Systemic lupus erythematosus
	Inguinal region
	Lower extremity infections
	Sexually transmitted diseases
	Lymphogranuloma venereum
	Chancroid
	Herpes simplex
	Syphilis
	Iliac region
	Bacterial adenitis
	Streptococcus pyogenes
	S. aureus
	Appendicitis
	Urinary tract infection
	Lymphoma
	Popliteal region: infections of distal areas
	Foot
	Lateral lower leg
	Knee joint

ALL = acute lymphoblastic leukemia.

mended. For bacterial infections, parenteral antibiotics are usually warranted. Diffuse lymphadenopathy due to viral infection is usually managed by observation after obtaining a CBC and appropriate viral titers or cultures. In such viral infections, resolution of lymphadenopathy usually occurs within 1 month. Children with suspected malignancy should be referred to a pediatric hematologist–oncologist; the care of such children is relatively urgent.

CANCER

The diagnosis of a malignancy in children or adolescents is most definitely a life-changing event, although the long-term outcome for these young patients has dramatically improved over the last 30 years. By implementing randomized clinical trials and providing multidisciplinary care, effective therapies have been identified, and the outlook for children with malignancy continues to improve. The remainder of this chapter will review the clinical presentation, differential diagnosis, management, and outcome for both common and uncommon malignant diseases seen in the pediatric age group.

Every year cancer develops in 15 of every 100,000 children between birth and 21 years of age, resulting in approximately 12,000 new cases

of cancer in this age group in the United States. The incidence of disease varies among racial groups. Cancer is more prevalent in the Caucasian population than in African Americans and Hispanic Americans. Although pediatric malignancies are curable in over 70% of cases, cancer is still the most common cause of death from disease in the U.S. population between the ages of 1 and 15 years. The Surveillance, Epidemiology, and End Results (SEER) Program of the National Cancer Institute presents the most recent data concerning the incidence of different types of cancer in children (Table 16.9).

Pediatric Pearl

As more children with cancer are cured, long-term side effects of therapy such as infertility and secondary malignancy have become more common.

Pathophysiology

Cancer is the result of uncontrollable cellular proliferation (hyperplasia). By the time of diagnosis, one transformed neoplastic cell can multiply and become over 10 billion cells. Cancer cells may be either localized or disseminated throughout the body. The disease is frequently identified by the presence of a mass that can be palpated or im-

TABLE 16.9 Cancer in Children 1–15 Years of Age (1975–1995)

Tumor Type	Relative Incidence (%)
All leukemias	31.5
Acute lymphoblastic leukemia (ALL)	24.5
Acute myeloid (AML)	3.2
Other leukemias	3.8
All lymphomas	10.8
Hodgkin disease	4.4
Non-Hodgkin lymphoma (including Burkitt lymphoma, miscellaneous lymphoreticular neoplasms)	5.8
Unspecified lymphomas	0.6
All central nervous system tumors	20.5
Neuroblastoma	7.5
Retinoblastoma	3.1
Wilms tumor and other renal tumors	6.3
All bone tumors	4.5
Osteosarcoma	2.4
Ewing Sarcoma	1.7
Other bone tumors	0.4
All soft-tissue sarcomas	7.0
Rhabdomyosarcoma, embryonal sarcoma	3.4
Fibrosarcoma	1.7
Other sarcomas	1.6
All other tumors	9.1
TOTAL	100.0

aged. Solid tumors may interfere with organ function, often causing pain. When the bone marrow is replaced by leukemia or metastatic tumors, loss of marrow function can occur. One or more of the following findings may indicate this loss: anemia, leukocytosis, leukopenia, or thrombocytopenia. In children, solid tumors are usually derived from mesenchymal tissues and called sarcomas, whereas in adults, the majority of solid tumors are derived from epithelial tissues and called carcinomas. In children, the percentage of cases classified as carcinomas and other malignant epithelial neoplasms is approximately 14%; in adults, the percentage is over 90%.

Just what initiates clonal expansion is unknown in most childhood cancers. Epidemiologic studies indicate that as few as 5% of cancers in children are linked to known genetic abnormalities (Table 16.10). Germline and somatic mutations of tumor-suppressor genes are associated with a variety of inherited cancer-susceptibility syndromes and sporadic neoplasia, respectively. Experts once believed that alterations in the structural DNA sequence alone could account for the etiology and pathogenesis of most cancers, but a growing body of evidence currently supports the hypothesis that **epigenetic** events may play a prominent role, particularly in leukemia. Epigenetic inheritance is defined as the acquisition of heritable change in gene expression that occurs without a change in DNA sequence. Examples of epigenetic events that appear to be involved in the process of cancer cell transformation are DNA methylation, histone deacetylation, and changes in chromatin organization. Little evidence suggests that exposure to environmental carcinogens plays a major role in pediatric cancer.

HEMATOPOIETIC MALIGNANCIES, LEUKEMIAS, AND LYMPHOMAS

Eighty percent of the cases of acute leukemia that present in childhood are **acute lymphocytic leukemia (ALL)**. On the basis of immunophenotype, 84% are B-cell subtype, 14% are T-cell subtype, and 2% are mature B-cell subtype (Burkitt) leukemia. Approximately 20% of leukemias are **acute myelocytic leukemia (AML). Chronic myelocytic leukemia (CML)** and **juvenile myelomonocytic leukemia (JMML)** together make up only 1%–2% of cases. Children with CML present most commonly with leukocytosis and splenomegaly. Their leukemia cells contain the pathognomonic chromosomal translocation t(9:22) known as the **Philadelphia chromosome**. Leukemia cells from approximately 3% of children with ALL share the same chromosomal translocation. JMML usually presents in children younger than 5 year of

TABLE 16.10 Inherited Syndromes Associated with Childhood Cancer

Brain tumors

Neurofibromatosis type I (NF I) [TS]: neurofibroma, sarcoma, pilocytic astrocytoma
Neurofibromatosis type II (NF II) [TS]: acoustic neuroma, meningioma
Tuberous sclerosis TSC1 and TSC2 (TS): subependymal giant cell astrocytoma
Gorlin syndrome: medulloblastoma, basal cell carcinoma
Turcot syndrome: colon carcinoma, medulloblastoma
Von Hippel-Lindau syndrome, hemangioblastoma, renal cell carcinoma, pheochromocytoma

Leukemia (as many as 5% of cases associated with inherited genetic syndromes)

Down syndrome (10–20-fold increase in ALL and AML)
Bloom syndrome
Neurofibromatosis
Shwachman syndrome
Ataxia-telangiectasia (*ATM* [DNA repair gene])
Fanconi anemia
Kostmann syndrome

Solid tumors

Multiple endocrine neoplasia (MEN type II A and B) [OG]: thyroid/parathyroid cancer, pheochromocytoma
Li-Fraumeni syndrome (p53) [TS]: sarcoma, breast cancer, brain tumor, leukemia
Adenomatous polyposis coli (APC [TS]: intestinal polyposis colorectal cancer, hepatoblastoma
Hereditary retinoblastoma (RB1 [TS] retinoblastoma and secondary cancer

ALL = acute lymphocytic/lymphoblastic leukemia; AML = acute myeloid leukemia, OG = oncogene;
TS = tumor suppressor gene.

age with leukocytosis of less than 100,000 cells/ mm^3, abnormally elevated hemoglobin F, and hepatosplenomegaly. **JMML** is not associated with the Philadelphia chromosome.

Clinical and Laboratory Evaluation

The diagnostic evaluation of children with suspected leukemia begins with a careful review of the medical history, a thorough physical examination, and laboratory studies (Table 16.11).

History and Physical Examination

It is important to pay attention to the family history, medication history, and any indication of exposure to ill individuals or report of recent international or other travel. Children may exhibit pallor and give a history of persistent fever, fatigue, and bone or joint pain. Involvement of the bone marrow with an expanding population of cells may also lead to petechiae, ecchymoses, epistaxis, and a multitude of other signs and symptoms (Table 16.12). The clinical findings are a re-

TABLE 16.11 Diagnostic Evaluation of Leukemia

Medical history and physical examination
Review of blood smear
CBC (hemoglobin, WBC differential, platelets)
Uric acid, BUN, total bilirubin, LDH, calcium, phosphorus, electrolytes, glucose, amylase, ALT (to identify hepatic, renal or metabolic abnormalities)
Urinalysis: infection, uric acid crystals, specific gravity
PT, PTT and fibrinogen: DIC
Immunoglobulins, varicella titer
Imaging: chest radiograph (posteroanterior and lateral) [mediastinal mass]; radiography of kidneys or renal ultrasound (if abnormal renal function)
Bone marrow aspirate for cell morphology with cytochemical stains, immunophenotype, cytogenetics and storage for future studies
Lumbar puncture (to identify presence of CNS leukemic involvement)
Blood culture (if febrile and neutropenic)

ALT = alanine aminotransferase; BUN = blood urea nitrogen; CBC = complete blood count; CNS = central nervous system; DIC = disseminated intravascular coagulopathy; LDH = lactate dehydrogenase; PT = prothrombin time; PTT = partial thromboplastin time; WBC = white blood count.

TABLE 16.12 **Presenting Clinical and Laboratory Features in Newly Diagnosed Childhood Cases of Acute Lymphoblastic Leukemia**

Clinical Feature	Percent of Children Affected (%)
Symptoms	
Fever	53
Fatigue	50
Bone or joint pain	40
Bleeding	38
Anorexia	19
Abdominal pain	10
Signs	
Liver edge > 5 cm below coastal margin	30
Anterior mediastinal mass	10
Laboratory findings	
Leukemic cells in spinal fluid	5
Leukocyte count	
< 10 × 10^9 cells/L	24
> 50 × 10^9 cells/L	23
Hemoglobin	
< 8 g/dl	52
>10 g/dl	22
Platelet count	
> 100 × 10^9 cells/L	32
< 10 × 10^9 cells/L	9

sult of marrow replacement and extent of spread. Often the history of illness is days to weeks in acute leukemia or months in chronic leukemia.

As Table 16.12 indicates, children with ALL present most commonly with fever, fatigue, bone or joint pain, and evidence of bleeding. Complaints of pain in the legs and joints and difficulty walking often indicate periosteal infiltration, elevation, and bone necrosis secondary to leukemia. On physical examination, lymphadenopathy is frequent, and hepatosplenomegaly occurs in over 50% of patients. Rarely, skin infiltration (leukemia cutis) and ocular involvement may be evident. An anterior mediastinal mass with or without adenopathy may be present in T-cell ALL, making it necessary to perform a careful initial history and examination that pays particular attention to respiratory symptoms such as cough or orthopnea. Superior vena cava syndrome and tracheal compression may be a presenting feature of ALL, particularly in adolescents.

Although the presenting features of children with AML and ALL are similar, gingival hyper-

trophy and subcutaneous or periosteal tumor infiltrates (**chloroma**) are found only in AML.

Pediatric Pearl

Chloromas are masses of myeloid leukemia cells found only in patients with AML and may be present with or without involvement of the bone marrow.

Rarely, subcutaneous masses, but not chloromas, can be found in patients with pre–B-cell ALL. Children with Down syndrome, who are at increased risk for leukemia, are more likely to have AML if younger than 4 years of age. Children with leukemia who have skin infiltrates (leukemia cutis) are more likely to have AML, except those younger than 1 year of age, when leukemia cutis can be seen with either ALL or AML.

Laboratory Evaluation

Children with leukemia most commonly present with increased numbers of WBCs or immature or primitive cells (blasts) circulating in the blood, so it is necessary to scrutinize the blood smear carefully for circulating blasts. In addition, coexisting anemia or thrombocytopenia is often present. A new patient who has abnormal values of any two of the three blood cell lines (i.e., RBCs, WBCs, platelets) should undergo a bone marrow aspirate. The bone marrow study determines whether the marrow has been replaced with undifferentiated cells (leukemia), has been infiltrated with clumps of tumor cells (solid tumors metastatic to the marrow), or demonstrates evidence of abnormal marrow function (myelodysplasia or aplasia).

Lymphoma should be suspected when enlarged lymph nodes or any tumor mass is found. To make a diagnosis, samples of the tumor are taken in addition to a bone marrow aspirate to check for marrow involvement. Sometimes the diagnosis can be made by identifying malignant cells in pleural fluid removed by thoracentesis. By arbitrary convention, if the bone marrow contains 25% or more blast forms, the patient is considered to have leukemia, if less than 25% blast forms, the diagnosis is considered to be lymphoma with marrow involvement.

Differential Diagnosis

After a thorough review of the medical history; a physical examination; and a laboratories studies, including a CBC; the clinician should consider the many possible differential diagnoses before concluding that leukemia is present (Table 16.13).

Acute Lymphocytic Leukemia (ALL)

Since the advent of chemotherapy in 1948, the outlook for children with ALL has improved greatly; the cure rate is over 80%. The improved survival seen over the past 30 years has been generated by advances in the design of clinical trials, the addition of tumor molecular markers to the standard classification of acute leukemia, the development of new chemotherapeutic agents, new and improved uses of antibiotics for infectious complications, safer supportive care with blood products, and BMT.

The availability of genetic and molecular information from the leukemic cells of each patient allows for a biological subtyping of leukemia. Different cure rates are noted for patients with certain cellular biologic differences. Current laboratory research is helping investigators design treatments that are selectively targeted at different subtypes of leukemia. Treatment is then based on the clinical and biological characteristics of each patient at the time of diagnosis. Criteria used to classify and risk-stratify leukemia include age at diagnosis, initial WBC, CNS involvement, leukemia cell immunophenotype, leukemia cell karyotype, and molecular abnormalities.

The **Children's Oncology Group** is a worldwide organization of institutions and physicians, nurses, and allied health professionals from the United States, Canada, Europe, and Australia who are committed to the development of new therapies for malignant disease in adolescence and childhood. Investigators from this group and others have developed specific trial protocols for children based on leukemia classification. These treatment protocols, which take into account differences in risk of relapse and long-term drug toxicities among patients, are used by member institutions. Patients are monitored for expected and unexpected effects of treatment to provide state-of-the-art care and a source of ideas for improvement of future therapy.

At the present time, the protocols for different categories of lymphoid leukemia are based on presenting features. For patients with B-precursor ALL, there are four levels of treatment regimens depending on clinical and biologic prognostic factors. Separate regimens exist for those children with infant leukemia (< 12 months of age at presentation), mature B-cell ALL, and T-cell ALL. Aside from the important clinical features of initial WBC, age, sex, and CNS involvement, the biologic features of immunophenotype, molecular abnormalities, classical cytogenetics, and DNA index are used to qualify and stratify children for treatment regimens. Certain nonrandom chromosomal and molecular abnormalities have independent prognostic importance. Four subsets of children with ALL have a very poor prognosis de-

---

TABLE 16.13 **Differential Diagnosis of Acute Leukemia**

Differential Diagnosis	Specific Disease
Decrease in two or more cell lines	
Infection	CMV, EBV, leishmaniasis, severe overwhelming infection, hepatitis, HIV
Bone marrow failure	Aplastic anemia, Fanconi anemia, Shwachman-Diamond syndrome
Marrow replacement or infiltration	Neuroblastoma, Ewing sarcoma, rhabdomyosarcoma
Hemophagocytic syndrome	Familial hemophagocytic lymphohistiocytosis, possibly associated with viral disease or leukemia, medulloblastoma
Decrease in single cell line	
Anemia	Transient erythroblastopenia of childhood, hemolytic anemia, Diamond-Blackfan anemia, dyserythropoietic anemia (congenital)
Thrombocytopenia	ITP, thrombocytopenia absent radii, Wiskott-Aldrich syndrome, DIC, HUS, Kasabach-Merritt syndrome
Neutropenia	Familial neutropenia (Kostmann syndrome), chronic idiopathic neutropenia, splenic trapping
Liver/spleen enlargement	Infections, liver disease, lymphoma, Gaucher disease (other storage diseases), myeloproliferative disease, polycystic disease with liver fibrosis, Langerhans histiocytosis

CMV = cytomegalovirus; DIC = disseminated intravascular coagulation; EBV = Epstein-Barr virus; HIV = human immunodeficiency syndrome; HUS = hemolytic-uremic syndrome; ITP = idiopathic thrombocytopenic purpura.

spite intensive chemotherapy: Ph+ ALL, hypodiploid (< 45 chromosomes), infants with t(4j11) and those who fail their initial induction therapy.

CHEMOTHERAPY. There are three phases of chemotherapy for ALL: induction, intensification/consolidation, and maintenance. In each phase, multiple drug combinations are used. The total duration of therapy is usually 2 $^1/_2$ years. Studies have shown that treatment for a longer period does not improve prognosis, and treatment for a shorter period leads to more frequent relapses.

Leukemia may involve the brain and meninges at the time of diagnosis, and treatment of the CNS is part of therapy. During induction, patients receive intrathecal administration of chemotherapy. To prevent CNS involvement, all patients receive high doses of systemic chemotherapy, which crosses the blood–brain barrier.

In general, children with ALL achieve remission after a 4- to 6-week period of **induction therapy**. The chemotherapeutic agents used during this phase usually include a steroid (prednisone or dexamethasone), vincristine, and asparaginase with or without daunomycin.

After completion of the induction phase, more than 97% of children are in **remission,** which is defined as 5% or fewer blasts when the bone marrow has returned to normal (no leukemia cells can be seen in the marrow). To be in remission, the blood count should have recovered to more than 1000 neutrophils/mm³ and more than 100,000 platelets/mm³. In addition, no infection should be evident.

Once remission is achieved, the **intensification/consolidation therapy** that follows is designed to destroy leukemia cells that cannot be seen with the microscope. In some patients in remission, small numbers of leukemia cells (1 in 1000–1 in 100,000 nucleated marrow cells), which remain undetected morphologically, can be detected by using sensitive immunologic or molecular biologic techniques. The prognostic importance of identifying small numbers of leukemia cells in the marrow in children in early remission is an important topic that is currently undergoing study in clinical trials. It is estimated that as many as 10⁸ leukemia cells can remain following induction therapy.

Currently, the duration of the intensification/consolidation phase is 6–8 months. Often, patients are admitted to the hospital for administration of chemotherapy or treatment of fever and neutropenia. The chemotherapeutic drugs involved are usually high-dose methotrexate and standard-dose methotrexate, 6-mercaptopurine, cyclophosphamide, and the agents used during induction. The intensity of this phase varies depending on the risk group of the individual patient.

The final phase of treatment is called **maintenance therap**y. The duration of this phase is 1–2 years, depending on the duration of the consolidation phase. During maintenance therapy, chemotherapy is less intensive, usually with daily 6-mercaptopurine and weekly methotrexate with periodic vincristine and steroid pulses. The maintenance phase is commonly outpatient-based and well tolerated.

Following completion of therapy, patients are examined regularly to monitor for relapse and identify any late effects of the therapy. If patients are still in initial complete remission 5 years after the end of therapy or 7 $^1/_2$ years after diagnosis, they are considered cured and free of leukemia. Particular areas of concern to clinicians following children after they have completed chemotherapy include growth and development, cognitive ability, fertility, cardiac and hepatic function, and surveillance for second malignancies.

SUPPORTIVE CARE. To ensure that children pass through therapy without significant morbidity, issues relating to supportive care are of paramount importance. During induction, children need aggressive fluid management as successful therapy can result in rapid tumor cell lysis. The breakdown of leukemia cells releases intracellular contents into the systemic circulation, which are excreted through the kidneys. To prevent complications of **tumor lysis syndrome,** high volumes of fluid (often > 2 L/m²), alkalinization of the urine, and allopurinol (a xanthine oxidase inhibitor) are necessary.

Frequently, infectious complications may develop during therapy due to neutropenia- or therapy-induced immunosuppression. Both bacterial and systemic fungal infections may occur. *Pneumocystis carinii* is a pathogen of particular importance; infection can be prevented by administration of a combination of trimethoprim and sulfamethoxazole, given daily for three consecutive days each week. This prophylactic regimen is given throughout the duration of therapy and continued several months after therapy has been completed. Patients on therapy are followed closely with weekly monitoring of CBCs. Those who develop a temperature above 38°C and have an ANC less than 500/mm³ are admitted to the hospital for therapy with appropriate broad-spectrum antibiotics.

BMT. Chemotherapy alone results in long-term disease-free survival in over 80% of children with ALL, so BMT is considered early during the first remission only for children who are likely to have a very poor prognosis—a **disease-free survival (DFS)** of less than 40%. (The DFS is the period of time from the achievement of complete remission to the time of relapse.) Patients with Ph+ ALL, hypodiploid ALL, infants less than 12 months of age with t(4;11) and those who have failed initial induction therapy are considered to have a DFS of less than 40%. Children with these characteristics should be considered for an allogeneic marrow transplant during first remission because current reports indicate that following BMT, these high-risk patients have a DFS of 67%–80%. Otherwise, BMT is used only when patients have suffered a relapse and are in second remission.

Acute Myelocytic Leukemia (AML)
A heterogeneous disease, AML is classified based on the morphology of the blasts and by the presence or absence of specific cytogenetic abnormalities. The outlook for children with AML has gradually improved, although the rate of improvement in prognosis is slower than for ALL.

CHEMOTHERAPY. Following one or two courses of an intensive induction regimen using aggressive combinations of several agents [usually high-dose cytosine arabinoside, daunorubicin (or idarubicin, mitoxantrone), etoposide, 6-thioguanine, dexamethasone], over 80% of children are in remission.

However, the morbidity and mortality of this myelosuppressive induction is quite high. Approximately 5% of children are resistant to induction therapy, and 10%–15% die during induction from infectious or toxic causes. Although as many as 80%–85% of children achieve remission, just over 50% are cured of their disease with chemotherapy alone. The risk of severe toxicity and death associated with the therapy is significant.

Once children achieve remission, the next phase of therapy is aggressive consolidation/maintenance with chemotherapy or BMT. Identifying the most effective chemotherapy regimens for children once they achieve complete remission is still under active investigation. Currently, repeated courses of intensive myelosuppressive chemotherapy are given over 4–6 months.

This treatment is associated with frequent hospitalization because children are at great risk for bacterial and fungal infections. Less toxic postinduction therapy is not effective.

BMT may also be useful. The 15%–20% of patients with a **human leukocyte antigen** (HLA) identical sibling donor are transplanted soon after achieving complete remission and have a 65% 4-year **event-free survival** (EFS), which is from the time of diagnosis until failure of remission, death in remission, or relapse of any kind. At the present time, autologous BMT or matched, unrelated donor BMT has no role for children in first remission.

UNIQUE AML SUBTYPES. In pediatric AML, certain morphologic and karyotypic abnormalities have prognostic importance. The morphology and karyotype of the myeloid leukemia cell at the time of diagnosis can be used to identify children whose leukemia cells contain specific chromosomal translocations that have therapeutic and prognostic importance. Using the French-American-British (FAB) system, pediatric AML can be generally subtyped from MO (undifferentiated AML) to M7 (megakaryocytic AML).

Information at diagnosis helps plan therapy for three particularly important AML subtypes. One is **promyelocytic leukemia (APL),** which is designated as M3 AML by the FAB system. The APL leukemia cells frequently contain numerous granules and Auer rods (pathognomonic of AML). Clinically, patients with APL (about 8% of AML in children) present with low WBCs, and not infrequently DIC occurs when therapy is initiated. The diagnosis of this subtype of myeloid leukemia is associated with a specific chromosomal translocation, t(15;17). Most importantly, children with APL can be successfully treated and achieve remission with all–*trans* retinoic acid therapy. At the present time, the best outcome is found when chemotherapy is used in combination with the vitamin A analog all–*trans* retinoic acid therapy. A new strategy adds arsenic trioxide (As_2O_3) to this combination in an attempt to improve on the current 70% EFS.

The second subtype is AML in children with **Down syndrome,** who are at increased risk for acute leukemia. Approximately 1 in 150 children with Down syndrome develops leukemia, and when a child with Down syndrome under the age of 4 years is diagnosed with leukemia, it is usually AML, frequently the M7 type. Newborns with Down syndrome may manifest a self-limited **transient myeloproliferative disorder (TMD)**. This "pseudoleukemia," which presents with circulating blasts, leukocytosis, and organomegaly, usually resolves with only supportive care within 6 weeks to 3 months. It is estimated that 25%–30% of infants with Down syndrome and TMD will subsequently develop AML 1–3 years following resolution of the TMD. Children with Down syndrome exhibit a relatively low tolerance for high-dose chemotherapy. Due to the frequent association with other defects associated with Down syndrome, aggressive therapy should be given very carefully. With current chemotherapy regimens utilizing anthracyclines and cytosine arabinoside for induction, AML-affected children with Down syndrome have a better EFS and a decreased relapse rate compared to children without Down syndrome. In recent studies, EFS, for children with Down syndrome and AML is over 80%.

The third subtype of AML involves children with monosomy 7, who may present with AML in a subacute myelodysplastic phase or de novo AML. Monosomy 7 and partial deletion of the long arm (7q-) is seen in myeloproliferative disease, **myelodysplastic syndrome,** and AML. This cytogenetic finding usually is a sign of poor response to chemotherapy and a rapidly progressive course. Although initial chemotherapy is essential for achievement of remission, children with monosomy 7 have a better EFS when treated with early BMT.

BMT. In AML, children in first remission (except those with Down syndrome) should undergo a BMT if they have an HLA-identical sibling donor. In Down syndrome–affected children, BMT should be avoided, because the prognosis is best with chemotherapy alone. For patients in first relapse or failing induction therapy, a matched unrelated BMT should be considered. Studies have not shown that autologous BMT is better than chemotherapy alone in patients in first remission; however, it warrants consideration in second remission if the first remission occurred over 12 months previously.

Non-Hodgkin Lymphoma and Hodgkin Disease

Lymphomas, a heterogeneous group of diseases arising from B or T lymphocytes, are the most common cancer seen in older adolescents—in the 15–19-year age group. **Non-Hodgkin lymphoma (NHL)** predominates in younger children, and **Hodgkin disease** predominates in adolescents. The risk of lymphoma is increased in children with congenital and acquired immune deficiencies. Currently, most children with lymphoma are curable; the 5-year overall survival rates for NHL and Hodgkin disease are 72% and 92%, respectively.

Lymphoma should be suspected in children with any significantly enlarged lymph node or mass lesion. The diagnostic evaluation always includes a bone marrow aspirate to rule out leukemia and imaging studies to identify the extent of disease. Both NHL and Hodgkin disease are pathologically classified, once adequate diagnostic material has been obtained and then staged (a determination of the extent of disease) so that appropriate therapy may be given. Patients who have extensive disease require more intensive therapy than children with less extensive disease.

Lymphomas in children are particularly sensitive to chemotherapy. All patients with NHL receive chemotherapy alone, while patients with Hodgkin disease are treated with radiation therapy to the area where tumor masses were present at the time of diagnosis in addition to three to five cycles of chemotherapy.

SOLID TUMORS

Clinical and Laboratory Evaluation

History

A solid tumor in a child is by definition a mass lesion. Most frequently, parents note an abdominal mass or a lump on the trunk or extremity in a young child during a bath; the mass continues to enlarge and may cause pain. Severe back pain, extremity weakness, or ataxia are symptoms that need immediate evaluation by a health care provider. A thorough review of the clinical history, with signs and symptoms, is mandatory. A detailed family history can be quite helpful for those diseases frequently linked to known genetic abnormalities (see Table 16.8). With solid tumors, the history of illness is usually longer than with hematologic malignancies. A history of symptoms and signs for 3–9 months is not unusual. Occasionally hemorrhage into a tumor (e.g., Wilms tumor) may lead to an earlier diagnosis. There appears to be no relationship between time to diagnosis and extent of disease.

Physical Examination

Physical evaluation may aid in the diagnosis. The tumor can often be identified directly by palpation (e.g., Wilms tumor, soft tissue sarcoma, Ewing sarcoma, osteosarcoma) or indirectly because the tumor interferes with normal functioning (e.g., CNS tumors, germ cell tumors). Occasionally, solid tumors (e.g., neuroblastoma, rhabdomyosarcoma, Ewing sarcoma) may partially infiltrate bone marrow and cause signs not unlike leukemia (i.e., anemia, neutropenia, thrombocytopenia).

Laboratory Evaluation

A chronic limp or extremity pain that does not resolve after a few days may be an indication for a radiograph to rule out tumor as a cause. Several laboratory studies are necessary in the diagnostic evaluation of children with suspected solid tumors (Table 16.14).

Differential Diagnosis

The presenting signs and symptoms associated with solid tumors in children can also be seen with several benign conditions and tumors (Table 16.15).

Brain Tumors

Brain tumors, which are the most common category of solid tumor in children in the United States, occur at a rate of 2.5 to 3.6/100,000 children 15 years of age and younger. In general, boys are affected more often (ratio, 1.2:1), and the median age at time of diagnosis is 6½ years. About one half of all CNS tumors in children are located in the cerebellum (25%) or brainstem (23%). **Astrocytomas,** which account for about 50% of childhood brain tumors, are the common solid tumor seen in individuals less than 20 years of age. Other tumors include **primitive neuroectodermal tumors** (e.g., **medulloblastomas** and other embryonal tumors) [20%], ependymomas (9%), and craniopharyngiomas (< 5%). As many as 80% of brain tumors in children require surgical intervention, either for diagnosis or as primary treatment; 60% require radiation therapy; and 40% need chemotherapy.

Neuroblastomas

Neuroblastomas, the most frequent extracranial solid tumor in children, accounts for approximately 8% of all malignancies in patients younger than 15 years of age. These tumors are the most frequent malignancy diagnosed in infants, and over 80% of cases occur in patients younger than 4 years.

Neuroblastomas may originate anywhere along the sympathetic nervous system chain from the organs of Zuckerkandl to the stellate ganglion. Over 65% of primary tumors arise in the abdomen. Adrenal tumors are more common in children, whereas thoracic and cervical primary tumors are more common in infants. Unlike other solid tumors in children, neuroblastomas are associated with metastatic disease at the time of diagnosis in 60%–70% of patients.

Pediatric Pearl

Common sites of metastasis are the bone marrow, bone, liver, and skin.

At the time of diagnosis, children older than 1 year of age are more likely than infants to have disseminated disease. The presenting signs and symptoms of neuroblastoma relate to the primary and metastatic sites involved, as with all solid tumors. For example, abdominal distention and hepatomegaly may occur in an abdominal primary tumor with liver metastases, whereas ptosis or eye swelling may indicate a metastatic or primary neuroblastoma of the head or neck.

TABLE 16.14 **Diagnostic Evaluation of Solid Tumors**

Clinical history and physical examination
CBC (hemoglobin, differential, platelets)
BUN, LDH, ALT, total bilirubin, creatinine, calcium
PT, PTT, fibrinogen (prior to biopsy, identify DIC)
Varicella titer (may need periodic varicella-zoster immune globulin or acyclovir)
Imaging studies of the primary tumor (to look for distant spread and appropriate staging) [plain radiographs, CT scan, MRI, ultrasound]
Bone marrow aspirate and biopsy (to look for tumor involvement, particularly in Ewing sarcoma, primitive neuroectodermal tumor, rhabdomyosarcoma, neuroblastoma)
Tumor markers, such as α-fetoprotein (hepatoblastoma, germ cell tumor) and β-human chorionic gonadotropin (germ cell tumor)

ALT = alanine aminotransferase; BUN = blood urea nitrogen; CBC = complete blood count; CT = computed tomography; DIC = disseminated intravascular coagulation; LDH = lactate dehydrogenase; MRI = magnetic resonance imaging; PT = prothrombin time; PTT = partial thromboplastin time; WBC = white blood count.

TABLE 16.15	Differential Diagnosis of Solid Tumors	
Sign or Symptom	**Benign Condition**	**Tumor**
Abdominal mass	Polycystic liver or kidneys, constipation, hydronephrosis, hepatomegaly, splenomegaly, nephroblastomatosis	Wilms tumor, neuroblastoma, lymphoma, germ cell tumor, PNET, soft tissue sarcoma, hepatoblastoma, intra-abdominal desmoplastic round cell tumor of the abdomen
Thoracic mass Anterior mediastinum	Thymoma, thymic cyst, dermoid	Lymphoma (NHL), germ cell tumor, thyroid carcinoma
Middle mediastinum	Sarcoidosis, tuberculosis, aspergillosis, vascular anomaly	Lymphoma (Hodgkin disease), metastatic disease
Posterior mediastinum	Esophageal duplication, ganglioneuroma, neurofibroma	Neuroblastoma, Ewing sarcoma/PNET,
Chest wall	Osteoma, Langerhans histiocytosis, scoliosis,	Ewing sarcoma/PNET, osteosarcoma
Head and neck mass	Infectious adenitis, hemangioma, cystic hygroma	Lymphoma, rhabdomyosarcoma, nasopharyngeal carcinoma, neuroblastoma
Extremity mass	Fracture, trauma, eosinophilic granuloma, osteoid osteoma, enchondroma	Lymphoma, Ewing sarcoma/PNET, osteosarcoma, rhabdomyosarcoma
Pelvic area mass	Bladder distention, constipation	Rhabdomyosarcoma, neuroblastoma, Ewing sarcoma/PNET, osteosarcoma
Intracranial mass	Dysplastic tissue, abscess, hemorrhage	Medulloblastoma/PNET, low- and high-grade astrocytoma, brainstem glioma, craniopharyngioma, germ cell tumors, ependymoma

NHL = Non-Hodgkin lymphoma; PNET = primitive neuroectodermal tumor.

Several paraneoplastic syndromes are associated with neuroblastoma: (1) opsoclonus–myoclonus–myoclonic jerking and conjugate, shooting eye movements, and (2) intractable secretory diarrhea, hypokalemia, and dehydration.

During initial evaluation, patients with suspected neuroblastoma should undergo bone marrow aspiration and biopsy, tumor mass biopsy, and collection of urine for catecholamines to confirm the diagnosis. Imaging studies, including computed tomography (CT) and magnetic resonance imaging (MRI), are used for staging, along with other biologic, radiographic, and pathologic information prior to initiating therapy. Therapy involves surgery to confirm the diagnosis and usually to remove residual disease following aggressive chemotherapy. In selected high-risk patients, autologous BMT in addition to surgery and chemotherapy has improved survival. Studies of the effectiveness of autologous BMT for all high-risk patients are as yet incomplete.

Among children with neuroblastoma, a unique category of disease called **stage IV-S neuroblastoma** may affect children younger than 1 year of age. These children present with a limited primary tumor (stage I or II) and have evidence of distant spread to the liver, skin, or bone marrow (but not actual bone involvement). These patients, who have an exceptionally good prognosis, most often require only observation. It is important to obtain adequate tissue for biological studies in these children, because a few manifest poor prognostic features such as N-*myc* amplification and require chemotherapy.

Wilms Tumors

Wilms tumors, which are only slightly less common than neuroblastomas, account for 7% of childhood malignancies. They are almost exclusively a tumor of young children, with 80% of cases occurring before the age of 5 years. Exclusive to the kidney, Wilms tumors arise out of persisting immature renal tissue termed nephrogenic rests, which are considered tumor precursor lesions. The classic presentation is a silent abdominal mass; however, as many as one-third of patients complain of pain. Parents usually discover the mass accidentally during bathing or pediatricians identify it incidentally during a physical examination performed for other reasons. The mass is usually limited to one side of the abdomen. Occasionally, acute hemorrhage into the tumor occurs, which is manifested as anemia and an acutely enlarging abdominal mass. Hematuria or hypertension are found in more than 20% of patients.

Histologic variants in Wilms tumor differ based on the presence of anaplasia, and these variants have prognostic importance. The two histologic variants that are associated with the kidney but are no longer called Wilms tumor are now distinct tumor types: (1) clear cell sarcoma and (2) rhabdoid tumor. They have much poorer prognoses than Wilms tumor and require a different chemotherapeutic regimen.

Wilms tumor occurs in hereditary and nonhereditary forms. It is frequently associated with the following congenital anomalies: WAGR syndrome (**W**ilms tumor, **a**niridia, **g**enitourinary abnormalities, mental **r**etardation), with a 30% likelihood of developing Wilms tumor; Beckwith-Wiedemann syndrome (gigantism, macroglossia), with a 5% incidence of Wilms tumor; sporadic aniridia; and hemihypertrophy. When children have one of these anomalies, they should undergo routine surveillance (approximately every 3 months) with renal ultrasound until either Wilms tumor develops or they reach the age of 8 years, at which time the risk of Wilms tumor decreases significantly.

Over many years, children with Wilms tumor have been treated by a succession of clinical protocols developed by the National Wilms Tumor Study Group. At the present time, over 90% of children with Wilms tumor are cured with a combination of surgery, less than 6 months of chemotherapy using vincristine, actinomycin D with or without doxorubicin, and radiation therapy for patients with more advanced disease.

Bone Tumors, Osteosarcomas, and Ewing Sarcomas

Approximately 5% of all childhood cancers are malignant bone tumors. Almost two-thirds are osteosarcomas, and one-third are Ewing sarcomas. Each tumor type is more frequent in adolescent patients; the peak occurrence coincides with the adolescent growth spurt. The incidence of osteosarcoma is slightly higher in African-

American children; the occurrence of Ewing sarcoma in African-American children is very rare. A few cases of osteosarcoma have been associated with ionizing radiation and the Li-Fraumeni syndrome. Ewing sarcoma is not associated with any such predisposing conditions.

Although **osteosarcomas** may develop in any bone, they are most often seen in the metaphysis of long bones. Fifty percent of cases involve the distal femur or proximal tibia. Parents usually seek medical attention for affect children because of pain, a mass, or swelling around a joint. Radiographs demonstrate a lytic or sclerotic lesion associated with a soft tissue mass. Staging studies indicate that approximately 25% of patients have metastatic disease. The most frequent site of metastases is the lungs. Therapy involves aggressive chemotherapy and resection of the primary tumor, with limb salvage therapy if possible. Radiation therapy is not used as primary therapy; osteosarcoma is resistant to radiation. With current therapy, as many as 75% of patients with nonmetastatic disease may be cured; in contrast, about 30% of those with metastatic disease at diagnosis may be long-term survivors.

As with osteosarcoma, **Ewing sarcoma**, a **primitive neuroectodermal tumor,** frequently occurs as pain or swelling around a bone or joint in a child or young adult. On presentation, the primary tumor is as likely to be in a long as a flat bone. With long bone involvement, the diaphysis is more likely to be affected, with bony destruction, a soft tissue mass, and an "onion skin" appearance. The pelvis and the femur are the most frequently involved bones. Approximately 20% of patients have pulmonary or bony metastatic lesions at diagnosis. Therapy initially involves intensive chemotherapy and is followed by surgery, radiation, or both for local tumor control. A recent clinical trial found that patients with no metastasis at diagnosis had an EFS of 80% and those who had metastatic disease at diagnosis had an EFS of 25%.

Soft Ttissue Sarcomas and Rhabdomyosarcomas

Of the soft tissue sarcomas, rhabdomyosarcomas are identified in slightly more than 3% of children with cancer; they are the most common soft tissue sarcomas, representing over 50% of cases. Fibrosarcomas and embryonal sarcomas, which are examples of other soft tissue sarcomas, occur much less frequently and are much less sensitive to chemotherapy. Rhabdomyosarcomas may occur anywhere in the body, either as a clearly visible mass lesion or an occult mass interfering with a body function (e.g., bowel or bladder control, vision or hearing loss). A few cases occur in patients with Li-Fraumeni syndrome. On histology there are alveolar and embryonal varieties. In general, the alveolar type of rhabdomyosarcomas occurs in the extremities of older children or adolescents and has a worse prognosis, while the embryonal type develops in the genitourinary or head and neck region of younger children and has a good prognosis.

The tumor may be primarily resected in 35% of cases, with metastatic lesions found approximately 15% of the time. Metastatic disease may occur as enlarged lymph nodes and pulmonary or bone lesions, and bone marrow infiltration is not uncommon. The site, presence of metastasis, and initial resectability of the tumor, in addition to histology, have significant prognostic import and form the basis for a risk-group stratification. With up to 1 year of aggressive therapy, long survival and cure is likely for more than 90% of patients with low-risk disease, 70%–80% of those with intermediate-risk disease, and 20% of those with high-risk disease.

Germ Cell Tumors

Approximately 900 children, adolescents, and young adults are diagnosed with germ cell tumors yearly in the United States. One half of pediatric germ cell tumors occur in adolescents from the ages of 15–19 years. This group of tumors can be separated into three general categories: benign teratomas (55%), immature teratomas (10%), and malignant tumors (35%). The malignant germ cell tumors are yolk sac tumors (known as endodermal sinus tumors), choriocarcinomas, embryonal carcinomas, and germinomas (seminoma, dysgerminoma).

Clinically, these tumors are usually very large when diagnosed and present as palpable or visible masses usually in the sacrococcygeal, testicular, or head and neck region. Germ cell tumors can cause constipation, urinary obstruction, respiratory difficulty, or neurologic dysfunction. Metastases from non-CNS primary tumors are usually pulmonary or nodal. Typically, ovarian tumors occur in children older than 4 years of age, whereas testicular tumors develop in infancy or adolescence. Tumor markers in the serum are useful for diagnosis and for following patients during and after completion of therapy. Serum α-fetoprotein is elevated in yolk sac tumors, and human chorionic gonadotropin (HCG) is elevated in choriocarcinoma and embryonal carcinoma.

The management of germ cell tumors depends on site and initial resectability. Benign teratomas require surgical resection only. For control of sacrococcygeal tumors, coccygectomy is warranted to prevent malignant degeneration at a later date. Follow-up involves imaging of the tumor area and monitoring of tumor markers for a 3-year period. Using this follow-up, more than 90% of patients with benign teratomas show no tumor recurrence. Surgery is usually effective for stage I germ cell tumors, while platinum-based adjuvant chemotherapy with etoposide and bleomycin is notably effective for higher stage testicular disease and for all ovarian primary tumors and patients with extragonadal tumors. Complete surgical resection of the tumor should be attempted whenever feasible. At present, the EFS for those with germ cell tumors requiring chemotherapy is greater than 80%.

SUGGESTED READINGS

Hematology

Adams RJ, McKie VC, Hsu L, et al: Prevention of a first stroke by transfusions in children with sickle cell anemia and abnormal results on transcranial Doppler ultrasonography. *N Engl J Med* 339:5–11, 1998.

Hathaway WE, Goodnight SH (eds): *Disorders of Hemostasis and Thrombosis*. New York, McGraw-Hill, 1993.

Miller DJ, Baehner RL: *Blood Diseases of Infancy and Childhood*. St. Louis, Mosby, 1995.

Nathan DG, Orkin SH (eds): *Nathan and Oski's Hematology of Infancy and Childhood,* 5th ed. Philadelphia, WB Saunders, 1997.

Rapaport SI: *Introduction to Hematology,* 2nd ed. Philadelphia, Lippincott Williams & Wilkins, 1987.

Sadler JE, Mannucci PM, Berntorp E, et al: Impact, diagnosis and treatment of von Willebrand disease. *Thromb Haemost* 84:160–174, 2000.

Web sites

http://www.tigc.org/eguidelines/hypercoagstates.htm

Oncology

Pizzo PA, Poplack DG (eds): *Principles and Practice of Pediatric Oncology*. Philadelphia, JB Lippincott, 1998.

Pui CH (ed): *Childhood Leukemias*. New York, Cambridge University Press, 1999.

Ries LAG, Smith MA, Gurney JG, et al (eds): Cancer incidence and survival among children and adolescents: United States SEER Program 1975–1995, National Cancer Institute, SEER Program. NIH Pub. 99–4649. Bethesda, MD, 1999.

Schwartz CL: Long-term survivors of childhood cancer: The late effects of therapy. *Oncologist* 4:45–54, 1999.

Web sites

http://seer.cancer.gov/Publications/childhood/index.html

Chapter 17

Allergy and Immunology

Elizabeth C. TePas and Dale T. Umetsu

ALLERGIC DISORDERS

Allergies are caused by untoward, inappropriate immunologic responses to "foreign" substances. Although any individual can have an allergic reaction, **atopic** individuals have a propensity to develop specific types of allergic reactions. Atopic individuals are not allergic to all foreign substances but tend to develop three specific diseases: **allergic rhinitis, asthma** (see Chapter 18, Pulmonology), and **atopic dermatitis** (eczema) [see Chapter 22, Dermatology]. Atopic children often first present with **food allergy**. Anaphylactic reactions, which are also discussed in this chapter, can occur in both atopic and nonatopic individuals.

Pathophysiology

"Immediate" or type 1 responses are triggered by antigen binding to immunoglobulin E (IgE) molecules on the surface of mast cells, resulting in mast cell degranulation and release of mediators such as histamine and eosinophil chemotactic factors. These mediators can cause urticaria, sneezing, and wheezing (due to increased vascular permeability and bronchial smooth muscle contraction). Persistence of symptoms occurs as a result of the later production of mast cell mediators such as leukotrienes, prostaglandins, platelet-activating factor (PAF), and cytokines [tumor necrosis factor-α (TNF-α), interleukin-4 (IL-4), IL-5].

In addition, persistent allergic symptoms may be due to the development of an **allergic inflammatory response** resulting from the influx of basophils, eosinophils, monocytes, lymphocytes, and neutrophils. These cell types interact extensively and amplify the allergic response by producing factors that increase synthesis of allergen-specific IgE (e.g., IL-4, IL-13) and factors that increase the influx and growth of eosinophils, basophils, and mast cells (e.g., granulocyte-macrophage colony-stimulating factor, IL-3, IL-5, IL-9, IL-10, RANTES). The infiltration of such cells characterizes the allergic inflammatory response associated with **late-phase responses** and bronchial or nasal **hyperreactivity.**

Children of parents with atopic disease are at higher risk for the development of allergies. Early exposure to allergens is thought to enhance the development of atopic disease, whereas breast-feeding for 6 months or more may prevent or delay the development of allergy in such infants. Because antigens from foods ingested by the mother are excreted into breast milk, breastfeeding decreases but does not eliminate exposure of the infant to food allergens, and only if the quantity of allergenic foods (e.g., cow's milk, egg, fish) has been reduced in the maternal diet during lactation. If breastfeeding is not possible, infants at risk may be fed hydrolyzed milk-based formulas (e.g., Alimentum, Pregestimil, or Nutramigen). Patients with severe food allergies may require free amino acid formulas (e.g., Neocate). Some clinicians recommend that egg and fish should be avoided in high-risk infants until 12 months of age and peanuts until 3–4 years of age.

ALLERGIC RHINITIS

Allergic rhinitis (hay fever) is a very common disorder, affecting as many as 10%–20% of children. Unless it is associated with asthma, allergic rhinitis is generally not a life-threatening disorder. However, it remains a significant problem in terms of morbidity and health care costs.

Pathophysiology

Allergic rhinitis is caused by a type 1 allergic response. Reaction to wind-borne pollens of grasses, trees, and weeds leads to **seasonal allergic rhinitis,** and reaction to house dust mite allergen, pet dander, or mold spores results in **perennial allergic rhinitis.**

Clinical and Laboratory Evaluation

History
A careful history regarding the nature, frequency, seasonality, duration, location (e.g., indoors or outdoors, home or school), and intensity of the symptoms is required to assess the problem. Exposure to nonspecific irritants (e.g., perfumes,

smoke, air pollution, or solvents) may also result in significant symptoms in patients with hyperreactive nasal mucosa.

Symptoms of allergic rhinitis include chronic recurrent sneezing, nasal congestion, clear rhinorrhea, and pruritus of the nose, eyes, ears, and soft palate. Patients frequently rub their nose with the palm of their hands (**allergic salute**) or rub the soft palate with their tongue, producing clucking sounds. Usually, allergic symptoms immediately follow (within 20 minutes) exposure to the offending allergen. In addition, severe reactions with nasal congestion, sneezing, and rhinorrhea may reoccur 6–12 hours after exposure (**late-phase reactions**). Perennial allergic rhinitis, with chronic rather than intermittent exposure to allergen, results in significant chronic nasal congestion, sniffing, and snoring but less sneezing than in seasonal rhinitis (occurs mainly in the morning on awakening). Associations between exposure and onset of symptoms are often less clear in perennial allergic rhinitis. In severe cases, an "allergic facies" with mouth breathing and dental malocclusion or overbite is observed.

Family history may be important. Often, patients with allergic rhinitis have a personal or family history of asthma or atopic dermatitis. An evaluation of clinical responses to medications and an environmental history, recording the place and type of residence, type of indoor heating, and the presence of pets and of cigarette smokers, is also warranted.

Physical Examination
The physical examination is often remarkable for the presence of **clear nasal discharge** and for **enlarged, often pale turbinates**. A transverse nasal crease may be present, secondary to the chronic practice of the allergic salute. Nasal polyps (gray, glistening membranous tissue, often with fine blood vessels) are very uncommon and are seen mainly in older children, adults, and in patients with cystic fibrosis. The sclera may be injected and, rarely, edematous, and the lower eyelids may be darkened (**allergic shiners**) from venous stasis and creased (**Dennie-Morgan lines**) from intermittent edema. When **vernal conjunctivitis** is present, the palpebral conjunctiva has a cobblestone appearance. A **geographic tongue** is also common in atopic patients. The middle ear may contain fluid or evidence of infection, and examination of the chest may reveal wheezing, rales, or rhonchi. Signs of asthma and atopic dermatitis may be present. Digital clubbing, which occurs in patients with severe chronic lung diseases (e.g., cystic fibrosis), does not generally occur in patients with allergy.

Laboratory Evaluation
Specific allergens to which patients are allergic can be identified by (immediate) skin tests or by in vitro serum testing (RAST). For inhalant allergens, skin testing is more sensitive, is less costly, and gives results in minutes rather than weeks, compared with RAST. However, skin testing can provoke significant anxiety in young children. Skin testing and RAST for food allergens are also available, but these are less reliable than for inhalants. Identification of specific offending allergens is critical if specific environmental control measures are to be implemented or if immunotherapy is contemplated (see allergen immunotherapy).

Other relevant laboratory studies include nasal cytology, which may show eosinophils (instead of neutrophils as in sinusitis). A complete blood count (CBC) with differential may show eosinophilia. Elevated serum IgE suggests the presence of allergic disease. Because there is considerable overlap between the values of normal and allergic individuals, however, the total IgE test has low sensitivity and low specificity and is useful mainly as a screening test when the presence of allergic disease is not clear. Total IgE is also elevated in parasitic infections, infectious mononucleosis, allergic bronchopulmonary aspergillosis, and various immunodeficiencies and neoplastic diseases.

Differential Diagnosis

Several conditions may be confused with allergic rhinitis (Table 17.1). Upper respiratory viral infections and chronic sinusitis are often very difficult to distinguish from allergic rhinitis, which is generally associated with sneezing and pruritus of the nose and eyes.

Management

The treatment for allergic rhinitis must be individualized. Disease severity varies greatly, and the clinician must assess its impact on patients before embarking on therapy, especially because some children (and adults) with severe allergic rhinitis often refuse prescribed medical therapy. Treatment modalities include avoidance of allergens, pharmacologic therapy (systemic and topical therapy), and allergen immunotherapy. Environmental controls may be sufficient for treatment of less severe disease, but a combination of therapeutic measures is necessary for more severe disease.

Environmental Control and Avoidance of Allergens
Environmental measures play a very important role in the treatment of allergic rhinitis and are often overlooked (Table 17.2).

TABLE 17.1 Differential Diagnosis of Rhinitis

Diagnosis	Character of Nasal Discharge	Comments
Allergic rhinitis		Both seasonal and perennial rhinitis are associated with nasal pruritus, sneezing, and allergic conjunctivitis
Seasonal rhinitis	Clear	Symptoms are more acute than in perennial rhinitis
Perennial rhinitis	Clear	Chronic nasal congestion and allergic shiners are prominent
Viral URI	Clear	Symptoms last only 7–10 days, may be associated with sore throat, fever, poor appetite, and exposure to others with URI
Sinusitis	Purulent or clear	Symptoms, often lasting > 10 days, are associated with cough, headache, halitosis, and abnormal sinus radiographs or computed tomography (CT) scans
NARES	Clear	Skin tests are negative but eosinophils are present on nasal smear
Vasomotor rhinitis	Clear	Perfuse nasal discharge is triggered by exercise, heat, cold, and strong smells
Hormonal rhinitis	Clear	Nasal congestion can result from hypothyroidism or pregnancy
Other		
Nasal polyps	Purulent or clear	Nasal polyps are associated with cystic fibrosis, aspirin triad (asthma, aspirin sensitivity, nasal polyps with chronic sinusitis), or symptoms of chronic rhinitis
Foreign body	Purulent	Condition primarily occurs in children < 2 years of age
Tumors	Purulent or clear	Condition is rare in children

NARES = nonallergic rhinitis with eosinophilia syndrome; URI = upper respiratory infection.

Pharmacologic Therapy

Antihistamines (H_1 antagonists), which are safe and effective medications for the treatment and prevention of allergic reactions, are particularly useful in controlling the symptoms of sneezing, nasal pruritus, and rhinorrhea. A large number of different antihistamines are available, but for simplicity, the physician should become familiar with only a few. Although diphenhydramine (Benadryl) and hydroxyzine (Atarax) are extremely effective in relieving acute allergic reactions, these should be avoided in patients with allergic rhinitis because they are especially sedating. Second-generation antihistamines include loratadine (Claritin) and fexofenadine (Allegra), which are nonsedating, and cetirizine (Zyrtec), which has a low rate of sedation (5%–10%). Loratadine and cetirizine are available in pill and liquid forms, and all are available in combination with a decongestant, although only in dose formulations suitable for older children and adults. Although these second-generation antihistamines are effective and have fewer side effects, they are expensive and still require a prescription in the United States.

For patients who have infrequent symptoms, first-generation antihistamines such as chlorpheniramine and brompheniramine, alone or in combination with decongestants (e.g., phenylephrine or

TABLE 17.2 Environmental Control Measures

1. Prohibit smokers from entering house.
2. Do not keep pets indoors if patient is allergic to cats or dogs.
3. Avoid using paints, solvent-based glues, or insect sprays while patient is home.
4. Use dust mite control measures, including covering pillows, mattresses, and box springs with special encasements. Keep humidity relatively low, as mites thrive in humid environments. Wash bedding weekly. Keep stuffed animals off bed and to a minimum. Discourage use of upholstered furniture.
5. Discourage use of carpets as floor coverings, because they greatly increase the level of dust mite antigen compared with hardwood floors.
6. Use air conditioners, which are beneficial in hot summer weather because windows can be kept closed to exclude airborne pollen allergens and humidity can be controlled. (This is true not only for houses but also for automobiles.)
7. Use air cleaners with high-efficiency particle arresting (HEPA) filters, which are able to remove 99.97% of particulate matter and are beneficial in bedrooms (effective for pollen, mold spores, and animal dander but not dust mite allergens).

pseudoephedrine), may be options for the treatment of allergic rhinitis (and upper respiratory infections). Although the older antihistamines can be sedating and may cause problems during the daytime in school-age children, they are often preferred by parents for use in young children at night.

Systemic adrenergic drugs (decongestants) are effective treatment for nasal congestion, but they do have significant potential side effects and so should be used judiciously. Topical preparations such as oxymetazoline hydrochloride (Afrin) or xylometazoline hydrochloride (Otrivin) should not be used for the treatment of allergic rhinitis, because after prolonged use (> 3–5 days) they can cause severe rebound edema **(rhinitis medicamentosa).**

Cromolyn (Nasalcrom), which is available as a nasal spray without prescription, is a weak anti-inflammatory agent. It inhibits mast cell degranulation, but has other antiallergic effects and is effective in relieving symptoms of allergic rhinitis. Because it has virtually no side effects, it is safe for use in children, although it must be used 2–6 times/day to be effective.

Topical nasal steroids [mometasone (Nasonex), fluticasone (Flonase), budesonide (Rhinocort), beclomethasone (Vancenase, Beconase)] are the most effective pharmacologic agents for the treatment of allergic rhinitis. They provide the greatest benefit for the broadest range of symptoms and are especially useful in patients who have prominent symptoms of nasal congestion. In general, patients receive only minute doses. However, at higher doses systemic effects may occur in some patients, possibly affecting growth and bone mineralization. Therefore, topical nasal steroids should be used with some caution. There is no indication for the use of systemic corticosteroids in the treatment of allergic rhinitis.

Allergen Immunotherapy

Allergen immunotherapy, which involves the subcutaneous administration of increasing doses of allergen, is highly effective and safe in patients with allergic rhinitis (and patients with asthma) in whom specific allergens (inhalant allergens and bee venom) are identified. Immunotherapy alters the underlying immune response to allergens by decreasing the production of allergen-specific IgE and of allergen-induced T_H2 cytokines such as IL-4. It is the only treatment currently available that alters the natural course of, and potentially cures, allergic disease. Because of the cost in terms of time and pain, allergen immunotherapy is generally reserved for patients older than 5–6 years of age with moderate-to-severe allergic rhinitis. However, because reports indicate that immunotherapy

prevents polysensitization and also prevents the progression toward asthma, more liberal use particularly in young children should be considered. The administration of allergen immunotherapy must take place in a physician's office where treatment for systemic reactions is readily available because of a small but real risk of anaphylaxis.

ATOPIC DERMATITIS

Atopic dermatitis or eczema, a very common childhood skin disorder, affects about 5%–10% of children. The prognosis in most affected patients is extremely good, with a tendency for remission at 3–5 years of age and with approximately 75% of patients outgrowing the problem by adolescence.

Clinical Evaluation

There is no pathognomonic feature or laboratory marker of atopic dermatitis, and therefore the diagnosis is a clinical one. The condition is characterized by the following features:

- Skin lesions that are pruritic, dry, scaly, and often erythematous
- Skin lesions that have a typical distribution
- A chronic relapsing course
- A positive family medical history for atopic disease

Differential Diagnosis

Any "eczematoid" lesion may have the appearance of atopic dermatitis, and these conditions must be distinguished from atopic dermatitis (Table 17.3). Because the term "eczematoid" is often used to describe the response of the skin to a sensitizing agent, it is important that the specific sensitizing agent be identified (where possible) for proper management. If a specific offending agent is identified (contact antigen or chemical), then part of the preventive approach obviously is avoidance of the particular agent or agents.

The most useful clue in making the diagnosis of atopic dermatitis is the distribution of the lesions, which is very typical but varies with age. In the **infantile form,** the face, extensor surface of the arms, and the chest are affected; the diaper area is spared. In older children, the lesions appear in the antecubital and popliteal fossae and on the wrists and dorsal surface of the hands. In the **adult form,** the dorsal surfaces of the hands and feet are affected. Associated findings include pityriasis alba (scaly, hypopigmented patches of skin, worse with sun exposure), keratosis pilaris (keratinized

TABLE 17.3 **Differential Diagnosis of Atopic Dermatitis**

Disorder	Comments
Seborrheic dermatitis	Usually begins on scalp (cradle cap) and sides of nose, with greasy, scaly lesions
Diaper dermatitis	Sparing of diaper area with atopic dermatitis
Contact dermatitis	Generally not chronic and recurring; does not occur with typical distribution but rather on exposed sites
Tinea	Usually found in skin folds (neck, diaper area) rather than with typical distribution of atopic dermatitis
Histiocytosis X	Generally hemorrhagic (petechia)
Psoriasis	Raised plaques with sharply demarcated, irregular borders and silvery scales, occurring mainly on scalp, knees, elbows, and genitalia
Pyoderma	Generally pustular
Scabies	Usually in intertriginous areas; can have generalized rash with Id reaction; often several family members affected

Other conditions
   Immunodeficiency disorders (Wiskott-Aldrich, SCID, hyper–IgE syndrome)
   Metabolic disorders
   Phenylketonuria, histidinemia
   Acrodermatitis enteropathica
   Ectodermal dysplasia
	Unusual presentation; poor response to steroids

SCID = severe combined immunodeficiency disease.

papules at the mouths of hair follicles, usually on the extensor surfaces of arms and thighs), elevated serum IgE, and food allergies.

Management

As with other atopic diseases, patients with atopic dermatitis often experience a chronic relapsing course, which can be frustrating to both parents and children. The focus of treatment should be on assessing the severity of the problem, which will vary with time, and on providing measures appropriate for the disease severity to control the symptoms. Excellent control can almost always be achieved.

General measures in the treatment of atopic dermatitis include avoidance of irritants such as soap, detergents, solvents, chemicals, and wool or acrylic clothing. The patient should dress with loose-fitting clothing and avoid overheating. Fingernails should be trimmed often.

Pediatric Pearl

Because pruritus is a significant feature of the disease and injury to the skin from scratching aggravates the condition, it is important to provide measures that reduce pruritus.

Skin hydration is a major part of the treatment plan because it greatly reduces pruritus. Frequent baths with water can result in drying of the skin, and this has led some physicians to recommend limitations on bathing. However, improved skin hydration can be achieved by short baths or showers 1–3 times/day followed immediately by the application of lubricants to trap moisture in the skin. Depending on the severity of the problem, fragrance-free creams, mineral oil, or petroleum jelly (Vaseline) can be used. More severe disease requires greater occlusion, but occasionally greater occlusion may result in folliculitis, especially in hot weather. Conversely, increased occlusion is required in winter months when drying of the skin is worse as a result of the use of indoor heat.

Treatment of atopic dermatitis involves the use of topical steroids on affected skin (generally, only on erythematous areas). Topical steroids decrease pruritus, reduce inflammation, and cause vasoconstriction. Topical steroids are available in different strengths and with different vehicles (Table 17.4). Ointments and gels provide better penetration, and therefore increased potency, compared with creams. Only low-potency steroids should be used on the face to avoid skin atrophy. High-potency steroids should be avoided except for limited periods of time and in restricted areas, because systemic side effects may occur with treatment of large areas of the body. Generally, systemic steroids are not necessary for the treatment of atopic dermatitis.

Oral antihistamines, which are effective in decreasing pruritus, are another component in the treatment of atopic dermatitis. Antihistamines such as hydroxyzine (Atarax or Vistaril), diphenhydramine (Benadryl), and cetirizine (Zyrtec) are often used. Nighttime doses are particularly important, because pruritus and scratching are often worse at night.

Because topical corticosteroids, especially high-potency formulations used for long periods, have potential local and systemic side effects, alternative treatments are promoted. Topical tacrolimus (Protopic) ointment and pimecrolimus (Elidel) are the most promising of these new therapies. These agents have a broad range of anti-inflammatory activities and are highly effective in treating atopic dermatitis. They do not cause skin atrophy because they do not affect collagen synthesis. In addition, at prescribed doses, they do not appear to have any systemic side effects.

Most patients with atopic dermatitis respond to treatment with good skin care, topical steroids, and antihistamines, but in those who are resistant to such care, food allergies must be considered. Recent studies indicate that as many as 30%–50% of young children with severe atopic dermatitis have food allergies. The diagnosis and the management of patients allergic to food are described in the next section.

Disease severity in atopic dermatitis tends to wax and wane. Acute exacerbations, caused by increased scratching, stress, heat, or infection, are characterized by increased pruritus and development of new skin lesions and should be treated with more aggressive skin care, including more frequent baths followed by emollients. When lesions become crusted, weepy, or vesicular, infection with *Staphylococcus aureus* or herpes

simplex (**eczema herpeticum**) should be suspected. Discontinuation of steroid medications and emollients is necessary at the involved sites, and cool, wet compresses to the skin are appropriate. Staphylococcal infections warrant topical povidone and topical or systemic antibiotics if necessary, whereas herpes simplex infections need topical or systemic acyclovir.

Pediatric Pearl

Patients with atopic dermatitis are also prone to superficial fungal skin infections. Therefore, scaly erythematous lesions without the usual distribution of atopic dermatitis and unresponsive to the usual therapy for eczema should be scraped and examined for hyphae and treated with antifungal medications.

FOOD ALLERGY

Adverse reactions to foods are relatively common in both children and adults. Because of the confusion regarding adverse reactions to food, as many as one-third of adults believe they have food "allergies," although the true incidence is estimated to be less than 2%–5% of the general population. In this discussion, the term "food allergy" refers to an abnormal response to a food that is triggered by an **IgE-mediated immunologic reaction.**

Pathophysiology

When severe reactions such as anaphylaxis occur immediately after ingestion, it is usually not difficult to identify the offending food. When symptoms are more vague (headache, fatigue, increased irritability, behavior disorders, colic, diarrhea, vomiting) and do not occur immediately after ingestion of the food, identification of the cause can be extremely difficult. Much of this difficulty is due to the fact that reactions to foods can occur via several mechanisms (Table 17.5), some of which are poorly understood.

Clinical Evaluation

The symptoms of food allergy vary considerably and range from rash (often urticaria or hives, or exacerbation of atopic dermatitis) to nausea, vomiting, abdominal pain, and diarrhea to wheezing, nasal congestion, and sneezing. Anaphylaxis, with respiratory and cardiovascular collapse, is the most severe reaction following ingestion (or sometimes occurring simply after touching or

---

TABLE 17.4 Some Topical Steroid Preparations

Low-potency agents
   Hydrocortisone 1%
Moderate-potency agents
   Betamethasone valerate 0.1% (Valisone)
   Triamcinolone 0.1% (Kenalog)
   Fluocinolone acetonide 0.025% (Synalar)
   Mometasone furoate 0.1% (Elocon)
High-potency agents
   Fluocinonide 0.05% (Lidex)
   Halcinonide 0.1% (Halog)

smelling the food in extremely sensitive individuals) [see ANAPHYLAXIS]. In young children, other reactions such as colitis may occur, in which case the mechanism may include T cells or immune complexes rather than IgE. In infants, food allergies may cause colic, vomiting, feeding problems, or growth failure. Most food allergies in young children resolve with time, although allergies to peanuts, which can be particularly severe, often remain for life.

Food reactions are difficult to diagnose because reliable tests are not widely available, except perhaps for IgE-mediated reactions. The diagnosis of food allergy is based on a careful history with regard to the reproducibility of the reaction, timing of the reaction (reactions occurring soon after ingestion are more likely to be confirmed), response to treatment (antihistamines should relieve urticaria), and response to elimination of the food from the diet. Adverse reactions resulting from food poisoning, pharmacologic effects, and gastrointestinal disorders (see Table 17.5) must be ruled out. A positive family history of food allergy or atopic dermatitis is common, and IgA deficiency may be present.

Skin tests (or RAST tests) for foods can be performed to confirm IgE-mediated food allergies. Food skin testing has a relatively **low specificity,** in that positive tests may occur in patients not experiencing allergic reactions to the particular food. However, the tests have a relatively **good sensitivity;** a negative test makes the presence of IgE-mediated allergy unlikely. A more definitive, although more time consuming, test for food allergies and food intolerance is the double-blind placebo-controlled food challenge in which the patient is given increasing oral doses of the suspected food in a blinded fashion.

The most common foods causing IgE-mediated reactions are milk, eggs, peanuts, shellfish, soy, and wheat. It is important to identify the specific problematic food(s) so that specific dietary recommendations can be made.

Management

Once food allergies have been identified, the treatment is dietary avoidance of the offending food or foods. Some foods, such as celery, are easily eliminated from the diet. Avoidance of other foods such as milk or wheat, which are added to several products such as bread, cakes, and cookies, requires careful dietary planning. Patients or their parents must read food product labels carefully and communicate closely with restaurants and schools in order to avoid the offending foods. Overzealous restriction of the diet frequently causes malnutrition and failure to thrive. Therefore substitute foods must be recommended. In infants, allergy to cow's milk or soy products (estimated frequency of 2%–5% of all infants) is often blamed for vomiting and feeding problems, prompting multiple formula changes over short periods of time. In such instances, diagnostic testing is useful, as is the switch to hypoallergenic formulas such as Pregestimil, Nutramigen, Alimentum, or Neocate. Once the feeding problem is under control and the offending food or foods have been identified, substitution of a less costly (and more palatable) formula can be attempted.

Because accidental ingestion of offending foods still may occur in spite of precautions, antihistamines and bronchodilators for mild reactions and epinephrine for more severe reactions (see ANAPHYLAXIS) should be available for administration. Patients with a history of food-induced anaphy-

TABLE 17.5	Mechanisms for Developing Adverse Reactions to Food
Mechanism	**Example**
IgE–mediated allergy	Anaphylaxis, urticaria (e.g., peanuts, eggs)
Delayed allergic responses	Atopic dermatitis
Immune (non–IgE-mediated)	Celiac disease, cow's milk protein enteropathy, eosinophilic gastroenteropathy
Food poisoning	Botulism, *Staphylococcus* enterotoxins
Infected food	Reaction to viruses or bacteria (e.g., *Salmonella, Shigella, Escherichia coli*)
Pharmacologic effect	Reaction to caffeine, alcohol, tyramine, histamine
Gastrointestinal disorders	Peptic ulcer disease, lactose deficiency, cholelithiasis, inflammatory bowel disease
Reactions to additives	Headaches (sodium nitrate), headache/flushing (monosodium glutamate), diarrhea (sorbitol), acute airway obstruction (metabisulfite)

laxis should be taught how to self-administer epinephrine using an Epipen or ANAkit and to wear a Medic-Alert bracelet.

ANAPHYLAXIS

Anaphylaxis is an acute, severe, life-endangering situation caused by an immunologic reaction. Risk factors include asthma, food allergy, and multiple antibiotic allergy; use of beta-blockers; and a history of prior reactions.

Pathophysiology

Most anaphylactic reactions are IgE- and mast cell–initiated processes and can occur in atopic as well as nonatopic individuals. Virtually any foreign substance, including foods or latex-associated proteins, can induce IgE synthesis and therefore induce an anaphylactic reaction (Table 17.6). As in other IgE-mediated reactions, mast cells are activated and release the contents of their granules, including histamine; tryptase; TNF; IL-1, IL-4, and IL-6; and lipid mediators such as prostaglandin D_2, leukotriene C4, and PAF. Histamine, TNF, and PAF cause the production of nitric oxide, resulting in vascular dilation and leakage. Depending on the allergen, mast cells can release some mediators but not others, resulting in clinical variants of anaphylaxis.

Pediatric Pearl

An **anaphylactoid reaction** is clinically similar to anaphylaxis, but it is not immunologically mediated. Mast cell degranulation occurs in the absence of an antigen–antibody interaction (e.g., with radiocontrast material, opiates, or complement components), and these agents do not cause late-phase reactions.

Clinical Evaluation

The symptoms of anaphylaxis include generalized urticaria, inspiratory stridor, laryngeal edema, difficulty swallowing, wheezing, nasal congestion, abdominal cramps, diarrhea, hypotension (decreased systemic vascular resistance, increased vascular permeability), and vascular collapse. Sneezing, pruritus (especially of hands and soles), a feeling of impending doom, or hoarseness in the throat and dysphonia may initiate the episode. Some clinicians have classified the degree of severity of anaphylaxis in the following manner:

- Grade 1: involving skin only (generalized urticaria)
- Grade 2: involving skin with nausea and hypotension

TABLE 17.6	Causes of Anaphylaxis

Drugs and medications
    Penicillin, cephalosporins
    Chymopapain, L-asparaginase
    Blood products
Foods
    Peanuts, seafood, eggs, milk
Stinging insects (Hymenoptera)
    Honey bee
    Wasp, vespid
    Fire ant
Allergen immunotherapy (allergy shots)
Latex (especially in patients with meningomyelocele)
Anaphylactoid reactions (not IgE-mediated)
    Immune complex
    Aspirin
    Preservatives (e.g., metabisulfite)
    Anesthetic agents
    Radiocontrast media
    Idiopathic exercise induced
    Direct mast cell degranulation
        Opiates
        Vancomycin
        Ciprofloxacin
        Complement components C5a, C3a

- Grade 3: involving shock
- Grade 4: involving respiratory arrest

It is now recognized that although anaphylaxis (like other allergic reactions) is an acute problem caused by an explosive release of mediators, in many cases anaphylaxis can be protracted or biphasic, due to the development of late-phase responses. Therefore, patients with anaphylaxis who symptomatically improve rapidly with treatment must be observed closely for recurrence for at least an additional 8–12 hours after the initial episode. Concurrent illness, underlying asthma, or use of β-adrenergic blockers [propranolol (Inderal)] can also predispose to a more severe episode of anaphylaxis.

Differential Diagnosis

Vasovagal reactions, hypoglycemic reactions to insulin, and cardiac arrests can mimic anaphylaxis. These types of episodes are not associated with skin manifestations (except diaphoresis).

Angioedema without urticaria can be caused by **C1 esterase inhibitor deficiency,** an autosomal dominant disorder. Patients have attacks of swelling (angioedema) that can involve any part of the body, including the airway, extremities, and GI tract. Minor trauma may trigger an attack. The disorder, which is not associated with urticaria or pruritis, is diagnosed by low serum level of C4, even when a patient is asymptomatic, and the C1 esterase inhibitor level will also be low or its function abnormal. Traditional treatments for anaphylaxis, such as epinephrine and antihistamines, are not effective. C1 esterase inhibitor replacement appears to be only marginally effective, and the only treatment for attacks is supportive measures. Treatment with androgen derivatives such as danazol and stanozolol are effective in preventing symptoms. However, these drugs can have unwanted side effects, especially in children and females.

Management

Successful treatment requires the prompt recognition of anaphylaxis and the institution of appropriate therapy as soon as possible. The causative agent should be identified and discontinued (e.g., intravenous antibiotics). The treatment of choice is epinephrine 0.01 ml/kg (up to 0.3–0.5 ml) SQ or IM. If anaphylaxis is due to an insect sting or allergy shot, another dose of epinephrine is indicated at the site of the sting or allergy shot, and a tourniquet should be placed around the involved extremity. Supplemental oxygen should be administered if necessary, and an airway should be established and maintained. Intubation or tracheotomy may be required. If the blood pressure is reduced, intravenous fluids (10–20 ml/kg of normal saline) should be administered (see Chapters 4 and 24). In addition, diphenhydramine, 1–2 mg/kg IM, IV, or PO, should be given. Cimetidine 4 mg/kg, an H_2 receptor antagonist, may also help. Corticosteroids (methylprednisolone/Solu-Medrol 1–2 mg/kg IV or prednisone 1–2 mg/kg PO), when given early, may help limit late-phase or prolonged responses. Inhaled bronchodilator therapy (albuterol sulfate) or aminophylline may also benefit patients with wheezing. For prevention, patients with a history of severe bee sting anaphylaxis benefit from immunotherapy with bee venom and from appropriate measures to avoid insects. Patients with a history of food, bee sting, or latex allergy and anaphylaxis should also

be taught how to self-administer epinephrine using an Epi-Pen or ANAkit and should wear a Medic-Alert bracelet.

IMMUNOLOGIC DISORDERS: RECURRENT INFECTION

Most children have frequent minor infections, including an average of 8–10 upper respiratory infections per year and at least one, if not many, episodes of otitis media in the first years of life. Thus, a high proportion of visits to pediatricians are for the evaluation and treatment of infection.

Pathophysiology

Several mechanisms are involved in host defense against infection. These mechanisms may be divided into three groups (Table 17.7). The anatomic–mucociliary compartment is an important part of host defenses and is frequently overlooked in the evaluation of recurrent infection. Innate immunity is the first line of defense against pathogens, occurs relatively rapidly, and it is antigen-nonspecific but can influence the subsequent development of the adaptive immune response. In contrast, adaptive immunity is antigen-specific and is more versatile, although its response is slower than innate immunity, especially with the first exposure to a particular antigen. All of these compartments interact with each other, and defects can occur in one or more of them. These defects result in frequent or unusually severe infections that are the hallmarks of primary immunodeficiency. Autoimmune disorders and malignancies may also occur in these patients.

Anatomic–Mucociliary Defenses

The body interfaces with its environment via the skin and the mucous membranes of the respiratory tract. Breaks in the integument or obstruction of normal drainage at these sites can lead to recurrent infection. Several defects in the anatomic–

TABLE 17.7 Mechanisms Involved in Host Defense

Anatomic–mucociliary barrier mechanisms
Innate immunity
    Cellular components: phagocytes, dendritic cells, and natural killer cells
    Soluble factors: complement, acute-phase proteins, and cytokines
Adaptive immunity
    B-cell compartment: humoral immunity
    T-cell compartment: cell-mediated immunity

mucociliary system may lead to recurrent infection (Table 17.8).

Innate Immunity

CELLULAR COMPONENTS. Phagocytic cells engulf and digest foreign antigens and microorganisms. **Polymorphonuclear neutrophils** are the predominant phagocytic cells in the blood. Their major function is to ingest pyogenic bacteria and some fungi, particularly *Aspergillus* spores. Neutrophils have cell surface receptors for the Fc portion of immunoglobulin and complement, which enhance recognition and phagocytosis of foreign material. Phagocytosis triggers the NADPH oxidase system that generates superoxide and hydrogen peroxide, which aid in the killing of ingested organisms.

Macrophages are long-lived phagocytic cells that develop from monocytes in the blood and are particularly effective in killing facultative intracellular organisms (e.g., mycobacteria, *Toxoplasmosis gondii, Legionella pneumophila*). Macrophages present antigen to T cells and secrete cytokines such as IL-1, IL-6, and IL-12.

Natural killer (NK) cells mediate cytotoxic activity against virally infected cells and tumor cells. NK cells also have Fc receptors, which allow them to recognize antibody-coated cells and kill them by antibody-dependent cellular cytotoxicity. In addition, NK cells recognize their targets through killer-activating and killer-inhibitory receptors. The activating receptors recognize several ubiquitous cell surface molecules and the inhibitory receptors recognize major histocompatibility complex (MHC) class I. Normally both molecules are present on the target cell surface and the kill order is overridden. However, when MHC class I expression is suppressed (e.g., by viral infection), limited inhibitory signaling is generated and the target cell is lysed.

Bacteria, fungi, and viruses contain conserved molecular motifs called pathogen-associated molecular patterns (PAMPs), which are recognized by pattern recognition receptors on cells of the innate immune system. There are three different types of pattern-recognition receptors: endocytic, signaling, and secreted. The first type of receptor (e.g., mannose receptor and macrophage scavenger receptor, which recognize microbial carbohydrates) enhances phagocytosis. The second type of receptor (e.g., Toll-like receptor) leads to increased production of cytokines and costimulatory molecules. Binding of pathogen-associated molecular patterns to both of these types of cell surface receptors leads to enhanced antigen presentation and T cell activation. A third type of pattern recognition receptor, a soluble factor (e.g., mannan-binding lectin), binds to microbial cell walls, flagging them for recognition by complement and phagocytes.

SOLUBLE FACTORS. The major soluble factors in the immune system are part of **complement,** a system consisting of about 30 plasma and cell membrane proteins that act in a sequential cascade to amplify

---

TABLE 17.8 **Anatomic–Mucociliary Defects That Result in Recurrent Infection**

Anatomic defects in upper airways
    Aspiration syndromes (gastroesophageal reflux, poor gag reflex, ineffective cough)
    Cleft palate, eustachian tube dysfunction
    Adenoidal hypertrophy
    Nasal polyps
    Obstruction of paranasal sinus drainage (osteomeatal complex disease)
    Encephaloceles, sinus tracts
Anatomic defects in tracheobronchial tree
    Tracheoesophageal fistula
    Pulmonary sequestration, bronchogenic cysts, vascular ring
    Tumor, foreign body, or enlarged nodes
Physiologic defects in upper and lower airways
    Primary ciliary dyskinesia syndromes, Young syndrome
    Cystic fibrosis
    Allergic rhinitis (causing congestion, obstruction, and abnormal secretions)
    Chronic smoke exposure (resulting in congestion, obstruction, and abnormal secretions)
Other defects
    Chronic atopic dermatitis
    Ureteral obstruction/reflux
    Poor vascular perfusion
    Central venous lines, artificial heart valves

immunologic stimuli in an antigen-nonspecific manner. The alternative and lectin pathways are antibody-independent, whereas the classic pathway is antibody-dependent. Activated complement components have potent opsonizing, chemotactic, vasoactive, and lytic activity and can activate neutrophil respiratory burst activity.

Several other soluble factors are important in innate immunity. Acute-phase proteins have both pro- and anti-inflammatory activity. They are involved in recognition of damaged cells and pathogens, activation of complement, induction of cytokine production, and promotion of wound healing. Chemokines are produced by antigen-presenting cells, endothelial cells, and B and T cells. They are involved in recruitment and activation of inflammatory cells. Cytokines serve as the messengers of the immune system and are also produced by inflammatory cells as well as epithelial and endothelial cells.

Adaptive Immunity

The adaptive immune system is composed of B cells and T cells, which generate extremely diverse yet specific receptors against pathogens and proteins.

B CELLS. **Antibodies** or **immunoglobulins** are serum proteins produced by B cells that bind specifically to **antigens** (e.g., glycoproteins, carbohydrates, or toxins). This interaction results in the inactivation or **agglutination** of the antigen, in **opsonization** of the antigen for **phagocytosis,** or in the binding and activation of **complement,** leading to **cytolysis** of the pathogen. Immunoglobulin (Ig) molecules can be divided into five major isotypes based on differences in their heavy-chain components: IgG, IgM, IgA, IgD, and IgE. Infants produce only small amounts of immunoglobulin before 4–6 months of age and receive virtually all of their immunoglobulin transplacentally from their mothers. Normal levels of serum immunoglobulin reach a nadir at around 4–6 months of age and then increase slowly over the next several years (Figure 17.1). Because the immune system matures over a period of several years, the ability to respond to bacterial polysaccharide antigens is not consistently acquired until after approximately 2 years of age. Adult levels of IgG are not present until about 5–7 years of age, whereas adult levels of IgA are not acquired until 10–14 years of age.

IgG, the major immunoglobulin in serum, is the major immunoglobulin produced in **secondary immune responses.** It diffuses well into tissues and crosses the placenta. IgG can be subdivided into four subclasses based on differences in the heavy chain: IgG1, IgG2, IgG3, and IgG4. In general, the IgG2 subclass accounts for antibody responses to polysaccharide antigens, whereas the IgG1 and IgG3 subclasses account for responses to protein antigens.

IgM in the first antibody produced after primary antigenic stimulation. It is involved in complement activation and opsonization. Secretory IgA is the primary immunoglobulin of the mucosa. IgD serves as an antigen receptor on B cells. IgE is the principal mediator of immediate hypersensitivity reactions.

T CELLS. T lymphocytes are involved in many immune mechanisms, including the cytolysis of virus-infected cells; stimulation of B-cell activation and differentiation; and recruitment of macrophages, neutrophils, eosinophils, basophils, and mast cells. T cells are the major cell type responsible for immunity to intracellular organisms (viruses, mycobacteria, *Toxoplasma gondii, Legionella, Brucella*), fungal organisms (e.g., *Candida*), and protozoa; for immune surveillance for cancer cells; and for causing **graft-versus-host disease** in patients after bone marrow transplantation.

T cells can be divided into two major subsets: CD4+ and CD8+. **CD4+ T cells** produce **cytokines** and play a central role in helping and regulating immune responses. CD4+ helper T (T$_H$) cells can be further subdivided into T$_H$1 cells, which secrete cytokines such as interferon-γ and IL-2, and T$_H$2 cells, which secrete cytokines such as IL-4, IL-5, and IL-13. T$_H$1 cells are important in activating macrophages and in cell-mediated immunity, and T$_H$2 cells are critical for the activation and differentiation of B cells (humoral immunity) and in downregulating immune responses. Development of T$_H$ cells expressing inappropriate cytokine profiles can exacerbate infection and cause allergy (T$_H$2), autoimmunity (T$_H$1), and graft-versus-host disease. **CD8+ T cells** are involved in killing virus-infected cells or tumor cells and possibly in suppressing or limiting immune responses.

Clinical and Laboratory Evaluation

History

A careful history of the frequency, type, location, and severity of infections is required to assess the severity of the problem and determine the extent of the immunologic workup that is necessary. Appropriate clinical judgment is essential so that the immunologically normal child is not burdened with unnecessary tests but the rare child with a true immunodeficiency is not missed. De-

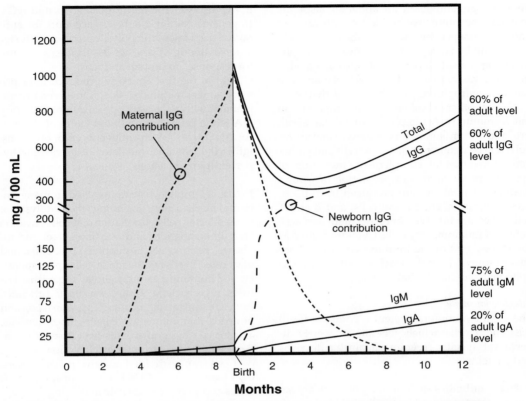

FIGURE 17.1. Immunoglobulin (IgG, IgM, IgA) levels in the fetus and infant in the first year of life. The IgG of the fetus and newborn infant is solely of maternal origin. Maternal IgG disappears by 9 months of age, by which time endogenous synthesis of IgG is well established. IgM and IgA in the neonate are entirely endogenously synthesized, because maternal IgM and IgA do not cross the placenta.

termining the number of infections is an important part of the assessment. Separate episodes must be differentiated from recurrence of single episodes, which often occurs when episodes of otitis media or sinusitis are inadequately treated. **With upper respiratory infection or otitis media, individuals who have more than 6–10 episodes per year may require investigation.** However, there is wide variation in the number of such infections occurring in immunologically normal children, and the frequency can increase with increased exposure, as in day-care centers or schools and during the winter months. **With more severe infections such as meningitis or sepsis, individuals with two or more such infections may warrant investigation.**

The site(s) of infections must also be determined. Patients with antibody deficiency disorders or with ciliary dyskinesia develop infections at multiple sites (e.g., ears, sinuses, lungs). Individuals with T-cell deficiencies or neutrophil dis-

orders such as chronic granulomatous disease develop infections at multiple mucous membrane sites (skin, nails, mouth, and groin). In contrast, individuals with anatomic problems (e.g., sequestered pulmonary lobe or ureteral reflux) develop infections confined to a single anatomic site (e.g., a single pulmonary lobe or the urinary tract).

The history must also include determination of the type(s) of infections that have occurred. Infection with encapsulated bacteria suggests antibody, complement, or neutrophil deficiency disorders. Multiple infections with fungi suggest T-cell deficiency. Invasive pulmonary infection with *Aspergillus fumigatus* suggests **chronic granulomatous disease (CGD).** Infections with *Neisseria* suggest a complement disorder. Severe infection after administration of live viral vaccines indicates severe immunodeficiency (e.g., reaction to oral polio vaccine suggests the diagnosis of **X-linked agammaglobulinemia**). Finally, development of opportunistic infections caused by uncommon organisms such as *Pneumocystis carinii* or *Pseudomonas aeruginosa* suggests severe impairment of the immune system.

Another important aspect of the history is the assessment of the severity and consequences of the infections. Clearly, recurrent life-threatening infections such as meningitis or sepsis are worrisome and require extensive investigation. However, recurrent otitis media or sinusitis may occur in immunologically normal children and require only limited studies. In such cases, full recovery is achieved after each infection without the accrual of morbidity. In contrast, recurrent infection in immunologically deficient children is associated with incomplete recovery at the sites of infection (e.g., tympanic membranes, skin, and lung), resulting in scarring, abnormal hearing, persistent drainage, chronic lung disease (CLD), failure to thrive, or anemia of chronic disease. In these cases, the accrual of substantial morbidity from repeated infections (including minor infections) suggests the presence of significant immunologic deficiency.

Other important aspects of the history include (1) family history of infants dying from infection and (2) human immunodeficiency virus (HIV) risk factors such as history of blood transfusions, intravenous drug use, or family history of HIV infection. A history of the particular conditions suggests certain immunodeficiency disorders. Infection associated with persistent atypical rashes indicates graft-versus-host disease; persistent eczema and a history of thrombocytopenia, Wiskott-Aldrich syndrome; presence of petechiae or telangiectasia, ataxia telangiectasia; neonatal tetany, cardiac disease, or micrognathia, DiGeorge syndrome; delay in umbilical cord detachment, leukocyte adhesion deficiency; chronic atypical diarrhea and malabsorption, graft-versus-host disease; and chronic viral gastrointestinal infection, a possible specific immunologic diagnosis. Finally, because **primary immunodeficiency** is rare, a history of diseases causing **secondary immunodeficiency** should be sought (Table 17.9).

Physical Examination

The physical examination should focus on the extent to which recurrent infection has disturbed normal growth and development and on the presence of features specific for certain immunodeficiency syndromes. The clinician should search for evidence of persistent infection (e.g., evidence of thrush in the mouth, purulent nasal or otitic discharge, or persistent rales). It is essential to check the tympanic membranes for scarring and the skin for scarring or rashes. It is also important to exam-

TABLE 17.9 Causes of Secondary Immunodeficiency
Viral infection
Measles
Rubella
Epstein-Barr virus (EBV)
Cytomegalovirus (CMV)
Human immunodeficiency virus (HIV)
Metabolic disorders
Malnutrition
Uremia
Diabetes
Sickle cell disease
Protein-losing disorders
Nephrotic syndrome
Protein-losing enteropathy
Prematurity
Immunosuppressive agents, including corticosteroids
Malignancy

ine lymphoid tissue such as the tonsils and lymph nodes. Absence of tonsils suggests **severe combined immunodeficiency disease (SCID)** or **X-linked agammaglobulinemia,** whereas increased size of lymphoid tissue suggests **common variable immunodeficiency (CVID)** or **HIV infection.** Examination of the extremities may show clubbing or cyanosis.

Laboratory Evaluation

Initiation of laboratory tests for recurrent infection is appropriate if the history and physical examination indicate an immunologic diagnosis. The history and physical examination may also suggest which of the five host defense compartments is defective, and the laboratory evaluation should be approached accordingly. The extent of the evaluation also depends on the assessment of the severity of the problem. If the severity of the problem is relatively low, screening tests alone may be necessary; more severe disease requires more sophisticated testing to search for a specific diagnosis (Table 17.10).

Pediatric Pearl

Children with recurrent mycobacterial infections should be evaluated for deficiencies of IFN-γ production, IL-12 production and reduced IL-12 receptor function.

TABLE 17.10 **Screening Laboratory Examinations***

GENERAL

Complete blood count, including hemoglobin, white blood cell count with differential and morphology, and platelet count

Radiographs to document infection in chest, sinus, mastoids, long bones, if indicated by clinical history

Culture, if appropriate

Erythrocyte sedimentation rate

ANTIBODY-MEDIATED IMMUNITY

Quantitative immunoglobulin levels: IgA, IgG, IgM, IgE

Isohemagglutinin titers (anti-A, anti-B): measures IgM function

Preexisting antibody levels: **diphtheria, tetanus,** polio, rubella, *Haemophilus influenzae, Streptococcus pneumoniae* (check pre- and post-titers if applicable)

CELL-MEDIATED IMMUNITY

Lymphocyte count and morphology

Delayed hypersensitivity skin tests (*Candida,* tetanus toxoid, tuberculin, mumps): measures T-cell and macrophage function

T- and B-cell subset enumeration by FACS analysis

T-lymphocyte function analyses: measures proliferation to mitogens and antigens

PHAGOCYTOSIS

Neutrophil cell count and morphology

Nitroblue tetrazolium dye test

Staphylococcal killing, chemotaxis assay

Myeloperoxidase stain

COMPLEMENT

Total hemolytic complement (CH50): measures complement activity

C3, C4 levels: measure important pathway components

*Initial screening tests for less severe disease are in **boldface** type.
   FACS = fluorescence-activated cell sorter.

Management

Several measures are appropriate in the management of immunocompromised children (Table 17.11). Immediate culture and aggressive antibiotic therapy is necessary for fever or other manifestations of infection because infection may rapidly disseminate and become life-threatening. Continuous prophylaxis with antibacterial, antiviral, or antifungal agents may also be warranted in certain instances where infection is difficult to control. Children with immunodeficiency contract infections with uncommonly encountered organisms. Therefore, poor response to commonly used antibiotics suggests the presence of a resistant or atypical pathogen, which must be specifically

TABLE 17.11 **General Management of Patients With Immunodeficiency**

Avoid transfusions with blood products unless they are irradiated and cytomegalovirus-negative

Avoid live virus vaccines, especially in patients with severe T-cell deficiencies or severe agammaglobulinemia and in household members

Follow pulmonary function in patients with recurrent pneumonia

Use chest physiotherapy and postural drainage in patients with recurrent pneumonia

Use prophylactic antibiotics, because minor infections can quickly disseminate

Examine diarrhea stools for *Giardia* and *Clostridium difficile*

Avoid unnecessary exposure to individuals with infection

Use intravenous immunoglobulin for severe antibody deficiency states at a dose of 400–500 mg/kg every 3–4 weeks identified by culture or biopsy and antibiotic sensitivities determined.

When examination and laboratory tests show children with recurrent infections to be immunologically normal, the goals of management are to eradicate infection already present and to reduce the frequency of reinfection. The use of **prophylactic antibiotics** is often helpful in children with **recurrent otitis media or sinusitis.** In children who have recurrent otitis media or sinusitis resistant to a long course (6–8 weeks) of antibiotics, other treatment methods are necessary (e.g., placement of pressure equalization tubes, adenoidectomy, or endoscopic sinus surgery to improve sinus drainage). **Recurrent streptococcal pharyngitis** is generally not associated with immunodeficiency. Recurrence may be secondary to poor compliance with antibiotic regimens, presence of streptococcal strains resistant to penicillin, or exposure to family members who are carriers.

Pediatric Pearl

Tonsillectomy may be indicated after the failure of effective prophylactic antibiotics and after seven or more episodes of streptococcal pharyngitis in 1 year.

IMMUNOLOGIC DISORDERS: IMMUNODEFICIENCY DISEASES

Primary immunodeficiencies may be classified in four ways; they involve of B-cell defects, T-cell defects, phagocytic defects, and complement defects. Specific disorders are considered in the following sections.

B-CELL DEFECTS

Deficiencies of antibody production are the most common primary immunodeficiency disorders (50%) [Tables 17.12 and 17.13]. These defects result in recurrent sinopulmonary infections (otitis media, sinusitis, pneumonia, and bacteremia) with encapsulated bacteria such as *Streptococcus pneumoniae, Haemophilus influenzae,* and staphylococci. Infections with fungal or viral pathogens (except enterovirus) do not generally pose problems. Classically, antibody deficiency states do not become manifest until after 6 months of age, when transplacentally acquired maternal antibody has been depleted. Deficiency of IgG synthesis can be observed in the first year of life (e.g., **X-linked agammaglobulinemia**) or may develop

TABLE 17.12 **Predominant Antibody Defects (B Cell Defects): Pathophysiologic Aspects**

Disorder	Genetics	Onset	Pathogenesis
Bruton agamma-globulinemia	X-linked (Xq22)	Infancy (6–9 months; 20% of cases present at >12 months, up to 3–5 yr)	Arrest in B-cell differentiation (pre-B level); mutation in the Btk gene
Common variable immunodeficiency (CVID)	AR, AD (6p21.3)	> 2 years of age (usually second to third decade)	Arrest in B cell to plasma cell differentiation
Transient hypo-gammaglobulinemia	Unknown	Infancy (3–7 months)	Delayed development of plasma cell maturation
IgA deficiency	X-linked, AR, ? (6p21.3)	Variable	Failure of IgA expressing B-cell differentiation
IgG subclass deficiency	AR (2p11, 14q32.3)	Variable	Defect in isotype IgG production
IgM deficiency	AR	First year	Defective helper T cell–B cell interaction
Immunodeficiency with increased IgM (hyper-IgM syndrome)	X-linked (Xq26), AR	2–3 years	Defect in IgG and IgA synthesis, due to CD40 ligand (CD154) deficiency
	AR	2–3 years	Defects in CD 40, and activation-induced cytidine deaminase (AID)

AD = autosomal dominant; AR = autosomal recessive; Btk = Bruton tyrosine kinase; Ig = immunoglobulin.

Disorder	Manifestations	Associated Features	Laboratory Evaluation	Treatment
Bruton agammaglobuline-mia	Recurrent high-grade infections (sinusitis, pneumonia, meningitis) with *Streptococcus pneumoniae*, *Haemophilus influenzae*, *Staphylococcus aureus*, and *Pseudomonas aeruginosa* Poliomyelitis with polio vaccine	Lymphoid hypoplasia (no tonsils)	Decreased CD19 or CD20+ B cells, Btk mutation or absent mRNA or protein, agamma-globulinemia, absent isohemagglutinins	IVIG, antibiotics
Common variable immunodeficiency (CVID) or common variable agammaglobulinemia	Sinusitis, bronchitis, pneumonia, chronic diarrhea	Autoimmune disease (RA, SLE, Graves disease, ITP), malignancy	Decreased IgG and IgA, absent isohemagglutinins	IVIG, antibiotics
Transient hypogamma-globulinemia	Recurrent viral and pyogenic infections	Frequently in families with immunodeficiencies	Decreased immunoglobulins, often have normal titers to tetanus and diphtheria toxoids and normal iso-hemagglutinins	Antibiotics (no IVIG)
IgA deficiency	Sinopulmonary and GI infections; may be normal	IgG subclass deficiency, common variable immuno-deficiency, autoimmune disease	Serum IgA < 7 mg/dl with normal IgG and IgM, normal response to immunizations	Antibiotics
IgG subclass deficiency	Variable (normal to recurrent sinopulmonary and GI infections)	IgA deficiency, ataxia telangiectasia	IgG subclass deficiency (IgG 1, 2, 3, or 4); whether patient responds to protein, polysaccharide and viral antigens is more relevant	Antibiotics (IVIG if has antibody deficiency to many antigens)
IgM deficiency	Recurrent septicemia, pneu-mococcus, *H. influenzae*	Whipple disease, regional enteritis, lymphoid hyper-plasia	Decreased IgM	Antibiotics, IVIG
Immunodeficiency with increased IgM (hyper-IgM syndrome)	Recurrent pyogenic infections (otitis media, sinusitis, tonsillitis, pneumonia), *Pneumocystis carinii* pneumonia, chronic diarrhea	Hematologic autoimmune disease	CD40L mutation, decreased IgG and IgA and normal to increased IgM, normal numbers of B cells but no antigen-specific antibodies	IVIG

Btk = Bruton tyrosine kinase; GI = gastrointestinal; Ig = immunoglobulin; ITP = idiopathic thrombocytopenia purpura; IVIG = intravenous immunoglobulin; RA = rheumatoid arthritis; SLE = systemic lupus erythematosus.

later in childhood or adulthood (e.g., **common variable immunodeficiency**). **Isolated deficiency of IgA** is associated with recurrent infection, although many individuals with low IgA levels are asymptomatic. Similarly, isolated IgG2 subclass deficiency is usually associated with a propensity to develop recurrent sinopulmonary infection.

A classic example of a B-cell deficiency is X-linked agammaglobulinemia, which is a congenital immunodeficiency in males. The characteristic profound deficiency of B cells results in severe hypogammaglobulinemia and absence of lymphoid tissue. The defect is limited to the B-cell linkage and is caused by mutations of the Bruton tyrosine kinase (Btk) gene on chromosome Xq22. Other B-cell deficiencies are listed in Tables 17.12 and 17.13.

Laboratory Evaluation

Patients with B-cell disease have decreased serum immunoglobulin levels, which must be interpreted in the context of the patient's age (see Table 17.12). An association of low albumin with low immunoglobulin levels suggests a low synthetic rate (due to poor nutrition) or an increased loss of proteins (e.g., from protein-losing enteropathy or through skin disease). High levels of immunoglobulin suggest intact B-cell immunity (e.g., in CGD, immotile cilia syndrome, or cystic fibrosis).

> ### Pediatric Pearl
> Very high levels of immunoglobulin suggest HIV infection.

Because the level of total immunoglobulin may be within the normal range even in the face of abnormal B-cell function, it is also important to determine if antibodies to specific antigens are present. Titers may be examined for specific antigens to which the patient has been exposed through routine immunizations (e.g., tetanus). If titers are low, the patient can be reimmunized, and the titers can be reexamined 2–4 weeks later. Inadequate responses to polysaccharide antigens such as *S. pneumoniae* generally occur before 2 years of age. Low responses in older children are associated with IgA deficiency and IgG subclass deficiency. Patients with absent immunoglobulin and absent antibody responses to antigens often do not have circulating B cells, which can be confirmed by B-cell enumeration on flow cytometry.

Management

The treatment for such B-cell disorders as X-linked agammaglobulinemia and common variable immunodeficiency (CVID) is intravenous

immunoglobulin (IVIG) and prophylactic courses of antibiotics with a low threshold for use (see Table 17.13). Patients with other antibody deficiency disorders benefit from prophylactic antibiotics, but intravenous immunoglobulin should be used only if prophylactic antibiotics fail or if B-cell function (responsiveness on antigen challenge) is impaired.

T-CELL DEFECTS

Patients with disorders of T-cell immunity (30% of primary immunodeficiencies) develop infections with fungi or intracellular pathogens (e.g., viruses, mycobacteria, *T. gondii, Leishmania*) that proliferate in somatic cells and macrophages [Tables 17.14 and 17.15]. Such patients may lack cytotoxic CD8+ cells and CD4+ helper T cells that activate macrophages. In severe T-cell deficiency, B-cell function may also be impaired, because it requires the assistance of T cells.

A classic example of T-cell deficiency is **Di-George syndrome**. This immunodeficiency syndrome varies markedly from severe T-cell deficiency to normal immune function. In the complete absence of T-cell function, B-cell function fails, resulting in severe combined immunodeficiency disease (SCID). Other diseases with abnormal T-cell function are listed in Tables 17.14 and 17.15.

Laboratory Evaluation

Immunologic findings in T-cell disorders include lymphopenia and the absence of delayed-type hypersensitivity reactions (e.g., to tetanus, diphtheria, or *Candida albicans*) [see Table 17.14]. Negative delayed-type hypersensitivity reactions may be apparent in 10%–20% of normal individuals. Therefore, patients with a negative test should receive a booster of tetanus or diphtheria toxoids and have repeat skin tests 2–4 weeks later. Analysis of T- (and B-) cell subsets may enumerate total numbers of CD4+ and CD8+ cells, NK cells, and monocytes and evaluate for the expression of human leukocyte antigens (HLAs). In addition, functional T-cell studies such as in vitro proliferation of T cells to mitogens (phytohemagglutinin, concanavalin A, or pokeweed mitogen) or to antigens (tetanus toxoid or *Candida*) are also appropriate.

Management

The treatment for severe T-cell disorders is bone marrow or stem cell transplantation (see Table 17.15). Intravenous immune (γ-globulin) replace-

TABLE 17.14 **Predominant Defects of Cell-Mediated Immunity (T-Cell Defects): Pathophysiologic Aspects**

Disorder	Genetics	Onset	Pathogenesis
DiGeorge anomaly (velocardiofacial syndrome or CATCH 22 syndrome)	AD (22q11.2, 10p13)	Early infancy	Hypoplasia of third and fourth pharyngeal pouch (thymic hypoplasia)
Wiskott-Aldrich syndrome	X-linked (Xp11.22)	Early infancy	53-kD protein (WASP) defect (impaired response to polysaccharide antigens)
Ataxia-telangiectasia (AT)	AR (11q22.3)	2–5 years	AT gene mutation (PI3 kinase) [involved in chromosomal repair].
Nijmegen breakage syndrome	AR (8q21)	Infancy	Defect in Nibrin protein (involved in chromosomal repair)
Cartilage-hair hypoplasia (short-limbed dwarf)	AR (9p13–21)	Birth	Unknown
Severe combined immuno-deficiency (SCID)			
Common γ-chain deficiency	X-linked (Xq13.1-q21.1)	1–3 months	Common γ chain (γc) mutation → IL-2Rγ depletion → severe T-cell depletion
ZAP-70, Jak-3 kinase, or IL-7Rα chain	AR (2q12, 19p13.1, or 15p13)	1–3 months	ZAP-70, Jak-3 kinase, or IL-7Rα deficiency
ADA deficiency	AR (20q13.11)	1–3 months	ADA deficiency results in dATP-induced lymphocyte toxicity
PNP deficiency	AR (14q13.1)	1–3 months	PNP deficiency results in dGTP-induced T cell toxicity
Reticular dysgenesis	AR	1–3 months	Defective maturation of common stem cell affecting myeloid and lymphoid cells
Omenn syndrome	AR (11p13)	1–3 months	Mutations of recombinase activating genes (RAG-1 and RAG-2)
Bare lymphocyte syndrome			
MHC class I	AR (6p21.3)	First decade	TAP1 and TAP2 mutations (transporters associated with antigen processing)
MHC class II	AR (1q, 13q, 16p13)	Early infancy	Mutations in RFX-5, RFXAP, CIITA, and RFX-B (DNA-binding factors)
Chronic mucocutaneous candidiasis (CMCC)	AR	3–5 years	Unknown
Lymphoproliferative syndrome (Duncan syndrome)	X-linked (Xq24–26); AR (10p14–15)	Variable	SLAM-associated protein (SAP) defect IL-2Rα defect

AD = autosomal dominant; ADA = adenosine deaminase; AR = autosomal recessive; CATCH 22 = cardiac anomalies, abnormal facies, thymic hypoplasia, cleft palate, hypocalcemia with 22q11.2 deletion; Ig = immunoglobulin; IL = interleukin; MHC = major histocompatability complex; PNP = purine nucleosidase; WASP = Wiskott-Aldrich syndrome protein.

TABLE 17.15 Predominant Defects of Cell-Mediated Immunity (T-Cell Defects): Clinical Aspects

Disorder	Manifestations	Associated Features	Laboratory Evaluation	Treatment
DiGeorge anomaly (velo-cardiofacial syndrome or CATCH 22 syndrome)	Variable	Hypoparathyroidism → hypo-calcemia, cardiac anomalies (truncus arteriosus, inter-rupted aortic arch type B, transposition, atrial septal defect), dysmorphic features (micrognathia, hypertelorism, low-set ears, bifid uvula, short philtrum), esophageal atresia	Decreased CD3 T cells (< 500/mm³ in severe cases), chromosome 22q11.2 deletion	No treatment needed for partial form, BMT or thymic epithelial explant for severe form
Wiskott-Aldrich syndrome	Recurrent otitis media, pneumonia, meningitis with encapsulated organisms; infection with *Pneumocystis carinii* and herpesviruses	Atopic dermatitis (also asthma and allergies), platelet dys-function, thrombocytopenia, autoimmune cytopenias and vasculitis, malignancy	< 70,000/mm³ platelets, mutation in WASP or absent mRNA or protein	Bone marrow transplant (BMT), splenectomy
Ataxia-telangiectasia (AT)	Sinopulmonary infections	Neurologic and endocrine dysfunction, malignancy, telangiectasia, sensitive to radiation, decreased IgA	Increased radiation-induced chromosomal breakage in cultured cells, mutation in ATM	Antibiotics, IVIG
Nijmegen breakage syndrome	Sinopulmonary, urinary tract, and gastrointestinal infections; bronchiectasis	Sensitivity to ionizing radia-tion, microcephaly with mild neurologic impairment, malignancy	Increased radiation-induced chromosomal breakage in cultured cells, mutation in Nibrin gene	Antibiotics
Cartilage-hair hypoplasia (short-limbed dwarf)	Variable	Metaphyseal or spondyloepi-physeal dysplasia → short extremities, short stature, fine sparse hair, short fingernails, redundant skin folds	Decreased numbers of T cells and decreased proliferation to antigens	BMT for severe forms
Severe combined immuno-deficiency (SCID) Common γ chain]	Candidiasis, all types of infections (bacterial, viral, fungal, protozoal)	Severe graft-versus-host disease from maternal fetal transfusions, failure to thrive	< 20% CD3+ T cells, absolute lymphocyte count < 3000/mm³, and detected gene mutation or decreased enzyme activity (depending on defect)	BMT or stem cell transplant

(continued)

TABLE 17.15 Predominant Defects of Cell-Mediated Immunity (T-Cell Defects) : Clinical Aspects *(Continued)*

Disorder	Manifestations	Associated Features	Laboratory Evaluation	Treatment
ZAP-70, Jak-3 kinase, or IL-7Rα chain	Candidiasis, all types of infections (bacterial, viral, fungal, protozoal)	Severe graft-versus-host disease from maternal fetal transfusions, failure to thrive	< 20% CD3+ T cells, absolute lymphocyte count < 3000/mm³, and detected gene mutation or decreased enzyme activity (depending on defect); absence of CD8 cells in ZAP-70 patients	BMT or stem cell transplant
ADA deficiency	Candidiasis, all types of infections (bacterial, viral, fungal, protozoal)	Multiple skeletal abnormalities, chondro-osseous dysplasia	< 20% CD3+ T cells, absolute lymphocyte count < 3000/mm³, and detected	BMT or stem cell transplant, polyethylene glycol-modified bovine ADA (PEG-ADA) if transplant not an option
PNP deficiency	Candidiasis, all types of infections (bacterial, viral, fungal, protozoal)	Neurologic disorders, severe graft-versus-host disease from transfusions	< 20% CD3+ T cells, absolute lymphocyte count < 3000/mm³, and detected	BMT or stem cell transplant
SCID (reticular dysgenesis)	Candidiasis, all types of infections (bacterial, viral, fungal, protozoal)	Agammaglobulinemia, alymphocytosis, agranulocytosis	< 20% CD3+ T cells, absolute lymphocyte count < 3000/mm³, and detected	BMT or stem cell transplant
Omenn syndrome	Candidiasis, all types of infections (bacterial, viral, fungal, protozoal)	Exfoliative erythroderma, eosinophilia, elevated IgE, lymphadenopathy, hepatosplenomegaly	< 20% CD3+ T cells, absolute lymphocyte count < 3000/mm³, and detected	BMT or stem cell transplant

Bare lymphocyte syndrome			
MHC class I	Sinopulmonary infections	Chronic lung inflammation	CD8+ T cell deficiency, no MHC class I antigens, TAP mutation	Variable
MHC class II	Respiratory tract infections, chronic diarrhea, CNS viral infections (polio, enterovirus, herpes)	Autoimmune disease, failure to thrive, sclerosing cholangitis	CD4+ T cell deficiency, no MHC class II antigens on B cells and monocytes, decreased immunoglobulins, normal lymphocyte proliferation to mitogens but not to antigens	Variable
Chronic mucocutaneous candidiasis (CMCC)	Candidal infections of mucous membranes, skin, and nails	Autoimmune endocrinopathies	No delayed type hypersensitivity or lymphocyte proliferation to Candida	Systemic antifungal therapy, transfer factor +/− fetal thymus transplant
Lymphoproliferative syndrome (Duncan syndrome)	Variable decrease in T-, B-, and natural killer cell function and hypogammaglobulinemia following EBV infection	Life-threatening EBV infection, lymphoma or Hodgkin disease, aplastic anemia, lymphohistiocytic disorders	SAP or IL-2Rα mutation, decreased antibody titers to EBV nuclear antigen (EBNA)	BMT

ADA = adenosine deaminase; AR = autosomal recessive; BMT = bone marrow transplant; CATCH 22 = cardiac anomalies, abnormal facies, thymic hypoplasia, cleft palate, hypocalcemia with 22q11.2 deletion; CNS = central nervous system; EBV = Epstein-Barr virus; Ig = immunoglobulin; IL = interleukin; IVIG = intravenous immunoglobulin; MHC = major histocompatability complex; PNP = purine nucleosidase; WASP = Wiskott-Aldrich syndrome protein.

ment (IVIG) is also useful. In other forms of SCID, transfer of the normal gene into the patient's stem cells (gene therapy) is currently being studied and may soon be a common therapeutic modality for these diseases.

PHAGOCYTIC DEFECTS

Disorders of the phagocytic defenses can be divided into those of deficient cell numbers and those of insufficient function (Tables 17.16 and 17.17). These disorders are characterized by mucous membrane infections (e.g., gingivitis, ab-

scesses in the skin and viscera), lymphadenitis, poor wound healing, delayed umbilical cord separation, and absence of pus (in disorders of cell numbers or of leukocyte movement). Microorganisms involved in these infections include *S. aureus*, fungi, and gram-negative bacteria.

Laboratory Evaluation

Evaluation for neutrophil disorders begins with a CBC and the examination of neutrophil number and morphology (see Table 17.16). Further studies are more complex and not always avail-

TABLE 17.16	Phagocytic Defects: Pathophysiologic Aspects		
Disorder	**Genetics**	**Onset**	**Pathogenesis**
Chronic granulomatous disease (CGD)	X-linked (66%) (Xp21.1), AR (33%) (1q25, 16q24)	First year of life for X-linked, later for AR	gp91^{phox} deficiency (X-linked) gp22^{phox}, gp47^{phox}, and gp67^{phox} deficiencies (AR)
Chédiak-Higashi syndrome	AR (1q42–43)	Infancy	Defect in vesicle membrane component → defective bactericidal function and chemotaxis, also poor natural killer and cytotoxic T cell function
Hyper-IgE (Job syndrome)	? AD with incomplete penetrance	Infancy	Decreased cell-mediated immunity and humoral immune responses to specific antigens with near-normal IgG, IgA, and IgM levels, and markedly elevated IgE, impaired chemotaxis, and opsonization
Myeloperoxidase deficiency	AR	Variable	Impaired bactericidal and fungicidal activity
Glucose-6-phosphate dehydrogenase (G6PD) deficiency	X-linked (highly polymorphic)	Variable (depends on level of enzyme activity)	Impaired bactericidal activity
Leukocyte adhesion deficiency	AR (21q22.3)	Infancy	Mutations in CD18 (β_2 integrin), a β-chain shared by three α-chains (LFA-1, Mac-1, and CR3) on chromosome 16; all four molecules are not expressed; defects in adherence, chemotaxis, and phagocytosis; reduced lymphocyte cytotoxicity

AD = autosomal dominant; AR = autosomal recessive; gp = glycoprotein; Ig = immunoglobulin.

TABLE 17.17 Phagocytic Defects: Clinical Aspects

Disorder	Manifestations	Associated Features	Laboratory Evaluation	Treatment
Chronic granulomatous disease (CGD)	Osteomyelitis, adenitis, and abscesses caused by *Staphylococcus aureus*, *Burkholderia cepacia*, and *Aspergillus fumigatus*	Granulomas (respiratory, gastrointestinal, and genitourinary tracts), failure to thrive, hepatosplenomegaly, lymphadenopathy)	Negative nitroblue tetrazolium (NBT) test, gene mutation or absent mRNA	Antimicrobial therapy (with granulocyte transfusion for fungal infections), IFN-γ, BMT
Chédiak-Higashi syndrome	Recurrent respiratory tract and other types of infections	Oculocutaneous albinism, neuropathy, giant neutrophilic cytoplasmic inclusions, malignancy	Gene mutation, giant lysosomal granules in neutrophils, neutropenia, abnormal chemotaxis assay with control serum	BMT
Hyper-IgE (Job syndrome)	Staphylococcal abscesses of the skin, lungs, joints, and viscera; infections with *Haemophilus influenzae*, *Candida*, and *Aspergillus*	Eczema, eosinophilia, coarse facial features, osteopenia, giant pneumatoceles, red hair, malignancy	Increased IgE and IgD; normal IgG, IgA, and IgM; eosinophilia; decreased T cell proliferation to antigens; low antibody titers	Anti-staphylococcal drugs
Myeloperoxidase deficiency	Mild immune dysfunction with increased susceptibility to infection with *Candida* (especially with coexisting disease such as diabetes)	Persistent candidiasis in diabetics	Decreased myeloperoxidase in leukocytes, decreased granulocyte count (when automated counter identifies granulocytes by myeloperoxidase content)	Antifungal therapy
Glucose-6-phosphate dehydrogenase (G6PD) deficiency	Phenotypically similar to chronic granulomatous disease (CGD)	Hemolytic anemia	Abbreviated O_2 production on superoxide assay, decreased G6PD	Antimicrobial therapy
Leukocyte adhesion deficiency	Staphylococcal, gram-negative enteric bacterial, and fungal infections (periodontitis, omphalitis, gingivitis, recurrent skin infections, repeated otitis media, pneumonia, septicemia, ileocolitis, peritonitis, perianal abscesses)	Delayed separation of the umbilical cord, impaired wound healing, leukocytosis (WBC count > 25,000/mm³) neutrophilia, absence of pus	Flow cytometry for CD18 or CD11a, CD11b, or CD11c (absent); abnormal chemotaxis assay with control serum	BMT for severe form

BMT = bone marrow transplant; gp = glycoprotein; IFN = interferon; Ig = immunoglobulin; WBC = white blood cell.

TABLE 17.18	Deficiency of Complement and Associated Disease
Deficient Protein	**Associated Disease**
C1q, C1r	SLE, glomerulonephritis
C2	SLE, arthritis, JRA, recurrent infections in some patients
C3	Recurrent infections, glomerulonephritis
C4	SLE-like disease
C5	Recurrent *Neisseria* infections
C6	Recurrent *Neisseria* infections
C7	Recurrent *Neisseria* infections, Raynaud phenomenon
C8	Recurrent *Neisseria* infections
C9	Autoimmune disease in some patients
Properdin C1 inhibitor	Recurrent infections, meningococcemia
Factor D	Hereditary angioedema
Factor H	Glomerulonephritis
Factor I	Recurrent infections
C4-binding protein	Collagen-vascular disease
C5a inhibitor	Familial Mediterranean fever
C3b receptor	SLE
C1 inhibitor	Hereditary angioedema

JRA = juvenile rheumatoid arthritis; SLE = systemic lupus erythematosus.

able, including the nitroblue tetrazolium test for CGD and in vitro tests for neutrophil phagocytosis, chemotaxis, and bacterial killing. In addition, tests for expression of CD18 and CD11 antigens (leukocyte adhesion deficiencies) and for myeloperoxidase activity by flow cytometry can be performed.

Management

Frequent courses of antibiotics are required for the treatment of neutrophil disorders (see Table 17.17). The frequency of infection in CGD is also decreased by treatment with subcutaneous recombinant interferon-γ. Recombinant granulocyte-macrophage colony-stimulating factor also appears to be effective in the treatment of some forms of neutropenia.

COMPLEMENT DEFECTS

Deficiency of some components results in recurrent pyogenic infection, whereas deficiency of other components results in lupus-like disease or vasculitis (Table 17.18). The literature contains reports of patients with the absence of each complement component.

Laboratory Evaluation

The total hemolytic activity of serum (CH_{50}) is a widely available test that is dependent on the presence of normal levels of the major compo-

nents of complement. If the CH_{50} is abnormal, individual components must be analyzed in specialized laboratories.

Management

Specific therapy with component replacement is not available, and frequent and long courses of antibiotics are the current treatment of choice for complement deficiencies. Immunization of patients and their close contacts with pneumococcal and meningococcal vaccines may be useful.

SUGGESTED READINGS

Fleisher TA, Ballow M: Primary immune deficiencies: Presentation, diagnosis, and management. *Pediatr Clin North Am* 47(6):2000 (entire issue).

Leung DYM: Atopic dermatitis: New insights and opportunities for therapeutic intervention. *J Allergy Clin Immunol* 105(5):860–876, 2000.

MacKay IR, Rosen FS (eds): "Advances in Immunology" series. *N Engl J Med* (beginning in July 2000).

Middleton Jr E, Reed CE, Ellis EF, et al: *Middleton's Allergy: Principles & Practice*, 5th ed. St. Louis, Mosby-Year Book, 1998.

Sampson HA: Food allergy. Part I: Immunopathogenesis and clinical disorders. *J Allergy Clin Immunol* 103(5):717–728, 1999.

Sampson HA: Food allergy. Part II: Diagnosis and management. *J Allergy Clin Immunol* 103(6):981–989, 1999.

TePas EC, Umetsu DT: Immunotherapy of asthma and allergic diseases. *Curr Opin Pediatr* 12(6):574–578, 2000.

Chapter 18

Pulmonology

Carol Conrad

Respiratory failure, the most frequent cause of life-threatening cardiorespiratory illness in children, indicates that there is a failure of gas exchange. Among the many causes of respiratory failure are infection, structural airway abnormality, aspiration into the airway and lungs, pulmonary embolus, exposure to noxious substances (e.g., smoke inhalation), and cardiac failure with pulmonary edema.

Maintenance of normal carbon dioxide homeostasis requires normal lung mechanics, circulation, and ventilatory drive. The principal causes of respiratory failure in children are **pulmonary disease** (pneumonia, acute respiratory distress syndrome, pulmonary edema), **airways disease** (mucous plugs, foreign bodies, anatomic abnormalities, compressions), **restrictive disease** (chest deformity, flail chest, abdominal ascites), and **neuromuscular disease** (myasthenia, botulism, tetanus, intoxication, head injury).

GENERAL PRINCIPLES OF PULMONARY DISEASE IN CHILDREN

Alveoli are few in number at birth at full-term, and maturation of the gas exchange area as well as the supporting cartilaginous structures affects the results of illness much differently in premature infants than in term infants. In turn, respiratory disease in toddlers is different than in older children or adults.

BASIC CONCEPTS IN PULMONARY PHYSIOLOGY

The basic function of the respiratory system is to supply oxygen to the body and to remove excess carbon dioxide from the body. The basic steps involved in this process are as follows:

1. **Ventilation,** which is the exchange of gas between the atmosphere and the alveoli
2. **Diffusion** of gases across the alveolar–capillary membranes
3. **Transport** of gases in the blood

4. **Diffusion** of oxygen from the capillaries of the systemic circulation to the cells of the body
5. **Internal respiration,** which is the use of oxygen and production of carbon dioxide within the cells

These processes cannot occur efficiently if there is a mismatch of airflow (ventilation) and blood flow (perfusion) to the alveoli. This is termed a ventilation–perfusion defect, or a $\dot{V}/\dot{Q}$ mismatch.

Various disorders of the pulmonary system affect the first three steps. Decreased ventilation may be due to an absence or occlusion of a conductive airway. If the airways are obstructed physically [e.g., due to a congenital defect such as stenosis or severe malacia (softness of the cartilage) of the airways], this can affect ventilation of the alveolar units. Similarly, obstruction of the bronchi and bronchioles occurs in diseases such as asthma and cystic fibrosis that are characterized by increased mucous production.

Abnormalities in perfusion can occur in instances of hypoxic or hypercarbic vasoconstriction of the arterioles and capillaries of the alveoli. The presence of an abnormal vascular pathway through the lungs (**arteriovenous malformation**) can also alter $\dot{V}/\dot{Q}$. Conditions that can inflame the alveolar epithelium (alveolitis) or cause fibrosis and thickening eventually create a decreased diffusion of gases across the alveolar wall. Acute inflammation affects gas diffusion more than blood perfusion, but progressive fibrosis affects perfusion eventually.

Gas transport in the blood takes place in two primary ways: by dissolving in plasma or by combining with hemoglobin. Approximately 98% of oxygen transport in the blood occurs by an oxygen–hemoglobin interaction. The binding of hemoglobin to oxygen is not a linear process; the avidity of hemoglobin for oxygen changes as the heme molecule becomes more "loaded" with oxygen. This relationship is the basis of the sigmoidal shape of the oxyhemoglobin dissociation curve.

Conformational changes in the hemoglobin molecule are essential within muscles and organs to allow for the release of oxygen and the uptake of carbon dioxide. Normal physiologic changes in the blood pH such as acidosis allow for the release of oxygen from the hemoglobin molecule to the tissues, which is essential for proper homeostasis during times of stress, including exercise and disease states such as sepsis. Another example involves fetal hemoglobin, which binds oxygen more avidly than adult type hemoglobin; this gives a growing fetus the ability to extract oxygen from the mother's blood cells.

Certain disease states confer an abnormally high or low affinity of the hemoglobin molecule for oxygen. With sickle cell disease, the hemoglobin molecule has low oxygen-binding affinity, and this worsens as the hemoglobin becomes less saturated with oxygen. As sickle cell hemoglobin starts to release oxygen molecules from its binding sites, it collapses, and the cells become "sickled" in appearance. The red blood cells (RBCs) become lodged in capillaries and produce the vaso-occlusive events typical of sickle cell disease.

When interpreting the meaning of arterial oxygen saturation measurements, it is vital to understand the correlation between the **oxygen saturation (SaO$_2$)** and the **arterial oxygen content (PaO$_2$)**. The PaO$_2$ reading measured with an arterial blood gas determines the amount of oxygen dissolved in plasma, which is in equilibrium with the oxygen bound to hemoglobin. The SaO$_2$ is a measure of how many available oxygen binding sites of the hemoglobin molecule are saturated by oxygen.

☀ Pediatric Pearl

To remember an approximate correlation between the PaO$_2$ and the pulse oximetry reading, a useful memory aid is: PaO$_2$ readings of 40 mm Hg, 50 mm Hg, and 60 mm Hg correlate with pulse oximetry readings of 70%, 80%, and 90%, respectively. Two rules of thumb properly evaluate SaO$_2$ readings and blood gas measurements:

1. A PaO$_2$ value below 80 mm Hg, which indicates hypoxia, is abnormal.
2. An SaO$_2$ value of 94% or less indicates hypoxia and is abnormal.

It is important to understand that poorly perfused limbs may produce low or inaccurate transcutaneous measurements of oxygen saturation. Shock, vasopressor administration, severe edema, or peripheral edema may cause erroneous readings. Finally, pulse oximeters are not calibrated to read accurately below a saturation of 70%; therefore reported values less than 70% are difficult to interpret.

Oxygen and Carbon Dioxide Imbalance

Hypoxemia refers to a decreased delivery of oxygen from the atmosphere to the blood, whereas **hypoxia** refers to decreased delivery of oxygen to the tissues. Arterial hypoxia may result from hypoventilation, absolute shunting, diffusion defects, or relative shunting (Table 18.1). Several conditions may lead to hypoxemia (Table 18.2).

Hypoventilation is a physiologic state in which the patient is neither breathing a sufficient tidal volume or an adequate number of breaths/minute (minute volume). This results in elevated levels of carbon dioxide in the blood and also in the alveolar gas. When the alveolar carbon dioxide content increases significantly (**hypercapnia**), the volume available for oxygen to diffuse through to the alveolar capillary bed is reduced and creates arterial hypoxemia (Table 18.3).

An **absolute shunt** is defined as blood passing from the right the left side of the heart without being oxygenated. A shunt diverts blood away from oxygenated alveoli, and the blood cannot receive oxygen. An absolute shunt can occur due to an **anatomic shunt** with persistent fetal circulation (see Chapter 10), idiopathic or secondary pulmonary hypertension, arteriovenous malformation, and congenital heart defects (see Chapter 13).

A **relative shunt** may develop at the level of the alveolus if the alveolus is blocked (pneumonia), collapsed (atelectasis), or filled with fluid (pulmonary edema). Decreased diffusion of oxygen and carbon dioxide across the alveolar epithelium to the pulmonary capillary bed is characteristic of disease states in which the alveolar and bronchiolar epithelium are thickened due to inflammation or fibrosis. This phenomenon is termed a **diffusion defect** and occurs in disease states such as cystic fibrosis, systemic lupus erythematosus, juvenile rheumatoid arthritis, and Wegener granulomatosis.

Many conditions may result in hypercapnia (see Table 18.3). These conditions can be divided into two broad physiologic categories, resulting in carbon dioxide imbalance: increased carbon dioxide production and decreased carbon dioxide clearance.

Respiratory Measurements

Blood Gas Analysis

A blood gas determination consists of four important measurements, pH, PO$_2$, PCO$_2$, and base excess, which provide information about the respiratory, circulatory, and metabolic condition of the patient.

TABLE 18.1 Types of Hypoxia	
Cause	**Underlying Problem**
Hypoxemic hypoxia	Lower-than-normal P_{AO_2} (hypoxemia)
Anemic hypoxia	Decreased hemoglobin or red blood cell count
	Carboxyhemoglobin
	Hemoglobinopathy
Circulatory hypoxia	Decreased cardiac output
	Decreased local perfusion
Affinity hypoxia	Decreased release of oxygen from hemoglobin to the tissues
Histotoxic hypoxia	Cyanide poisoning

A sample of blood from arteries, veins, or capillaries may be used for blood gas determination. Arterial puncture is the one measure that most accurately reflects the level of oxygen being delivered to the tissues. A venous blood gas can be used instead of an arterial blood gas but tends to reflect local tissue oxygenation and carbon dioxide clearance. However, a venous blood gas is a reasonable estimate of arterial acid–base status in a patient who is well hydrated and well perfused.

Pediatric Pearl

When perfusion of the circulatory system is adequate, the venous pH is 0.04 units lower than the arterial pH, because the venous P_{CO_2} is 5–7 mm Hg higher than the arterial P_{CO_2}.

Carbon dioxide is transported more readily than oxygen in the blood because it is highly lipid soluble. Due to the higher solubility and diffusivity of carbon dioxide, $\dot{V}/\dot{Q}$ mismatches lead more frequently to measured abnormalities of the P_{aO_2}.

Respiratory acidosis develops from an imbalance between metabolic carbon dioxide production and pulmonary carbon dioxide excretion. This most often arises from decreased efficiency of carbon dioxide elimination in the lung—**alveolar hypoventilation.** Alveolar hypoventilation results in carbon dioxide retention and **hypercapnia.** A new balance between carbon dioxide production and removal may be corrected by short-term chemical buffering and more long-term renal adaptations. Hypoxemia usually accompanies respiratory acidosis.

TABLE 18.2 Clinical Causes of Arterial Hypoxemia	
Problem	**Example**
Low P_{IO_2} (partial pressure of inspired oxygen	Low F_{IO_2}, altitude
Alveolar hypoventilation (low alveolar P_{O_2} with increased alveolar P_{CO_2})	Central nervous system depression
	Pulmonary disease (pneumonia, pulmonary edema)
	Obstructive lung disease (cystic fibrosis, asthma)
	Restrictive chest wall disease (Jeune syndrome)
	Neuromuscular disease (muscular dystrophy)
Diffusion block	Pulmonary fibrosis (systemic lupus erythematosus, juvenile rheumatoid arthritis, vasculitides)
	Alveolitis
	Pulmonary hypoplasia (congenital lung hypoplasia syndromes)
	Pulmonary resection (lobectomy, pneumonectomy)
$\dot{V}/\dot{Q}$ mismatch, poor distribution of ventilation	Pulmonary embolism
	Mucous plugging
	Bronchospasm
Shunt	Congenital heart disease (persistent patent ductus arteriosus, ventricular septal defect with right-to-left shunt, pulmonary arteriovenous malformation)
	Pneumonia
	Atelectasis
	Pulmonary hypertension

TABLE 18.3	Causes of Hypercapnia
Problem	**Example**
Increased production	Increased body temperature
	Excessive muscular activity
	Physiologic stress
	Sepsis
	Parenteral nutrition with glucose
Decreased clearance	Tissue gas exchange
	Increased tissue CO_2 production
	Poor tissue perfusion (ischemia)
	Disrupted diffusion (edema)
	Loading
	Capillary shunt from peripheral vasodilation (septic shock)
	Transport
	Low hemoglobin level
	Low cardiac output
	Unloading
	Venous-to-arterial shunts (right-to-left cardiac shunts)
	Pulmonary gas exchange
	Decreased ventilation (asthma, cystic fibrosis, emphysema, respiratory depression, neuromuscular disorder)
	Increased dead space (asthma)
	Disruption of alveolar–capillary diffusion (alveolitis, pulmonary edema, pneumonia)

Blood pH changes in response to acute respiratory events in expected ways (Tables 18.4 and 18.5). The tables are a guide to determine the direction in which the pH, P_{CO_2}, and the HCO_3^- should vary in different clinical circumstances.

Pediatric Pearl

A tip for rapid analysis of blood gas values: For every 10-mm Hg change in carbon dioxide, the pH changes by 0.08 units in the opposite direction.

Estimating Oxygenation

The Pa_{O_2}, the partial pressure of oxygen dissolved in serum, is used as a measure of the adequacy of oxygenation (assuming that there is an adequate amount of hemoglobin present to bind the oxygen, and that the hemoglobin binds oxygen normally). The **alveolar gas equation,** which is the amount of oxygen that should be present in the alveoli (Pa_{O_2}) based on a known temperature and F_{IO_2} (fraction of inspired oxygen), reflects the efficiency of gas exchange.

$$PA_{O_2} = PI_{O_2} - PA_{CO_2}\left[\frac{F_{IO_2} + 1 - F_{IO_2}}{R}\right]$$

where PA_{O_2} = partial pressure of oxygen at the alveolar level, PI_{O_2} = partial pressure of inspired oxygen, Pa_{O_2} = partial pressure of oxygen in arterial blood as measured by arterial blood gas, F_{IO_2} = fraction of inspired oxygen, and R = respiratory quotient (0.8). For most clinical applications, the alveolar gas equation can be closely es-

TABLE 18.4	Rules of Acute Respiratory Compensation	
Change	**Rule**	**Example**
↑ P_{CO_2}	For every increase of 10 mm Hg, pH decreases by 0.08	P_{CO_2}: 40 → 60 mm Hg; pH: 7.40 → 7.24
↓ P_{CO_2}	For every decrease of 10 mm Hg, pH increases by 0.07	P_{CO_2}: 40 → 20 mm Hg; pH: 7.40 → 7.54

TABLE 18.5 Acid-Base Disturbances as Measured by Arterial Blood Gas

Condition	pH	Pco_2	HCO_3^-
Uncompensated respiratory acidosis	↓↓	↑↑	↑
Uncompensated respiratory alkalosis	↑↑	↓↓	↓
Uncompensated metabolic acidosis	↓↓	—	↓↓
Uncompensated metabolic alkalosis	↑↑	—	↑↑
Partially compensated respiratory acidosis	↓	↑↑	↑↑
Partially compensated respiratory alkalosis	↑	↓↓	↓↓
Partially compensated metabolic acidosis	↓	↓↓	↓↓
Partially compensated metabolic alkalosis	↑	↑↑	↑↑
Respiratory and metabolic acidosis	↓↓	↑↑	↓
Respiratory and metabolic alkalosis	↑↑	↓↓	↑

timated with the following modified formula and thus stated more simply:

$$PAO_2 = [760 \text{ mm Hg} - 47 \text{ mm Hg}] \times$$
$$FIO_2 - PaCO_2(1.25)$$

where 760 mm Hg = barometric pressure at sea level and 47 mm Hg = vapor pressure in airway. $PaCO_2$ is measured from arterial blood gas, which can be used to approximate the alveolar carbon dioxide.

Subtracting the PAO_2 measured on arterial blood gas from the calculated PAO_2 gives the **alveolar–arterial oxygen gradient**. Calculation of the alveolar–arterial oxygen gradient while a patient is breathing room air can differentiate hypoventilation from shunting.

Arterial oxygen values can be altered by the fraction of inspired oxygen (FIO_2), the condition of the alveolar air–blood barrier, and the amount of pulmonary blood flow. At sea level, an arterial PO_2 of 97 mm Hg (range, 80–105) is normal for a patient breathing "room air." A patient with normal lungs receiving supplemental oxygen should have an arterial PO_2 approximately 5 times the FIO_2 (Table 18.6).

TABLE 18.6 Predicted Effect of Fraction of Inspired Oxygen (FIO_2) on Blood Oxygen Content

FIO_2	Predicted Arterial PO_2 (mm Hg)
0.30	150
0.40	200
0.50	250
0.80	400
1.00	500

CLINICAL APPROACH TO THE CHILD WITH PULMONARY DISEASE

When a pediatrician is faced with a child with acute or chronic respiratory illness and worried parents, it is essential to obtain a complete history and perform a comprehensive physical examination.

History

In general, the pulmonary history should include questions that establish the age of onset of the problem and factors that appear to initiate cough, breathlessness, or "noisy" breathing. It is necessary to inquire about the duration of symptoms and if the problem has persisted despite medical interventions. The vast majority of referrals to pediatric pulmonologists are for recurrent or chronic cough, and the second most frequent reason for referral is for noisy breathing. A significant proportion of children referred with a chronic cough receive the diagnosis of asthma. Other conditions are possible; the history may provide specific clues to the diagnosis of cough (Table 18.7).

Pediatric Pearl

It is important to remember that history-taking primarily involves the ability to listen carefully. However, some caution is indicated. Parents may use words that have an entirely different meaning to them than to the health professional. "Bronchitis," "wheeze," and "croup" are some of the most frequently misused words in the pediatric lexicon.

It is essential to determine the nature of the child's problem. For example, is a cough dry or

| TABLE 18.7 | Clues to Diagnosis in Children With Chronic Cough |

History	Disease
Cough starts when child is supine	Gastroesophageal reflux, postnasal drip
Paroxysmal cough	Pertussis, chlamydia, foreign body
Recurrent cough with wheeze	Asthma, foreign body, mediastinal tumor, cystic fibrosis
Cough associated with swallowing	Gastroesophageal reflux, aspiration due to dysfunctional swallow, tracheoesophageal reflux
Cough with aphonia	Foreign body in larynx, papillomatosis, croup, or psychoneurosis
Ringing, brassy cough	Tracheitis
Barking cough	Croup or subglottic disease
Cough in early A.M.	Asthma
Cough with exercise	Exercise-induced bronchospasm

wet? Has the child's primary care physician heard the child wheeze? The child may have associated symptoms or signs with the cough (e.g., pale, boggy mucosa that indicate allergic rhinitis with postnasal drip). Other important factors to consider include the timing of the symptoms, which can lead to rapid diagnosis (e.g., nighttime cough in patients with gastroesophageal reflux disease, which worsens when patients are sleeping or supine); knowledge of response to previous medication regimens, which can help determine the nature of the disease; and any occurrences of allergies to medicines or foods, which could account for the child's current problem or may affect treatment.

The history should also include details of the antenatal and perinatal periods. Decreased fetal motion may indicate a neuromuscular disorder that leads to alveolar hypoventilation and restrictive chest wall disease. **Oligohydramnios** may indicate the presence of pulmonary hypoplasia, because much of the amniotic fluid produced by the fetus is generated from lung epithelium. Oligohydramnios may also be a sign of a renal anomaly and the presence of other congenital anomalies. Knowledge of any perinatal resuscitation efforts, including the reason for their use, is helpful. It is crucial to know the gestational age at birth and if intubation and mechanical ventilation or supplemental oxygen was necessary to determine whether **respiratory distress syndrome** occurred. Any history of cyanosis in the absence of cardiac anomalies should lead to an investigation of possible tracheal or bronchial stenosis or malacia, decreased alveolar volume (pulmonary hypoplasia), and pulmonary vascular malformations (see Chapter 10).

When evaluating respiratory difficulties, family history is important. A family history of asthma is significant. The family history is also helpful in determining the likelihood of other disorders such

as cystic fibrosis; however, the majority of children diagnosed with cystic fibrosis have no family history of the disease. A history of multiple unusual infections that include the sinopulmonary tract or the skin, as well as recurrent candidiasis or delayed umbilical cord disconnection could lead to a suspicion of chronic granulomatous disease, immunoglobulin G (IgG) deficiency, or other lymphocytic disorders that predispose children to recurrent infection (see Chapter 17).

Pediatric Pearl

All details of the past medical history are important to elicit. A history of multiple admissions to the hospital or repeated trips to the emergency department can provide information about the adequacy of the regimen of medications children are receiving.

Physical Examination

Before beginning the physical examination, it is necessary to scrutinize the vital signs and anthropometrics. As a general rule, children with chronic illness such as cystic fibrosis or immunodeficiency syndromes present with growth failure. In contrast, children with asthma rarely have problems maintaining their weight.

Examination of the head and neck is an essential part of the pulmonary examination and can guide the differential diagnosis. The structures of the upper respiratory tract warrant careful inspection for signs of sinusitis (edematous, erythematous nasal mucosa; purulent or clear nasal discharge); nasal polyps (present in cystic fibrosis and asthma); allergic shiners (darkness under the eyes); cobble stoning of posterior pharynx (chronic postnasal drip); allergic rhinitis (pale, edematous mucosa); and a nasal crease (or a history of the "salute sign" in which the patient rubs the nose with the palm of the hand). It is also important to look for signs consistent with **obstructive sleep apnea syndrome** when evaluating a history of snoring or gasping during sleep. Children with large tonsils and adenoids are often mouth-breathers who snore loudly while asleep. Enlarged tonsils and signs of enlarged adenoids (poor palatal elevation with phonation) are regions of possible airflow obstruction.

Examination of the chest involves observation of the breathing pattern and assessment of the respiratory effort initially. A normal inspiratory-to-expiratory ratio (I:E) is 1:2. Children with **obstructive** types of illness (e.g., cystic fibrosis, asthma) breathe with a prolonged expiratory phase, and the I:E increases to 1:3 or 1:4. In addition, they may have a hyperinflated thorax. Patients with **restrictive** breathing patterns breathe rapidly and shallowly. Inspection of the chest wall for symmetry, pectus deformity, and the size of the thorax is warranted. Retractions can be more difficult to appreciate in infants than in older children; they are not seen in the intercostal spaces. More often, the lower part of the rib cage is actually pulled inward as the diaphragm contracts when the infant inspires due to the high compliance of the chest wall. "Head-bobbing," a result of the use of the suprasternal accessory muscles of respiration, is a sign of increased resistance of the small airways in infants. It is important to evaluate how much effort the patient expends to achieve sufficient airflow. Percussion of the thorax can reveal either hyper-resonance due to localized air trapping or dullness to percussion if consolidation of a lobe or segment is present.

When auscultating breath sounds, it is necessary to listen for crackles, wheezing, and stridor. Crackles and wheezes originate from lower airway disease (Table 18.8). Do these sounds occur during inspiration or expiration? The resistance to airflow caused by obstructing lesions depends on the location of the obstruction (intra- or extrathoracic) and

on the phase of respiration. Noise that occurs on both inspiration and expiration suggests a **fixed stenosis** of the airway (i.e., a lesion in which the internal diameter, and hence, the airway resistance does not change with the phase of respiration). Such a lesion could be either intrathoracic or extrathoracic in origin.

It is also important to determine the distribution, pitch, and quality of sounds to differentiate between upper (extrathoracic) and lower (intrathoracic) airway pathology (Table 18.9). Airways are distended or compressed during the phases of respiration. The occurrence of an expiratory wheeze in the absence of inspiratory stridor (or vice versa) indicates a **variable stenosis.** When a variable obstruction is **intrathoracic,** it is primarily appreciated on **expiration,** because the lesion is dilated on inspiration by the negative intrathoracic pressure surrounding the airway at that point. When a variable obstruction is **extrathoracic,** obstruction worsens on **inspiration** and improves during expiration, because the positive intraluminal pressures distend this portion of the airway.

Other signs to note on physical examination include heart murmurs; a loud snapping P_2 (the portion of the second heart sound that indicates closure of the pulmonic valve, which when loud indicates pulmonary hypertension); digital clubbing (present in cystic fibrosis, cyanotic heart disease, bronchiectasis, inflammatory bowel disease); signs of atopy (eczema, Dennie lines, pale nasal mucosa, edema of mucosa), and enlargement of the abdominal organs.

Laboratory Evaluation

Pulmonary Function Tests

Pulmonary function tests are well characterized in young infants and toddlers as well as in older children. Clinicians have traditionally performed spirometry and lung volume measurements on patients who can accomplish a coordinated, forced

---

TABLE 18.8 **Sounds Produced by Lower Airways**

Sound (ATS)	Frequently Used Synonym	Acoustic Characteristics
Crackle		Usually inspiratory sound
-coarse	Rhonchi	Loud, low in pitch
-fine	Rale	Softer and shorter in duration, higher in pitch
Wheeze		Usually expiratory sound
-high-pitched		Long, musical
-low-pitched		Loud, long, sonorous

ATS = American Thoracic Society.

TABLE 18.9	Sounds Produced by Upper Airway Obstruction	
	Type of Pathology	
Type of Obstruction	**Intrathoracic**	**Extrathoracic**
Fixed	Noise on both inspiration and expiration	
Variable	Expiration: Wheeze predominates	Inspiration: Stridor dominates

expiratory maneuver (i.e., children > 5 years of age). More recently, techniques have been developed in which these maneuvers can be performed with sedated infants, but standard values are still being collected and the technique refined. Results are more readily obtainable in children older than 5 years of age. Uses for pulmonary function tests include (1) differentiating between restrictive and obstructive lung pathology, and (2) answering questions about respiratory function. Clinicians most commonly perform these pulmonary tests to assess the response to bronchodilator treatment and to determine whether a disease is improving or progressing in response to therapy. It is necessary to obtain results both before and after bronchodilator use.

Two basic methods are useful for the determination of lung volume and function. **Spirometry** measures "active" lung volumes (i.e., air volumes that a patient actively blows into the spirometer). A pneumotachometer simultaneously measures the rate of airflow. Use of these values allows the clinician to characterize the type of lung disease that affects a particular child. **Plethysmography** measures the actual volumes of air contained within the thorax. The patient sits in the plethysmograph and performs breathing maneuvers that result in measurable pressure changes inside the device. Using the ideal gas law, it is possible to calculate the volume at which the maneuver began. By convention, the maneuver begins when the patient has exhaled to the **functional residual capacity (FRC)**. Once this volume is known, the calculation of all other lung volumes is possible.

The use of spirometry and plethysmography is reliable in children of all ages. However, the technique used for infants and toddlers is different from that used for more cooperative older children, who can consistently follow instructions and perform repeated and prolonged exhalation maneuvers.

ABSOLUTE LUNG VOLUMES. Total lung capacity (TLC), **FRC,** and **residual volume (RV)** are determined using plethysmography (Figure 18.1). A lung capacity is simply the addition of two or more lung volumes; a lung volume is defined as the smallest

unit measure of the additive volumes within the thorax (Table 18.10). TLC, FRC, and RV are useful for following the course of chronic lung disease such as cystic fibrosis or restrictive lung disease.

SPIROMETRY. The most basic maneuver in spirometry is the slow **vital capacity (VC)** maneuver. To obtain a volume–time spirogram (see Figure 18.1), a child should first breathe quietly into the spirometer. After two or three tidal breaths are recorded, the child slowly inspires to **RV.** When the same maneuver is repeated, but with a forced exhalation [a forced vital capacity (FVC)], the rate of airflow rises quickly to its maximum value immediately after exhalation is initiated. As the lung volume decreases, the intrathoracic airways narrow, airway resistance increases, and the rate of airflow progressively falls. The standard time for exhalation is 6 seconds. Shorter exhalation times may be insufficient for detection of lung dysfunction and lead to underestimation of abnormalities. The volume exhaled in 1 second **[forced expiratory volume in 1 second (FEV$_1$)]** is obtained during this maneuver.

It is essential to obtain maximal efforts to differentiate restrictive and obstructive lung disease. The two types of lung disease produce different spirometric patterns (Table 18.11).

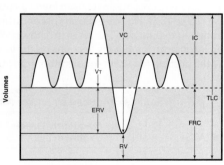

FIGURE 18.1. Volume–time spirogram. ERV = expiratory reserve volume; FRC = functional reserve capacity; IC = inspiratory capacity; TLC = total lung capacity; RV = residual volume; VC = vital capacity; Vt = tidal volume.

TABLE 18.10 Definitions of Lung Volumes and Measures Used in Spirometry and Plethysmography

Term	Acronym	Definition
Forced expiratory flow rate	FEF	Rate at which exhaled air flows; by convention, FEF is measured at 25%, 50%, and 75% of FVC
Forced expiratory volume in 1 second	FEV_1	Amount of air released after 1 second during a maximal exhalation
Functional residual capacity	FRC	Usual point at which exhalation ends; reflects balance of forces between expansile nature of chest wall and contractile nature of lung parenchyma
Residual volume	RV	Least volume of air remaining in lung after maximal expiratory maneuver (after SVC or FVC)
Tidal volume	V_T	Amount of air inhaled during breath
Total lung capacity	TLC	Total amount of air that can be contained within thorax after maximal inspiratory maneuver Sum of RV and VC
Vital capacity (slow and forced)	SVC, FVC	Amount of air released when exhaling from TLC to RV

Pediatric Pearl

The relation of the FEV_1 to the FVC is the key to differentiating obstructive lung disease from restrictive lung disease.

Obstructive lung disease (e.g., asthma, cystic fibrosis) is characterized by a reduction in airflow and trapping of air inside the thorax behind tight, plugged airways. This physiologic abnormality lowers the FEV_1. Because the FEV_1 is more reduced than the forced vital capacity (FVC), obstruction results in a low FEV_1/FVC ratio [FEV_1 (%)]. On the flow–volume curve, the exhalation limb has a scalloped shape.

Restrictive lung disease is characterized by a low FEV_1 and a proportionate reduction in the FVC. Thus, the FEV_1/FVC ratio is unchanged from normal ($> 80\%$). Children with pulmonary fibrosis (secondary to chemotherapy for cancer, systemic lupus erythematosus, or Wegener granulomatosis) typically have spirometric abnormalities of this type.

DIFFUSING CAPACITY (DLCO). $\dot{V}/\dot{Q}$ relationships within the lung and the function of the pulmonary capillary bed primarily affect gas transfer in the lungs, which is measured as the diffusing capacity for CO (DLCO). Any factor that affects the alveolus or the hemoglobin molecule alters the uptake of CO. Anemia and the lung volume at which it is measured affect the measurement of the DLCO. Decreased DLCO is most commonly seen in interstitial lung disease, sickle cell disease, and pulmonary vascular disease (pulmonary hypertension). DLCO is useful for monitoring the effects of chemotherapeutic agents and radiation on the lung parenchyma in children.

TABLE 18.11 Plethysmographic and Spirometric Patterns of Obstructive and Restrictive Lung Disease

Plethysmographic/ Spirometric Value	Obstructive Lung Disease	Restrictive Lung Disease
FVC	↓ or normal	↓
FEV_1	↓	↓
FEV_1/FVC	↓	$> 80\%$
TLC	Normal or ↑	↓
FRC	↑	↓
RV	Normal or ↑	↓
RV/TLC	↑	Normal

FVC = forced vital capacity; FEV_1 = forced expiratory volume in 1 second; FEV_1 (%) = FEV_1/FVC; TLC = total lung capacity; FRC = functional residual capacity; RV = residual volume.

Measurement of DLCO is usually performed as a single breath maneuver. The patient inhales a low concentration of CO mixed with a tracer gas such as helium. Any reduction in the concentration of the CO as it is exhaled and measured by the detecting sensor relates to its diffusion throughout the alveolar membrane and into RBCs as they circulate through the pulmonary capillaries.

Additional modalities for assessing pulmonary function, including **arterial blood gas measurement** and **oxygen saturation measurement,** are discussed in the section on respiratory physiology (see BLOOD GAS ANALYSIS and ESTIMATING OXYGENATION).

Radiologic Procedures

The reasons for obtaining plain chest films in children are numerous. All children with chronic coughs should have a recent chest radiograph (Figure 18.2). Sudden chest pain is an indication for radiography (Figure 18.3). Children with suspected pulmonary infections are obvious candidates for radiography. It is necessary to read films carefully and systematically (Table 18.12).

Computed tomography (CT) is a noninvasive procedure, which offers many advantages. CT scans of the sinuses are more sensitive and specific than plain radiographs, and such sinus films may be appropriate in patients with chronic purulent nasal secretions. In addition, CT allows assessment of the fine detail of the pulmonary parenchyma. Several patterns of CT abnormalities correspond with specific histologic diseases (Table 18.13).

High-resolution CT (HRCT), which combines the technique of obtaining frequent "slices" of images through the chest with high-frequency resolution, can provide the detail of structures as small as 0.5 mm. With HRCT, it is possible to stage disease severity and more readily follow response to therapy. Situations in which HRCT provides new or important information include airspace disease, complicated infections, empyema, evaluation of loculated effusions, immunocompromise, tuberculosis, pulmonary hemorrhage, pulmonary edema, interstitial disease, bronchopulmonary dysplasia, histiocytosis, sarcoid disease, bronchiectasis, cystic fibrosis (Figure 18.4), bronchiolitis obliterans, and bronchial obstruction. HRCT is also used as a guide for percutaneous biopsy or for open lung biopsy.

Barium studies (contrast esophagrams) may be warranted in infants who have cough associated with feeding or frequent large emesis after feedings. These procedures, which detect **vascular rings** or mediastinal lesions that impinge on the trachea and **tracheoesophageal fistulae,** are useful in the evaluation of swallowing dysfunction, esophageal anatomy, and intestinal obstructive defects.

Noncontrast use of fluoroscopy is helpful in assessing diaphragmatic excursion and upper

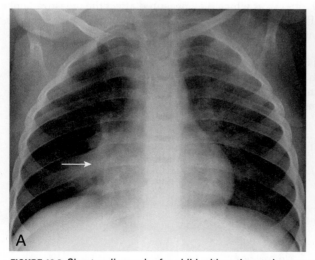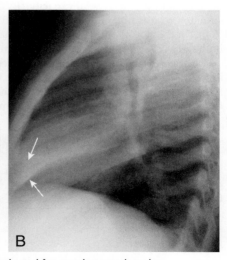

FIGURE 18.2. Chest radiograph of a child with asthma who was evaluated for ongoing cough and recurrent "pneumonia." A. This anteroposterior view clearly shows an area of atelectasis of the medial segment in the right middle lobe. This film demonstrates the classic "silhouette" sign, in which consolidation of the medial segment of the right middle lobe obscures the normal silhouette of the heart on the right border. B. This lateral view demonstrates the classic wedge-shaped opacity of right middle lobe atelectasis.

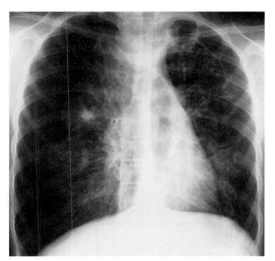

FIGURE 18.3. Chest radiograph showing a right-sided pneumothorax. This 11-year-old girl with severe lung disease due to cystic fibrosis complained of a sudden onset of chest pain. The right side of the chest film demonstrates a sickle-shaped area of a dark lucency at the apex of the thorax indicative of a pneumothorax.

airway and pharyngeal anatomy. Diagnosis of infants with stridor due to **laryngomalacia** or infants with wheezing and **tracheobronchomalacia** may involve fluoroscopy.

Tests for Specific Situations

Immunology studies (total IgG, IgM, and IgA titers, IgG subclass titers, antibody titers to previous vaccinations) warrant consideration in the evaluation of children with recurrent otitis, bronchiectasis, or productive cough unresponsive to antibiotics. Serum IgE levels and radioallergosorbent or skin testing are necessary for evaluation of atopic disease (see Chapter 17).

Ciliary function studies may be warranted in patients with purulent otitis unresponsive to antibiotics or patients with an association of sinusitis, otitis, pneumonia, bronchiectasis, with or without situs inversus anomaly. Such tests involve nuclear scans, which use technetium-99–labeled inhalant and real time imaging to evaluate mucociliary clearance time, or electron microscopy to evaluate ciliary structure.

Sweat chloride iontophoresis is used to diagnose cystic fibrosis. This test is indicated in all patients with an abnormal chest radiograph, failure to thrive, steatorrhea or constipation, a cough unresponsive to bronchodilator use and routine antibiotic courses, and sputum cultures previously positive for *Haemophilus influenzae*, *Staphylococcus aureus*, and *Pseudomonas aeruginosa*.

Pediatric Bronchoscopy

The direct visual examination of children's airways is an important diagnostic tool. Airway structure and anatomy can be directly visualized while the child is spontaneously breathing; the appearance of the airway mucosa can provide information about certain pathologic processes. Sampling tissues with biopsy or brushing or lavage of airway secretions can help establish specific diagnoses. Determination of the dynamic changes occurring in the airways may lead to diagnoses of laryngo-, tracheo-, or bronchomalacia. There are several indications for bronchoscopic evaluation, which have a variety of causes (Table 18.14). A pulmonologist may often perform a bronchoscopy to remove airway obstructions such as foreign bodies, inspissated secretions, or tissue masses. A bronchoscope may also be useful in the delivery of therapeutic agents to the lower airways.

Two types of bronchoscopes exist. The original bronchoscopes were rigid metal tubes passed through the mouth. Over the last 15 years, flexible fiberoptic instruments more suitable for use in very small infants and children have been developed. In general, rigid bronchoscopy is the procedure of choice for removal of foreign bodies, some dynamic studies of the airways, and for other therapeutic purposes. Flexible bronchoscopy is the preferred modality for cases that require diagnosis and lower airway (alveolar) sampling. The major advantage of using a rigid broncho-

TABLE 18.12	**Approach to the Chest Film: ABCS**
A	**A**bdomen: visceral situs, masses, free air, calcification, bowel loops, diaphragmatic contours
B	**B**ones: fractures, anomalies, masses
C	**C**hest
	Airway: patency, position, size, shape, peribronchiolar cuffing
	Mediastinum: position, size, shape
	Lungs: Volume, vascularity, density-opacity (linear markings, nodules, cysts vs. alveolar filling defects)
S	**S**oft tissue swelling, foreign body

TABLE 18.13	Patterns of Abnormalities Found on Computed Tomography (CT)
Abnormality	**Disease Entity**
Irregular linear pattern	Idiopathic pulmonary fibrosis
	Lymphatic tumor (lymphangiomatosis)
Cystic pattern	Cystic fibrosis
	Lymphangiomatosis
Nodular pattern	Cystic fibrosis
	Histiocytosis X
	Hypersensitivity pneumonitis
	Sarcoidosis
	Fungal infection
Ground glass pattern	Alveolar proteinosis
	Eosinophilic pneumonia
	Bronchiolitis obliterans with organizing pneumonia

scope lies in the fact that the inner diameter of the scope is usually large enough for the passage of instruments. In addition, it doubles as an endotracheal tube during the procedure, thus establishing and maintaining control of the airway and facilitating the delivery of oxygen and anesthetic gases. The primary drawback is that the bronchoscope must be passed through the patient's mouth to reach the trachea; the bronchoscopist must be able to open the mouth and extend the neck to provide a straight pathway. Certain congenital defects of the head and neck may obviate this method. General anesthesia is always required for rigid bronchoscopy.

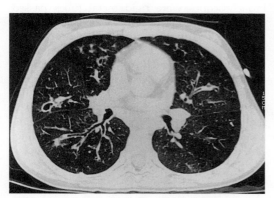

FIGURE 18.4. High-resolution computed tomography (HRCT) scan from the same girl described in Figure 18.3. Note that the definition of airway disease and areas of consolidation are more readily apparent, and the disease process is much more advanced than appears on the chest film. The airway walls are thickened, both the central and peripheral airways exhibit bronchiectatic changes, and opacifications are present where mucous plugs and lung consolidation exist.

SPECIFIC PULMONARY DISORDERS

STRIDOR

Stridor, a form of a wheeze, is frequently loud and harsh in quality. It is primarily described as an inspiratory sound. Children who exhibit difficulty breathing in the form of stridor are described as being **stridulous.**

Pathophysiology

In stridor, sound is generated by increased turbulent airflow from obstruction at the level of the larynx, the subglottic region of the larynx, and the extrathoracic trachea. The pitch is related to the degree of obstruction as well as to the velocity of airflow through the obstructed area. As a rule, the higher the pitch, the more severe the obstruction.

Clinical and Laboratory Evaluation

The previous discussion of the components of the history and physical examination allows the clinician to differentiate between intrathoracic and extrathoracic obstruction lesions of the airway (see CLINICAL APPROACH TO THE CHILD WITH PULMONARY DISEASE).

Laboratory Evaluation

Many diagnostic tools are available to evaluate the upper and lower airway for causes of stridor (Table 18.15). The test with the highest yield is **flexible fiberoptic bronchoscopy.** However, this procedure is invasive and not without risk (see PEDIATRIC BRONCHOSCOPY). **Fluoroscopy** of the airways, which is quicker and less invasive, can

TABLE 18.14	Indications for Bronchoscopy
Symptom	**Cause**
Stridor (recurrent or chronic)	Congenital laryngomalacia
	Cricoid ring
	Complete tracheal rings
	Mass lesion compressing trachea
Persistent wheezing	Tracheomalacia
	Bronchial or tracheal compression
	Foreign body aspiration
Pneumonia (acute)	Bacterial, fungal, or viral pathogen
Pneumonia (chronic or recurrent)	Tracheoesophageal fistula
	Recurrent aspiration
	Congenital airway anomaly
	Foreign body
	Pulmonary hemorrhage
	Alveolar proteinosis
Persistent cough	Anatomic abnormalities (tracheoesophageal fistula, tracheal bronchus)
	Foreign body aspiration
	Tracheomalacia
	Bronchomalacia
	Chronic infection (immune deficiency, cystic fibrosis)
Atelectasis	Mucous plugging unresponsive to medical therapy
	Foreign body
	Anatomic abnormality
Radiographic abnormalities	Localized hyperinflation (congenital lobar emphysema, bronchial stenosis, foreign body)
Hemoptysis	Acute pulmonary hemorrhage
Tracheostomy	Routine endoscopic evaluation of airway
	Evaluation of development of granulation tissue
	Bleeding, acute
	Evaluation of resolution of tracheo- or bronchomalacia
Vocal cord dysfunction	Vocal cord paralysis
	Vocal cord tethering
	Paradoxical vocal cord movement
Aid in endotracheal intubation	Congenital deformities of the airway

provide good dynamic visualization of the airway. However, this method may "miss" certain pathologies such as subglottic stenosis or intraluminal hemangioma, so if doubt still exists, bronchoscopy should be undertaken.

Differential Diagnosis

The differential diagnosis of stridor varies with the age at presentation, the type of noise, and the acuity of the presentation (see Table 18.15).

Management

Most causes of stridor require some form of medical or surgical intervention. The only type of stridor that might not require treatment is **congenital laryngomalacia.** Most infants are born with some degree of softness of the cartilage of the larynx; as they mature, this cartilage becomes stiffer. If the laryngomalacia is severe, the infant may suffer growth failure, develop a pectus excavatum deformity, or suffer chronic aspiration if the pressure generated during a vigorous gasp causes gastroesophageal reflux. These extreme and rare cases may require treatment with uvulopalatoplasty or with tracheostomy until the child is older.

ASTHMA

Asthma is defined as a disease of the bronchial airways characterized by hyperresponsiveness to inhaled allergen. The application of smooth muscle relaxants reverses the resulting bronchoconstrictive response. A heterogeneous disease, asthma has different clinical pictures and different pathogenic mechanisms.

Asthma occurs in about 4%–8% of the population, but urban areas have far higher reported rates, estimated at 20% in some areas. The inci-

TABLE 18.15 Diagnostic Evaluation of Stridor			
Condition	**Infants**	**Older Children/ Adolescents**	**Diagnostic Studies**
Acute onset			
Viral croup (laryngotracheobronchitis)	X	X	Anteroposterior neck radiograph
Spasmodic croup		X	History
Foreign body aspiration	X	X	Inspiratory and expiratory films, right and left lateral decubitus films, fluoroscopy, barium esophagram, rigid bronchoscopy
Epiglottitis		X	Lateral neck or direct visualization in operating room with qualified surgeon
Abscess: retropharyngeal, peritonsillar		X	Lateral neck radiograph
Allergic reaction		X	History
Trauma		X	History
Angioneurotic edema (C1 esterase deficiency)		X	History, C1 esterase level
Chronic onset			
Laryngomalacia	X		History, fluoroscopy, flexible bronchoscopy
Vocal cord dysfunction	X	X	Flexible bronchoscopy, history
Subglottic stenosis	X	X	History, pulmonary function test, flexible bronchoscopy
Laryngeal cyst, hemangioma, web, papilloma	X	X	Flexible bronchoscopy
Epiglottic cyst	X		Flexible bronchoscopy
Laryngotracheoesophageal cleft	X		Suspension laryngoscopy
Retained foreign body		X	Flexible bronchoscopy, rigid bronchoscopy

dence is highest during the first 3–4 years of life, with more than 80% of cases starting before 4 years of age. During these early years, both the immune system and the respiratory system undergo growth and maturation, which subsequently determine the pattern of future response of these systems to environmental exposure. Asthma is a developmental disease with a strong genetic component. The basic abnormality consists of an altered development of the patterns of immune and airway response to external stimuli; this abnormality probably persists for life.

Males are more likely than females to have asthma, and the disease clusters in certain regions of the United States such as the South and the West. However, the most striking clusters are in urban areas, where air pollutants may play a role. The incidence is also higher in the African-American population.

Pathophysiology

Various clinical conditions can be associated with lower airway obstruction during childhood, depending on age, gender, genetic background, and environmental exposure. Which of these conditions leads to the chronic asthmatic condition is poorly understood. The most important environmental factors in the development of asthma are the intensity, timing, and mode of exposure to aeroallergens that stimulate the production of IgE. Atopy and an increased predisposition to form IgE antibodies on exposure to common environmental antigens are present in the majority of patients with asthma (see Chapter 17). Exposure to high levels of inhaled allergens, especially dust mites, at an early age is an important determinant in the development of asthma. Additional environmental determinants are concurrent exposure to cofactors such as cigarette smoke. The role of food allergens in the pathogenesis of asthma is controversial. In general, pulmonary reactions to ingested foods are rare, and the correlation of hyperreactivity to food allergens with radioallergosorbent testing and abnormal IgE levels is low.

Two phases represent the pathophysiology of the inflammatory response in asthma: the early and late asthmatic reactions (Figure 18.5). In the **early asthmatic reaction,** rapid bronchoconstriction usually occurs, after bronchial provocation

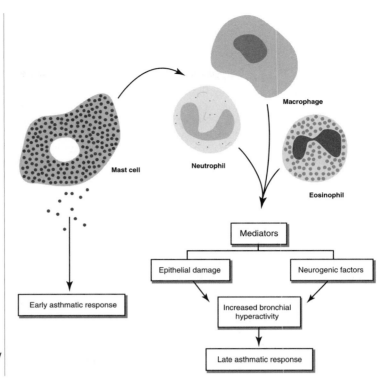

FIGURE 18.5. Asthma inflammatory cascade.

with an allergen to which the subject is sensitized; this lasts for about 1 hour. The cause of the acute inflammation of the airways is the release of mediators from a variety of effector cells such as mast cells and eosinophils. Mast cell degranulation leads to release of mediators including prostaglandins, leukotrienes, and other mediators which lead to signs of the late asthmatic reaction and result in increased vascular permeability, mucus hypersecretion, and smooth muscle contraction.

The **late asthmatic reaction,** a more prolonged phase of airway narrowing that follows the early asthmatic reaction, starts 2–3 hours after exposure, reaches a maximal airway response by 4–8 hours, and resolves in 12–24 hours. An overall increase in hyperresponsiveness marks this late asthmatic reaction; this increase may persist for days after the late asthmatic reaction appears to have resolved. Pathologic examination of asthmatic airways has shown a highly cellular infiltration into the bronchial epithelium of neutrophils, eosinophils, and lymphocytes. These cellular infiltrations are associated with destruction of bronchial epithelium, the expansion and activation of fibroblasts, and hypertrophy and hyperplasia of the smooth muscle. In fact, after airway inflammation has been established, airway hyperresponsiveness and symptoms can persist despite the removal of the responsible allergens, because structural and functional alterations remain.

Clinical and Laboratory Evaluation

Establishing the diagnosis of asthma in children may be challenging due to the extreme difficulty of testing airway reactivity to inhaled allergens. This procedure is usually not performed because of safety issues, especially in infants and small children. The nature of asthma is episodic. A thorough history and physical examination as well as knowledge of the child's response to bronchodilators and anti-inflammatory medications may suffice until the child is old enough to cooperate with spirometric testing procedures.

History
Knowledge of precipitating factors is valuable. Do the symptoms have a recurrent nature, suggesting environmental or seasonal factors? In older children, the most common triggers of asthma are dust or other aeroallergens, whereas in younger children, viral respiratory infections usually trigger asthma. Many families live in older homes that drain poorly during the winter and rainy seasons. This situation can lead to growth of molds in the home, which may lead to

development of allergic bronchopulmonary aspergillosis or mold hypersensitivity. For many children with a chronic cough, eliciting a history of a sudden appearance of cough, wheezing, or stridor may guide the diagnosis toward foreign body aspiration, especially in toddlers. Travel history and any recent history of immigration is important, too. Tuberculosis is endemic in several countries. Therefore, it is necessary to determine a family's country of origin and whether a tuberculosis skin test was administered on entry to the United States.

Other key questions that the pediatrician should ask during history-taking have been mentioned previously (see CLINICAL APPROACH TO THE CHILD WITH PULMONARY DISEASE, HISTORY). If a sibling has previously been diagnosed with asthma, the child in question is seven times more likely of being diagnosed with asthma. After elucidating the character of the disease, the physician should attempt to classify the asthma into one of four types (Table 18.16). Is it mild, mild persistent, moderate persistent, or severe? Because asthma can present in many different subtypes, this classification is somewhat arbitrary.

Physical Examination

Most children with asthma present with recurrent episodes of wheezing and dyspnea. Several different clinical syndromes may be apparent (Table 18.17).

Laboratory Evaluation

Pulmonary function testing before and after bronchodilator therapy is the most specific means of evaluation. These tests can be reliably performed in most clinics that treat children 5 years of age or older (see PULMONARY FUNCTION TESTS).

Management

Convincing evidence suggests that untreated asthma results in chronic inflammation that may induce structural changes in the asthmatic airway, leading to irreversible abnormalities in lung function. This knowledge has led to significant changes in both the short- and long-term management of the disease.

As previously described, recurrent bouts of asthma may lead to cellular infiltration into the airways, and fibrotic remodeling of the airways

---

TABLE 18.16 **Classification of Asthma Subtypes**

| Characteristics | Asthma Subtype | | |
	Mild Persistent	Moderate Persistent	Severe
Frequency of exacerbations	1–2 times/week	2 times/week <3 ED visits/year	Daily wheezing Sudden, severe exacerbations >3 ED visits/year >2 hospitalizations/year
Frequency of symptoms	Few between exacerbations	Cough/low-grade wheeze frequent	Continuous low-grade cough Wheezing always present
Exercise tolerance	Good	Diminished	Very poor; limited activity
Nocturnal asthma	1–2 times/month	2–3 times/week	> 3 times/week
School attendance	Good	Occasional absence	Frequently absent
Pulmonary function			
• Peak expiratory flow rate	80% predicted; variability < 20% A.M. to P.M.	60%–80% of predicted; variability ≤ 30%	< 60% predicted; variability > 30%
• Spirometry	Minimal obstruction; > 15% response to bronchodilator	Obstruction at low lung volumes; > 15% response to bronchodilator	Scalloped flow–volume loop ≤35% predicted flow in small airways
• Methacholine sensitivity*	$PC_{20} > 20$ mg/ml	$PC_{20} = 2$–20 mg/ml	$PC_{20} < 2$ mg/ml

ED = emergency department.

*Sensitivity to methacholine is measured by the PC_{20}, of the dose of methacholine inhalation challenge that results in a decrease in the FEV_1 by 20% from baseline.

TABLE 18.17	Clinical Appearance of Asthma
Clinical Syndrome	**Symptoms/Signs**
Classical episodic asthma	Episodes of coughing and/or wheezing that occur intermittently
	Between episodes, no overt symptomatology
Persistent asthma	Daily symptoms
	Acute, severe exacerbations
Cough-variant asthma	Cough only
Hypersecretory asthma (common in infants and children, especially after viral infections)	Recurrent cough with bronchitis
Recurrent "pneumonia"	Similar to pneumonia in radiologic appearance, with excessive, tenacious mucous secretions blocking larger airways, causing atelectasis of segments and subsegments
Exercise-induced asthma	Severe bouts of bronchospasm triggered only by exercise and/or cold air
	Seemingly well between episodes
Severe episodic asthma	Life-threatening attacks
	Symptom-free and quite well between episodes
Persistent wheezing (infants known as the "fat, happy wheezers")	Usually without much respiratory distress
	Often due to chronic aspiration from gastro-esophageal reflux

develops in severe asthma. While it is not currently known whether these pathophysiologic changes eventually occur in patients with all levels of severity of asthma, the currently available medications have been refined and proven safe for long-term use in children.

A written treatment plan may also help patients with asthma. The **Asthma Action Plan,** commonly used by physicians, is a method for asthma management and monitoring that patients take home and use to help modify their medication regimen based on changes in their clinical status (e.g., shortness of breath, cough, chest tightness).

Medical Treatment

In general, any child with persistent asthma should receive preventive daily treatment with an anti-inflammatory therapy (Table 18.18). The purpose of anti-inflammatory treatment is to decrease the number of exacerbations experienced by a particular child. It is hoped that this will lead to a more normal lifestyle as well as greater participation in usual childhood activities. Additional therapy may be necessary depending on the type of asthma the child has (Table 18.19).

Children with only seasonal symptomatology may require daily use of anti-inflammatory medications, starting several weeks before the expected antigen exposure. For patients with exercise-induced asthma, inhaled cromolyn sodium or salmeterol, taken 15–30 minutes before exercise, can offer effective prophylaxis against bronchospasm.

Children with asthma who experience more frequent symptoms should receive daily prophylaxis with anti-inflammatory therapy. β-agonists can be used in conjunction, based on peak flow rates and the asthma action plan. The medication most commonly prescribed to achieve effective anti-inflammatory treatment is generally an inhaled corticosteroid (ICS) such as beclomethasone, fluticasone, or budesonide. Fluticasone has the highest topical-to-systemic ratio of drug absorption, is rapidly metabolized by the liver, and is very potent compared to other ICSs. Therefore, it is often the ICS drug of first choice. A trial of an inhaled form of a nonsteroidal anti-inflammatory drug (NSAID) [cromolyn sodium] is warranted in children with mild asthma, given the extremely low level of adverse reactions and lack of systemic uptake of the drug. If this is not helpful, and breakthrough episodes of wheezing still occur frequently, then replacement with an ICS is necessary. Both ICSs and cromolyn sodium may require several weeks of daily use before the beneficial effects are realized.

Pediatric Pearl

Corticosteroids are the most efficacious treatment currently available for the long-term management of asthma.

The anti-inflammatory effects of corticosteroids are likely to be via directly inhibiting the binding

TABLE 18.18 Medications Used for Treatment of Asthma				
Medication	Mild Intermittent	Mild Persistent	Moderate Persistent	Severe
β-agonist				
Short-acting	As needed	As needed	As needed	As needed
Long-acting	No	No	Daily	Daily
Anti-inflammatory				
Cromolyn sodium	Seasonal use for extrinsic asthma	Trial of 2 months may be considered	No	No
Inhaled corticosteroid	No	Yes	Yes	Yes
Leukotriene receptor antagonist or synthesis inhibitor	No	Yes, but not as monotherapy	Yes	Yes
Anticholinergic	No	Consider	Yes	Yes
Theophylline	No	No	Consider	Yes

of certain transcription factors to cellular DNA that are activated by signals from inflammatory cells. Corticosteroids also up-regulate the number of β-adrenergic receptors on bronchial smooth muscle. Within the respiratory epithelium, corticosteroids decrease the numbers of inflammatory cells such as eosinophils, basophils, and polymorphonuclear cells. However, it may take as long as 6 months to reverse the histologic changes present in asthma-affected airways.

Children with severe, uncontrollable asthma, which is diagnosed in less than 10% of cases, require a medication regimen that "brings out the big guns" quickly and effectively. The use of two or three types of bronchodilators may be necessary, along with large doses of inhaled steroids.

Leukotriene receptor antagonists and leukotriene-synthesis inhibitors provide new mediator-specific therapy for asthma. These agents block the inflammatory airway response to inhaled aeroallergen challenge. In chronic asthma, they lead to improved lung function, reduced symptoms, and they frequently can allow for reduced doses of ICSs. Because several studies reported that these medications are less effective than steroids, it is not recommended that they be used as monotherapy.

In addition, the use of long-acting β-agonists such as salmeterol is often indicated. These drugs bind more tightly to the β-agonist receptor and have a duration of action of up to 12 hours. Oral β-agonists are effective, along with sustained-release theophylline preparations. However, systemic side effects such as jitteriness, hyperactivity, headache, and emesis are frequent when serum levels exceed the therapeutic range (for theophylline and other xanthine derivatives).

Unfortunately, children with asthma are often undertreated, based on the perception by both parents and physicians that long-term treatment with ICSs is deleterious. Much investigation has taken place concerning the possible association of long-term use of ICSs and bone growth delay as well as other side effects such as adrenal suppression, behavioral changes, blood glucose elevation, and cataracts. Side effects are rare with ICSs, but can occur, primarily when high doses are used. It is necessary to regularly monitor children who receive long-term treatment with ICSs for elevation in blood pressure, serum blood sugar, lag in growth, and cataract development (i.e., yearly ophthalmologic examinations). However, recent studies have shown only a 1-cm difference in height between moderate asthmatics treated with 400 µg/day of budesonide and their healthy cohorts, with no occurrence of side effects consistent with adrenal suppression or corticosteroid excess. In addition, ICSs have been associated with dysphonia and thrush, but it is possible to avert these conditions by using spacer devices.

Methods of Drug Delivery

In asthma therapy, inhalation tends to be the preferred mode of drug delivery. Not only does it allow for more rapid onset of action and lower dosage requirements, but it also eliminates systemic side effects of drugs that are also available in ingestible form. Three inhalation systems are currently available for the delivery of aerosolized medications: metered-dose inhalers, dry-powder inhalers, and nebulizers used with liquid preparations.

Metered-dose inhalers have the advantage of being portable, lightweight, and less expensive

TABLE 18.19 Medications Used in Asthma

Medication	Action	Dose	Side Effects
Albuterol Salbutamol	β-agonist Bronchodilator	MDI (90 μg/puff): 2 puffs per dose q4–6hr; can be used q1hr in monitored setting DPI (200 mg/capsule): 1 inhalation q4–6hr Neb solution (0.5%): 0.25–0.5 ml in 2 ml diluent Neb solution premix (0.083%): 1 vial q4–6hr	Tachycardia, jitteriness, hyperactivity
Salmeterol	β-agonist, bronchodilator, long acting	MDI (25 μg/puff): 2 puffs bid DPI (50 μg/puff): 1 puff bid	Tachycardia, jitteriness, hyperactivity
Ipratropium bromide	Anticholinergic, inhibits bronchospasm	MDI (18 μg/puff): 2 puffs q4hr prn	Dry mouth or respiratory secretions
Beclomethasone dipropionate	ICS, preventive, anti-inflammatory	MDI (42 μg/puff): 2 puffs bid DPI (100 μg/puff): 1 puff bid	Thrush, adrenocortical suppression (very high doses)
Fluticasone	ICS	MDI (44, 110, 220 μg/puff): 1–2 puffs bid	Thrush, adrenocortical suppression (very high doses)
Flunisolide	ICS	MDI (250 μg/puff): 1–2 puffs bid	Thrush, adrenocortical suppression (very high doses)
Budesonide	ICS	DPI (100, 200 μg/puff): 1–2 puffs qd-bid Neb solution premix (250, 500 μg/ml): 0.5–1 ml qd–bid	Thrush, adrenocortical suppression (very high doses)
Montelukast	Leukotriene receptor antagonist	4 mg chewable tablet qhs for children 2–4 years of age 5 mg chewable tablet qhs for children 5–11 years of age 10 mg tablet qhs for children ≥ 12 years of age	Headache, gastritis
Zileuton	Leukotriene synthesis inhibitor	10 mg PO bid for children ≥ 12 years of age	Headache, gastritis, liver enzyme elevation
Cromolyn sodium	Mast cell stabilizer	20 mg MDI or neb solution tid or 15 min before exercise	None

DPI = dry-powder inhaler; ICS = inhaled corticosteroid; MDI = metered-dose inhaler; neb = nebulizer; q = every; bid = twice a day; prn = as needed; qhs = every night before sleep.

than the liquid nebulizer forms of medications. The disadvantage of using a metered-dose inhaler is the high speed of delivery; when the inhaler is actuated, the medication is dispensed from the canister at a speed approximating 400 miles/hour! This leads to impaction of nearly 99% of the med-ication on the oropharynx; only 1% of the medication reaches the lungs. The prescription of a spacer device, which ameliorates this problem, is warranted in all children. It is necessary to inhale one puff of medication at a time. The medication can be inhaled either through the mouth as a single breath or with panting tidal maneuvers with equal effect. Spacers can be used in infants; they are available with masks that fit around the nose and mouth for a tight seal. Older children can use spacers fitted with a mouthpiece.

Because of environmental concerns, the availability of metered-dose inhalers will be severely limited by 2005. **Dry-powder inhalers** are breath-actuated devices designed to eliminate the use of fluorocarbons (the propellant used in metered-dose inhalers) and to obviate the need for spacer devices. Dry-powder inhalers, like metered-dose inhalers, are also portable, lightweight, and less expensive than the liquid nebulizer preparations. However, not all medications are yet available in dry-powder inhalant form.

Nebulizers are used for two reasons: (1) they are effective, and (2) even the most cooperative child may not receive adequate amounts of medication by metered-dose inhalers or dry-powder inhalers. In addition, the breathing pattern of infants or children have a great effect on intrapulmonary deposition of medication. Nebulizers may thus be more effective in children with tachypnea and cough in the setting of an acute asthma attack.

CYSTIC FIBROSIS

Cystic fibrosis is a chronic, multisystem, lethal recessive disorder that results from defective epithelial chloride transport with major manifestations affecting the respiratory, gastrointestinal (GI), and reproductive systems. The primary morbidity results from progressive obstructive lung disease. In addition, a very large percentage of patients with cystic fibrosis are pancreatic insufficient, which manifests as malabsorption and insulin deficiency. Nearly 100% of affected patients also have chronic sinusitis and nasal polyposis. Male infertility results from congenital bilateral absence or eventual obstruction and scarring of the vas deferens. Other less common problems encountered in patients with cystic fibrosis include cirrhosis of the liver, cholelithiasis, recurrent pancreatitis, gastroesophageal reflux, and GI hypomotility.

In the past, the prognosis in patients with cystic fibrosis was quite grave, and most infants and children did not survive past the age of 5 years. Due to the advent of supplemental enzymes to aid in food digestion and absorption, refined methods of chest physiotherapy, and improved antibiotics, the median survival age for individuals with cystic fibrosis in the United States is now approximately 31 years. Associated symptoms and the rate of decline in pulmonary function vary widely in severity, and many patients are now living into their 40s and 50s. It is difficult to predict the life expectancy of a child born in 2001 with cystic fibrosis because of the time delay of the impact of changes in therapy on life expectancy.

Pathophysiology

Cystic fibrosis is inherited in an autosomal recessive pattern; both parents are usually asymptomatic carriers of the gene mutation. The most common lethal genetic disease affecting Caucasians, cystic fibrosis has an incidence of approximately 1 in 2500 live births, with a corresponding carrier frequency of 1 in 32. In Mexican Americans, the incidence is approximately 1 in 4500 live births. In African Americans, the incidence is approximately 1 in 17,000. Cystic fibrosis is extremely rare in persons of native African or Asian descent.

Mutations in the cystic fibrosis transmembrane conductance regulator (CFTR), located on chromosome 7, are responsible for cystic fibrosis. The gene, which was cloned in 1989, is quite large, containing over 250,000 base pairs; it encodes a chloride channel protein of 1480 amino acids. To date, scientists have identified over 1000 mutations. The ΔF508 mutation is a three-base pair deletion that results in deletion of a phenylalanine at position 508 of the protein. This mutation, which most commonly occurs in persons of Anglo-Saxon descent, is found in approximately 75% of patients with cystic fibrosis. The large number of mutations described so far limits the usefulness of DNA analysis as a screening test for cystic fibrosis.

Some CFTR mutations are associated with more severe disease expression than others, and ΔF508 is one of the mutations most commonly associated with the "severe" phenotype. Conversely, patients with mutations correlated with normal pancreatic function tend to have a "milder" cystic fibrosis phenotype. Although there is a correlation between genotype and pancreatic status, there is no correlation between specific mutations and pulmonary phenotype, implying the presence of modifier genes that impact on the expression of the disease.

In cystic fibrosis, the characteristic defect involves a reduced ability of epithelial cells in the airways and pancreas to secrete chloride in response to cAMP-mediated agonists. The decrease in chloride secretion into the airway leads to decreased fluid in the airways, which is thought to lead to relatively dehydrated respiratory (and intestinal) secretions, abnormal mucociliary clearance, and eventually, lung disease. The exact pathophysiologic mechanism of altered ion and water transport across the epithelia of these organs is not completely known, and the understanding of how CFTR dysfunction leads to organ dysfunction is a matter of much debate. Whatever the mechanism is, it is clear that the CFTR defect eventually leads to inflammation and chronic obstruction of the lungs (Figure 18.6).

Colonization with certain strains of bacteria, usually *Staphylococcus aureus, Haemophilus influen-*

Pathogenesis of CF lung disease

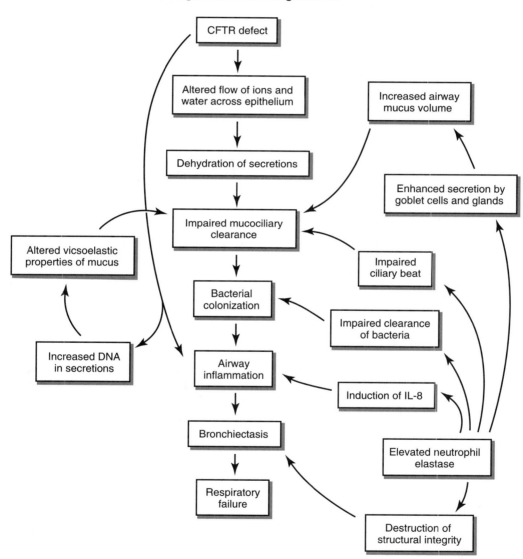

FIGURE 18.6. Pathogenesis of lung disease in cystic fibrosis. Airway secretions, being dehydrated and viscous, obstruct the airway. Pathologic changes include inflammatory cell infiltration of the airways, goblet cell hyperplasia, and submucosal gland hypertrophy. Bacterial colonization may occur. Chronic infection and inflammation leads to bronchiectasis and peribronchial fibrosis. Mucociliary clearance is also greatly impaired. CFTR = cystic fibrosis transmembrane conductance regulator; IL-8 = interleukin 8.

zae, and *Pseudomonas aeruginosa* eventually occurs in cystic fibrosis. Scientists believe that bacterial colonization is due to increased adherence of these organisms to the airway epithelia. Colonization with *S. aureus* and *H. influenzae* is common in infants and younger children with cystic fibrosis. *P. aeruginosa* colonizes approximately 75% of children by 10 years of age. After colonization with *P. aeruginosa*, lung function deteriorates more rapidly.

Another classic pathologic feature of the cystic fibrosis airway is the infiltration of inflammatory cells into the airways, even in early lung disease and in patients who are not yet colonized by bacteria. Neutrophil elastase appears to be a major player in the pathogenesis of cystic and bronchiectatic changes.

Clinical and Laboratory Evaluation

History

Cystic fibrosis has many clinical manifestations (Table 18.20). Meconium ileus of the newborn is the most common manifestation in infants. Respiratory symptomatology becomes the more common presenting sign in older infants, toddlers, and children with cystic fibrosis.

Intestinal obstruction is common in patients with cystic fibrosis. Meconium ileus is a presenting sign in about 20% of infants with cystic fibrosis immediately after birth and may lead to intestinal perforation. In older patients, a meconium ileus "equivalent" syndrome results in distal intestinal obstruction due to the bulkiness of the stools. Episodes of rectal prolapse occur because of this condition and should serve as a "red flag" for the practitioner. The incidence of intussusception is high for this reason as well. Children with a history of slow growth or failure to thrive, even in the absence of respiratory problems, should also be evaluated for cystic fibrosis.

Physical Examination

Some of the many findings discovered by the physical examination in cystic fibrosis are "classic," and their presence may be a strong indication for cystic fibrosis testing. Children with cystic fibrosis are frequently at the 25th percentile on growth charts. However, it is important to note that 20% of children with cystic fibrosis have normal pancreatic function for the first 5 years of life, and therefore, may not present initially with failure to thrive.

Physical examination in children with cystic fibrosis should begin with the head—the nose in particular. Virtually all patients with the disease have inflamed erythematous nasal mucosa. One of the most classic findings is nasal polyps, which are often growing from the epithelium of the nasal turbinates. These opaque–white structures are composed of mucus-secreting epithelium and glisten in the light of the otoscope. They are similar to a small bunch of grapes in appearance.

Although sinusitis and rhinitis are universal, signs such as pain to palpation or frequent headaches are most often absent. In addition, the maxillary sinuses of affected patients are small, and the frontal sinuses often are hypoplastic or completely absent. If this is evident on a sinus CT, it is nearly always an indication of cystic fibrosis.

The examination of the chest in patients with moderate or severe disease may reveal signs of air trapping, including the use of the suprasternal accessory muscles of respiration, some bowing of the sternum, or kyphosis of the superior thoracic spine, which all cause an evident increase from the normal anterior–posterior dimension of the chest. Crackles and wheezes are not unusual, but in infants, the most common finding is only wheezing or a slightly prolonged expiratory phase.

Examination of the abdomen may reveal the presence of firm but ill-defined stool masses in the colon. Hepatomegaly is rare, but splenomegaly may be present in patients with significant biliary cirrhosis. Palpation of the spermatic cord in boys may reveal the absence of the vas deferens.

The fingers and toes show changes associated with clubbing early in the disease process. There are four grades of clubbing (Table 18.21). Signs such as cardiac abnormalities consistent with cor pulmonale are rare.

Laboratory Evaluation

The gold standard for diagnosis of cystic fibrosis is the sweat test or pilocarpine iontophoresis test. Because cystic fibrosis affects the sweat glands, affected patients are less able to reabsorb chloride from sweat than normal individuals. This leads to a very high level of chloride in the sweat and a reliable method of diagnosis. Premature infants lack fully developed, mature sweat glands, but usually by the time a term infant is 9 weeks of age, the test can be performed successfully.

Pediatric Pearl

False-positive sweat tests do occur. Causes include adrenal insufficiency, ectodermal dysplasia, nephrogenic diabetes insipidus, glycogen storage disease type 1, anorexia nervosa, hypoparathyroidism, familial cholestatic syndromes, malnutrition, hypothyroidism, mucopolysaccharidoses, and fucosidosis.

TABLE 18.20 | **Clinical Manifestations and Treatment of Cystic Fibrosis**

Symptom	Treatment
Upper Respiratory Tract	
Nasal polyposis	Nasal saline rinses, topical corticosteroid, polypectomy
Sinusitis	Maxillary antrostomy and ethmoidectomy, antibiotic flushes
Pulmonary	
Bronchiolitis, bronchiectasis	ICS, high-dose ibuprofen, chest physiotherapy, oral corticosteroids, antibiotic
Atelectasis	Chest physiotherapy, ICS, antibiotic, oral corticosteroids
Bronchitis	Chest physiotherapy, antibiotic, ICS, oral corticosteroids, mucolytics
Hemoptysis	Arterial embolization, transfusion
Pneumothorax	Chest tube, fibrin glue, surgical stapling, pleurodesis
Pneumonia	Intravenous, inhaled, or oral antibiotic, chest physiotherapy
Reactive airway disease	ICS, oral corticosteroids, β-agonist, anticholinergic agents
Respiratory failure	Oxygen, noninvasive mechanical ventilation, endotracheal intubation with mechanical ventilation, lung transplant
Gastrointestinal	
Gastroesophageal reflux	Antacid, intestinal prokinetic agent, fundoplication
Intussusception	N-acetylcysteine enema, Gastrografin or hypaque enema, surgery
Meconium ileus	N-acetylcysteine by nasogastric tube, lactulose, surgery
Meconium ileus equivalent (distal intestinal obstruction syndrome)	N-acetylcysteine by nasogastric tube, lactulose, laxative, hypaque enema
Pancreatic exocrine deficiency	Pancreatic enzyme replacement, antacid, gastrointestinal promotility agents
Pancreatitis	NPO, fluid, low-fat diet, surgery
Peptic ulcer disease	Antacid
Rectal prolapse	Enhanced nutrition and optimized pancreatic enzyme replacement, surgical treatment rarely necessary
Hepatobiliary	
Cholecystitis	Antibiotic therapy
Cholelithiasis	Ursodeoxycholic acid, cholecystectomy
Cholestasis	Ursodeoxycholic acid, pancreatic enzyme, gastrointestinal prokinetic agent
Cirrhosis/portal hypertension	Liver transplant, lactulose, ursodeoxycholic acid, splenectomy
Nutritional/Metabolic	
Diabetes mellitus	Insulin, oral hypoglycemics
Hypoprothrombinemia	Vitamin K
Iron deficiency anemia	Iron
Salt depletion syndrome	High-salt diet, liquid intake
Protein-calorie malnutrition	High-calorie, high-protein diet with pancreatic enzyme replacement therapy
Vitamin A deficiency	5000–10,000 IU/week supplement
Vitamin E deficiency	400–800 IU/day supplement
Failure to thrive	Nutritional support, pancreatic enzyme, intravenous lipids
Malnutrition	Nutritional support, pancreatic enzyme
Growth retardation	Nutritional support, pancreatic enzyme
Osteoporosis	Calcium replacement, pamidronate, high-dose vitamin D replacement
Miscellaneous	
Arthritis/arthropathy	Analgesics, pamidronate
Clubbing of the digits	
Absence of the vas deferens	
Decreased female fertility	
Delayed puberty	
Erythema nodosum	Oral corticosteroid therapy

ICS = inhaled corticosteroid; NPO = nothing by mouth.

TABLE 18.21	Stages of Clubbing

Stage	Description
0	Normal
1+	Obliteration of notch at fingernail cuticle
2+	Slight rounding of base of nail
3+	Involvement of soft tissues of finger pad
4+	Most extreme amount of clubbing, described as a "parrot's beak"

Management

The management of patients with cystic fibrosis can be very complicated because of the multisystem involvement and a high frequency of complications. For these reasons, a comprehensive and intensive therapeutic program is essential. A physician experienced in cystic fibrosis and its manifestations should follow all affected patients at intervals of 2–3 months. A team approach, including nursing, nutrition, physical therapy, respiratory therapy, and counseling personnel, is most beneficial. A variety of therapeutic measures are useful (see Table 18.20).

Treatment of Pulmonary Problems

Treatment of pulmonary complications of cystic fibrosis, which occurs on a daily basis, focuses on clearance of excess mucus from the tracheobronchial tree. There are several modes of clearance: flutter device; positive expiratory pressure device; manual chest physiotherapy; intrapulmonary percussive ventilation; percussion vest; active cycle of breathing; and autogenic drainage. These are forms of airway clearance that center on meditation and airways clearance maneuvers rather than assistance with mechanical devices. No studies have found that one particular method provides more optimal clearance than the others, and individual patients have different experiences with each of the different modes. Clinicians should educate patients about the importance of daily clearance of mucus and expect them to perform twice-daily airways clearance sessions once a mode of treatment has been selected.

It is necessary to use aggressive antibiotic therapy when patients begin to experience "the dwindles"—a characteristic slow deterioration of pulmonary function that usually presents as an increase in baseline cough, sputum production, wheezing, crackles, and weight loss. When available, the patient's most recent sputum or throat culture guides antibiotic therapy. A recent addition to the routine regimen for patients colonized with *P. aeruginosa* has been twice-daily dosing with inhaled tobramycin, given for 28-day cycles every other month.

If hospitalization for cystic fibrosis–associated pneumonia is necessary, double antibiotic therapy is used in the treatment of a gram-negative bacillus such as *P. aeruginosa* to achieve a synergistic bactericidal effect. The most common antibiotic regimens use an aminoglycoside such as tobramycin combined with a third-generation semisynthetic penicillin or a cephalosporin that has adequate antipseudomonal activity (ceftazidime or cefepime).

No clinical trials have found that corticosteroids are effective in slowing the rate of pulmonary deterioration in cystic fibrosis. These agents do not diminish chronic airway inflammation. However, NSAIDs appear to slow the progression of lung disease significantly. Some patients with cystic fibrosis who are older than 5 years of age have received high-dose ibuprofen as an addition to their daily drug regimen. Doses are 20–30 mg/kg/dose twice daily.

Because of the high concentration of DNA released from dead leukocytes, the sputum of patients with cystic fibrosis is more abundant and has increased viscosity. Recombinant human DNAse (rhDNAse) is effective in decreasing sputum viscosity, increasing expectorated quantity, and minimizing the number of pulmonary exacerbations.

In most patients with cystic fibrosis who have severe, end-stage lung disease, lung transplantation is an option. Since 1985, more than 750 patients with cystic fibrosis in the United States have undergone lung transplantation. The 2-year survival rate is approximately 65%. The survival rate of cystic fibrosis patients after transplant is no different than for non–cystic fibrosis patients who undergo heart–lung or double-lung transplantation.

Treatment of Gastrointestinal Problems

GI symptomatology is typical in patients with cystic fibrosis. However, treatment with oral pancreatic enzyme replacement therapy is often all that is needed to improve and maintain adequate nutritional status and minimize malabsorption, steatorrhea, constipation, and diarrhea. Pancreatic enzymes are available in many forms (powder, capsule, gel). Most patients are maintained on lipase 500—5000 U/kg/meal. Infants often require the powdered form added to their formula. The capsules contain small microencapsulated enzymes, which are protected from acid digestion in the stomach, and are most active in the duodenum and ileum, where the pH is alkaline. Because patients with cystic fibrosis tend to be pancreatic insufficient, they may require concomitant doses of antacid to maximize the activity of the pancreatic enzyme in the small intestine.

Treatment of Complications

HEMOPTYSIS. Patients often experience blood streaking of their sputum, which is probably due to rupture of surface capillaries secondary to vigorous coughing. A larger danger exists if bleeding occurs due to erosion of a bronchus into a bronchial artery; this most often occurs in association with a pulmonary exacerbation. Massive hemoptysis, a serious complication in patients with advanced disease, results in significant mortality. Although the condition occurs in less than 10% of adults and rarely in children, an estimated 1% of all patients with cystic fibrosis die from massive hemoptysis. The majority of patients who experience this complication and survive will suffer a recurrence.

For significant bleeding, a procedure known as arterial embolization is used to control the rupture. It involves a procedure similar to cardiac catheterization, in which the femoral artery is entered and the catheter passed up the aorta to the point of branching of the bronchial arteries. Abnormal arterialization to the lung from the aorta, the internal thoracic artery, and the thyroid artery are most often the culprits; they can be embolized with fibrin beads or springs placed in the blood vessel.

PNEUMOTHORAX. Pneumothorax, which occurs in 8%–23% of older patients with cystic fibrosis, may affect children with severe disease. The mortality rate is about 4%, and the recurrence rate is 50%–70%. Rupture of subpleural blebs are the progenitors of pneumothorax in most patients.

Treatment for pneumothorax varies. If the area is small and the patient is stable, treatment with 100% oxygen by mask is preferred. However, a bronchopleural fistula may persist, and treatment with fibrin glue to obliterate the pleural space may be necessary. Partial pleurectomy has the highest success rate, but if the patient is a lung transplant candidate, intercostal drainage, chemical pleurodesis, ligation of bullae, or limited surgical pleurodesis should be performed in preference to pleurectomy.

RESPIRATORY FAILURE AND COR PULMONALE. Hypertrophy of the right ventricle is common in adults with severe cystic fibrosis. However, progression to overt cardiac failure is not, and once it develops, survival time is short. Before cor pulmonale develops, oxygen therapy may begin, initially for nocturnal use.

Intubation and mechanical ventilation are considered futile in most patients with severe lung dysfunction unless there is an acute reversible problem (e.g., hemoptysis, pneumothorax); after its resolution, removal of the mechanical ventilation may occur. However, nasal mechanical ventilation with bilevel positive airway pressure (BiPAP) supports many patients nocturnally or as a bridge to eventual lung transplantation.

BRONCHOPULMONARY DYSPLASIA/CHRONIC LUNG DISEASE

Previous clinical observations and investigations suggest that **bronchopulmonary dysplasia (BPD)** is the chronic phase of neonatal lung damage caused by oxidant injury and barotrauma in susceptible premature infants. Over 30 years ago, BPD was described as a progression of characteristic radiographic findings that correlate with pathologic changes of acute and chronic inflammation, fibrosis, and bronchial smooth muscle hypertrophy in premature respiratory-dependent infants. Despite the improved survival of extremely low birth weight infants (< 1000 g) since the introduction of exogenous surfactant, BPD remains a major cause of morbidity in neonatal intensive care units (NICUs).

Diagnosis

In the absence of formal diagnostic criteria, practitioners use the following clinical standards to define BPD.

1. Need for positive pressure ventilation for at least 3 days
2. Signs of respiratory distress such as tachypnea, wheezing, and retractions
3. Need for supplemental oxygen to maintain PaO_2 at greater than 50 mm Hg at 28 days of life
4. Presence of typical radiographic changes (see Chapter 10, Neonatology)

However, these criteria are insufficient; most infants who weigh less than 1000 g at birth are still oxygen-dependent after 4 weeks. A modified criterion suggests that BPD can be diagnosed if an infant requires oxygen therapy at 36 weeks' gestational age, regardless of age at birth.

The term **chronic lung disease (CLD)** refers to the complex interaction of antenatal and postnatal factors that lead to ongoing symptomatology and need for treatment for respiratory problems in infants. CLD describes a wide variety of disorders that affect the upper and lower respiratory tract, including BPD.

CLD is frequently accompanied by other disorders, such as cardiovascular problems, gastroesophageal reflux, congenital anomalies, growth impairment and nutritional difficulty, and sensory and neurodevelopmental handicaps. The pediatrician must follow these conditions closely. It is important to realize that many affected infants will require ongoing respiratory treatment for the first 2 years of life, if not longer.

A large proportion of children with CLD have concomitant reactive airways disease. Bronchodilators improve gas exchange and decrease the resistance of the airways such that the work of breathing is reduced after bronchodilator administration. Anti-inflammatory agents such as inhaled corticosteroids (see asthma) are also commonly used as a means to decrease airway reactivity and also to hasten the resolution of inflammatory status of the airway epithelium and avoid fibrotic remodeling of the airways. No controlled trials have demonstrated that long-term use of corticosteroids leads to an improvement in pulmonary function in older children or adults.

In CLD, there is evidence of a disturbance in water balance and chronic peribronchiolar edema. Diuretics are frequently used to decrease interstitial fluid, increase pulmonary compliance, and minimize small airway obstruction. However, there is no convincing evidence that this medication is effective for long periods of time, and infants are often allowed to "outgrow" their disease after they are discharged from the NICU.

Management

Adequate oxygenation is the cornerstone of CLD management. However, controversy exists about how low oxygen levels should be before infants are considered hypoxic, and thus, what PaO_2 level to attain once supplemental oxygen is prescribed. Chronically hypoxemic children exhibit growth failure, developmental delays, and they may have pulmonary hypertension. Too much oxygen promotes the formation of oxygen radicals in airways where an inflammatory process is occurring; this leads to poor lung function in the long run.

APNEA AND THE CONTROL OF BREATHING

The problem of infantile apnea is difficult for pediatricians, it is impossible to establish an underlying cause in many cases. Parents want to be reassured that their child is not at risk for **sudden infant death syndrome (SIDS; crib death).** Unfortunately, no predictive tools are available to assess the risk of SIDS in any individual infant. In this section, SIDS will be discussed, and the approach to the conditions of **apnea of infancy** and **apparent life-threatening event (ALTE)** will also be addressed. Each of these terms has a particular meaning for pediatricians (Table 18.22).

SUDDEN INFANT DEATH SYNDROME

Sudden infant death syndrome (SIDS) is the sudden death of an infant younger than 1 year of age that remains unexplained after completion of a postmortem investigation, including an autopsy, examination of the scene of death, and review of the clinical history. In 1998, SIDS was the third leading cause of infant mortality (8.9%) in the United States after congenital anomalies (22%) and short gestation/low birth weight (14%).

Deaths from SIDS follow a recognizable epidemiologic pattern. They are most likely to occur in the colder months and in the second to fourth months of life. The risk for SIDS in siblings of SIDS victims is approximately four times greater than in the general population. The rates of SIDS in the United States are higher for black infants than for white, Hispanic, and Asian infants.

In California, SIDS-related public health measures were initiated during the early 1990s. To help standardize the diagnosis of SIDS, autopsy and death scene protocols, including medical history, were developed by an expert committee and implemented after legislative mandate.

Pathophysiology

No single mechanism for SIDS has been established. It is likely that several distinct pathophysiologic mechanism may contribute to SIDS. A brainstem abnormality related to neuroregulation of cardiorespiratory or other autonomic functions is a compelling hypothesis that is currently being investigated. Autopsy studies indi-

TABLE 18.22   Disorders of Control of Breathing

Condition	Definition
Apnea	Cessation of airflow Central (no respiratory effort) or obstructive May be normal at all ages [short (< 15 seconds)]
Periodic breathing	Three or more respiratory pauses of > 3 seconds with < 20 seconds of respiration between pauses May be normal
Apparent life-threatening event (ALTE)	Episode that is frightening to observer Characterized by some combination of apnea, color change, marked change in muscle tone, choking, or gagging In some cases, fear the infant has died
Apnea in infancy	Unexplained episode of apnea (> 20 seconds) or shorter respiratory pause associated with bradycardia, cyanosis, pallor, and/or marked hypotonia Infants in whom no specific cause for an ALTE can be identified.
Sudden infant death syndrome (SIDS)	Sudden death that is unexplained by history Thorough postmortem evaluation fails to demonstrate adequate cause of death

cating preexisting, chronic, low-grade hypoxemia attributed to sleep-related hypoventilation support this hypothesis. Environmental factors associated with an increased risk for SIDS include prone positioning for sleep, exposure to cigarette smoke during gestation or after birth, overheating, and not breastfeeding.

Clinical Evaluation

No autopsy finding is pathognomonic for SIDS, and no finding is required for the diagnosis. However, some features are common to many victims. Petechial hemorrhages are found in more than 70%–90% of cases. Pulmonary edema is often found, and it may be substantial. Some unexpected deaths may be "misdiagnosed" as pneumonia or other natural conditions based on minimal findings at autopsy that are insufficient to explain sudden death; this relates to the lack of uniform criteria among pathologists.

Management

The American Academy of Pediatrics (AAP) Task Force on Infant Positioning and SIDS issued its first recommendation on the nonprone positioning of infants in June 1992—the "Back to Sleep" program. Public education campaigns focused on reduction of environmental risk factors for SIDS such as prone positioning and exposure to cigarette smoke. Changes in the rate and epidemiologic patterns of SIDS in California from 1990 through 1995 demonstrated drastic changes in the patterns of SIDS. The SIDS postneonatal mortality rate declined 38.9% from 118 deaths/100,000 live

births in 1991 to 72/100,000 in 1996 ($P < .001$), thus indicating the impact of ongoing strategies to reduce SIDS mortality.

APPARENT LIFE-THREATENING EVENTS*

Apparent life-threatening event (ALTE), a term used to describe the clinical presentation of infants who have an a seemingly life-threatening event, is not a diagnosis. The etiology is known in 49%–62% of cases (Table 18.23). Having an ALTE is a risk factor for SIDS. However, less than 7% of SIDS victims have a prior history of ALTE. Infants who have experienced ALTE are at particular risk for SIDS, including those who have had repeated episodes requiring mouth-to-mouth resuscitation, especially if they are siblings of SIDS victims or have a seizure disorder. Although the reported recurrence rate for ALTE based on parental observation is 41%–63%, recent data based on occurrence of actual events suggest that these values are overestimates. This lack of agreement between parental observation and recorded events underscores the difficulty in defining groups at risk for SIDS.

Pathophysiology

During active sleep, the tone of upper airway and intercostal muscles decreases, possibly leading to upper airway narrowing or closure. Increased resistance to airflow and hypoventilation may result. Reduction in tone of upper airway and in-

---

The section on apparent life-threatening events was contributed by Jeff Ewig, M.D.

TABLE 18.23 Differential Diagnosis of Apparent Life-Threatening Event (ALTE)

Normal Events

Periodic breathing

Infection

TB
Sepsis
Meningitis
RSV
Pertussis

Chronic Conditions

Gastroesophageal
    Reflux/Aspiration
Seizures (cause vs. effect)
Cardiac disease
    Cardiomyopathy
    Arrhythmia
    Prolonged QT syndrome
Upper airway obstruction
Metabolic (rare cause)
Central nervous system
    Tumor
    Structural lesion (i.e., Arnold-Chiari II), central
        hypoventilation
Anemia (premature infants)
Vasovagal
    Breath-holding spell
Miscellaneous
    Suffocation
    Medication effect
    Accidents
    Munchausen by proxy

Apnea of Infancy

Idiopathic (diagnosis of exclusion)

RSV = respiratory syncytial virus; TB = tuberculosis.

tercostal muscles may lead to severe reductions in FRC, providing a lower reserve of oxygen and putting the infant at risk for rapid development of hypoxemia during apnea.

Clinical and Laboratory Evaluation

History

The clinician must decide if an ALTE truly occurred and if an underlying condition caused the episode. The history obtained from the parents or caregiver is the most important part of the evaluation of an infant who presents with ALTE. The infant's state of consciousness (i.e., asleep or awake) at the time of the event should be ascertained. Awake events are atypical for apnea of infancy and suggest other causes. The timing of feeding in relation to the event is important. Any evidence of prior sleep disturbance, noisy breathing, or feeding difficulties is noteworthy. Vomiting or choking suggest **gastroesophageal reflux** or **aspiration**. Noisy respirations suggest **upper airway obstruction**. Abnormal movement or rigidity suggest occurrence of a **seizure**. A seizure may be the cause of the ALTE, or it may be secondary to prolonged hypoxemia. The duration of the episode and any change in skin color (pallor or cyanosis) or muscle tone are important.

A history of recent illness suggests infection as the cause of the event. The type of intervention (stimulation versus resuscitation) and the time to recovery give clues as to the severity of the event. Repeat events always in the presence of the same witness may suggest a diagnosis of **Munchausen syndrome by proxy**. A perinatal history of asphyxia or sepsis is frequently seen in ALTE of neurologic origin. Any medications given to the infant should be noted. A family history of unexplained deaths or syncopal episodes warrants consideration of rare metabolic disorders (especially if occurring outside the normal age range for SIDS), seizure disorders, cardiac rhythm disturbances, or child abuse.

Physical Examination

It is important to note the temperature, cardiac and respiratory rate, and rhythm. The pediatrician should look for features that might indicate increased risk for upper airway obstruction such as micrognathia, Pierre Robin anomaly, midface hypoplasia, and large tonsils and adenoids. The rate and depth of breathing, retractions, or unusual pauses are noteworthy. Signs of upper and lower respiratory tract infection should be noted. Respiratory syncytial virus (RSV) is frequently a cause of apnea in infants. A careful cardiac, neurologic, and developmental assessment is mandatory.

Laboratory Evaluation

For patients whose history does not suggest a significant event, a limited diagnostic evaluation is warranted (Table 18.24). A bicarbonate level should be obtained as soon as possible after the event; a low value suggests a significant insult. The clinician may obtain additional studies according to the index of suspicion (Table 18.25).

Management

Infants who present after having a significant ALTE should be hospitalized for at least 48 hours for diagnostic evaluation and cardiorespiratory monitoring. After testing is complete (see LABORATORY EVALUATION), it is necessary to decide whether home monitoring or pharmacologic ther-

TABLE 18.24 Laboratory Evaluation of Apparent Life-Threatening Event (ALTE)

Test	Comments
CBC, hematocrit	Low hematocrit (anemia), high WBC count (infection)
Bicarbonate	Low: significant event
	High: chronic hypoventilation
Electrolytes	Low yield
Calcium	Low yield
Glucose	Low yield
Cultures (blood, urine, CSF)	Positive culture → infection
Chest radiograph	Infection, aspiration, cardiomegaly
ECG	Dysrhythmia, prolonged QT interval
EEG (for seizure)	Spike-wave pattern
pH probe (for gastroesophageal reflux)	Abnormal values, which differ depending on the age of infant
Nasopharyngeal swab for direct viral examination (DVE)	Rapid detection of RSV, influenza A and B, parainfluenza

CBC = complete blood count; CSF = cerebrospinal fluid; ECG = electrocardiogram; EEG = electro-encephalogram; RSV = respiratory syncytial virus; WBC = white blood cell.

apy is appropriate. Specific causes of ALTE require treatment. However, it should not be assumed that identification of a cause eliminates future risk. Pneumograms should not be used as a screening tool to determine future risk as normal pneumograms do not imply absence of risk for SIDS. The National Institutes of Health (NIH) recommends monitoring for the following groups of patients: (1) infants who have had one or more severe ALTEs requiring mouth-to-mouth resuscitation or vigorous stimulation, (2) siblings of two or more SIDS victims, and (3) infants with central hypoventilation. Monitoring may be considered on an individual basis for siblings of one SIDS victim and infants with less severe ALTE episodes.

Because of the low incidence of SIDS and the low incidence of ALTE in infants who subse-quently die of SIDS, it is difficult to demonstrate the effectiveness of monitoring in preventing SIDS. The decision to monitor an infant at home requires multiple support systems to be in place, including nursing and physician support, psychosocial support, and periodic visits from the supplier to inspect the equipment. Patients are not discharged from the hospital until all caretakers can effectively perform cardiopulmonary resuscitation (CPR). Parents must understand that home monitoring is not a guarantee against SIDS. Criteria for discontinuing monitoring are: (1) no event requiring vigorous stimulation or resuscitation in 2–3 months, (2) no observed prolonged apnea or bradycardia for 2 months, (3) no alarms with stress (i.e., upper respiratory infection, immunization), and (4) normal event recording.

TABLE 18.25 Other Tests to Consider in Evaluating an Apparent Life-Threatening Event (ALTE)

Test	Comment
Airway films	Adenoidal and tonsillar hypertrophy, subglottic stenosis
Computed tomography (head)	Concussion, areas of bleeding, brainstem compression
Polysomnography	Hypoventilation, abnormal periods of apnea, bradycardia
Metabolic workup	Urine organic acids, serum long-chain fatty acids
Barium swallow	Assessment for aspiration or tracheoesophageal fistula
Echocardiography	Right ventricular hypertrophy, arrhythmias
Cranial ultrasound	Bleeding, periventricular leukomalacia
Bronchoscopy	Hemorrhage, culture of lavage fluid, foreign body aspiration

SUGGESTED READINGS

General References

Albert R, Spiro S, Jett J (eds): *Comprehensive Respiratory Medicine,* St. Louis, Mosby, 1999.

Loughlin GM, Eigen H: *Respiratory Disease in Children: Diagnosis and Management.* Baltimore, Williams & Wilkins, 1994.

Taussig L, Landau L, Le Souef P, et al (eds): *Pediatric Respiratory Medicine,* St. Louis, Mosby, 1999.

Asthma

Doull IJ, Freezer NJ, Holgate ST: Growth of prepubertal children with mild asthma treated with inhaled beclomethasone dipropionate. *Am J Respir Crit Care Med* 151:1715–1719, 1995.

Gelb AF, Zamel N: Lung elastic recoil in acute and chronic asthma. *Curr Opin Pulm Med* 8:50–53, 2002.

Message SA, Johnston SL: Viruses in asthma. *Br Med Bull* 61:29–43, 2002.

Rubin BK, Marcushamer S, Priel I, et al: Emergency management of the child with asthma. *Pediatr Pulmonol* 8:45, 1990.

Strachan DP, Wong HJ, Spector TD: Concordance and interrelationship of atopic disease and markers of allergic sensitization among adult female twins. *J Allerg Clin Immunol* 108:901–907, 2001.

Welliver R, Wong D, Sum M, et al: The development of respiratory syncytial virus specific IgE and the release of histamine in nasopharyngeal secretions after infection. *N Engl J Med* 305:841–846, 1981.

Yunginger FW, Reed CE, O'Connel EF, et al: A community-based study of the epidemiology of asthma. Incidence rates 1964–1983. *Am Rev Respir Dis* 146:888–894, 1992.

Cystic Fibrosis

FitzSimmons SC: The changing epidemiology of cystic fibrosis. *J Pediatr* 122:1, 1993.

Konstan MW, Byard PJ, Hoppel CL, et al: Effect of high-dose ibuprofen in patients with cystic fibrosis. *J Pediatr* 127:501, 1995.

Ramsey BW, Pepe MS, Quan JM, et al: Intermittent administration of inhaled tobramycin in patients with cystic fibrosis. *N Engl J Med* 340:23–30, 1999.

Schidlow D, Taussig LM, Knowles MR: Cystic Fibrosis Foundation Consensus Conference Report on pulmonary complications of cystic fibrosis. *Pediatr Pulmonol* 15:187, 1993.

Tizzano EF, Buchwald M: Cystic fibrosis: Beyond the gene to therapy. *J Pediatr* 120:337, 1992.

Apnea and the Control of Breathing

Brooks JG: Sudden infant death syndrome. In *Respiratory Disease in Children: Diagnosis and Management.* Edited by Loughlin G, Eigen H. Baltimore, Williams & Wilkins, 1994.

Consensus Statement: National Institute of Health Consensus Development Conference on Infantile Apnea and Home Monitoring, Sept. 29–Oct. 1, 1986. *Pediatrics,* 79:292, 1987.

Hoffman HJ, Damus K, Hillman L, et al: Risk factors for SIDS: Results of the National Institutes of Health and Human Development SIDS Cooperative Epidemiological Study. *Ann N Y Acad Sci* 533:13–30, 1988.

Hunt CE: Cardiorespiratory control hypothesis for sudden infant death syndrome. *Clin Perinatol* 19:757, 1992.

Hunt CE: Sudden infant death syndrome and other causes of infant mortality: Diagnosis, mechanisms, and risk for recurrence in siblings. *Am J Respir Crit Care Med* 164:346–347, 2001.

Peterson DR, Sabotta EE, Daling JR: Infant mortality among subsequent siblings of infants who died of sudden infant death syndrome. *J Pediatr* 108:911, 1986.

Spitzer AR, Gibson E: Home monitoring. *Clin Perinatol* 1992, 19:907.

Steinschneider A: Prolonged apnea and sudden infant death syndrome: Clinical and laboratory observations. *Pediatrics* 50:646, 1972.

Chapter 19

Neurology

Alfred J. Spiro

Infants and children often present to pediatricians with certain problems that appear to have a neurologic basis. This chapter discusses neurologically based situations frequently encountered by pediatricians and outlines approaches to the understanding and management of these problems. It is in no way intended to provide a complete summary of neurologic disorders encountered in practice or be a complete manual for diagnosis and therapy.

EVALUATION OF THE FLOPPY INFANT

Floppiness, also known as hypotonia, is defined as diminished resistance to passive movement around a joint. Floppiness may be graded as mild, moderate, or severe, all subjective assessments; the degree may vary when the baby is rested, content, hungry, or irritable.

Pathophysiology

Floppiness is an excellent operational term, because the condition may result from many varied lesions of the central nervous system (CNS) or motor unit. Infants with floppiness related to lesions of the motor unit are also generally weak; however, weakness and floppiness may be difficult to distinguish. Floppiness may also result from secondary involvement of the nervous system from systemic disorders. The occurrence of one lesion does not necessarily exclude the coexistence of an additional lesion elsewhere. For example, in the neonatal period, an acutely ill infant suffering from asphyxia, sepsis, intraventricular hemorrhage, meningitis, or marked hyperbilirubinemia may be floppy.

Clinical and Laboratory Evaluation

History

It is important to determine whether evidence of an intercurrent illness was apparent when the floppiness was first noted. The clinician should also ascertain when the floppiness began (i.e., was it present at birth or acquired at a later date?) as well as the course of the floppiness (i.e., is it in-creasing or diminishing with advancing age?). Other questions to ask include: Are the legs, arms, or all limbs floppy? Is there any other evidence of lack of motor control? (A history of sleeping with open eyelids indicates facial muscle weakness.) What is the infant's general health? What are the details concerning the infant's acquisition of motor, language, and social milestones?

In addition, the clinician should obtain details of the pregnancy, including the mother's perception of fetal movements, and information concerning delivery, birth weight, and the presence of hyperbilirubinemia or neonatal seizures. A detailed family history with special emphasis on neuromuscular disorders is important. The occurrence of any consanguinity hints at an autosomal recessive problem. Many of the motor unit disorders in which floppiness or weakness are prominent are genetically determined.

Physical Examination

A general examination to rule out systemic disorders and to check for dysmorphic features is imperative. A search for scoliosis, seen in many neuromuscular disorders, is also warranted. It is important to plot the head circumference of an infant on an appropriate graph. If it exceeds the 95th percentile, the head circumference of both parents should be measured. (In infants who have large heads from various causes, hypotonicity is frequently an associated finding.)

The examiner should assess the degree of floppiness (i.e., reduced resistance to passive movement) when infants are quiet and not crying (Table 19.1). Characterization and documentation of floppiness may require several evaluations. If infants are weak in addition to being hypotonic, a paucity of spontaneous movements (in a young infant) or inability to move an extremity against gravity may be observed. It is possible to test functional strength by ascertaining whether an infant can hold the head erect or pull the neck up in the traction response, roll over, sit up, crawl, or stand with support or independently at the appropriate time.

Developmental assessment may be a source of information about the normalcy of gross and

TABLE 19.1 Physical Examination in Hypotonic Infants

Site of Disorder	Degree of Hypotonia	Deep Tendon Reflexes	Other Findings
Cerebral hemisphere	Varied	Present to hyperactive	Possible obtundation; developmental retardation, seizures common
Anterior horn cell	Marked	Absent	Alert and responsive; paucity of movements; fasciculations of tongue
Peripheral nerve	Moderate	Absent ankle jerks	
Myoneural junction	Varied	Present	Extraocular muscle and respiratory involvement
Muscle	Moderate	Hypoactive	Facial weakness; check mother for myotonia

fine motor, language, and social–adaptive milestones. In hypotonia due to cerebral lesions, a delay in all spheres of development often occurs, although motor system abnormalities may be the most obvious. Examination of the cranial nerves should focus on the extraocular muscles, because certain disorders of the myoneural junction and rare myopathies can cause external ophthalmoparesis in addition to floppiness. The clinician should examine the tongue (with the baby not crying) for fasciculations, which are frequently observed in infantile progressive spinal muscular atrophy.

Deep tendon reflexes warrant attention. Generally, reflexes are maintained or hyperactive in floppiness of cerebral origin and reduced to absent in most motor unit disorders (see Table 19.1).

Laboratory Evaluation

Laboratory studies should be goal-directed (Table 19.2). In infants with dysmorphic features and hypotonia such as observed in Down syndrome, chromosomal studies might be diagnostic. If hypothyroidism is suspected, thyroid function studies are appropriate, and in many states, these are part of the routine neonatal screening. If the history and physical examination are suggestive of a cerebral lesion, an imaging study such as computed tomography (CT), or, preferably, magnetic resonance imaging (MRI), of the brain might be indicated. An electroencephalogram (EEG) may be necessary if seizures are present. Electrodiagnostic studies and muscle biopsy are very useful procedures in selected instances when noninvasive testing is not confirmatory. Genetic studies

TABLE 19.2 Laboratory Studies in Hypotonic Infants

Site of Disorder	Serum Genetic Studies	Muscle Enzymes	Electrodiagnostic Studies	Muscle Biopsy	Other
Cause outside CNS	Can be helpful	Normal	Normal	Not helpful	Thyroid tests
Cerebral hemisphere	Important in stigmatized infants	Normal	Normal	Not helpful	Imaging
Anterior horn cell disease	Diagnostic	Normal	Not mandatory	Not mandatory	
Peripheral nerve	May be helpful	Normal	Very important	Not necessary	
Myoneural junction	Not helpful	Normal	Very important	Not necessary	Edrophonium
Muscle	Careful pedigree	Elevated	Useful	Diagnostic	
	Degree of hypotonia	Deep tendon reflexes	Other		

CNS = central nervous system.

(DNA testing to document a specific deletion on chromosome 5) to confirm a diagnosis of anterior horn cell disease in infants and children (spinal muscular atrophy of varying types) are available in specialized laboratories. Nerve conduction velocity determinations can usually document peripheral nerve disorders. An edrophonium (Tensilon) test and specialized electrodiagnostic tests can be extremely useful in a suspected myoneural junction disorder or in a clinically involved newborn of a mother with myasthenia gravis. Muscle biopsy, using specialized analytical techniques, may be diagnostic when myopathy is suspected; serum muscle enzyme levels are very frequently elevated in myopathies.

Differential Diagnosis

Several conditions must be considered in the differential diagnosis of a floppy infant.

Primary Lesions Outside of the Nervous System

CHROMOSOMAL DISORDERS. Infants with **Down syndrome** are mildly to moderately floppy. Infants with **Prader-Willi syndrome** are severely floppy and obtunded early in infancy. Developmental retardation is noted in both conditions.

HYPOTHYROIDISM. Hypotonia is associated with other signs of thyroid dysfunction.

EHLERS-DANLOS SYNDROME. This syndrome may simulate nervous system or motor system disorders because of the association of hypotonicity and lax joints.

HYPERMAGNESEMIA. Previous magnesium sulfate therapy for toxemia in the mother may relate to hypermagnesemia in newborns with hypotonia. The hypotonia is generally transient.

Cerebral Disorders

Hypoxic–ischemic encephalopathy (HIE) and intraventricular hemorrhage in low-birth-weight infants are frequently associated with marked hypotonia. These infants might develop features of cerebral palsy or other neurologic manifestations later in infancy or early childhood.

Anterior Horn Cell Disease

In **infantile progressive spinal muscular atrophy, type I** (formerly referred to as Werdnig-Hoffmann disease), infants are bright and alert as well as weak and floppy. Onset occurs in the first 6 months of life, with areflexia, normal central recognition of pain, and fasciculations of the tongue. Inheritance is autosomal recessive. In type II disease, infants are able to sit; weakness and hypotonicity begin after they learn to sit, but the children will not be able to walk independently. In type III disease, weakness begins only after children have learned to walk. In all types of the disorder, cognition is completely normal.

Pediatric Pearl

In a floppy infant with normal cognition, absent deep tendon reflexes and fasciculations of the tongue, spinal muscular atrophy is the most likely diagnosis.

Peripheral Nerve Disorder

Most peripheral neuropathies in children are hereditary sensorimotor neuropathies. Clinical manifestations are very rare in newborns but appear in childhood or later. Rare CNS disease such as the leukodystrophies (e.g., adrenoleukodystrophy or metachromatic leukodystrophy) are characterized by peripheral nerve involvement but are associated with dementia and spasticity.

Myoneural Junction Disorders

Passively acquired **myasthenia gravis** is an autoimmune disorder that may occur in newborns of mothers with myasthenia gravis. Recovery from this disorder usually occurs within the first few weeks, but some infants require therapy for only a few days. Actively acquired autoimmune myasthenia gravis is very rare in infants but can be seen in older children. Nonautoimmune myasthenic syndromes and botulism are also rare.

Myopathies

MYOTONIC DYSTROPHY. Floppiness may be severe at birth, with obtundation, difficulty with sucking and respirations in the neonatal period, areflexia, clubfoot, and weakness of facial muscles. The mother should be examined for myotonia (autosomal dominant disorder); DNA studies can confirm the diagnosis. Myotonic dystrophy is a triplet repeat disorder.

CONGENITAL MUSCULAR DYSTROPHY AND MYOPATHIES WITH CHARACTERISTIC MORPHOLOGY. Congenital muscular dystrophy and myopathies with characteristic morphology (nemaline myopathy, central core disease, fiber-type disproportion, glycogen storage disease due to acid maltase deficiency) are hereditary disorders, with varying degrees of floppiness, weakness, and respiratory and sucking problems in early life. Infants with glycogen storage disease due to acid maltase deficiency have enlarged hearts on radiography. Diagnosis is made by muscle biopsy.

MITOCHONDRIAL ENCEPHALOMYELOPATHIES. Involvement of muscle or the nervous system is variable in mitochondrial encephalomyelopathies. Lacticacidemia is frequent, and the test for elevated serum lactate is useful for screening. DNA studies performed on blood samples can be useful in the diagnosis. Specialized studies on muscle mitochondria obtained from a skeletal muscle biopsy may also provide a specific diagnosis in selected cases.

Management

Specific therapy depends on diagnosis, but in general, it is essential to provide respiratory and nutritional requirements and supportive therapy. Some neonates or infants require temporary ventilatory support and gavage feedings or a feeding gastrostomy. Many disorders with hypotonia as a prominent feature are genetically determined, which usually makes an exact diagnosis imperative, even if no specific therapy is available. However, in some instances, careful observation is the only necessary treatment.

Cerebral Disorders
Physical therapy may be necessary.

Anterior Horn Cell Disease
In **infantile progressive spinal muscular atrophy,** treatment is supportive. No specific medical therapy is available. Genetic counseling is warranted, because prenatal diagnosis is readily available if the parents desire it.

Myoneural Junction Disorders
Neonates with symptomatic passively acquired **myasthenia gravis** may receive treatment with pyridostigmine (Mestinon). After several days the dose can be reduced or stopped and, if necessary, restarted. Prognosis is good.

Myopathies
MYOTONIC DYSTROPHY. Most infants with this disorder are developmentally delayed in all spheres. Supportive therapy, such as tube feeding and respiratory support, may be necessary. Genetic counseling is warranted, because prenatal diagnosis is available if the parents desire it. Orthopedic surgeons should treat clubfoot.

CONGENITAL MYOPATHIES. Genetic counseling is appropriate because many myopathies are hereditary, although prenatal diagnosis is not yet available. Supportive therapy may be necessary, depending on the severity of respiratory and swallowing problems. Therapy is needed for congestive heart failure in infants with glycogen storage disease due to acid maltase deficiency.

BENIGN FEBRILE SEIZURES

Benign febrile seizures in infancy or childhood are associated with fever of extracranial origin and without acute neurologic illness.

> **Pediatric Pearl**
> Benign febrile seizures are not a form of epilepsy, which is defined as recurrent nonfebrile seizures.

Approximately 2%–5% of all children experience one or more benign febrile seizures, making them the most common type of childhood seizures. Benign febrile seizures occur in infants and children from 6 months to 5 years of age but are most frequent between 18 and 22 months of age.

Pathophysiology

Maturational differences at the neuronal level probably account for the susceptibility of young children to seizures provoked by fever, but the exact mechanism remains an enigma. There may be a genetically determined predisposition for benign febrile seizures.

Benign febrile convulsions are tonic–clonic, self-limited, brief, and without residual neurologic deficits. Any illness accompanied by high fever, such as an upper respiratory infection, acute otitis media, acute gastroenteritis, influenza, or roseola, and fevers following administration of immunizations can provoke febrile seizures, which **occur most commonly during the onset of fever.** The seizures may be the first sign of an unrecognized underlying illness. **There is no clearly documented proof that seizures cause brain damage.**

Clinical and Laboratory Evaluation

History
The examiner should question parents about the underlying illness responsible for the fever. For example:

- Did the child have an ear infection, immunization, respiratory tract infection, rash (suggesting an exanthema), diarrhea, or vomiting before the seizure?

- Was the convulsion the first indication of illness, or had fever been present before the seizure?
- What was the degree of temperature elevation (if known) before the seizure, or did the child feel warm?
- Did the fever develop suddenly or rise rapidly?

It is important to obtain as accurate a description as possible of the seizure itself, but parents may find this an emotion-laden experience, and the examiner should not press them too hard for details. Questions should relate to the duration and the generalization or possible focality of the seizure, if it was repeated or clustered, and when it began in relationship to the fever, if known. Other necessary questions concern the presence of a postictal phase or the presence or absence of paralysis, breathing difficulty, respiratory problem, aspiration, or cyanosis.

Questions to ask include: Has the child had anything suggesting a febrile seizure in the past? If so, how many, and what were the circumstances (i.e., degree of fever, duration of convulsions)? Family history of seizures, febrile or afebrile, is noteworthy. Medication history should be ascertained, especially if anticonvulsants were given. After the acute febrile seizure is over, the clinician should obtain other detailed information about the child's past medical history and developmental history (gross motor, fine motor, language, social, and adaptive elements).

Physical Examination

If the child is actively having a seizure, it should be timed. By definition, benign febrile convulsions are limited to less than 15 minutes. Prolonged benign febrile seizures are uncommon. The child is in status epilepticus, by definition, if the seizure lasts more than 30 minutes with no regaining of consciousness, and requires appropriate management.

After termination of the seizure, measurement of vital signs is important, and frequent assessment of the patient's level of consciousness is necessary. It is important to search for the origin of a child's temperature elevation judiciously; otitis media, upper respiratory infections, roseola, and pneumonia are common causes of high fevers associated with febrile seizures.

In a preliminary evaluation after the seizure, the most important features of the basic general and neurologic examination include **assessment of the anterior fontanelle (in an infant) and assessment for meningismus (neck stiffness).** Evaluation of meningismus involves testing passive

flexion of the neck with the quiet child in the supine position; stiffness of the neck in an otherwise cooperative patient or flexion of the knees is abnormal **(Brudzinski sign)**. Funduscopy is necessary to exclude papilledema, but increased intracranial pressure may be present in infants and children with no evidence of abnormalities in the optic disks, because cranial sutures can separate at an early age. The clinician should look for focality; hints of paralysis or weakness on one side of the body, for example, may be present transiently (Todd paralysis) and may be found by noting differences in tone or strength between the right and left arms and legs. Similarly, differences in reflexes and toe (Babinski) responses may also suggest focality.

After the child has been stabilized, the remainder of the neurologic assessment may proceed. The clinician should note any dysmorphic features and plot the head circumference, as in every examination. It is essential to check the skin for evidence of any of the many neurocutaneous disorders. Mental status assessment is necessary, and as noted above, early and periodic assessment of level of consciousness is important. Remember that the child may sleep deeply after a seizure or may have taken anticonvulsants that alter the mental status. This fact is noteworthy, and the examiner should reevaluate the mental status when the child becomes fully alert and is "back to normal."

Complete assessment of the motor system is necessary with regard to strength, tone, coordination, and dysmetria to attempt to assess the normalcy of the nervous system or to detect any possible abnormalities. The gait, deep tendon reflexes, and toe responses need rechecking. Tests for sensation (central recognition of pain, touch) may occur in accordance with the age level of the child.

Laboratory Evaluation

If a brief febrile seizure occurs early in an infectious illness accompanied by a high fever, and if infants or children awaken after the seizure alert and with no noted neurologic abnormalities, usually observation and a very simple workup directed at the cause of the fever are all that is necessary. Thus, in most cases, when attempting to ascertain the cause of the fever, a complete blood count (CBC), appropriate cultures, and a urinalysis are appropriate.

Careful examination of the cerebrospinal fluid (CSF) is necessary in several conditions (Table 19.3). The clinician should obtain pressure (when possible), cell count, culture, and determination

TABLE 19.3 **Criteria for Cerebrospinal Fluid (CSF) Studies in Febrile Seizures**

Any hint of meningitis or meningismus
No explanation for fever or with sickness out of proportion to illness apparently responsible for fever
No explanation for a high-pitched cry or sick-appearing infant
No explanation for petechiae
Stiff neck
Coma, paresis, or paralysis

of glucose and protein levels. In children who do not have increased intracranial pressure, a lumbar puncture is completely safe. CSF protein levels are lower in infants and children than in adults (usually < 20 mg/dl).

An EEG is *not* necessary after a first benign febrile seizure. However, parental pressure to perform the study may be strong. If the physician acquiesces, the EEG should be performed several days after the seizure, because spurious "abnormalities" may be seen during the immediate postseizure period, and the tracing will only have to be repeated.

Imaging studies are unnecessary following benign febrile seizures. Workup in afebrile seizures is usually more complex and involved.

Differential Diagnosis

The single most important practical consideration in the differential diagnosis of febrile seizures is bacterial meningitis or any other forms of meningitis. In the past, people tended to consider febrile seizures as a form of epilepsy. This seizure condition is no longer in the differential diagnosis.

Management

The major principles of management of febrile seizures include:

- Safely terminating the seizure (if the child is actually having one)
- Establishing the diagnosis by prudently excluding meningitis, if this disorder is being considered in the differential diagnosis
- Explaining the benign nature of febrile seizures to the parents

In addition, it is necessary to lower the body temperature and treat the acute infection that resulted in the temperature elevation, if possible.

With the first febrile seizure, observation in the emergency department on an outpatient basis is optimal. **If a child is having a prolonged seizure that does not seem to be stopping spontaneously, intravenous lorazepam (0.1 mg/kg, with a maximum of 4 mg) may be required.** Generally, the seizure stops within a few minutes; sometimes, however, an additional dose of lorazepam is necessary. Respiratory depression is a possible side effect, and careful observation for respiratory problems and the need for assisted ventilation is essential. The likelihood of the need for ventilatory assistance rises sharply in proportion to the duration of the seizure.

Other drugs are useful in the treatment of febrile seizures that do not stop spontaneously. Intravenous diazepam (0.3 mg/kg) is also effective in the termination of febrile seizures. Although diazepam frequently stops a seizure more rapidly than does lorazepam, the duration of its effective anticonvulsant action is shorter. Frequently, repeat administration is necessary, and because of its relatively short duration (30–45 minutes), it sometimes requires an additional anticonvulsant such as phenobarbital. Intravenous phenobarbital (10 mg/kg) may be warranted if diazepam administration has not resulted in a cessation of the seizure after 20–30 minutes. If phenobarbital must be used after the diazepam, respiratory depression is common, and the child should be intubated. Because of the possibility of respiratory depression, extreme caution is required when administering diazepam to a child with a febrile seizure if the child is known to have been taking phenobarbital chronically. (This illustrates the extreme importance of a correct history!)

Reduction of body temperature generally involves evaporative cooling and administration of acetaminophen in appropriate dose and by the best route. Obviously, if an acute infection causing the fever is identified, appropriate treatment is required. As noted earlier, if there is any hint of meningitis, a lumbar puncture with careful examination of the CSF is necessary. Certainly it is better to err on the side of safety. Some experts advocate routine lumbar puncture in the event of a first seizure, because it takes a great deal of clinical experience and judgment to decide whether a child is more ill than appearance and well-being might suggest.

Any seizure can be a terribly frightening experience for a child's parents and family, who will be afraid of the complications of the lumbar puncture and its long-term effects on their child. It is imperative to give them reassurance. Despite what the parents may have heard or read to the contrary, lumbar puncture is a benign procedure. When a child recovers quickly to full function after a brief febrile seizure, parental reassurance is generally easy to provide; in these circumstances, the benign nature of the condition is clearly evident.

With a prolonged febrile seizure (status epilepticus), the parents are reasonably concerned about the prognosis. **In a recent long-term follow-up study of patients with febrile status epilepticus, no child without prior neurologic deficits or without prior evidence of afebrile seizures or acute CNS infection died or developed any new neurologic deficit following the seizure.** This is not true for children with neurologic impairment prior to the episode of febrile status epilepticus; these children have a higher risk for recurrent afebrile or febrile seizures or recurrent febrile status.

In a recent prospective study of recurrent febrile seizures, investigators concluded that an increased risk of recurrent febrile seizures was associated with children younger than 18 months and a family history of febrile seizures. A family history of epilepsy, complex febrile seizures, and neurodevelopmental problems do not increase the risk of recurrent febrile seizures, but they do serve as predictors of later epilepsy in children who have febrile seizures. Children who have a short duration of fever prior to the seizure and those who experience a seizure associated with a lower temperature elevation have an increased risk of recurrence of a febrile seizure.

Benign febrile seizures are just that—benign. Because daily phenobarbital used in an attempt to prevent recurrence of febrile seizures is probably ineffective and may be detrimental to children's cognitive development, this drug is generally no longer used for that purpose. **Similarly, phenobarbital given just at the time of a temperature elevation in a child with benign febrile seizures is ineffective.** The parents of children with febrile seizures should receive an explanation of these facts.

EPILEPSY

Epilepsy can be defined as recurrent convulsive or nonconvulsive seizures. The disorder is much more common in children than in adults but can occur at virtually any age.

Pathophysiology

Epileptic seizures are generated by abnormal synchronization of neuronal pool discharges caused by numerous acquired or genetic, structural, metabolic, and idiopathic conditions. The exact mechanism responsible for the onset or the cessation of a seizure is still unclear. Excitatory and inhibitory neurotransmitters probably play a major role, as do changes in the intracellular and extracellular environment.

Seizures can be classified into two major groups: generalized and focal. In **generalized seizures,** the abnormal discharge is generated in deep midline structures of the brain. Thus, there is no aura (warning), and no focal features are apparent during the seizure. However, many seizures begin focally and generalize rapidly, so that the focal onset goes unnoticed. In this situation, an EEG can frequently define the focal onset; the seizure is then classified as focal with secondary generalization.

In **focal (or partial) seizures,** the discharge that generates the seizure arises from a localized area in the brain and is manifested by involvement of a limited portion of the body (e.g., hand or arm). This type of seizure usually is a result of localized pathology such as mesial temporal gliosis (sclerosis of the hippocampus), trauma, tumor, vascular abnormalities, or hamartoma. If consciousness is not impaired, the seizure is classified as a **simple partial seizure,** but if consciousness is impaired, the seizure is classified as a **complex partial seizure.**

Clinical and Laboratory Evaluation

History

In most cases, the examiner has not had the opportunity to observe the child having a seizure, so the event has to be reconstructed by obtaining as accurate a history as possible. Commonly, observers of a convulsion are so emotionally involved with the event that they have difficulty recalling details and even major characteristics. The questioner should make every effort to respect this human condition.

Nevertheless, the historical record should be as reliable as possible, and this involves asking several questions (Table 19.4). Care should be used in asking leading questions or trying to retrieve an answer from a patient or observer who has unclear recall of the event. The examiner should also determine the child's and the family's understanding about the seizure and explore their fears and anxieties.

Physical Examination

Examination during a seizure is limited. However, once the seizure has stopped, and the child is stabilized, it is possible to perform a general examination, with special emphasis on assessing

TABLE 19.4	**Questions to Ask When Taking the History of Children with Seizures**

Questions concerning one particular seizure

How and where did the seizure begin (i.e., focal or generalized)?

Did a particular event precipitate the seizure?

Was there an aura or warning?

What was the condition of the head, eyes, and arms at the onset of the seizure, especially if they turned to one side or the other?

Were any behavioral manifestations such as automatisms associated with the seizure?

How long did the seizure last?

Did a postictal phase (e.g., excessive sleepiness) follow the seizure?

Did staring spells occur during the seizure?

Does the child's language and speech (dysphasia) change during the seizure, or is there a lack of speech (aphasia)?

Did the seizure result in incontinence?

Questions concerning general seizure pattern

How often do the seizures occur?

Have there been any sudden pattern changes in the seizures, which might suggest an expanding or changing lesion?

Is there a family history of seizures?*

At what age did the seizures begin?[†]

Have any medications been taken on a regular basis? If so, history of previous medications, doses prescribed, their effects on the seizures, and their side effects should be obtained.

Has there been any recent trauma or previous neurologic or other illnesses?

---

*Family history, best recorded in a pedigree diagram, with specific emphasis on the family history of seizures, is important to obtain.

[†]Age of onset is important, because various types of seizure disorders are more common at certain ages.

any features of focality. Postictal paralysis (Todd paralysis) can last for several hours or more. Deep tendon reflex asymmetry and frank hemiparesis may provide a clue to focality, as can the everted posture of one foot. During a seizure, extensor plantar responses may be present, but after the seizure stops, asymmetrical responses may also offer a clue to focality. The clinician should be sure to assess mental status and cranial nerve function, with particular emphasis on funduscopy and on asymmetries of extraocular and facial muscular function.

In addition, it is important to examine the skin carefully, looking for evidence of a neurocutaneous disorder (e.g., neurofibromatosis, tuberous sclerosis), which may be associated with seizures. Listening over the head with the bell of a stethoscope sometimes reveals the bruit of an underlying arteriovenous malformation. Careful assessment for evidence of trauma should also occur, and if the history is suspicious, the clinician should consider the possibility of child abuse.

Laboratory Evaluation

So-called routine blood studies are generally of no help in establishing a particular metabolic cause for seizures in children unless the history suggests one. The exception is in neonates with seizures in whom routine measurements of glucose, calcium, and electrolytes are performed because neither the history nor the physical examination alone is sufficient to hint at a metabolic etiology.

The **EEG,** a recording of brain electrical activity, is extremely useful in the assessment of children with seizures, although a normal EEG in the interictal period does not exclude the diagnosis of a seizure disorder. A routine EEG is a recording of less than 1 hour of brain activity. When necessary, so-called activation procedures can be used to document an abnormality not seen in a routine study; activation procedures include sleep, sleep deprivation, photic stimulation at various frequencies, and hyperventilation. In specialized situations, the EEG may be recorded over a prolonged period of time (e.g., for several days, if necessary), often with simultaneous closed circuit TV monitoring of the patient. Clinicians must always assess EEG recordings with the history and physical examination in mind; an EEG request should, therefore, include a clinical summary and list any anticonvulsants or other medications the child is taking, because these may affect the tracing.

The EEG can be very helpful in distinguishing partial from generalized seizures and in diagnosing seizures that begin focally and become generalized secondarily. In some instances, the pattern of EEG abnormality may raise the possibility of the presence of an underlying structural lesion; in other cases, it may eliminate this possibility. The EEG interpretation takes into account the level and type of sleep and the maturity of the brain.

Neuroimaging studies, namely MRI or CT scanning, are indicated in the following circumstances:

- When seizures are focal
- When the EEG interpretation suggests an underlying focality in the presence of abnormal neurologic findings on examination
- When seizures accompany a neurocutaneous disorder

Imaging studies are unlikely to be positive in children with generalized seizures, and as a rule, the performance of these tests is unnecessary.

Differential Diagnosis

Epileptic seizures can sometimes be mistaken for **psychogenic seizures.** One of the most characteristic features of psychogenic seizures is the maintenance of consciousness during a generalized tonic or tonic–clonic attack and the usual lack of a postictal phase. Similarly, in psychogenic seizures the EEG fails to show epileptic discharges during an attack. Other episodic disorders that can mimic seizures include breath-holding spells, syncope, and night terrors (Table 19.5).

Classification of true epileptic seizures is based on their clinical and EEG features (Table 19.6).

Generalized Seizures

TONIC–CLONIC CONVULSIONS. These seizures, which are common in children, involve all extremities and have tonic (rigid) and clonic (jerking) components. In many cases, the generalization is secondary and the onset is focal; it is possible to determine this using an EEG and from the history of an aura or behavioral or other changes prior to the seizure onset. If an aura is present, it may be followed by sudden loss of consciousness and rolling up of the eyes, with tonic contraction of all muscles following rapidly. Apnea and cyanosis may occur, after which the clonic contraction and relaxation may begin rapidly and subsequently diminish with varying duration for the entire event. After the convulsion has ended, a postictal phase is common, with deep sleep and confusion for a prolonged period of time.

Primary or secondary generalized seizures may occur at any time, frequently at night or before or after children fall asleep or awaken. Numerous potential precipitating factors may result in a generalized convulsion, including fever, fatigue, or sleep deprivation, phenobarbital withdrawal when the drug is used as an anticonvulsant, and alcohol consumption.

NONCONVULSIVE SEIZURES (ABSENCE OR PETIT MAL SEIZURES). Children who have nonconvulsive seizures, which may occur innumerable times during the day, are frequently misdiagnosed as having staring spells. Each episode lasts only a few seconds, and there is no aura. Body movements are minimal or nonexistent, and the attacks stop abruptly. Hyperventilation may precipitate the attacks and therefore documents them. Children are unaware

TABLE 19.5	**Nonepileptic Paroxysmal Events**	
Psychogenic seizures	Consciousness not lost
	Normal EEG during attack
	No postictal behavior
	Frequently combative during attack
	Can occur in patients with seizures
Breath-holding spells	Mainly between 1 and 2 years of age
	Precipitating event before attack
	Breath-holding after crying
	Pallor or cyanosis, then limpness
Syncope	Usually follows emotional episode
	May have orthostatic hypotension
	EEG is normal
Night terrors	Paroxysmal sleep disturbance
	EEG normal during attacks

EEG = electroencephalogram.

TABLE 19.6 Childhood Seizure Disorders	
Seizure Disorder	**Associated Characteristics**
Generalized tonic–clonic convulsions	Involve all extremities Tonic and clonic components Loss of consciousness Postictal phase common
Absence or petit mal seizures	Last a few seconds No aura Body movement unusual Child unaware of occurrence
Juvenile myoclonic epilepsy	Genetically determined Generalized seizures with myoclonic jerking in morning
Complex partial seizures	Blunted consciousness Aura Strange behavior and speech (chewing and lip-smacking)
Simple partial seizures	Localized motor or sensory symptoms No impairment of consciousness May become generalized
Infantile spasms	Brief sudden muscular contractions Begin at 3–9 months of age Associated with retardation

of the existence of the seizures. The occurrence of many attacks may jeopardize school performance.

In an EEG taken during a nonconvulsive seizure, generalized, three-per-second spike and wave complexes are recorded. The EEG in the interictal period is usually normal.

JUVENILE MYOCLONIC EPILEPSY. In this genetically determined form of epilepsy, attacks occur in the morning after waking and are characterized by absence attacks with myoclonic jerking of an extremity. The EEG is characteristic.

Pediatric Pearl

In juvenile myoclonic epilepsy, children often will not volunteer that they have jerking of their hands; it is important to obtain this history, because workup and management are different in this type of epilepsy.

Partial Seizures

COMPLEX PARTIAL SEIZURES. In this common type of childhood epilepsy, symptomatology is variable. Consciousness, although blunted and altered, is not lost completely. Children may experience an aura and may appear to be dazed or confused and staring. Speech can be irrelevant, incoherent, or absent, and children may exhibit strange behavior or movements, such as incoherently walking around the room. Chewing and lip-smacking movements and purposeless movements such as

picking at one's clothes are common. Drowsiness usually follows the seizure, and children may not have any recollection of the event or may recall a dream-like state. The attacks frequently last for several minutes, noticeably different from absence attacks.

Interictal EEGs may be completely normal in complex partial seizures. Activation procedures are very often necessary to provoke the EEG abnormality; however, hyperventilation does not induce an attack.

SIMPLE PARTIAL SEIZURES. In this relatively common form of childhood epilepsy, localized motor or sensory symptoms with no impairment in level of consciousness are characteristic. Although these seizures may remain localized (focal), they frequently become generalized. In so-called **rolandic seizures,** attacks begin with an aura in the tongue, cheek, or gums, followed by tonic or tonic–clonic movements of the face. The EEG most commonly shows a midtemporal spike focus. Prognosis is very good, and control is achieved readily with anticonvulsants.

Infantile Spasms

Attacks, which frequently begin between 3 and 9 months of age, consist of one or more brief, sudden muscular contractions in which the head is flexed (head nodding), the arms are extended, and the legs drawn up. Episodes are very brief and may be confused with colic or an exaggerated Moro response. These seizures may occur in large clusters, often more than 100/day. Very often, parents do not recognize the attacks as abnormal or as seizures until they occur in large numbers and are accompanied by retarded development, an extremely common feature in infantile spasms.

In most children, the EEG is very abnormal, with diffuse dysrhythmia accompanied by high-voltage slow waves and multiple spike wave discharges, a pattern called hypsarrhythmia. In cryptogenic infantile spasms, the cause is unknown, and in symptomatic forms, several factors such as developmental abnormalities of the brain, tuberous sclerosis, and metabolic, traumatic, and structural disorders, among others, may be the cause of the attacks. The prognosis for normal development is poor.

Management

When deciding whether and how to treat children with epilepsy, it is necessary to determine the type of seizure—generally on the basis of a meticulous history together with an EEG and the prognosis for children with this particular type of seizure. A single seizure does not constitute epilepsy and generally does not warrant treatment. The side effects of anticonvulsant medications are also important (Table 19.7). Several new anticonvulsant medications may now be used; their discussion is beyond the scope of this chapter. Among others, these include topiramate, tiagabine, levetiracetam, lamotrigine, gabapentin, and zonisamide.

As a general rule, treatment involves the medication most likely to be effective for the particular type of epilepsy involved. One medication at a time is used, and the dose is increased periodically, when necessary, to the point of good seizure control or until evidence of toxicity is apparent.

Pediatric Pearl

In the treatment of epilepsy, the goal should be to use the lowest effective dose of the least toxic anticonvulsant for the briefest period of time.

As with febrile seizures, providing reassurance to the child and family is paramount; they must understand that the seizures will not result in brain damage. The clinician should tell them that the dosage and type of medication may have to be changed frequently, depending on its side effects and effect on seizure control, and that the child should be able to lead as normal a life as possible. Adequate seizure control is possible in a high percentage of children with epilepsy, and when a child has been seizure-free for approximately 2 years, the anticonvulsant frequently can be tapered and stopped to test whether the child remains seizure-free without anticonvulsant medication.

Other modes of treatment may be necessary. In children with infantile spasms, a series of adrenocorticotropic hormone (ACTH) injections used daily over several weeks generally controls the actual seizures, but the prognosis with respect to normal development is poor. In some selected cases of focal seizure disorders, assessment for surgical intervention may be appropriate.

TABLE 19.7 **Anticonvulsants Used in the Treatment of Epileptic Seizures**

| Drug | Seizure Type | | | Usual Dose (mg/kg) | Cost | Side Effects |
	Tonic-Clonic	Partial	Absence			
Phenobarbital	+	+		4–6	Low	Drowsiness; hyperactivity, rash, cognitive changes
Valproic acid	+	+	+	15–100	Moderate	Liver and pancreatic abnormalities; hair loss; polycystic ovary; neural tube defects
Carbamazepine		+		10–30	Moderate	Drowsiness; hepatotoxicity; granulocytopenia; rash
Ethosuximide			+	20–40	Moderate	Gastrointestinal upset; granulocytopenia
Phenytoin	+	+		4–8	Low	Rash; gum hyperplasia; hirsutism

+ = useful.

HEADACHE

Virtually everyone has experienced a headache at some time, and even in children, headaches are one of the most common medical complaints. The vast majority of headaches are benign, and many are related to systemic infection with fever, such as "flu" or a sore throat, especially a streptococcal pharyngitis.

Pathophysiology

Headaches result from a variety of causes. Many headaches are related to **head trauma or increased muscular contraction.** Others may be due to disorders of other structures in the head such as **paranasal sinuses and the temporomandibular joint.** Some headaches are purely **psychogenic** in origin, as those associated with depression. **Increased intracranial pressure,** such as that occurring with brain tumor, with intracranial hemorrhage or infection, or idiopathically, also may account for headaches. **Infections such as meningitis,** with or without increased pressure, can also result in headaches. The **various varieties of migraine (with and without aura)** are very frequent causes of recurrent headaches in children.

Pediatric Pearl

Contrary to popular thinking, migraine is common, even in children.

Brain parenchyma is insensitive to pain. However, other intracranial structures such as the large arteries, the venous sinuses, and the dura at the base of the skull are sensitive to pain. Pain may result from various vascular changes and several abnormalities relating to the metabolism of serotonin and its metabolites. In migraine, serotonin metabolism is systemically abnormal both during and between attacks. Serotonin may lead to vasodilation or vasoconstriction of the intracranial vasculature; this forms the basis for some of the old and many of the new drugs used in patients with migraine, because many of these drugs affect serotonin metabolism.

Clinical and Laboratory Evaluation

History

In most children with headaches, the history alone may suggest the diagnosis. If at all possible, the examiner should obtain information directly from children, in order to judge their assessment of pain, not that of the parents or caretakers. Ob-

viously, the parents' impression is also important to consider, but the use of a direct approach to history-taking gains children's confidence. While obtaining this history, the examiner can assess its accuracy, often gaining insight into parent–child relationships. Frequently, the initial history is the most accurate, because subsequent histories may be biased by questions asked by prior examiners. Questions should not be leading.

A detailed history concerning the frequency of the headaches, the duration, dates of origin, character, and severity is necessary. Character and severity are subjective; occasionally, the examiner may obtain an assessment of severity by asking children to rate the severity on a scale of 1 to 10 or if the headache interferes with activities or necessitates absence from school or cessation of play. Remember that pain thresholds vary tremendously in different individuals. In the event of a severe headache of acute onset, the examiner may ask, if the information has not been volunteered, **whether this is the worst headache the child has ever experienced.** The examiner should ask about associated symptoms such as **aura;** is there a warning before a headache begins or do the parents perceive something different about a child's appearance or behavior? Other associated manifestations include **photophobia; annoyance or being bothered by loud noises; visual abnormalities such as changes in visual perception; nausea, vomiting, or associated abdominal pain; or vertigo.**

The clinician should ask what the child does when experiencing a headache. Does the child lie down in a quiet room and want to go to sleep? If so, does the child feel better on awakening? If there have been repeated headaches, questions about changes in the character of the headaches from prior episodes and what particular time of day the headache occurs are appropriate.

In addition, the examiner should inquire about any possible precipitating event, such as sudden or unexpected changes in the family dynamics. Questions also should concern any interrelated illness, fever, family history of headaches, and association with eating a particular type of food. Information concerning any prior self-medication attempts and the dosage and length of use of prescribed medication are important to obtain. Questions that relate to child and parental anxieties concerning the headache are also warranted. Is either the child or parents afraid that something may be seriously wrong with the child's brain, such as a tumor or stroke? Is the child afraid that this is something similar to another experience in the family or an event shown on TV? Children can hardly remain untouched by innumerable TV advertisements for headache remedies and their resulting influence.

Physical Examination

Although neurologic examination is normal in the vast majority of children with headaches, careful, detailed examination is important for many reasons. **Tests for meningismus, increased intracranial pressure, and associated illnesses,** such as **sinusitis,** that might explain the headache are necessary, and children should not receive the impression that the examiner is trivializing the complaints. The clinician should evaluate neck stiffness and assess meningeal signs, certainly if the headache is accompanied by fever. Checking for papilledema allows assessment of increased intracranial pressure. Reassurance is an important modality of treatment in headaches, and it is comforting to have the examiner give a diagnosis and tell children that they are normal.

Laboratory Evaluation

In children with chronic or recurrent headaches, when good current and past histories are coupled with normal physical and neurologic examinations, a diagnosis is generally possible with no laboratory work. If the history or abnormalities on physical examination make the examiner suspect an underlying disorder, then specific tests can be used to document that disorder. In the case of suspected meningitis, evaluation of the CSF is safe after the clinician has excluded the presence of increased intracranial pressure.

☀ Pediatric Pearl

If focal neurologic findings are present, neuroimaging studies are usually necessary to perform before lumbar puncture to check for possible cerebral herniation.

The clinician should order other laboratory tests judiciously. For example, **Lyme disease studies are certainly justified in a child who may have been bitten by a deer tick and has since developed headaches.**

Neuroimaging studies such as CT or MRI scans are not indicated or routinely needed in children with headaches. Both of these studies are being used at great public expense. EEG, another overused procedure, has no place in the assessment of such children. All of these procedures may be counterproductive in the management of children with headaches without neurologic abnormalities, because they place undue emphasis on the possibility of an abnormality in the brain. This makes reassurance, the major thrust of treatment, more difficult. In addition, the EEG is not a good investigative tool for detecting small lesions in the brain, and nonspecific meaningless abnormalities, which are difficult to explain to children, are common.

Differential Diagnosis

Common types of chronic headaches in children include **vascular headaches (migraine) and muscle contraction (tension) headaches;** tension headaches are more prevalent in adolescents and adults. In muscular contraction headaches, children may describe a perception of tightness or a feeling that a band is constricting the head. They may have difficulty localizing or pointing to the regions of the head that are painful. Although bothersome, muscular contraction headaches are not severe enough to interfere with usual activities such as school or play. Neurologic evaluation is unrevealing.

The most frequently encountered type of vascular headaches in children is migraine without aura. The headache may be bifrontal, generalized, bitemporal, or difficult for children to define, and it may be pounding or throbbing. Before the actual headache begins, children may volunteer some poorly defined complaints of dizziness or nausea. The duration ranges widely—from hours to an entire day or more. Autonomic dysfunction, such as pallor or nausea, is present in some cases. At times, children who can fall asleep awaken free of pain.

Migraine with aura is less common in children. However, it should be remembered that children must be adequately perceptive to be able to describe the aura. The aura is usually visual, such as flashing lights, scotomata (patchy losses of vision), or transient blindness. Auras are of short duration, and a rapidly developing severe one-sided pounding or throbbing headache follows. The affected side generally varies. Nausea and, less frequently, vomiting may accompany the headache. Some children experience a lessening or disappearance of the headache after vomiting. Photophobia is frequent, and children may want to lie down in a darkened quiet room and try to sleep.

Migraine headaches are paroxysmal, and their frequency is variable. Precipitating factors, which may differ from case to case, include various types of food, caffeine, stress, fatigue, emotional problems, head trauma, and menstrual periods. Neurologic examination reveals no abnormal features.

Migraine may be associated with certain transient neurologic deficits that depend on the area of the brain affected by vasoconstriction and ischemia. **This complicated form is variable. For example, it may manifest as transient hemiparesis or be associated with transient unilateral orbital or eye pain and paralysis of the third cranial nerve on the same side.** Neuroimaging procedures are usually indicated the first time children with complicated migraine visit a physician. MRI is the most useful study.

Brain tumors are uncommon causes of headaches in children. Headaches due to brain tumors are often chronic and progressive and are more frequent in the morning, although they may occur any time of day. Other symptoms and signs of increased intracranial pressure often accompany the headache, including diplopia (double vision due to sixth nerve involvement), ataxia, irritability, personality changes, papilledema, and focal neurologic findings.

With pseudotumor cerebri, headaches are accompanied by signs and symptoms of increased intracranial pressure. Focal signs are absent, and no mass lesion is seen on imaging.

Headaches related to **sudden onset of subarachnoid hemorrhage** are frequently associated with stiff neck, fever, change in mental status, signs and symptoms of increased intracranial pressure, and focal neurologic abnormalities. Children may describe them as the worst headache in their lives.

Management

With all chronic headaches, most of which are vascular in origin (migraine), reassurance of the affected child and family should be the first and foremost therapeutic measure. After a thorough explanation of the benign nature of the headache, favorable outcome, and absence of tumor or stroke, the clinician should discuss therapeutic options in detail with the child and family. An acceptable option is the use of no medication at all. Because many children are attuned to the dangers of drugs of all kinds, including those commonly used to treat headaches, the child may readily accept this option. During the parent–child discussion, the clinician should also suggest solutions to stressful situations at home or in school and other possible precipitating factors, such as anxiety, lack of sleep, and school-related stress. If certain foods appear to be direct precipitating factors, their elimination may be effective. Unconventional therapeutic methods, such as using biofeedback and relaxation techniques, may be appropriate in older children and adolescents. A headache diary may be useful.

At times, children have successfully treated their headaches on their own, with over-the-counter drugs. They frequently report relief with aspirin, acetaminophen, or small doses of ibuprofen. A clinician should caution children about the potential side effects of these drugs.

For children who have infrequent attacks of common migraine, the use of nonsteroidal anti-inflammatory drugs (NSAIDs), taken when the headache begins, is a reasonable option, if acetaminophen does not help. NSAIDs should be taken with food, which may be difficult when nausea or vomiting accompany a headache.

In older children who experience infrequent attacks of migraine, caffeine and ergotamine preparations (Cafergot) may be useful in aborting headaches if the medication is taken at the first perception of an aura. This is difficult because the aura may appear virtually at any time, and a child must have the medication at hand. In school, where there are many regulations to prevent children taking medication on their own, by the time a child gets to the school nurse it may be too late for the caffeine–ergotamine combination to abort the headache. During the past few years, drugs known as triptans have made an important addition to migraine therapy in older children. These are formulated for oral, intranasal, and subcutaneous administration in individuals free of cardiac disorders.

For children with debilitating and frequent migraine attacks, prophylaxis should be a topic of child–family discussion. Prophylaxis means that a patient will take daily medication whether headaches are present or not; this idea is sometimes difficult for children to comprehend, and compliance is frequently not ideal. Several classes of drugs may be used for migraine prophylaxis, including beta-blocking agents [e.g., propranolol (contraindicated in asthmatics)], antidepressant agents (e.g., amitriptyline), calcium channel blocking agents, and divalproex sodium. If one of these drugs is successful over a substantial period of time, an attempt at lowering the dosage or stopping the medication should be considered, because spontaneous remission may occur in children with chronic headaches. Each of these agents has potential side effects, which children need to understand. The long-term prognosis is generally favorable.

BRAIN TUMORS

Approximately 20% of all malignancies in childhood are brain tumors. About two-thirds of these brain tumors are **infratentorial** (below the dural partition that separates the cerebrum from the cerebellum); the remainder are **supratentorial.** The origin of many of these tumors is unclear, and the noncommittal term "primitive neuroectodermal tumor" has been used to describe many of them (Table 19.8).

Pathophysiology

Any intracranial mass, including a brain tumor, results in compression of the parenchyma and may result in obstruction of the normal CSF pathways, causing ventricular dilation. Because of very limited compressibility, intracranial pressure rises, with further compression on draining venous sinuses. This initiates and perpetuates a cycle resulting in reduction of cerebral blood flow, cerebral hypoxia, further vascular dilation, further increased intracerebral volume, and increased pressure. In infants and young children whose cranial sutures have not yet fused, the sutures may split and the head circumference may expand in the presence of increased intracranial pressure.

Brain tumors may produce neurologic abnormalities as a result of their infiltration of the particular portion of the brain in which this process is occurring. For example, infiltrative tumors in the brainstem will produce cranial nerve abnormalities by local encroachment on their nuclei. An expanding intracranial mass may also be a cause. Herniation of a section of the brain through various openings (e.g., herniation of the cerebellar tonsils through the foramen magnum) may result in further dysfunction of brainstem structures and diminished blood flow.

TABLE 19.8 **Brain Tumors in Children**

Infratentorial
    Cerebellar astrocytoma
    Medulloblastoma
    Ependymoma
    Brainstem glioma
Supratentorial
    Astrocytoma
    Glioblastoma
    Oligodendroglioma
Intraventricular
    Choroid plexus papilloma
    Ependymoma
Craniopharyngioma
Optic glioma
Pinealoma

Clinical and Laboratory Evaluation

History

Because brain tumors may lead to increased intracranial pressure, questions should primarily elicit information regarding symptoms associated with increased pressure, which include vomiting, headache, and visual dysfunction. **Vomiting** is a very common feature in the presence of increased pressure, and nausea may also be present. Both nausea and vomiting are most prominent in the morning. Although there is no temporal relationship to food, children's appetite may also be diminished.

Headache, which is similarly more pronounced in the morning, is virtually a constant accompanying feature in children with increased intracranial pressure. Although the clinician should ask children and parents about the region of the head where the perceived headache occurs, the site of the headache is of poor localizing value. It is more important to ask about the duration of the headache. When increased intracranial pressure is initially present, headaches may last for just a short time in the morning, and children may be better the rest of the day. As the pressure increases with time, the headaches may become more severe and of longer duration. As noted, separation of cranial sutures in children younger than 12 years of age may provide temporary alleviation of symptoms.

The examiner should direct questions to elicit a history of diplopia (double vision), which may result from involvement of the cranial nerves, most commonly of the sixth (or abducens) nerve. This results in **diplopia** on attempts to look to either side. The degree of diplopia, which may vary, becomes more pronounced as the intracranial pressure rises. At times, children may compensate and develop a **head tilt.** However, it should be emphasized that papilledema resulting from increased intracranial pressure produces virtually no visual symptoms. Visual acuity is normal, although transient, and mild visual field obscuration occurs.

Additional questions should also attempt to elicit **personality changes, drowsiness, irritability,** or changes in level of consciousness, any or all of which may be associated with increased intracranial pressure or lesions encroaching on the brainstem and other regions of the brain such as the hypothalamus. Other questions should include those designed to obtain information about problems with motor dysfunction such as gait disturbances, loss of balance, or loss of normal function of the hands.

Physical Examination

It is important to check the skin for evidence of a neurocutaneous disorder. For example, if numerous **café au lait spots** or axillary freckles are present, the observer should consider **neurofibromatosis** type 1–related tumors. The presence of irregular depigmented areas on the skin should prompt the examiner to consider **tuberous sclerosis**–related intracranial lesions. Alterations of vital signs such as systemic hypertension, bradycardia, and irregular respirations **(Cushing effect)** sometimes accompany increased intracranial pressure but are usually late findings. The clinician should always measure head circumference and plot it on an appropriate graph.

Detailed assessment of mental status is always necessary, because somnolence and irritability, for example, may accompany increased intracranial pressure. It is important to examine cranial nerves carefully, placing special emphasis on assessment of extraocular muscle function and funduscopy. Checking for **papilledema,** an abnormal elevation of the optic nerve head, is an integral part of the assessment of any child with suspected increased intracranial pressure. In papilledema, the disk margins are blurred or obliterated, and loss of spontaneous venous pulsations is present. The veins may be tortuous, and frank hemorrhages may be seen in the retina. Despite these abnormalities, in early papilledema, visual acuity is preserved. A very high percentage of children with brain tumors have papilledema. Abnormalities of the peripheral fields of vision, which can be tested readily in cooperative children, may provide clues to anatomical localization, as in a suprasellar tumor.

Examination of the motor system is also important. Gait abnormalities, for example, may provide clues to the localization of a tumor. Ataxia, which is assessed by asking children to walk tandem forward and backward, is observed in infratentorial tumors. Unilateral weakness, evaluated by watching for drift of the outstretched arms, limping, or strength asymmetries and checked either functionally by observation or with manual muscle testing, may provide a clue to hemispheric or long tract involvement. [Similarly, asymmetries in tone or deep tendon reflexes, presence of dysmetria (past-pointing), presence or absence of extensor plantar responses, and sensory abnormalities may provide clues to the localization of a tumor.

Laboratory Evaluation

In children with suspected brain tumors, either CT scanning or MRI can be used to visualize the lesion. Each technique has certain advantages and disadvantages, but generally, MRI provides the most clinically useful information. However, MRI has certain disadvantages; expense, long testing time (much longer than with CT scanning), necessity for sedation (usually), and the possibility of claustrophobia in the apparatus.

Examination of the CSF by lumbar puncture in children suspected of having brain tumors should occur only *after* imaging studies have been completed and after consultation with a neurologist, because in the presence of a mass lesion, there is an increased risk of brain herniation when CSF is removed via the lumbar route. Under some circumstances, a neurosurgeon may remove ventricular fluid for cytology and glucose determination. In tumors in or near the ventricles, CSF may be xanthochromic (yellow), with a very high protein level. The CSF glucose level is generally normal in most brain tumors.

The value of skull radiographs is very limited in the diagnosis of brain tumors in children. Separation of the cranial sutures is visible in many children with increased intracranial pressure, but pressure must be elevated for a considerable period prior to splitting. Intracranial calcifications may also be detectable; calcifications are seen in some tumors and with several other clinical entities. In some children with seizures, an EEG may demonstrate a focal slow wave activity; this finding may prompt the electroencephalographer to report the suspicion of an underlying mass lesion, but the EEG is not used as a primary localizing tool.

Differential Diagnosis

Not all children with increased intracranial pressure have underlying brain tumors. For example, brain abscesses may occur in young children, especially those with congenital heart disease; MRI can be used to substantiate the diagnoses. In pseudotumor cerebri or so-called benign increase in intracranial pressure, neuroimaging studies are normal and document the absence of a structural lesion. Hydrocephalus and various CNS infections may also lead to increased intracranial pressure.

If the history, physical examination, and laboratory evaluation indicates a probable brain tumor, several types are possible. Three of the common brain tumors in children—**medulloblastomas, astrocytomas,** and **ependymomas**—arise in or near the cerebellum. Although these tumors arise from different structures, their clinical manifestations may be similar. In all tumors involving the cerebellum, the ventricular system may become obstructed, leading to increasing intracranial pressure. Vomiting, headache, and unsteadiness of gait (ataxia) are the most common manifestations and are generally present for several weeks before the diagnosis is established. Unsteadiness of gait results in children holding their feet far apart in an attempt to steady themselves while walking. They may fall and use objects or the wall for support. Cerebellar lesions may also lead to dysmetria and notable slowing when affected children attempt to perform rapid alternating movements. MRI generally substantiates the diagnosis. In children in whom medulloblastoma is identified, imaging of the spinal cord is routinely used to exclude seeding in that region.

Tumors of the **brainstem** are malignant, not only because of their biology but also because of their location. These tumors arise most commonly from the pons **(pontine glioma)** and result in gross enlargement of the brainstem, commonly caused by infiltration. Some tumors in this area result in signs and symptoms caused by torsion or pressure on the brainstem. Brainstem tumors are usually seen in children between 2 and 12 years of age.

Because of the tumor location, cranial nerve palsies are very common. In early stages, signs and symptoms of increased intracranial pressure may be absent. Facial muscle weakness, strabismus, and swallowing difficulties may be accompanied by gait disturbances, vomiting, or gradual onset of hemiparesis. Children may have a head tilt and evidence of extensor plantar responses. Involvement of one or more cranial nerves, especially when findings suggest long tract (corticospinal) involvement, should prompt the examiner to localize the lesion to the brainstem. The progression of symptoms and signs is often relentless, and children may experience involvement of several cranial nerves, increasing paralysis, and impaired consciousness. MRI is very useful in the diagnosis of brainstem tumors. Use of this imaging modality excludes rare problems such as vascular abnormalities of the brainstem or so-called brainstem encephalitis.

The most common midline tumor is the **craniopharyngioma.** Other midline tumors include **optic nerve gliomas** and **pinealomas.** Craniopharyngiomas are generally slow-growing tumors located in the suprasellar region; if they expand forward, they can press against the optic chiasm. With further expansion to other regions, they may compress the pituitary gland and the third ventricle. Because of the proximity to the optic chiasm, impaired vision or defects in the peripheral fields of vision such as unilateral or bitem-

poral field cuts are common. Routine school examination may lead to the discovery of diminished vision, frequently in one eye, in otherwise apparently asymptomatic children.

Craniopharyngiomas may also result in multiple pituitary hormone deficiencies. Thus, children may have diminished linear growth; the clinician should obtain prior height and weight measurements and plot these values on normal growth charts. Precocious puberty is occasionally seen in boys with midline tumors. Increased intracranial pressure can occur in children with craniopharyngiomas, but if it does, it is usually evident rather late in the course. MRI, which demonstrates the tumor, may provide information concerning its location and extent. A significant percentage of craniopharyngiomas in children contain calcifications, readily imaged in skull radiographs or CT scans.

Optic nerve gliomas are one of the most common intracranial tumors in neurofibromatosis type 1. Diminished vision in one eye (of which children may not be aware) is the most common finding; other findings are exophthalmos, strabismus, nystagmus, and optic atrophy. A clinician who may suspect a tumor in a child with cutaneous signs of neurofibromatosis type 1 can readily make the diagnosis with neuroimaging studies.

Hemispheric tumors account for approximately one-third of brain tumors in children, and most of these are malignant (e.g., **astrocytoma** or **oligodendroglioma**). Because of their location in the cerebral hemispheres, seizures, either generalized or with a focal component, are the most common presenting feature. The neurologic assessment may be completely normal. EEG performed when children present with seizures may show focal slowing, suggesting an underlying mass. These supratentorial tumors occur more commonly in older children and adolescents. Neuroimaging, preferably with MRI, establishes the diagnosis.

Management

Treatment of brain tumors in children, which depends on the biology and location of the particular tumor, usually involves a multidisciplinary team approach. In some tumors (e.g., unilateral confined optic glioma), careful observation and follow-up may be prudent. If intracranial pressure elevation is present, vigorous treatment, either surgically by ventriculostomy or medically with induced hypocarbia and diuretics, is essential, depending on circumstances. Surgical resection and radiation or chemotherapy may be appropriate in selected tumors. All therapeutic methods have major immediate and long-term side effects. See the Suggested Readings for a further discussion of treatment effects.

Unfortunately, the therapeutic situation has not improved over the past decade. Management, which is changing constantly, is very complex and specialized.

MYOPATHIES

Myopathies constitute a group of diverse disorders in which skeletal muscle is the organ system primarily involved. Several varieties of myopathies—**dystrophic, myotonic,** and **inflammatory**—are considered in this section. Dystrophic myopathies (the several types of **muscular dystrophies**) and **myotonic myopathies** are genetically determined disorders, whereas inflammatory myopathies (**polymyositis** and **dermatomyositis**) are autoimmune-related entities. Several other myopathies occur less frequently in children and are not discussed here (Table 19.9).

Pathophysiology

Skeletal muscle biopsy specimens from patients with myopathies reveal characteristic pathologic abnormalities. These include abnormal variability in fiber size, increased amount of endomysial connective tissue and fat, architectural changes in scattered fibers, and internally positioned nuclei. Inflammatory cells and vascular abnormalities are evident in inflammatory myopathies. Serum muscle enzymes, the most important of which is creatinine kinase, are generally elevated in the myopathies.

Clinical and Laboratory Evaluation

History

Because muscle is the target organ in myopathies, its major function (movement production) is disturbed. Depending on severity, this results in weakness that manifests in difficulty climbing or

---

TABLE 19.9 **Myopathies in Children**

Common
　　Dystrophic (muscular dystrophy)
　　Myotonic
　　Inflammatory (polymyositis and dermatomyositis)
Less common
　　Endocrine
　　Metabolic
　　Periodic paralysis
　　Congenital
　　Toxic

---

descending stairs; trouble or awkwardness in running (waddling like a duck); or other gait abnormalities, such as walking up on the toes or difficulty getting up from a sitting position or from the floor, raising the arms over the head, or carrying packages. The examiner should ask about these functional problems, and if present, about the duration of symptoms, whether there has been any worsening or improvement, and the presence or absence of pain and muscle tenderness. In young children, the history should ascertain whether the child has a worsening gross motor deficit. Has the child lost function after having attained a particular capability, such as walking, sitting, or running? Other questions to ask include:

- Is weakness accompanied by any signs or symptoms of systemic involvement such as a rash or fever, as seen in dermatomyositis?
- Has there been stiffness or weakness in the hands or difficulty in letting go of objects after holding them in the hand (myotonia)?
- Has there been any problem with swallowing or chewing, which would be present if pharyngeal muscles or muscles of mastication are weak?
- Are there any problems with the facial muscles, which would affect the child's ability to blow up a balloon, whistle with pursed lips, or close the eyelids completely during sleep?

Because dystrophic and myotonic myopathies are genetically determined, a careful family history with special emphasis on muscular and related problems is mandatory. Other necessary inquiries concern parental consanguinity (marriage to a close relative), which would suggest a greater possibility of an autosomal recessive disorder.

Physical Examination

A complete general and neurologic examination is necessary. Functional testing may be helpful, because the major complaint will most probably be **weakness**. The clinician should observe children walking, not in the confines of a small room, but in a corridor and up and down stairs, to see if there is a waddle, indicating weakness in the hip girdle, and to see if they need the support of a banister to pull themselves up while climbing stairs. If possible, the examiner should watch children run or try to rise from a prone position; they may have to use their arms to push themselves up if they have weakness of the large muscles around the hip girdle. It is necessary to see whether any muscle wasting (atrophy) or enlargement is present, especially large calves. The clinician should check whether children can walk on their toes, to document normalcy of the gastrocnemius–soleus group, and on their heels, to test function of the anterior tibialis muscles. It is necessary to check muscles supplied by the cranial nerves, with special emphasis on the extraocular, facial, palatal, lingual, sternocleidomastoid, and trapezius muscles.

Manual muscle testing (i.e., testing strength of individual muscles) takes a great deal of practice, but a few large muscles, such as deltoids, biceps, and quadriceps, are relatively easy to test, as is hand grasp strength. In place of testing neck flexor muscle strength, which also takes much practice, the examiner may ask the child to raise his or her head while in the supine position. It is also necessary to check deep tendon reflexes; they are reduced or absent in most genetic myopathies. However, their absence does not exclude a myopathy.

In addition, observation of children's skin for a subtle rash, particularly the skin over the eyelids, the interphalangeal joints and knuckles, and the extensor surfaces of elbows and knees areas is necessary. Skin involvement is evident in dermatomyositis.

To check for **myotonia,** the inability to relax after a voluntary contraction, the clinician may ask children to close their hands forcibly. If they have action (or reflex) myotonia, they will only be able to open their hands very slowly and may have to flex their wrists to perform this function. A sharp tap with a reflex hammer on the thenar mass may elicit myotonia, but this requires practice or demonstration by an experienced examiner.

Laboratory Evaluation

Genetic studies (DNA analyses) are currently available in many commercial laboratories for selected muscular disorders such as Duchenne or Becker muscular dystrophy and myotonic dystrophy. Serum muscle enzyme determinations [creatine kinase (CK), lactate dehydrogenase (LDH), aspartate aminotransferase (AST), and alanine aminotransferase (ALT)] usually reveal abnormal values in myopathies. **In Duchenne and Becker muscular dystrophy, the CK values are always markedly elevated.** However, with some of these disorders, abnormalities, if present, may be very modest.

In **electromyography (EMG),** an electrodiagnostic study, needle electrodes are inserted into the muscle, and extracellular recordings are made electronically. Certain abnormalities (e.g., short-duration single motor unit potentials) are apparent on minimal volition in cooperative children. The procedure is moderately uncomfortable, although sedation can be used, if necessary. In myotonia, characteristic EMG findings are seen and heard, among which is a sound described as similar to a dive bomber diving.

A properly performed muscle biopsy, either with a special needle or through a skin incision, can be helpful in the differential diagnosis of myopathies when specialized studies are used.

Differential Diagnosis

Several conditions must be considered in the diagnosis of myopathy.

Dystrophic Myopathies

The different types of myopathies (muscular dystrophies) each have characteristic patterns of inheritance, onset, clinical course, muscular involvement, and laboratory findings (Table 19.10).

Duchenne muscular dystrophy affects only boys, with very rare exceptions, because it is an X-linked disease. Toe-walking is frequently seen after the child learns to walk, attempts at running may be awkward, and waddling may become prominent by 5 years of age. Calf muscles appear large by that time. Because of slowly increasing weakness, children experience difficulty with stairs as they grow older. Weakness is relentlessly progressive, and all boys with Duchenne

---

TABLE 19.10 Muscular Dystrophies

Disorder	Inheritance	Onset	Course	Muscles Involved	Other Findings
Duchenne	X-linked recessive	< 5 years	Progressive	Pelvic and shoulder girdles; large calves	Mental retardation; cardiac involvement; absent dystrophin
Facioscapulo-humeral	Autosomal dominant	Early to late	Slow	Facial muscles; shoulder girdle	Cognition normal
Limb girdle	Recessive and dominant	Variable	Slow	Shoulder and pelvic girdles	Cognition normal

muscular dystrophy are wheelchair-bound by 12 years of age. Cardiorespiratory compromise leads to death in their 20s. All boys with Duchenne muscular dystrophy have markedly elevated serum CK levels even before developing overt muscle weakness. About two-thirds have a deletion on DNA testing; in the one-third who have no demonstrable deletion, a muscle biopsy specimen indicates characteristic pathologic findings without the muscle protein dystrophin. In a milder form of X-linked muscular dystrophy **(Becker type),** the onset is generally later, and the course is much more slowly progressive. Dystrophin is present in muscle biopsies, although in diminished amounts.

Limb girdle (LG) and **facioscapulohumeral (FSH) muscular dystrophies** are much more variable in their time of presentation of weakness and in their course. Genetic testing (DNA) is available when FSH muscular dystrophy is suspected. Serum CK elevation may be modest or absent. Similarly, muscle biopsies are much less specific than those in Duchenne muscular dystrophy; dystrophin content is normal. To distinguish the several forms of LG dystrophy, specialized testing of muscle biopsy specimens is necessary.

Myotonic Dystrophy

This autosomal dominant disorder exhibits marked variability in age of onset and progression. In addition to myotonia, which is most readily demonstrable by the inability to relax the hand after squeezing it shut tightly, children may complain of weakness of the hand muscles, may be retarded or have learning difficulties in school, and have hypernasal speech. Adolescent boys often have early onset of frontal baldness, and cataracts (seen with a slit lamp examination) are very common. An infantile form may be manifest with severe floppiness and clubfoot at birth; in this form, the mother, not the father, always has myotonic dystrophy, although signs and symptoms are so mild that neither she nor her physician is usually aware of the presence of the disease. Myotonic dystrophy is usually a clinical diagnosis, but in older children, the results of EMG are characteristic. Muscle enzymes are usually only minimally elevated, and muscle biopsies are unnecessary. DNA testing is now available.

Inflammatory Muscle Disorders

Weakness (more in the legs than in the arms), which can be documented on functional testing, is usually the presenting symptom in children. The onset of weakness is generally not as insidious as it is with dystrophy, although it is still most commonly subacute. The child or parents can usually date the onset of weakness, often a matter of weeks or a few months. Muscle, joint pain, or both sometimes accompany the weakness. In **dermatomyositis,** an inflammatory muscle disease of children that is more common than polymyositis, a violaceous rash may be present on the eyelids, and erythema may be present on the knuckle areas and extensor surfaces of the knees and elbows. Inflammatory myopathies are not genetically determined. Serum muscle enzymes are generally elevated, and EMG studies, although not specific, are helpful. A muscle biopsy specimen provides a tissue diagnosis in a large percentage of children.

Management

No specific medication to cure the dystrophin myopathies or myotonic dystrophy is available. Prednisone 0.75 mg/kg/day can slow the relentless progression of Duchenne muscular dystrophy. Gene replacement therapy, which may be a possibility, is not yet available. Physical therapy is indicated in most children with muscular dystrophy, and bracing and adaptive devices can be provided when necessary. It is essential to observe children for joint contractures, and treatment for scoliosis is necessary. The multidisciplinary approach available in Muscular Dystrophy Association–supported clinics is the best therapy for most children. Genetic counseling for families is indicated in most instances.

Prednisone or immunosuppressive agents such as azathioprine or methotrexate in appropriate doses, with the usual cautions regarding side effects, are also useful in inflammatory myopathies, because these conditions are immunologically mediated disorders with an inflammatory component. Physical therapy is also helpful.

SUGGESTED READINGS

General
Menkes JH, Sarnat HB (eds): *Child Neurology,* 6th ed. Philadelphia, Lippincott Williams & Wilkins, 2000.

Evaluation of the Floppy Infant
Dubowitz V: The floppy infant. *Clin Dev Med* 76:1–158, 1980.

Jones HR: EMG evaluation of the floppy infant: Differential diagnosis and technical aspects. *Muscle Nerve* 13:338–347, 1990.

Russell JW, Afifi AK, Ross MA: Predictive value of electromyography in diagnosis and prognosis of the hypotonic infant. *J Child Neurol* 7:387–391, 1992.

Vannucci RC: Differential diagnosis of diseases producing hypotonia. *Pediatr Ann* 18:404–410, 1989.

Wasiewski WW: Central nervous system disorders producing hypotonia. *Pediatr Ann* 18:412–419, 1989.

Benign Febrile Seizures

Baumann RJ, Duffner PK: Treatment of children with simple febrile seizures: The AAP practice parameter. *Pediatr Neurol* 23:11–17, 2000.

Camfield PR, Camfield CS: Management and treatment of febrile seizures. *Curr Probl Pediatr* 27:6–14, 1997.

Knudsen FU: Febrile seizures: Treatment and prognosis. *Epilepsia* 41:2–9, 2000.

Epilepsy

Engel J Jr, Pedley TA, Aicardi J, et al: *Epilepsy. A Comprehensive Textbook*. Philadelphia, Lippincott Williams & Wilkins, 2000.

Mizrahi EM, Kellaway P: *Diagnosis and Management of Neonatal Seizures*. Philadelphia, Lippincott Williams & Wilkins, 2000.

Wyllie E: *The Treatment of Epilepsy—Principles and Practice*, 3rd ed. Philadelphia, Lippincott Williams & Wilkins, 2001.

Headache

Barlow CF: Headaches and migraine in childhood. *Clin Dev Med* 91:1–288, 1984.

Bulloch B, Tenenbein M: Emergency department management of pediatric migraine. *Pediatr Emerg Care* 16:196–201, 2000.

Congden PJ, Forsythe WI: Migraine in childhood: A study of 300 children. *Dev Med Child Neurol* 21:209–216, 1979.

Hersh EV, Moore PA, Ross GL: Over-the-counter analgesics and antipyretics: a critical assessment. *Clin Ther* 22:500–548, 2000.

Brain tumors

Cohen ME, Duffner (eds): *Brain Tumors in Children. Principles of Diagnosis and Treatment*. New York: Raven Press, 1994.

Packer RJ: Brain tumors in children. *Arch Neurol* 56:421–425, 1999.

Pollack IF: Brain tumors in children. *N Engl J Med* 331:1500–1507, 1994.

Myopathies

Ashizawa T, Dunne CJ, et al: Anticipation in myotonic dystrophy. *Neurology* 42:1171–1177, 1877–1883, 1992.

Brooke MH: *A Clinical View of Neuromuscular Disease*, 2nd ed. Baltimore, Williams & Wilkins, 1986.

Darras BT: Molecular genetics of Duchenne and Becker muscular dystrophy. *J Pediatr* 117:1–15, 1990.

Griggs RC, Moxley RT, Mendell JR, et al: Prednisone in Duchenne dystrophy. A randomized, controlled trial defining the time course and dose response. *Arch Neurol* 48:383–388, 1991.

Harper PS: *Myotonic Dystrophy*. Philadelphia, WB Saunders, 1979.

Chapter 20

Nephrology

Juan C. Kupferman, Suroj Supavekin, and
Frederick J. Kaskel

EVALUATION OF KIDNEY FUNCTION

By convention, kidney function is usually interpreted as the degree of glomerular filtration. However, the kidneys have many other functions that may be assessed by both laboratory and imaging studies (Table 20.1).

Assessment of Renal Status and Evaluation of Parenchymal Damage

The first study in the evaluation of children with suspected renal disease is complete **urinalysis,** which yields information about the overall function of the urinary tract. The presence of **proteinuria** may be indicative of renal parenchymal damage. **Hematuria,** either macroscopic or microscopic, is an important manifestation of renal disease, although other urinary tract and systemic entities may present with hematuria. Furthermore, a urine dipstick that is positive for blood may reflect the presence not only of red blood cells (RBCs) but also of hemoglobin and myoglobin. Analysis of the urine sediment confirms the presence of RBCs or white blood cells (WBCs), different types of casts, crystals, and bacteria.

Assessment of Glomerular Filtration

The **glomerular filtration rate** (GFR) provides a broad reflection of the functioning nephron mass. In common clinical practice, GFR can be evaluated by measuring serum creatinine (SCr), blood urea nitrogen (BUN), and creatinine clearance, or by performing a renal radionuclide scan.

Serum Creatinine
Creatinine is synthesized predominantly in the skeletal muscle and is excreted exclusively through the kidneys. In general, the rate of creatinine synthesis remains constant, and its serum concentration reflects the rate of renal elimination. Therefore,

an elevated SCr concentration denotes a diminished renal clearance of creatinine and a decline in GFR. It is important to remember that **SCr is lower in children** than in adults. After the first days of life (with SCr higher, close to maternal levels), the normal SCr in infants is about 0.3–0.4 mg/dl and increases slowly up to 0.9–1.0 mg/dl in adolescence.

Blood Urea Nitrogen
BUN is the final product in the metabolism of proteins and is excreted by the kidneys. Urea is freely filtered by the glomerulus but is also reabsorbed in the renal tubules, **making the BUN a less reliable indicator of the GFR.** Furthermore, extrarenal factors may increase [e.g., gastrointestinal (GI) bleeding, dehydration, increased protein intake or catabolism] or decrease (e.g., decreased protein intake, malnutrition, liver disease) the concentration of BUN, independent of renal function.

Creatinine Clearance
Creatinine clearance is a relatively accurate test to assess GFR in pediatric patients. One disadvantage of this method is the need for a 24-hour urine collection, which may be difficult to obtain in young children. The following formula is useful:

$$\text{CCr (ml/min/1.73 m}^2) = \frac{\text{UCr (mg/dl)} \times \text{UV (ml/day)} \times 1.73 \text{ (m}^2)}{\text{SCr (mg/dl)} \times 1440 \text{ (min)} \times \text{BSA (m}^2)}$$

where CCr equals creatinine clearance, UCr equals urine creatinine concentration, UV equals urine volume, 1440 is the time of collection in minutes (24 hours), and BSA is the patient's body surface area. It is important to note that creatinine clearance is expressed in relation to BSA and that the normal range has been standardized to a BSA of 1.73 m². GFR is low at birth (20 ml/min/1.73 m²), increases to 60 ml/min/1.73 m² by the first month of life, and reaches normal adult levels by the second year of life.

TABLE 20.1 Laboratory and Imaging Studies Used to Evaluate Renal Status

LABORATORY STUDIES

Blood
- Serum sodium, potassium, chloride, bicarbonate, pH, Pco_2, anion gap
- Serum creatinine (SCr), blood urea nitrogen (BUN), creatinine clearance (CCr) [Schwartz formula for estimation of CCr]
- Calcium, phosphorus, alkaline phosphatase, magnesium, uric acid
- Hematocrit/hemoglobin, reticulocyte count, iron studies
- Hormone or enzyme serum levels: renin, aldosterone, vasopressin, parathyroid hormone, erythropoietin, vitamin D_3

Urine
- Urinalysis: specific gravity, pH, dipstick, protein, blood, urine sediment
- Urine electrolytes, fractional excretion of electrolytes, urinary anion gap
- Urine osmolality
- Calcium:creatinine ratio, protein:creatinine ratio
- Microalbuminuria
- Urine culture

Kidney
- Renal biopsy: histology, immunofluorescence, electron microscopy

IMAGING STUDIES
- Renal and bladder ultrasound
- Doppler ultrasound
- Radionuclide renal scan
- Contrast voiding cystourethrogram (VCUG), nuclear cystogram
- Intravenous pyelogram
- Computed tomography
- Magnetic resonance imaging, magnetic resonance arteriography
- Arteriography

 CASE 1

A 4-year-old boy has a SCr of 0.5 mg/dl, a UCr of 30 mg/dl, a UV of 1000 ml/day, and a BSA of 0.7 m². By using the formula for creatinine clearance, his GFR (by creatinine clearance) is:

$$\frac{30 \text{ (mg/dl)} \times 1000 \text{ ml} \times 1.73 \text{ m}^2}{0.5 \text{ (mg/dl)} \times 1440 \text{ min} \times 0.7 \text{ m}^2} =$$

$$103 \text{ ml/min/1.73 m}^2$$

The adequacy of the 24-hour collection can be determined by total creatinine content. An adequate 24-hour urine collection should have at least a total creatinine content of 15 mg/kg in a female or 20 mg/kg in a male. It is easier to estimate the GFR using a mathematical formula (Schwartz) without the need of a 24-hour urine collection. It requires only the patient's height and SCr, as follows:

CCr (ml/min/1.73 m²) =

$$\frac{\text{UCr (mg/dl)} \times \text{UV (ml/day)} \times 1.73 \text{ (m}^2)}{\text{SCr (mg/dl)} \times 1440 \text{ (min)} \times \text{BSA (m}^2)}$$

$$GFR = \frac{k \times \text{height (cm)}}{SCr \text{ (mg/dl)}}$$

where k (constant) equals 0.45 during the first year of life, 0.55 in children 2–13 years of age, 0.7 in adolescent males, and 0.57 in adolescent females. The result is expressed directly for 1.73 m² of BSA.

 CASE 2

A 5-year-old boy has a height of 110 cm and a SCr of 0.5 mg/dl. By using the Schwartz formula, his estimated GFR is:

$$\frac{0.55 \times 110}{0.5} = 121 \text{ ml/min/1.73 m}^2$$

Radionuclide Scan

In specific situations, it is necessary to evaluate each kidney GFR separately by radionuclide studies. Technetium-99m–labeled diethylenetriamine pentaacetic acid (^{99m}Tc-DTPA) is commonly used to measure GFR (see ASSESSMENT OF RENAL STRUCTURE).

Assessment of Renal Concentration and Dilution Capacity

The **renal concentration capacity** is commonly assessed by measuring the urine **specific gravity** and the urine **osmolality**. Urine specific gravity reflects the ratio between the weight of an amount of urine and the weight of the same amount of distilled water. Because the weight of urine is determined by the number of solutes dissolved, specific gravity indirectly reflects the urine concentration of the solutes. However, specific gravity has limitations; any solute in the urine (e.g., protein or glucose) may increase the urine weight and therefore be reflected in the specific gravity evaluation. The urine specific gravity may vary between 1.000 and 1.030, depending on the hydration status. **Urine osmolality is a more accurate method of assessing the renal concentration capacity** because it measures the number of osmotically active solutes present in a solution. If a renal concentration defect is suspected, a water deprivation test may be necessary for confirmation and for diagnosing either a renal or an extrarenal cause.

Assessment of Renal Acidification

To evaluate a renal acidification defect, the excretion of NH_4^+ should be assessed by the **urine net charge (or urinary anion gap).** (see RENAL TUBULAR ACIDOSIS). The appropriate renal response in metabolic acidosis should be the excretion of an acid urine. The **urine pH** is another tool to assess the renal acidification process. If the urine pH is high in a child with acidosis, it suggests a renal acidification defect. A complete evaluation may include other studies, including fractional excretion of bicarbonate (HCO_3^-) and urinary P_{CO_2}.

Assessment of Renal Handling of Electrolytes

The kidneys are important regulators of fluid and electrolyte balance, although other factors such as hormones (e.g., antidiuretic hormone, aldosterone, parathyroid hormone, vitamin D_3, insulin) also participate in the complex regulation of sodium, potassium, chloride, bicarbonate, calcium, phosphorus, and magnesium. The serum electrolytes may reflect the consequence of the interaction between extrarenal and renal factors. It is important to note that **the level of a particular electrolyte does not necessarily reflect the content of that electrolyte in the body.**

Urine electrolytes may be measured in a 24-hour urine collection or in a random urine sample.

The fractional excretion of an electrolyte expresses the amount excreted related to the amount filtered, as a percentage. The **fractional excretion of sodium** (FE_{Na}), a useful parameter in the evaluation of oliguria, can help differentiate between prerenal and renal causes of acute renal failure. The FE_{Na} is calculated as follows:

FE_{Na}:

$$\frac{Urine\ Na\ (mEq/L)/Serum\ Na\ (mEq/L)}{Urine\ Cr(mg/dl)/Serum\ Cr\ (mg/dl)} \times 100$$

In prerenal oliguria, the FE_{Na} is less than 1%. In acute tubular necrosis, the FE_{Na} is greater than 2%.

 CASE 3

A 1-year-old girl presents with decreased urine output. She has a history of vomiting and diarrhea. Serum Na is 136 mEq/L, SCr is 1.0 mg/dl, urine Na is 6 mEq/L, and urine Cr is 20 mg/dl. Her FE_{Na} is 6/136 ÷ 20/1.0 × 100 = 0.22%, consistent with a prerenal cause of oliguria (dehydration secondary to vomiting and diarrhea).

Assessment of Hormone Production

The kidneys also have important endocrine functions. Many different substances are produced or metabolized by the kidney. **Erythropoietin** production is impaired in children with renal failure, leading to chronic anemia. **Vitamin D_3** (1,25-dihydroxycholecalciferol) is also decreased in renal failure secondary to a decrease in the 1-hydroxylation of 25-hydroxyvitamin D_3, which normally occurs in the kidney. **Renin** is produced by the kidneys and is elevated in some forms of hypertension. The plasma renin activity level can be measured during the evaluation of hypertensive disease. The kidneys are also the target organs for substances produced elsewhere in the body (e.g., **aldosterone** and **antidiuretic hormone**), which may be measured in plasma.

Assessment of Renal Structure

Urinary tract (kidneys and bladder) ultrasonography is usually the first imaging study in the evaluation of a child with possible kidney disease. It provides excellent information about renal size, parenchymal texture, size of the collecting system, and anatomy of the bladder. It allows for the detection of hydronephrosis, cysts, calculi, duplicated kidneys, and ureterocele, although it cannot detect vesicoureteral reflux (VUR), and does not provide any information about renal function.

A contrast **voiding cystourethrogram** (VCUG) is a fluoroscopic study in which the contrast media is injected into the bladder via an indwelling catheter. Appearance of the dye above the level of the bladder indicates the presence of VUR. VCUG may not only confirm the presence of VUR but may also give information about bladder and urethral anatomy, including the presence of posterior urethral valves in males.

Radionuclide renal imaging is useful for assessment of the glomerular filtration and the relative contribution of each kidney to overall renal function, and for evaluation of urinary obstruction. ^{99m}Tc-DTPA is one of the agents most frequently used because it is excreted only by glomerular filtration. Technetium 99m–labeled mercaptoacetyltriglycine (^{99m}Tc-MAG-3) measures effective renal plasma flow and is more useful in very young children.

Radionuclide renal imaging has other uses such as for evaluation of renal parenchyma and VUR. Technetium 99m–labeled dimercaptosuccinic acid (^{99m}Tc-DMSA), which binds to cortical tubular cells, is the agent of choice for the evaluation of renal scarring and acute inflammation. Radionuclide voiding cystography (RVC) involves introducing a technetium 99m–labeled radiopharmaceutical in the bladder through a urethral catheter and filling the bladder to capacity with sterile normal saline. A gamma camera behind the patient provides continuous computer recording of bladder filling and voiding to detect VUR. Advantages of RVC are a lower radiation dose than with VCUG and continuous monitoring for reflux during the study. The major disadvantage of RVC is that it provides less anatomic information than VCUG. RVC does not provide any anatomic evaluation of the urethra, which is necessary to exclude posterior urethral valves in males.

The **intravenous pyelogram** (IVP) is useful for evaluation of the anatomy of the kidney and collecting system but is currently used less frequently, because less invasive and safer studies are available. In selected cases, computed tomography (CT), magnetic resonance imaging (MRI), or angiography may be needed.

Assessment of Renal Histology

A renal biopsy is sometimes necessary to establish a specific diagnosis in children with renal disease. It is a safe procedure, which can be done either percutaneously or by open surgery. The percutaneous technique is the most commonly used and can be guided by ultrasound or CT.

The sample is evaluated by histologic and immunologic staining methods and by electron microscopy.

PROTEINURIA AND NEPHROTIC SYNDROME

The occurrence of **proteinuria** in a single urine specimen in children and adolescents is relatively common. About 5%–15% of children have a random urine specimen showing proteinuria by urine dipstick. However, if urine collections are serially collected four times in each child, the total incidence falls to 0.1%.

The **nephrotic syndrome** is characterized by massive proteinuria, hypoalbuminemia, edema, and hyperlipidemia; the most common presenting symptom is edema. The primary renal abnormality is an increased glomerular permeability, a consequence usually of an immunologically mediated decrease in the anionic charge on the glomerular filtration barrier, resulting in proteinuria. The urinary protein loss generally exceeds 40 mg/hr/m^2 and is composed primarily of albumin (albuminuria).

Pathophysiology

The normal rate of protein excretion in the urine is less than 4 mg/m^2/hr throughout childhood. Approximately 50% of this small amount of protein consists of Tamm-Horsfall protein, a glycoprotein secreted by the renal tubules. Another 50% are plasma proteins filtered by the glomeruli, including albumin, β_2-microglobulin, and transferrin. Albumin comprises less than 30% of the total urinary protein excretion in normal individuals. The modest proteinuria that is normally present is usually not detected on routine dipstick testing. The low excretion rate of protein occurs because large serum proteins (e.g., albumin, immunoglobulins) are not filtered by the glomeruli and because the proximal tubules reabsorb most of the filtered low-molecular-weight proteins (e.g., insulin, β_2-microglobulin). Excess urinary protein losses may be caused by increased permeability of the glomeruli to the passage of proteins (glomerular proteinuria) or by decreased reabsorption of low-molecular-weight proteins by the renal tubules (tubular proteinuria).

As recent studies have shown, increasing levels of proteinuria are the best predictor of progressive renal damage in children with proteinuric renal disease. Persistent proteinuria seems to be both a marker of renal disease and a cause of progressive renal injury. Severe persistent proteinuria may also be a long-term risk factor for atherosclerosis in children. As the severity of proteinuria increases, it is associated with a variety of metabolic disturbances that contribute to cardiovascular disease, including hypercholesterolemia, and hypercoagulability.

Clinical edema usually appears when the serum albumin falls below 2.5 g/dl. The mechanisms for the development of edema include: (1) transudation of fluid from the intravascular space into the interstitium secondary to hypoalbuminemia, and (2) increased renal tubular reabsorption of sodium and water. The hyperlipidemia is secondary to both an increase in lipoprotein synthesis by the liver and a decrease in lipid catabolism resulting from reduced activity of the enzyme lipoprotein lipase and lecithin cholesterol acetyltransferase. Hepatic uptake of low-density lipoprotein also decreases.

Clinical and Laboratory Evaluation

Children with nephrotic syndrome may present with a history of mild puffiness around the eyes, especially in the morning. This sign is often confused with manifestations of allergy. The edema can progress further, resulting in ascites, pleural effusion, and scrotal or labial edema. When fever is present, it may reflect sepsis, pneumonia, or peritonitis.

History
The search for significant underlying renal disease begins with a careful history. Impairment in growth and development, unexplained polydipsia or polyuria, hearing loss, or visual problems increase the suspicion of a significant underlying renal disease. The medical history should include perinatal events such as oligohydramnios; a history of previous infections such as upper respiratory tract infection; symptoms of bladder dysfunction such as frequency or dysuria; and systemic symptoms such as headache, edema, and joint pain. A thorough inquiry into the patient's medication history is necessary. Family history of renal diseases or renal failure is important. Assessment of any changes in urine output warrant evaluation.

Physical Examination
In patients with proteinuria, the physical examination is usually unremarkable. The patient's height and weight should be plotted on a growth chart to assess the nutrition and growth status. In patients with established nephrotic syndrome, a careful physical examination is essential to assess severity of disease and to determine whether the child needs to be hospitalized. Examination findings help in distinguishing nonrenal causes of edema such as cardiac, hepatic, or nutritional factors and excluding the possible involvement of systemic diseases. The first step should be an assessment of the vital signs and of hemodynamic stability. Orthostatic changes in blood pressure along with decreased peripheral perfusion may indicate a decrease in the intravascular volume. Edema may appear in the extremities, in the abdomen, in the pleural space, in the scrotum or labia majora, or around the eyes. Auscultation of the lungs is important to evaluate for a pleural effusion or signs of consolidation. Palpation of the abdomen is necessary for the evaluation of ascites and to rule out peritonitis in patients with fever and abdominal pain.

Laboratory Evaluation
TESTING FOR PROTEINURIA. The urinary dipstick test, the most commonly used screening test for proteinuria, primarily detects urinary albumin. False-negative results may occur with very dilute urine. False-positive results may occur with concentrated or very alkaline urine (pH $>$ 8), gram-negative bacteria, detergents, or skin cleansers containing ammonium salts.

Evaluation of children with persistent proteinuria is complex (Figure 20.1). Several methods to test for proteinuria are available (Table 20.2). The most accurate method is the 24-hour urine collection. However, it is inconvenient and difficult to obtain in children. Therefore, a spot urine for protein and creatinine has become the most common method to quantify proteinuria in children. It should be obtained preferably in a first-morning urine specimen, as urine protein concentration can vary widely during the day. Studies have indicated that the urine protein:creatinine ratio accurately reflects 24-hour urine protein excretion. In addition, a renal sonogram should be obtained in children with persistent proteinuria.

In most children with nephrotic syndrome, a renal biopsy is not required for initial diagnosis, because the majority have minimal change disease. If nephrotic syndrome develops during the first year of life or during adolescence, or if they present with features that make the possibility of minimal change disease less likely (e.g., a decrease in renal function, hypertension, gross hematuria or hypocomplementemia), a biopsy should be considered before treatment. Children with nephrotic syndrome have a urine protein:creatinine ratio greater than 2.0 or a 24-hour urine protein ex-

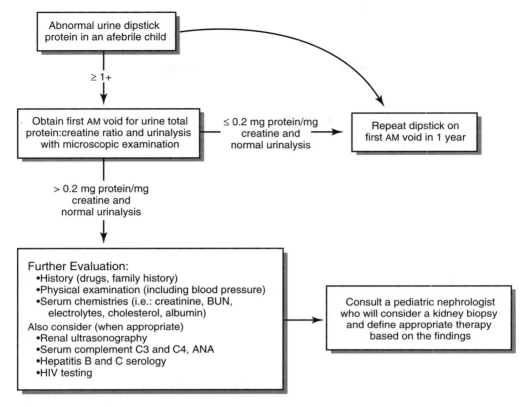

FIGURE 20.1. Evaluation of asymptomatic persistent proteinuria in children and adolescents. If the urinalysis is normal and the protein:creatinine ratio is less than 0.2, no additional studies are necessary. However, if the urinalysis shows other abnormalities or the first-morning urine protein:creatinine ratio is greater than 0.2, the blood level of albumin, cholesterol, creatinine, and electrolytes should be determined. A low serum albumin along with an increase in serum lipid levels confirms the diagnosis of nephrotic syndrome. Additional laboratory studies are indicated to rule out secondary causes. Antistreptolysin O and streptozyme levels may be useful to rule out previous streptococcal infection. Serum complement levels C3 and C4 and antinuclear antibodies (ANAs) assist in the diagnosis of systemic lupus erythematosus (SLE). Serologic studies for hepatitis B and C, and human immunodeficiency virus (HIV) should also be considered.

TABLE 20.2	**Laboratory Testing for Proteinuria**
Method	**Normal Range**
Dipstick	Negative
Protein:creatinine ratio	< 0.5 (mg protein/mg creatinine) in children 6–24 months of age
	<0.2 (mg protein/mg creatinine) in children > 2 years of age
24-hour urine for protein	< 4 (mg protein/m²/hr) or < 5 (mg protein/kg/day)
Microalbuminuria	< 30 (mg albumin/g Cr)

cretion of more than 40 mg/m^2/hr (or > 50 mg/kg/day, more than 10 times the normal range).

TESTING FOR ALBUMINURIA. Specific measurement of albumin in the urine (microalbuminuria) is a more accurate measurement than routine urinalysis dipstick in assessing the degree of albuminuria. Increased urine albumin excretion appears before other measurable changes in renal function. **Levels of urine albumin excretion below the sensitivity of the dipstick have been referred to as microalbuminuria, which is defined as urine albumin excretion between 30 and 300 mg per 24 hours.** To simplify testing, a first-voided urine can be analyzed for its albumin (mg) to creatinine (g) ratio. A ratio (albumin:creatinine) greater than 30 is considered abnormal.

Pediatric Pearl

It is important to note that children with microalbuminuria may have a normal urinalysis.

Studies have shown that the presence of microalbuminuria is a sensitive indicator of kidney disease in diabetes mellitus. Testing for microalbuminuria is indicated in children with diabetes to check for early kidney involvement.

Differential Diagnosis

When proteinuria is detected, it is important to determine whether it is transient, orthostatic, or persistent. **Transient proteinuria** (e.g., associated with fever, dehydration, stress, or exercise) is not considered to be indicative of underlying renal disease. **Orthostatic proteinuria,** which rarely exceeds 1 g/m^2/day, is defined as an elevated protein excretion in the upright position but normal during recumbency. It occurs in school-age children. Long-term follow-up studies have documented the benign nature of orthostatic proteinuria. However, there have been a few reports of renal disease identified later in life in children who were initially found to have orthostatic proteinuria. **Persistent proteinuria** is defined as proteinuria > 1+ by dipstick on multiple occasions and is abnormal and should be investigated.

Nephrotic syndrome can be divided into two major categories (Table 20.3). In **primary nephrotic syndrome,** the etiology is unknown and only the kidney is involved. In **secondary nephrotic syndrome,** a renal disorder appears during the course of another systemic disease or during drug treatment. The most common form of nephrotic syn-

---

TABLE 20.3 Etiologic Classification of Nephrotic Syndrome in Children

Primary nephrotic syndrome
  Minimal change nephrotic syndrome
  Focal and segmental glomerulosclerosis
  Membranous nephropathy
  Membranoproliferative glomerulonephritis
  Congenital nephrotic syndrome

Secondary nephrotic syndrome
  Diabetes
  Systemic lupus erythematosus
  Hepatitis B and C, syphilis, human immunodeficiency virus (HIV), malaria
  Henoch-Schönlein purpura
  Tumor
  Alport syndrome
  Amyloidosis
  Sickle cell disease
  Drug reaction (drug-induced nephrotic syndrome)

---

drome in childhood is **minimal change disease,** which accounts for 75% of cases.

Management

It is recommended that children with proteinuria receive the recommended daily allowance of protein for age. High dietary protein intake may worsen proteinuria and does not improve hypoalbuminemia.

Corticosteroids are the drugs of choice in childhood nephrotic syndrome (Figure 20.2). Oral prednisone or prednisolone (60 mg/m^2/day or 2 mg/kg/day; maximum: 80 mg/day) is given daily for 4–6 weeks. Then, the dose is tapered to 40 mg/m^2/day on alternate days for another 4–6 weeks to minimize side effects such as growth retardation. This form of therapy results in complete remission in more than 90% of patients. If the patient does not respond to steroids in 4–6 weeks, a renal biopsy is indicated for histologic diagnosis. Most children (60%–80%) experience a number of relapses of nephrotic syndrome. Treatment for relapses involves a short course of daily steroids at the initial higher dose until the urine is free of protein for 3 days, followed by the alternate-day schedule for 4–6 weeks at the lower dose. The edema improves in steroid-responsive patients as soon as the proteinuria decreases, the serum albumin increases, and the driving forces for edema formation disappear.

Intravenous pulse steroids (methylprednisolone) have been used with success in patients

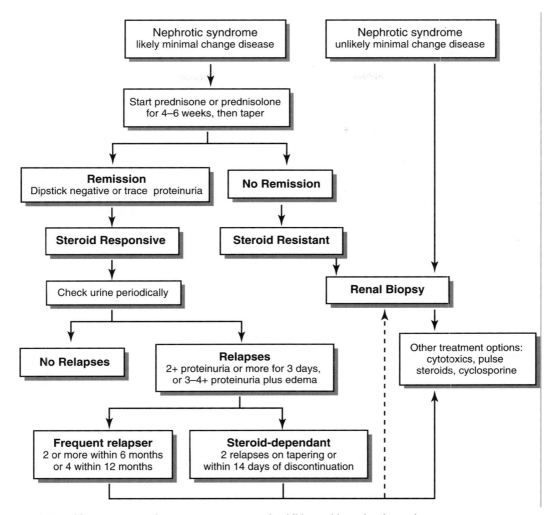

FIGURE 20.2. Management and response to treatment in children with nephrotic syndrome.

with steroid-resistant nephrotic syndrome. Cytotoxic agents are occasionally indicated in steroid-dependent nephrotic syndrome, when steroid side effects become a problem. Cyclophosphamide or chlorambucil, given for 8–12 weeks, may achieve long periods of remission and reduce the need of steroids. Both drugs have significant side effects that include infection, leukemia, gonadal dysfunction, hemorrhagic cystitis, and bone marrow suppression. As studies have shown, cyclosporine A also induces a remission in patients with steroid-dependent or steroid-resistant nephrotic syndrome. However, the remission does not persist for a prolonged period of time after discontinuation of the drug.

Adjunctive therapy with angiotensin-converting enzyme inhibitors in patients with steroid-resistant nephrotic syndrome is now being used more frequently. It may decrease the rate of protein excretion by as much as 50%.

In patients with severe edema, intravenous albumin (1 g/kg of 25% albumin) administered in conjunction with diuretics may be of help. It must be remembered that this is only a temporary therapy and carries the risk of inducing hypertension, fluid overload, and pulmonary edema. During chronic management of patients with nephrotic syndrome, fluid restriction is generally not necessary, although a low-sodium diet is indicated to counteract the alterations in sodium metabolism.

Complications in nephrotic syndrome may derive from the disease itself or from its treatment. As nephrotic children lose immunoglobulin G (IgG) in the urine, they are at increased risk for infections (e.g., cellulitis, peritonitis, pneumonia). Antibiotics with broad-spectrum coverage of both gram-positive and gram-negative organisms are appropriate until culture results are available. A serious complication is the risk of a thromboembolic event secondary to a hypercoagulability state. Avoidance of arterial punctures and of diuretics during periods of hypovolemia may be of help in preventing thrombosis. Growth retardation is one of the multiple side effects of long-term steroid therapy; however, administering steroids on alternate days may reduce this effect.

HEMATURIA AND GLOMERULONEPHRITIS

Hematuria may be gross (macroscopic) or microscopic. By definition, gross hematuria is the presence of enough blood in the urine to change its appearance to naked eye inspection, and therefore, easily recognized. In contrast, microscopic hematuria, an abnormal number of RBCs in the urine, should be defined more precisely to include all patients with disease and exclude patients without disease. By definition, microscopic hematuria is more than five RBCs per high power field (HPF) in three of three fresh urine specimens collected over a few weeks.

Pathophysiology

Glomerulonephritis is an important cause of hematuria in children. Glomerular disease may result from immunologic abnormalities, coagulation disturbances, biochemical defects, or direct toxic insults. Immunologic abnormalities appear to be the predominant mechanism for glomerular disease in humans. Renal injury may be due to one of several immunologic processes: circulating autoantibodies to glomerular antigens, deposition of circulating antigen–antibody complexes in the glomeruli, and cell-mediated processes damaging the glomeruli. The glomerular antigen may be a normal component of the glomerulus or an antigen that has been deposited in the glomerulus.

Clinical and Laboratory Evaluation

History

Children with hematuria may present in one of three ways: (1) onset of gross hematuria, (2) onset of urinary or other symptoms with the incidental finding of microscopic hematuria, or (3) incidental finding of microscopic hematuria during a health evaluation. It is important to inquire about activities and symptoms that preceded or were concomitant with the hematuria, as well as history of hematuria or other renal disease in family members (Table 20.4).

Children with acute glomerulonephritis present typically with hematuria, edema, and hypertension, with or without oliguria. Gross hematuria is the presenting symptom in many patients. However, affected children may be completely asymptomatic, and the disease may be discovered when a routine urinalysis reveals microscopic hematuria. Clinical edema, typically in the periorbital area, or a decrease in urine output are other significant presenting signs. Nonspecific symptoms such as fever, anorexia, weakness, or headache may accompany the disease. Respiratory symptoms and neurologic abnormalities may indicate a severe ongoing process. The presence of extrarenal manifestations such as a purpuric skin rash, joint involvement, GI bleeding, or pleuritis may be more indicative of a systemic disease with renal involvement.

Physical Examination

A complete physical examination is important for the assessment of disease severity and for diagnosis of a secondary cause. (In children with

TABLE 20.4 Personal and Family History in Children with Hematuria	
History	**Possible Cause of Hematuria**
Personal	
Streptococcal pharyngitis or impetigo	Poststreptococcal glomerulonephritis
Dysuria, urinary frequency	Lower urinary tract infection
Recurrent episodes of gross hematuria with viral illnesses	IgA nephropathy
Exercise	Exercise-related hematuria
Trauma	Trauma-related hematuria
Family	
Deafness and renal insufficiency	Alport syndrome
Urolithiasis	Hypercalciuria, urolithiasis
Hematuria, isolated	Thin basement membrane disease

asymptomatic microscopic hematuria, the physical examination is usually unremarkable.) Measurement of blood pressure and determination of growth pattern are the first steps. Hypertension and failure to thrive are commonly present in children with chronic renal disease. It is essential to address the presence and localization of edema. A sudden increase in weight gain may relate to the presence of edema. Abnormal physical features may indicate a congenital syndrome with renal disease. Eye fundi should be examined to detect changes related to chronic hypertension or systemic diseases. The presence of tonsillar hypertrophy or resolving exudates may be present in a child with recent streptococcal pharyngitis. Auscultation of the chest is important to rule out cardiac failure and pulmonary edema. Hepatosplenomegaly is not an expected finding in primary glomerulonephritis, and its presence may indicate another systemic illness. The presence of an abdominal or flank mass suggests a renal tumor, obstructive uropathy, or multicystic or polycystic kidney disease. Pain and tenderness over the costovertebral angle or the suprapubic area suggest a urinary tract infection. The external genitalia should be examined for trauma, infection, or bleeding. The skin should be examined for infection or rashes.

Laboratory Evaluation

The most common test for the detection of RBCs in the urine is the urine strip test for blood (dipstick test). The chromogen in the reagent strip specifically reacts with hemoglobin (or myoglobin) to produce an oxidized product, which has a green-blue color. These very sensitive strips can detect the presence of 2–5 RBCs/HPF (Table 20.5).

Urinalysis of family members may provide important information regarding the diagnosis and prognosis of the patient's underlying disease. A stable relative with hematuria may indicate a favorable prognosis.

The presence of RBC casts is characteristic of glomerulonephritis. Urine for calcium-to-creatinine ratio (Ca:Cr) should be obtained to identify hypercalciuria (> 0.8 in children younger than 6 months, > 0.6 in children 7–18 months, and > 0.2 in children $\geq$ 6 years). A 24-hour urinary calcium excretion greater than 4 mg/kg confirms the diagnosis. A urine culture should be obtained to exclude cystitis or pyelonephritis. Serum electrolytes, BUN, and SCr should be obtained to assess renal function; a complete blood count (CBC) for anemia and infection; hemoglobin electrophoresis if the patient is of African heritage and the sickle cell status is unknown; and prothrombin time and partial thromboplastin time for coagulopathy.

The diagnosis of postinfectious glomerulonephritis requires the detection of both the glomerulonephritis and the cause of infection. In poststreptococcal glomerulonephritis, the success rate in obtaining a positive culture during an epidemic varies between 10% and 70%. The diagnosis usually depends on serologic criteria. An increase in titers of antistreptococcal antibodies indicates recent infection, but not all of these tests are equally useful. Antistreptolysin O (ASO) titers are less frequently elevated than anti-DNAse B titers (streptozyme). Recent studies indicate that the antizymogen titer test is superior to both ASO and anti-DNAse B titers. An immune-mediated process should be suspected if there is any alteration in the serum complement level or the presence of autoantibodies (Figure 20.3). In the first week of poststreptococcal glomerulonephritis, the serum C3 and the total serum hemolytic complement are decreased in more than 90% of cases. Serum complement level should normalize after 6–8 weeks of onset in children with poststreptococcal glomerulonephritis.

If hypocomplementemia persists beyond 8 weeks, the possibility of other diagnosis should be considered (membranoproliferative glomeru-

TABLE 20.5 **Laboratory Testing for Hematuria**	
Urine Dipstick for Blood	**Interpretation**
Negative	*Rules out hematuria*
Negative (dark or red urine)	Foods, dyes, drugs, metabolites, or crystals in urine
Positive	
• No RBCs	Hemoglobinuria or myoglobinuria; presence of hematuria needs to be confirmed by microscopic examination of urine for presence of RBCs
• < 5 RBCs	Most likely normal; repeat periodically
• > 5 RBCs	*Confirms hematuria*

RBCs = red blood cells.

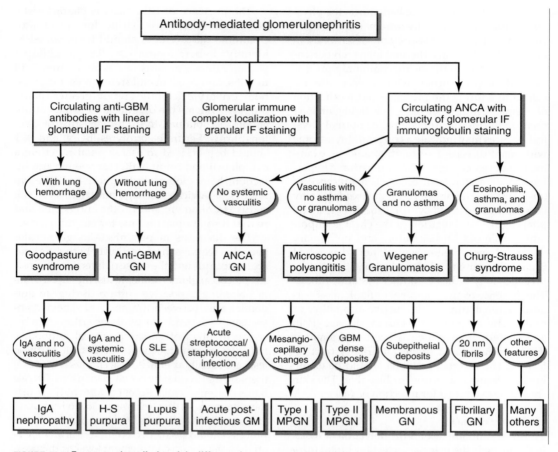

FIGURE 20.3. Features that distinguish different immunopathologic categories of antibody-mediated glomerulonephritis. ANCA = antineutrophil cytoplasmic autoantibodies; AntiGBM = anti-glomerular basement membrane; CBC = complete blood count; Cr = creatinine; GBM = glomerular basement membrane; GN = glomerulonephritis; IF = immunofluorescence microscopy; H-S = Henoch-Schönlein; MPGN = membranoproliferative glomerulonephritis; SCr = serum creatinine.

lonephritis, lupus nephritis). Antinuclear antibody (ANA) for systemic lupus erythematosus (SLE), hepatitis B titers for membranous nephropathy, and hepatitis B and hepatitis C for membranoproliferative glomerulonephritis should also be obtained. A formal neurosensory test for hearing loss is necessary in any child with persistent hematuria.

Imaging studies may also be indicated. Urinary tract ultrasonography, a noninvasive study, is useful for the evaluation of children with hematuria. Other imaging studies may also be necessary (VCUG, CT, radionuclide studies) in selected patients. A renal biopsy may be indicated in children with rapidly progressive glomerulonephritis for histologic diagnosis and for assessment of severity of disease.

Differential Diagnosis

The causes of gross and microscopic hematuria are extensive (Table 20.6). Glomerulonephritis is considered primary when the kidney is the only involved organ and secondary when the renal in-

TABLE 20.6 **Causes of Hematuria in Children**

Anatomical abnormalities (hydronephrosis; cystic disease)
Bladder and kidney infection (urinary tract infection)
Coagulation/hematology (sickle cell trait or disease; leukemia)
Drugs
Exercise
Familial hematuria (Alport syndrome; thin basement membrane disease)
Glomerulonephritis
Hypercalciuria–hyperuricosuria–urolithiasis
Interstitial nephritis
Trauma and tumors (Wilms tumor)

volvement is part of a systemic disease. It can be acute, chronic, or rapidly progressive according to its clinical presentation and prognosis. Acute glomerulonephritis has a tendency for spontaneous resolution. Rapidly progressive glomerulonephritis refers to a marked and rapidly progressive deterioration in renal function. Chronic glomerulonephritis involves a persistent abnormal urine sediment with a slow and progressive loss of renal function over time.

Specific types of glomerulonephritis include:

- **Poststreptococcal glomerulonephritis,** the most common type of glomerulonephritis in children, results, indirectly, through an immunologic process, from group A β-hemolytic streptococcus. Reported cases of acute glomerulonephritis following infection with many other bacteria and viruses have occurred. Gross hematuria mostly occurs 2 weeks after acute infection. Hypertension, edema, and impairment of renal function may develop.
- **Immunoglobulin A (IgA) nephropathy,** the most common variety of primary glomerulonephritis, is characterized by recurrent episodes of gross hematuria, usually 1–2 days after a viral respiratory or GI infection. Mesangial IgA deposition is the most prominent finding on renal biopsy specimens.
- **Alport syndrome** is a form of familial nephritis with neurosensory hearing loss and slow progression to renal insufficiency.
- **Familial benign hematuria** is defined by familial occurrence of persistent hematuria without proteinuria, progression to renal failure, or hearing defect. Thin glomerular basement membrane is commonly found on these patients.

Management

From the practical point of view, children with confirmed hematuria can be divided clinically in four groups: (1) gross hematuria, (2) microscopic hematuria with clinical symptoms, (3) asymptomatic microscopic hematuria (isolated), and (4) asymptomatic microscopic hematuria with proteinuria. The evaluation and management of children with hematuria is complex (Figure 20.4).

The general management of glomerulonephritis involves salt and water restriction. Treatment depends on the severity of the disease, degree of renal involvement, and presence of renal failure, hypertension, or other complications. A decrease in urine output, the presence of high blood pressure, or any sign of fluid overload may be an indication for hospitalization. Fluid restriction and close monitoring of electrolytes may be indicated in patients with acute renal failure. Dialysis may be necessary in patients with fluid overload or hyperkalemia unresponsive to conservative therapy. When hypertension is present, it is generally related to fluid overload. Loop diuretics such as furosemide may be useful in the management of both fluid overload and hypertension.

Specific treatment of glomerulonephritis depends on the etiology or severity of the disorder. Steroids and cyclophosphamide are indicated for severe lupus nephritis in an attempt to decrease the immunologic process. The use of plasma exchange may be indicated in severe cases to decrease the amount of circulating factors (e.g., immunoglobulins) involved in kidney damage (e.g., in Goodpasture syndrome).

HENOCH-SCHÖNLEIN PURPURA

Henoch-Schönlein purpura is the most common form of **vasculitis** in children. Vasculitis is a clinicopathologic process characterized by inflammation and damage to blood vessels, resulting in compromise of the vessel lumen and ischemic changes in the tissues supplied by the involved vessels.

The incidence of Henoch-Schönlein purpura is approximately 10 cases per 100,000 children per year. Seventy-five percent of all cases occur in children between 2 and 11 years of age; the disease is rare in adults and younger children. Males are affected twice as frequently as females.

Pathophysiology

Henoch-Schönlein purpura is an IgA-mediated vasculitis in the small vessels of involved organs. The etiology is unknown. Both bacterial (*Strepto-*

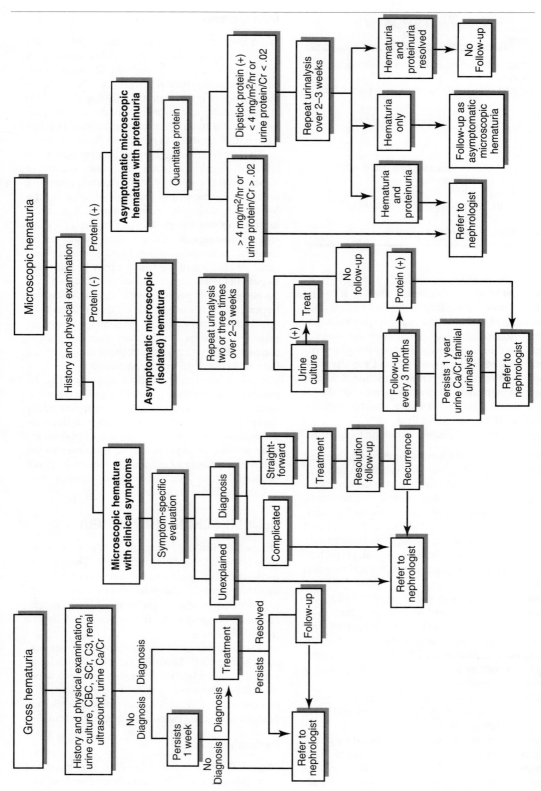

FIGURE 20.4. Algorithm for the practical evaluation and management of children with hematuria. Dx = diagnosis; F/U = follow-up; PE = physical examination; UA = urinalysis; US = ultrasonogram.

coccus, Yersinia, Mycoplasma) and viral infections (Epstein-Barr virus, varicella, parvovirus, and adenovirus) have been reported to precede Henoch-Schönlein purpura. Other reported preceding stimuli include immunizations, drugs, foods, and insect bites.

Clinical and Laboratory Evaluation

A preceding event (e.g., infection, medication, immunization) may be discovered in many children. The onset of Henoch-Schönlein purpura may be acute with the appearance of characteristic symptoms in any order or simultaneously.

History
Purpuric rash, arthritis, abdominal pain, and nephritis are the most typical findings. **Purpura** is the most common finding, but it may not be the presenting feature. It appears typically in the lower extremities and buttocks but may also be present in the upper extremities, trunk, and face. The rash may persist for weeks, be transient, or recur. **Arthritis** or **arthralgias** may also be manifest in the ankles, knees, or hands. In some cases, joint involvement may be the presenting feature. Although the arthritis may be incapacitating, it is self-limited and nondeforming. **GI symptoms** result from edema of the bowel wall and hemorrhage owing to vasculitis, and generally appear after the purpura, but rarely may precede it. Abdominal pain is the most common complaint. Vomiting, hematemesis, bloody diarrhea, or melena are common and may be severe. Intussusception is the most common surgical complication.

Renal manifestations generally appear within 3 months of the onset of the rash. In a few cases, gross hematuria is the presenting finding. The frequency of renal involvement (gross or microscopic hematuria) varies between 20% and 90%. Hematuria is the clinical hallmark of Henoch-Schönlein purpura nephritis. Approximately 80% of patients manifest nephritis within 4 weeks and 95% within 3 months of onset of other symptoms. There is no relationship between the severity of extrarenal organ involvement and the severity of nephritis.

Other complications include central nervous system (CNS) involvement (seizures, paresis, or coma), eye and cardiac involvement, and pulmonary or intramuscular hemorrhage. Pancreatitis and orchitis have also been described.

Physical Examination
Inspection of the skin may show the typical distribution and appearance of the rash. The classic lesions consist of urticarial, maculopapular, or palpable purpuric lesions. In some cases, different appearances or localizations may complicate the diagnosis. Vesicular eruptions and erythema multiforme have been described. Vital signs, blood pressure, and urine output should be monitored in patients who present with GI bleeding. Edema may be present in the scalp, extremities, back, and eyelids. Joint involvement tends to be periarticular, and joints may be swollen, tender, and painful on motion. A complete physical examination is important to rule out involvement of the pancreas, lungs, heart, testes, and CNS.

Laboratory Evaluation
An initial urinalysis is necessary to diagnose any renal involvement. The long-term prognosis is determined by the extent of renal involvement, which varies from mild to severe rapid progressive glomerulonephritis. The most common finding is **hematuria with or without proteinuria.** If the urine is abnormal, a SCr level and BUN need to be performed to assess kidney function. A kidney biopsy should be considered in patients with severe clinical manifestations of renal disease, nephrotic syndrome, or rapid progressive glomerulonephritis. Histologically the typical finding in Henoch-Schönlein purpura is the presence of mesangial deposits of IgA by immunofluorescence.

Laboratory studies are indicated depending on the clinical presentation. A CBC may show **anemia** in patients with GI bleeding. ANA, antineutrophilic cytoplasmic antibody (ANCA), and rheumatoid factor are usually negative. **Stool guaiac** examinations should be done to screen for occult GI bleeding. Serum IgA levels may be elevated or normal. Radiologic studies are indicated in patients with acute abdominal pain. A head CT scan may be useful in children with neurologic involvement to rule out other causes.

Differential Diagnosis

In the presence of an atypical rash, other vasculitides should be considered. Patients with microscopic polyarteritis, Wegener granulomatosis, and SLE may all present with nephritis. The associated clinical features with the presence of ANCA or ANA can help differentiate these conditions. Cytoplasmic ANCA (c-ANCA) is more commonly associated with Wegener granulomatosis, whereas perinuclear ANCA (p-ANCA) is more often associated with microscopic polyarteritis. A purpuric rash can be caused by sepsis or thrombocytopenia. The clinical picture, distribution of the rash, and hematologic studies should identify these patients.

Management

No specific treatment is available for Henoch-Schönlein purpura, and the management is supportive. Most patients with renal involvement show mild urine abnormalities but should be followed up for a prolonged period of time until the urinalysis becomes normal. Children with more severe presentations such as acute renal failure, hypertension, or nephrotic syndrome should be hospitalized and followed very carefully, **because of possible rapid progression to end-stage renal disease.**

Many drugs, including oral corticosteroids, intravenous pulses of methylprednisolone, cytotoxic agents, anticoagulants, and plasmapheresis, have been used to treat severe renal involvement. The available data suggest that patients with severe nephritis (decreased renal function and > 50% crescents on renal biopsy) should receive a combination of high-dose intravenous methylprednisolone plus an immunosuppressive agent, either azathioprine or cyclophosphamide. Plasmapheresis may be of benefit in a few patients with rapidly progressive Henoch-Schönlein purpura nephritis. Some studies have shown that oral prednisone may be effective in preventing the development of nephropathy, while others have shown no effect. However, prednisone is effective in alleviating the GI manifestations.

In the absence of nephropathy, recurrence of clinical manifestations may occur, but the prognosis of patients with Henoch-Schönlein purpura is excellent. Long-term follow-up is necessary in children with renal involvement for evidence of progression of disease. The presence of renal insufficiency or nephrotic syndrome at onset and the finding of crescentic glomerulonephritis on biopsy appear to increase the risk of progressive renal disease.

URINARY TRACT INFECTION

Urinary tract infections (UTIs) are common in children. UTIs are important because they cause acute morbidity and may result in long-term medical problems, including hypertension and reduced renal function.

Pathophysiology

UTIs usually occur as a consequence of colonization of the periurethral area by a virulent organism that subsequently gains access to the bladder. Only in the first 8–12 weeks of life, UTIs may be secondary to a hematogenous source. During the first months of life, uncircumcised male infants are at increased risk for UTIs, but thereafter UTIs predominate in females. An important risk factor in girls is previous antibiotic therapy, which disrupts the normal periurethral flora and fosters the growth of uropathogenic bacteria. Several factors predispose to UTIs (Table 20.7).

The most common organisms isolated from the periurethral area are members of the Enterobacteriaceae. *Escherichia coli* is the most common cause of infection. *Enterococcus* species, *Staphylococcus aureus,* and group B streptococcus are the most frequent isolated gram-positive bacteria. In adolescence, *S. saprophyticus* becomes a frequent pathogen. Adenovirus has been associated with acute hemorrhagic cystitis in school-age children. Additional organisms causing UTIs in patients with instrumented urinary tracts or urinary tract abnormalities include *Pseudomonas* species, *Candida* species, *Corynebacterium* species, and coagulase-negative staphylococci.

VUR, which may lead to UTIs, is considered a congenital anomaly of the ureterovesical junction in which there is a shortened submucosal tunnel with lateral placement of the ureteral orifice in the bladder. The longitudinal muscle is not able to adequately constrict the submucosal ureter, so the valve mechanism is defective and urine backflows into the ureter. VUR is graded according to degree of reflux from mild (limited to the ureter) to severe (associated with massive dilatation of calyces, pelvis and ureter). VUR is identified in 30%–50% of children who are evaluated after their first UTI. As they grow, the submucosal tunnel elongates and the valve mechanism becomes more effective. Therefore, the natural course of mild reflux is to resolve or improve with time. Patients with more severe reflux are less likely to have spontaneous resolution.

TABLE 20.7 Factors Predisposing to Urinary Tract Infection (UTI)
Urinary tract obstruction
Vesicoureteral reflux
Neurogenic bladder
Urolithiasis
Presence of foreskin
Voiding dysfunction
Constipation
Sexual abuse
Sexual intercourse
Uroepithelial deficiency with increased bacterial adherence
Antibiotic therapy
Poor perineal hygiene

Renal scarring, a potential consequence of UTIs, may be congenital or acquired. It has been recently shown that infants may have renal scarring at birth even without infection. In older children with UTIs, the infection itself, and not VUR, is the prerequisite for acquired renal scarring. However, there is a correlation between the degree of reflux and the severity of renal scarring. Furthermore, the risk of renal damage increases with the number of recurrences.

Clinical and Laboratory Evaluation

History

The spectrum of clinical manifestations of UTI in children is broad. The clinical signs and symptoms specific for UTIs commonly seen in adults such as dysuria, urgency, and flank pain are not generally identified in infants, although they may occur in older children (Table 20.8). Young infants with UTIs generally present with fever.

Pediatric Pearl

The possibility of UTI should be considered in any child younger than 2 years of age with unexplained fever.

A history of crying on urination or of foul-smelling urine increases the likelihood that UTI is the cause of fever. An altered voiding pattern may be recognized as a symptom of UTI as early as the second year after birth in some children. Nonspecific signs and symptoms, such as irritability, vomiting, diarrhea, and failure to thrive, may reflect the presence of UTI. Hematuria when associated with dysuria or pain with urination is most likely due to lower UTI. A detailed voiding and defecation history should be obtained in any child with recurrent UTIs.

Physical Examination

A complete physical examination is essential to assess the degree of illness or toxicity and to rule out other severe infections such as sepsis or meningitis. The presence of fever is important in young children with UTI, because it has been accepted as a clinical marker of renal parenchymal involvement (pyelonephritis). It is important to record vital signs, including blood pressure. Examination of the abdomen and back for costovertebral tenderness, flank or abdominal mass or tenderness, or a palpable bladder is appropriate, and inspection of the genitalia for signs of trauma or infection is warranted. It is also important to note whether the child has been circumcised, because uncircumcised boys have a higher chance of developing UTI in the first year of life than do circumcised boys. Physical examination should also include careful inspection of the lumbosacral area for signs of underlying dysraphism.

Laboratory Evaluation

In infants or children who are unable to void on request, catheterization or suprapubic aspiration should be used to obtain a specimen for urinalysis and culture. A midstream clean-catch specimen may be obtained from children with urinary control. A bagged urine specimen that shows no growth or fewer than 10,000 colony-forming units (CFU)/ml is evidence of the absence of a UTI. If children who have not yet achieved urinary control have symptoms that require immediate treatment, and a urinalysis obtained by urine bag shows pyuria, positive nitrites, or bacteriuria, a urine culture should be obtained by either suprapubic aspiration or bladder catheterization before the initiation of antibiotics, because of the high incidence of false-positive urine cultures obtained by urine bag.

The three most useful components of the urinalysis in the evaluation of UTI are the leukocyte esterase test, the nitrite test, and urine microscopy. A positive result on a leukocyte esterase test appears to be as sensitive as microscopy, with the identification of WBCs. The nitrite test has a very high specificity and positive predictive value. Urinalysis cannot substitute for a urine culture to document the presence of UTI, but it can be valuable

TABLE 20.8	**Signs and Symptoms of Urinary Tract Infection (UTI)**
Young Children	**Older Children**
Fever	Fever, chills, malaise
Crying on urination	Dysuria, urgency, pain on urination
Frequency	Frequency
Hematuria	Hematuria
Gastrointestinal symptoms	Flank pain
Poor growth	New-onset enuresis

in selecting patients for prompt initiation of therapy while waiting for the results of the urine culture. UTI is confirmed or excluded based on the number of CFUs that grow on the culture media. What constitutes a significant colony depends on the collection method and the clinical status of the patient; definitions of positive and negative cultures are operational and not absolute (Table 20.9).

The goals of performing imaging studies in children with UTIs are to detect urologic abnormalities (e.g., VUR, bladder dysfunction, obstructive uropathy) and to discover renal parenchymal damage. The current imaging workup consists of renal ultrasound and VCUG or RVC (Table 20.10). If significant hydronephrosis is discovered on renal ultrasound, a nuclear renal scan (with ^{99m}Tc-MAG-3 or DTPA) is used for evaluation of urinary tract obstruction. Renal cortical scintigraphy with ^{99m}Tc-labeled DMSA is sensitive and specific for the diagnosis of pyelonephritis in children. This renal test shows decreased uptake of radiotracer in areas of inflammation, which is secondary to decreased delivery of agent to the infected tissue (cortical ischemia) and decreased tubular function in areas of infection. CT imaging and MRI have also been utilized for diagnosis of pyelonephritis. CT may be useful in patients with a presentation that could be caused by some other illness (e.g., intra-abdominal abscess, appendicitis). Cost and the need of sedation are the major disadvantages of MRI.

Differential Diagnosis

The presentation of febrile infants who have positive results on urine cultures frequently poses a diagnostic question: do the infants have true UTIs or asymptomatic bacteriuria with fever from another source? Asymptomatic bacteriuria does not appear to present a danger to the host. It is considered to be a phenomenon whereby mucosal receptors permit attachment by *E. coli*, creating a carrier-state (colonization) rather than infection. Pyuria may be a possible marker to differentiate between UTI and asymptomatic bacteriuria. However, although the presence of pyuria increases the likelihood of true UTI, the absence of pyuria does not preclude the possibility of true UTI. Pyuria is particularly insensitive in neonates and very young infants. Therefore, it is prudent to consider that all young infants with significant bacteriuria and fever have true UTI.

Management

The goals of treatment of acute UTI are to eliminate the acute infection, to prevent urosepsis, and to reduce the likelihood of renal damage. Patients who are toxic-appearing, dehydrated, or unable to retain oral intake (including medications) should receive an antimicrobial parenterally. The clinical condition of most patients improves within 24–48 hours. Treatment can then be completed orally. For patients who do not appear toxic, options include administration of an antimicrobial parenterally on an outpatient basis, or receiving the antibiotic orally for 7–14 days.

Treatment of acute pyelonephritis or cystitis may be initiated based on clinical findings and urinalysis (Figure 20.5). However, the diagnosis of a UTI is not documented by urinalysis, and imaging studies of the urinary tract should not be obtained until the diagnosis of UTI is confirmed by a positive urine culture. The usual choices for treatment of UTI orally include a cephalosporin, trimethoprim–sulfamethoxazole, or amoxicillin. However, amoxicillin appears less effective due to emerging bacterial resistance. Cephalosporins are very effective antibiotics parenterally. Other antibiotics are useful in the treatment of UTIs (Table 20.11). Agents that are excreted in the

---

TABLE 20.9 **Interpretation of Urine Culture for Diagnosis of Urinary Tract Infection (UTI)**

Method of Collection	Quantitative Culture: Urinary Tract Infection Present
Suprapubic aspiration	Growth of urinary pathogens in any number (exception is up to $2–3 \times 10^3$ CFU/ml of coagulase-negative staphylococci)
Catheterization	Febrile infants or children usually have $\geq 50 \times 10^3$ CFU/ml of single urinary pathogen, but infection may be present with counts from 10×10^3–50×10^3 CFU/ml
Midstream clean-void	Symptomatic patients usually have $\geq 10^5$ CFU/ml of single urinary tract pathogen
	Asymptomatic patients need to have at least two specimens on different days with $\geq 10^5$ CFU/ml of same organism

CFU/ml = colony-forming units per milliliter.

TABLE 20.10 **Indications of Imaging Studies in Children with Urinary Tract Infections (UTIs)**

- RUS and VCUG or RVC in a child of any age with a febrile UTI
- RUS and VCUG or RVC in a young child with a well-documented UTI
- RUS only in an older child with symptoms of lower UTI
  VCUG or RVC if abnormal RUS or if recurrent UTI
  VCUG with history of dysfunctional voiding
- DMSA scan if RUS or voiding study are markedly abnormal, to detect renal scars, if this changes clinical management
- Radionuclide renal scan if urinary tract obstruction is considered

DMSA = dimercaptosuccinic acid; RUS = renal ultrasound; RVC = radionuclide voiding cystography; VCUG = voiding cystourethrogram.

urine but do not achieve therapeutic concentrations in the bloodstream (e.g., nitrofurantoin) should not be used to treat UTI in patients in whom renal involvement is likely.

Routine reculturing of the urine after 2 days of antimicrobial therapy is generally not necessary if the patient has had the expected clinical response and the bacteria isolated is determined to be sensitive to the antimicrobial being administered. If a patient does not improve, or the bacteria is resistant to the antimicrobial, a repeat urine culture is warranted after 48 hours of treatment.

Antibiotic prophylaxis is indicated in children with VUR. The antibiotics of choice are cephalexin or amoxicillin in children younger than 2 months

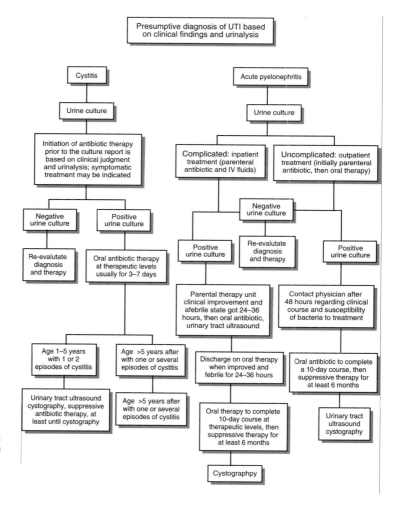

FIGURE 20.5. Algorithm for the evaluation and management of urinary tract infection (UTI) in children. IV = intravenous.

TABLE 20.11 Antimicrobials for Treatment of Urinary Tract Infection (UTI)

Parenteral

Cephalosporins
    Ceftriaxone
    Cefotaxime
    Ceftazidime
    Cefuroxime
    Cefazolin
Aminoglycosides
    Gentamicin
    Tobramycin
Penicillins
    Ampicillin

Oral

Cephalosporins
    Cefixime
    Cephalexin
    Cefuroxime
    Cefadroxil
Penicillins
    Amoxicillin
    Trimethoprim–sulfamethoxazole

of age and trimethoprim–sulfamethoxazole or nitrofurantoin in children older than 2 months of age. All agents should be given as a single daily dose (Table 20.12). Surgical reimplantation may be needed in children with severe VUR and breakthrough infections.

HYPERTENSION

Normal blood pressure in children and adolescents is defined as systolic and diastolic blood pressure readings that are less than the 90th percentile for age, sex, and height. **High normal blood pressure** is defined as average systolic or diastolic pressures readings between the 90th and the 95th percentile for age, sex and height. **Hypertension** is defined as average systolic or diastolic blood pressure readings, taken on at least three separate occasions, greater than or equal to the 95th percentile for age, sex, and height (Tables 20.13 and 20.14). **Hypertensive emergency** can be defined as an acute and severely elevated blood pressure that determines the occurrence of symptoms and signs directly attributable to high blood pressure.

It is important to remember that normal blood pressure in children increases with age. For example, a blood pressure of 130/80 mm Hg is normal for an 18-year-old adolescent but is definitely above the 95th percentile for a 5-year-old child.

Pathophysiology

Hypertension may be either primary, or essential, or secondary to another disease process. Primary hypertension is not a single disease entity but is probably secondary to several mechanisms. A genetic component is likely; normotensive children of hypertensive parents have greater increases in blood pressure in response to stress or sodium loading than children of normotensive parents. Racial differences in these blood pressure responses are present, with exaggerated hypertensive responses more likely in black than in white children.

As children grow older, their blood pressures tends to track along a given percentile. Thus, children and adolescents with blood pressures above the 90th percentile for age are more likely to become adults with hypertension. There are other maturational differences in the pathophysiology of hypertension. For example, adolescents with primary hypertension are more likely to have elevated cardiac output and normal systemic vascular resistance, whereas adults with primary hypertension are more likely to have normal cardiac output and elevated systemic vascular resistance.

TABLE 20.12 Antimicrobials for Prophylaxis of Urinary Tract Infection (UTI)

Children < 2 months
- Cephalexin
  10 mg/kg/day (single dose)
- Amoxicillin
  15–20 mg/kg/day (single dose)

Children > 2 months
- Trimethoprim—sulfamethoxazole
  2–4 mg/kg/day of trimethoprim, 10–20 mg/kg/day of sulfamethoxazole (single dose)
- Nitrofurantoin
  1–2 mg/kg/day (single dose)

TABLE 20.13 Blood Pressure Levels (90th and 95th Percentiles) for Boys 1–17 Years of Age by Percentiles of Height

Age (yr)	Blood Pressure Percentile	Systolic Blood Pressure By Percentile of Height (mm Hg)							Diastolic Blood Pressure by Percentile of Height (mm Hg)						
		5%	10%	25%	50%	75%	90%	95%	5%	10%	25%	50%	75%	90%	95%
1	90	97	98	99	100	102	103	104	53	53	53	54	55	56	56
	95	101	102	103	104	105	107	107	57	57	57	58	59	60	60
2	90	99	99	100	102	103	104	105	57	57	58	58	59	60	61
	95	102	103	104	105	107	108	109	61	61	62	62	63	64	65
3	90	100	100	102	103	104	105	106	61	61	61	62	63	63	64
	95	104	104	105	107	108	109	110	65	65	65	66	67	67	68
4	90	101	102	103	104	106	107	108	63	63	64	65	65	66	67
	95	105	106	107	108	109	111	111	67	67	68	69	69	70	71
5	90	103	103	104	106	107	108	109	65	66	66	67	68	68	69
	95	107	107	108	110	111	112	113	69	70	70	71	72	72	73
6	90	104	105	106	107	109	110	111	67	67	68	69	69	70	71
	95	108	109	110	111	112	114	114	71	71	72	73	73	74	75
7	90	106	107	108	109	110	112	112	69	69	69	70	71	72	72
	95	110	110	112	113	114	115	116	73	73	73	74	75	76	76
8	90	108	109	110	111	112	113	114	70	70	71	71	72	73	74
	95	112	112	113	115	116	117	118	74	74	75	75	76	77	78
9	90	110	110	112	113	114	115	116	71	72	72	73	74	74	75
	95	114	114	115	117	118	119	120	75	76	76	77	78	78	79
10	90	112	112	114	115	116	117	118	73	73	73	74	75	76	76
	95	116	116	117	119	120	121	122	77	77	77	78	79	80	80
11	90	114	114	116	117	118	119	120	74	74	75	75	76	77	77
	95	118	118	119	121	122	123	124	78	78	79	79	80	81	81
12	90	116	116	118	119	120	121	122	75	75	76	76	77	78	78
	95	120	120	121	123	124	125	126	79	79	80	80	81	82	82
13	90	118	118	119	121	122	123	124	76	76	77	78	78	79	80
	95	121	122	123	125	126	127	128	80	80	81	82	82	83	84
14	90	119	120	121	122	124	125	126	77	77	78	79	79	80	81
	95	123	124	125	126	128	129	130	81	81	82	83	83	84	85
15	90	121	121	122	124	125	126	127	78	78	79	79	80	81	82
	95	124	125	126	128	129	130	131	82	82	83	83	84	85	86
16	90	122	122	123	125	126	127	128	79	79	79	80	81	82	82
	95	125	126	127	129	130	131	132	83	83	83	84	85	86	86
17	90	122	123	124	125	126	128	128	79	79	79	80	81	82	82
	95	126	126	127	129	130	131	132	83	83	83	84	85	86	86

TABLE 20.14 Blood Pressure Levels (90th and 95th Percentiles) for Girls 1–17 Years of Age by Percentiles of Height

Age (yr)	Blood Pressure Percentile	Systolic Blood Pressure By Percentile of Height (mm Hg)							Diastolic Blood Pressure by Percentile of Height (mm Hg)						
		5%	10%	25%	50%	75%	90%	95%	5%	10%	25%	50%	75%	90%	95%
1	90	94	95	97	98	100	102	102	50	51	52	53	54	54	55
	95	98	99	101	102	104	106	106	55	55	56	57	58	59	59
2	90	98	99	100	102	104	105	106	55	55	56	57	58	59	59
	95	101	102	104	106	108	109	110	59	59	60	61	62	63	63
3	90	100	101	103	105	107	108	109	59	59	60	61	62	63	63
	95	104	105	107	109	111	112	113	63	63	64	65	66	67	67
4	90	102	103	105	107	109	110	111	62	62	63	64	65	66	66
	95	106	107	109	111	113	114	115	66	67	67	68	70	70	71
5	90	104	105	106	108	110	112	112	65	65	66	67	68	69	69
	95	108	109	110	112	114	115	116	69	70	70	71	73	73	74
6	90	105	106	108	110	111	113	114	67	68	69	70	71	71	72
	95	109	110	112	114	115	117	117	72	72	73	74	75	76	76
7	90	106	107	109	111	113	114	115	69	70	71	72	72	73	74
	95	110	111	113	115	116	118	119	74	74	75	76	77	78	78
8	90	107	108	110	112	114	115	116	71	71	72	73	74	75	75
	95	111	112	114	116	118	119	120	75	76	76	77	78	79	80
9	90	109	110	112	113	115	117	117	72	73	73	74	75	76	76
	95	113	114	116	117	119	121	121	76	77	78	79	80	80	81
10	90	110	112	113	115	117	118	119	73	74	74	75	76	77	77
	95	114	115	117	119	121	122	123	77	78	79	80	80	81	82
11	90	112	113	115	117	119	120	121	74	74	75	76	77	78	78
	95	116	117	119	121	123	124	125	78	79	79	80	81	82	82
12	90	115	116	117	119	121	123	123	75	75	76	77	78	78	79
	95	119	120	121	123	125	126	127	79	79	80	81	82	83	83
13	90	117	118	120	122	124	125	126	75	76	76	77	78	79	80
	95	121	122	124	126	128	129	130	79	80	81	82	83	83	84
14	90	120	121	123	125	126	128	128	76	76	77	78	79	80	80
	95	124	125	127	128	130	132	132	80	81	81	82	83	84	85
15	90	123	124	125	127	129	131	131	77	77	78	79	80	81	81
	95	127	128	129	131	133	134	135	81	82	83	83	84	85	86
16	90	125	126	128	130	132	133	134	79	79	80	81	82	82	83
	95	129	130	132	134	136	137	138	83	83	84	85	86	87	87
17	90	128	129	131	133	134	136	136	81	81	82	83	84	85	85
	95	132	133	135	136	138	140	140	85	85	86	87	88	89	89

Clinical and Laboratory Evaluation

History

Most children with hypertension are asymptomatic; their condition is detected as the result of a routine examination (e.g., a preschool or precamp "physical"). Many children and adolescents with blood pressure levels at or just greater than the 95th percentile are overweight and have family histories of hypertension.

It is important to enquire about inherited renal diseases (e.g., polycystic kidney disease), early cardiovascular disease, stroke, or hypercholesterolemia in other family members. A history of hematuria, proteinuria, polyuria, or frequent UTIs may suggest underlying parenchymal renal disease. The presence of weight loss, sweating, flushing, fevers, palpitation, or weakness may suggest an underlying endocrine problem. A thorough history should include the neonatal period, with emphasis on the use of umbilical catheters, present and past history of renal or urologic disorders and use of medications.

Initially, symptoms may include headache and blurry vision. With more severe and chronic hypertension, these may progress to seizures, stroke, coma, congestive heart failure, and renal failure.

Physical Examination

Accurate measurement of blood pressure is critical. It is important to reduce the level of patient anxiety and select a cuff of the proper size. The length of the cuff should cover at least two-thirds of the length of the upper arm, and the bladder of the pressure cuff should nearly encircle the upper arm with no overlapping of the ends.

A cuff that is too small yields an artificially elevated blood pressure. If the child's arm size seems to be between sizes of available blood pressure cuffs, the error in blood pressure measured with too large a cuff is smaller than the error in blood pressure measured with too small a cuff. Doppler and oscillometric techniques may be useful in infants and young children.

Blood pressure increases gradually with age, and reference standards must be used (see Tables 20.13 and 20.14). Blood pressure that is consistently above the 95th percentile for age on several repeated measurements over several weeks warrants further evaluation.

The physical examination should explore for evidence of secondary hypertension and end-organ damage (e.g., eyes, heart, vessels, kidneys, brain). Always measure blood pressure in all four extremities at least once to evaluate for the presence of coarctation of the aorta. Always palpate the femoral and radial pulses simultaneously when evaluating a patient with hypertension. A weak femoral pulse or a radial–femoral delay is an indication of coarctation of the aorta as the cause of the hypertension.

Other physical findings that may provide clues about secondary illnesses include abdominal bruits (**renal artery stenosis**); café au lait spots (**neurofibromatosis**); abdominal or flank masses (**renal conditions, tumors**); and striae and cushingoid features (**Cushing syndrome**).

It must be emphasized that blood pressure is not static but varies, and a more accurate representation of blood pressure may be determined by an average of multiple blood pressure measurements. To document blood pressure changes at home and at school, 24-hour ambulatory blood pressure monitoring may be useful. This helps determine nocturnal and diurnal variations and evaluate response to antihypertensive therapy.

Laboratory Evaluation

Severe blood pressure elevation warrants aggressive evaluation, regardless of age. In contrast, asymptomatic adolescents with mild blood pressure elevation may require only minimal studies.

Initial laboratory evaluation, including CBC, serum chemistries, BUN, serum creatinine, and urinalysis, may suggest the presence of an identifiable cause. Children with renal parenchymal disease may have abnormal urinalysis or elevated BUN and serum creatinine. Children with renovascular disease often have elevated plasma renin activity. If plasma renin activity is below normal, it may indicate the presence of mineralocorticoid excess. A lipid profile should be obtained, especially in overweight children and adolescents.

Imaging studies include chest radiography and renal ultrasound. Echocardiography is more sensitive than electrocardiography (ECG) for detecting left ventricular hypertrophy.

More sophisticated laboratory and imaging studies are necessary in selected patients. Captopril renal scan, magnetic resonance arteriography, or renal vein renin sampling may be useful for the evaluation of renovascular hypertension. Measurement of catecholamines in urine or plasma is indicated when pheochromocytoma is a strong clinical possibility.

Differential Diagnosis

Hypertension may be either primary (essential) or secondary to another disease process. The younger the patient, the greater the likelihood that the hypertension is secondary. Potential causes of secondary hypertension include abnormalities of renal, endocrine, cardiovascular, and neurologic systems as well as reactions to drugs or toxins (Table 20.15). Renal parenchymal disease accounts for 60%–80% of secondary hypertension in children.

Management

For patients with primary (essential) hypertension, initial treatment is usually nonpharmacologic unless blood pressure is dangerously high

or symptoms are present. Therapeutic measures include weight reduction, a decrease in dietary sodium intake, and initiation of a regular exercise program.

For patients with secondary hypertension, management is directed both at control of blood pressure and correction of the primary pathologic process, if possible. Treatment of renal artery stenosis may involve catheter angioplasty; surgical resection (e.g., for coarctation of the aorta); and appropriate pharmacologic therapy (e.g., for other primary diseases).

For those children with more severe or persistent hypertension and those with end-organ involvement (e.g., left ventricular hypertrophy, hypertensive retinopathy), the use of antihypertensive pharmacotherapy is warranted. Many different medications are now available (Table 20.16). In general, hypertension related to renal parenchymal disorders with elevated plasma renin levels responds well to angiotensin-converting enzyme (ACE) inhibitors, which decrease the formation of angiotensin II and aldosterone. Calcium

---

TABLE 20.15 **Differential Diagnosis of Secondary Hypertension**

Peripheral vascular causes
  Coarctation of the aorta
  Renal artery or vein thrombosis (premature infants with umbilical catheters)
  Renal artery stenosis
  Fibromuscular dysplasia
  Neurofibromatosis
  Arteritis
  Sarcoidosis

Renal causes
  Congenital lesions
  Obstructive uropathies
  Dysplastic or polycystic kidneys
  Acquired lesions
  Glomerulonephritis
  Henoch-Schönlein purpura
  Hemolytic-uremic syndrome
  Nephrotic syndrome
  Collagen vascular disease (systemic lupus erythematosus)
  Alport syndrome
  Vesicoureteral reflux
  Drugs (cyclosporine, steroids)
  Toxins (lead)

Endocrine causes
  Pheochromocytoma
  Neuroblastoma
  Adrenogenital syndrome
  Cushing syndrome
  Diabetic nephropathy
  Hyperparathyroidism
  Hyperaldosteronism
  Hyperthyroidism

Neurologic causes
  Neurofibromatosis
  Increased intracranial pressure
  Intracranial hemorrhage
  Encephalitis
  Guillain-Barré syndrome
  Riley-Day syndrome
  Quadriplegia

TABLE 20.16 **Oral Antihypertensive Agents for Chronic Hypertension in Children**

Angiotensin-converting enzyme (ACE) inhibitors
  Captopril
  Enalapril
  Lisinopril

Calcium channel antagonists
  Nifedipine
  Isradipine
  Amlodipine

Diuretics
  Hydrochlorothiazide
  Furosemide
  Spironolactone
  Triamterene

β-Adrenergic antagonists
  Propranolol
  Atenolol

α_2-Adrenergic agonist (central)
  Clonidine

Vasodilators
  Hydralazine
  Minoxidil

Angiotensin receptor antagonist
  Losartan

channel antagonists are effective antihypertensive agents. Other useful agents include diuretics, β-adrenergic antagonists, and vasodilators. Angiotensin receptor antagonists are a new group of antihypertensive drugs that may be more commonly used in children in the near future.

In hypertensive emergencies, the goal of therapy is to prevent hypertension-related adverse effects by a controlled reduction of blood pressure, allowing preservation of target organ function and minimizing complications of therapy. Placement on a cardiac monitor is essential, and establishment of intravenous access is appropriate. An arterial line to confirm the blood pressure cuff readings and to guide therapy may be necessary. Treatment should occur in an intensive care unit, where therapy should begin as soon as possible.

A reasonable objective in most hypertensive emergencies is to lower the blood pressure by approximately 25%–30% over a period of several minutes to several hours, depending on the clinical situation. It is important to avoid precipitous reduction in blood pressure and reductions to normotensive or hypotensive levels should be avoided, because they may provoke end-organ ischemia or infarction. Maintenance of an initial target blood pressure over several days and subsequent reduction to normotensive levels over the next several weeks is appropriate. Short-acting parenteral therapy is recommended for successful and safe management. Effective medications for the treatment of hypertensive emergencies in children include sodium nitroprusside, labetalol, and nicardipine. Once blood pressure is stabilized with intravenous drugs, oral antihypertensive agents should be gradually introduced.

RENAL TUBULAR ACIDOSIS

Renal tubular acidosis (RTA) is a clinical–biochemical syndrome characterized by impaired renal acidification. It involves the reabsorption of HCO_3^- or the excretion of H^+ and expression by hyperchloremic metabolic acidosis and minimal or absent renal insufficiency. There are three different types of RTA based on clinical and functional studies: (1) proximal RTA, or type 2; (2) distal RTA, or type 1; and (3) hyperkalemic RTA, or type 4.

Pathophysiology

Acidification of the urine can be viewed as a coordinated two-step process. The first step is the reabsorption of filtered HCO_3^- in the proximal tubule. The second step is excretion of fixed acids through the titration of urinary buffers and the excretion of NH_4^+ in the distal tubule.

In **proximal HCO_3^- reabsorption,** 80%–90% of the filtered load of HCO_3^- is reabsorbed in the proximal tubule. The primary processes that occur in this segment are H^+ secretion at the luminal membrane via a specific Na^+–H^+ exchanger and HCO_3^- transport at the basolateral membrane via a Na–HCO_3 cotransporter (Figure 20.6).

In **distal urinary acidification,** the primary processes are reclamation of the 10%–20% of the remaining HCO_3^- that escaped proximal reabsorption, titration of divalent basic HPO_4^{2-}, which is converted to the monovalent acid form or titratable acid, and accumulation of NH_3 intraluminally, which buffers H^+ to form nondiffusible ammonium (NH_4^+)[Figure 20.7].

Proximal RTA (type 2), which is caused by an impairment of HCO_3^- reabsorption in the proximal tubule, is characterized by a decreased renal HCO_3^- threshold. Distal acidification remains intact, and when plasma HCO_3^- concentration decreases to a level below the renal threshold, patients may lower urine pH below 5.5 and excrete adequate amounts of NH_4^+.

Distal RTA (type 1), which is caused by impaired distal acidification, is characterized by the inability to maximally lower urine pH (< 5.5) under the stimulus of systemic acidemia. The impaired excretion of NH_4^+ is secondary to this defect.

Hyperkalemic RTA (type 4), which involves an acidification defect that is primarily caused by impaired renal genesis of ammonia, is characterized by a normal ability to acidify the urine

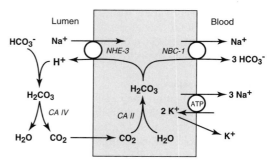

FIGURE 20.6. Schematic model of HCO_3^- reabsorption in the proximal tubule. The processes shown are H+ secretion at the luminal membrane via a specific Na^+–H+ exchanger (NHE-3) and HCO_3^- transport at the basolateral membrane via a Na^+–HCO_3^- cotransporter (NBC-1). Cytoplasmic carbonic anhydrase II (CA II) and membrane-bound carbonic anhydrase IV (CA IV) are necessary for reabsorption of HCO_3^-.

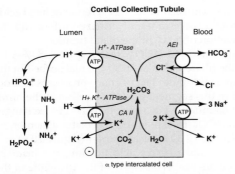

Cortical Collecting Tubule

FIGURE 20.7. Schematic model of H^+ secretion in the cortical collecting tubule. The process shown is luminal H^+ secretion in the α-type intercalated cell by a H^+-ATPase (main pump) and by a H^+,K^+-ATPase. Intracellularly formed HCO_3^- leaves the cell via Cl^--HCO_3^- exchange, facilitated by an anion exchanger (AE1). Cytoplasmic carbonic anhydrase II (CA II) is necessary for secretion of H^+.

after an acid load. However, net acid excretion remains subnormal due to a very low rate of NH_4^+ excretion. The decrease in NH_3 production is largely caused by hyperkalemia. Aldosterone deficiency or resistance may also play a role.

Clinical and Laboratory Evaluation

History
A pediatrician may suspect RTA during the workup of children with failure to thrive. Children may have a history of repetitive episodes of dehydration, with vomiting, anorexia, or constipation. Others may present with clinical manifestations of electrolyte depletion such as periodic paralysis secondary to hypokalemia. In some cases, symptoms and signs of kidney stones may precede the diagnosis of RTA. Renal deposition of calcium salts (nephrocalcinosis), thought to be the result of hypercalciuria and hypocitraturia, can occur.

Physical Examination
Physical examination may reveal only growth retardation. Other clinical findings may include signs of dehydration secondary to diarrhea or polyuria. In some cases, examination suggests a secondary cause of the RTA (e.g., cystine crystals in the cornea in patients with cystinosis, neurologic involvement in Lowe syndrome, jaundice in hepatic diseases).

Laboratory Evaluation
The first step in the evaluation of children with metabolic acidosis is calculation of the **plasma anion gap** (Figure 20.8). The plasma anion gap is

calculated by the difference between the sum of the major plasma cations ($Na^+ + K^+$) and the major anions ($Cl^- + HCO_3^-$). However, because of the relatively low and stable serum concentration of K^+, it has only a minor influence on the plasma anion gap.

$$\text{Plasma anion gap} = Na^+ - (Cl^- + HCO_3^-)$$

If the plasma anion gap is normal (12 ± 4 mEq/L), the possibility of GI losses of HCO_3^- or RTA should be considered.

URINARY ANION GAP. This value is an indirect index of urinary NH_4^+ excretion. It is estimated by using the measured concentration of electrolytes in the urine: Na^+, K^+ and Cl^-; NH_4^+ is not directly measured. A normal renal response to metabolic acidosis is an increase in the excretion of NH_4^+ in the urine, and NH_4^+ is usually excreted in the urine along with Cl^-. Any increase in the excretion of NH_4^+ during metabolic acidosis is accompanied by an increase in the excretion of Cl^-. Therefore, a negative urine anion gap ($[Cl^-] > [Na^+] + [K^+)$ reflects an increased excretion of NH_4^+. If urine NH_4^+ does not increase, the urine anion gap becomes positive ($[Cl^-] < [Na^+] + [K^+]$), which suggests a distal acidification defect.

URINE PH. This measurement has been used for diagnosis of distal RTA (type 1), the only type of RTA in which the urine pH cannot decrease below 5.5–6.0, regardless of the severity of the acidosis. A urine pH of more than 6.0 in the setting of metabolic acidosis suggests a defect in distal acidification. However, the urine pH may be misleading. Although urine pH of less than 5.5 rules out distal RTA (type 1), it does not ensure a normal distal acidification because it does not reflect the rate of NH_4^+ excretion.

It is important to assess the **plasma potassium** for characterization of RTA. Distal RTA is characterized by hypokalemia due to an increased excretion of potassium in the collecting duct. In hyperkalemic RTA (type 4), a low rate of NH_4^+ excretion is associated with hyperkalemia.

OTHER STUDIES. In specific cases, other tests may be necessary. Examples include fractional excretion of HCO_3^- to confirm the diagnosis of proximal RTA, urine Pco_2 to confirm distal RTA, and renin and aldosterone levels for hyperkalemic RTA. In addition, a kidney ultrasonogram aids in the diagnosis of nephrocalcinosis and urolithiasis, which may develop in children with RTA.

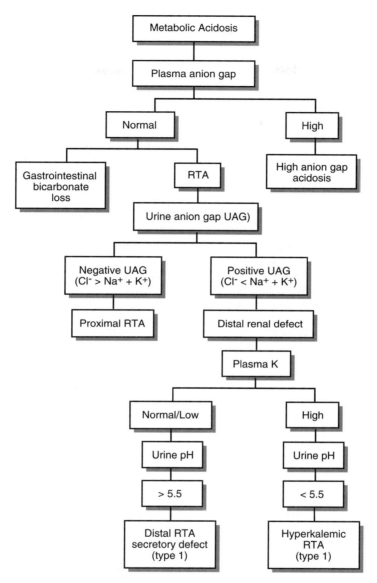

FIGURE 20.8. Algorithm representing the evaluation of children with renal tubular acidosis (RTA).

CASE 4

A 5-year-old girl presents with failure to thrive. She has no history of GI losses. Serum electrolyte values are: Na^+, 136 mEq/L; Cl^-, 111 mEq/L; and HCO_3^-, 13 mEq/L. Urine electrolyte values are: Na^+, 30 mEq/L; Cl^-, 40 mEq/L; and K^+, 20 mEq/L. Urine pH is 6.5.

Step 1: Calculation of plasma anion gap

$$\text{Plasma anion gap} = Na^+ - (Cl^- + HCO_3^-) = 136 - 124 = 12 \text{ mEq/L}$$

This value is consistent with normal anion gap acidosis.

Step 2: Calculation of urine anion gap

The serum electrolyte value for Cl^- (40 mEq/L) is less than the sum of the values for $Na^+ + K^+$ (50 mEq/L), which denotes a positive urinary anion gap.

This is consistent with low NH_4^+ excretion and a defect in distal acidification (type 1 versus type 4).

Step 3: Evaluation of plasma K

K^+ is normal. Therefore, this rules out hyperkalemic RTA (type 4).

Step 4: Evaluation of urine pH

The urine pH is 6.5, which confirms the inability to acidify the urine during acidemia and distal RTA (type 1).

Differential Diagnosis

Proximal RTA (type 2) is most commonly observed in children with Fanconi syndrome, which is a condition of global proximal tubule dysfunction, but it may also occur as a primary or inherited disease. In children, distal RTA (type 1) is almost always observed as a primary inherited entity. Hyperkalemic RTA (type 4) is associated with low aldosterone states such as congenital adrenal hyperplasia, with aldosterone-resistant states such as pseudohypoaldosteronism, and with medications such as spironolactone and ACE inhibitors.

Management

The first goal in the treatment of both proximal and distal RTA is the correction of the metabolic acidosis with the use of daily alkali supplementation. Generally, patients with proximal RTA need a larger dose of alkali than patients with distal RTA. The correction of the acidosis improves the growth rate significantly and may reduce the risk of nephrocalcinosis. Potassium abnormalities should be corrected. Hypokalemia is treated with potassium supplementation, whereas hyperkalemia may need a potassium-restricted diet, diuretics, or potassium-binding exchange resins.

ACUTE AND CHRONIC RENAL FAILURE

Acute renal failure (ARF) is defined as a rapid deterioration of renal function associated with the accumulation of nitrogenous waste products in the body. However, the urine volume in ARF may vary over a wide range. ARF can be classified according to the urine volume: oliguric (decreased) ARF and nonoliguric (normal) ARF.

Chronic renal failure (CRF) is characterized by a slow and progressive decrease in kidney function over time. CRF includes a broad spectrum of functional impairment, from a GFR of 80 mL/min per 1.73 m^2 to as low as 10 mL/min per

1.73 m^2. **End-stage renal disease** (ESRD) is present when the GFR is 10 mL/min per 1.73 m^2 or below and renal replacement therapy is needed to maintain life.

Pathophysiology

Several hypotheses regarding the pathophysiology of ARF have been suggested. The **vascular/hemodynamic theory** states that hemodynamic events are important factors in the pathogenesis. Three events may account for the decrease in glomerular filtration: (1) a constriction of the afferent arteriole; (2) a dilatation of the efferent arteriole; and (3) a decrease in permeability of the glomerular capillaries. Different hormones may be responsible for these hemodynamic abnormalities (e.g., angiotensin II, thromboxane A$_2$, endothelin). The **tubular obstruction theory** states that the glomerular filtration may be decreased secondary to a tubular obstruction by cellular debris, increasing the hydrostatic pressure within the Bowman capsule. The **back leak theory** states that the glomerular filtrate (including nonreabsorbable substances) may be reabsorbed because of disruption of the integrity of the tubular epithelium. In summary, the pathogenesis of ARF appears to be multifactorial and cannot be explained completely by any one of these theories alone.

The initial damage in CRF may be due to a wide spectrum of diseases that may present abruptly (as ARF) or insidiously. Different factors may be involved in the progressive deterioration of renal function. The **hyperfiltration theory** states that the surviving glomeruli can be damaged as a result of the increased filtered load to which they are exposed.

Clinical and Laboratory Evaluation

History

The history should focus on determining the probable cause of ARF. Hospitalized patients may develop ARF after a surgical procedure, especially complex cardiovascular surgery, or after administration of nephrotoxic medications such as aminoglycosides and radiocontrast material. Patients at risk for developing ARF in the hospital are children with severe burns, trauma, sepsis, or tumors. Bloody diarrhea, pallor, or seizures may suggest **hemolytic-uremic syndrome,** a common cause of ARF in infants. A history of skin or throat infection, hematuria, and edema is suggestive of a **poststreptococcal glomerulonephritis**. In neonates, the use of umbilical artery catheters may predispose the patient to **renal artery thrombosis** and ARF. Abnormal prenatal or postnatal ultrasound may suggest a **congenital urinary tract abnormality** as a predisposing factor.

A family history of genitourinary diseases is an important consideration in any kidney disease. A history of poor growth and development, polyuria, polydipsia, enuresis, hematuria, edema, and hypertension suggest an underlying chronic abnormality. A history of **recurrent UTIs** or recurrent episodes of fever diagnosed as "pharyngitis/ otitis" and treated with antibiotics could have been undiagnosed and undertreated UTIs. Anorexia, nausea, vomiting, headaches, and neurologic abnormalities may also be present but are nonspecific. A family history of deafness, ocular abnormalities, hypertension, or cystic kidney disease may be indicative of an inherited renal disorder.

Physical Examination

Assessment of the state of hydration and volume status help distinguish ARF from prerenal azotemia and establish the severity of the process. A height below the third percentile may be the first indicator of a kidney problem and by itself suggests an underlying chronic disorder. Vital signs, including blood pressure and weight changes, should be monitored closely. The blood pressure should be monitored periodically, and if elevated, funduscopic examination and an echocardiogram should be performed for evaluation of involvement of target organs. The presence of edema, purpura, or pallor should be assessed. Chest auscultation may be used to evaluate cardiac arrhythmias, tachycardia, or congested lungs. Hepatomegaly, palpable renal masses, or an abdominal bruit may be discovered on abdominal examination. It is important to rule out an enlarged bladder secondary to urinary retention. Signs of rickets and bone deformities may be present secondary to renal osteodystrophy.

Laboratory Evaluation

A urinalysis with renal tubular casts, tubular cells, and cellular debris suggests ARF. The absence of cellular elements and protein is most compatible with prerenal or postrenal azotemia. **Prerenal azotemia** is caused by diminished blood flow to a well-functioning kidney. **Postrenal azotemia** is a result of events occurring after urine formation, generally secondary to an obstruction to urine flow. In prerenal azotemia, as tubular function is preserved, urinary sodium concentration is low. As the concentration capacity remains intact, urinary osmolality is high. Normal tubular reabsorption results in the normal concentration of urinary nitrogenous waste products, increasing the urine: plasma creatinine ratio. On the other hand, when the tubules are damaged, as in acute tubular necrosis, the urinary sodium concentration is high and the urine:plasma creatinine ratio is low because of impaired concentration capacity.

Serum electrolytes should be monitored very closely, including calcium, phosphorus, and magnesium. Hemoglobin, hematocrit, and platelet count may be decreased, and reticulocyte and white blood cell counts may be increased in hemolytic-uremic syndrome. Uric acid may be increased as a result of **tumor lysis,** whereas lactic dehydrogenase and creatine phosphokinase may be elevated in **rhabdomyolysis** (traumatic or nontraumatic muscle destruction causing myoglobinuria and ARF). Serum complement levels may be decreased in both **SLE** and **poststreptococcal glomerulonephritis**. Elevated antinuclear antibodies are suggestive of SLE. A throat culture and ASO or streptozyme are indicated if poststreptococcal glomerulonephritis is a consideration. Blood and urine cultures are indicated if an infection is suspected. A toxicologic screening of urine may be of help in the diagnosis of ARF secondary to **nephrotoxins.**

A chest radiograph may reveal pulmonary congestion and increased heart size resulting from fluid overload. An ECG may show alterations related to hyperkalemia or other electrolyte abnormalities. Radiologic evaluation may include a kidney ultrasound to assess kidney size, the presence of hydronephrosis, or cystic disease. A DMSA renal scan is of help in the diagnosis of renal scarring secondary to **VUR** or **pyelonephritis.** Bone radiographs may show signs of osteodystrophy such as subperiosteal decalcification. A kidney biopsy may be necessary for the diagnosis of the primary disease in mild-to-moderate CRF, but it will show nonspecific chronic scarring, fibrosis, and atrophy in advanced disease, making it very difficult to determine the precise underlying etiology of the CRF.

Periodic follow-up for evaluation of the degree of renal function is necessary in children with CRF. Assessment of serum electrolytes and acid–base status is routine, followed by treatment for metabolic complications such as **acidosis, hyperkalemia, hyperphosphatemia, hypocalcemia,** and **hyponatremia.** It is important to monitor calcium, phosphorus, parathyroid hormone, and alkaline phosphatase to prevent or ameliorate the complications of osteodystrophy. Hematocrit, hemoglobin, reticulocyte count, serum iron, ferritin, and transferrin are necessary for evaluation of anemia.

Differential Diagnosis

The diagnosis of ARF is a diagnosis of exclusion. Both prerenal and postrenal factors may also cause alterations in renal function with retention of nitrogenous waste products. It is important to distinguish these entities because they are reversible with appropriate therapeutic intervention. Several conditions may cause ARF (Table 20.17).

It is important to make a specific diagnosis in children with CRF, even if the degree of renal failure is advanced and no specific therapy is available. Appropriate genetic counseling for families with hereditary or metabolic diseases and identification of potential living related donors for renal transplantation are facilitated by identifying the cause of CRF. Several diseases may cause CRF (Table 20.18).

Management

The management of ARF consists of supportive care until the kidneys recover from the acute renal insult. Patients with ARF require hospitalization, often in an intensive care unit. A careful balance of intake and output of fluids and electrolytes is extremely important. This approach may prevent or ameliorate the development of fluid overload (in oliguric ARF), of fluid depletion (in nonoliguric ARF), and of electrolyte abnormalities such as hy-

TABLE 20.17 Causes of Acute Renal Failure in Children

Prerenal azotemia
- Hypovolemia: dehydration, hemorrhage
- Hypotension: sepsis, heart failure
- Hypoxia: respiratory distress syndrome
- Renal vasoconstriction: drug effect

Intrinsic renal failure
- Ischemic disorders: hypovolemia, hypotension
- Nephrotoxins: aminoglycosides, radiocontrast agents, myoglobin, hemoglobin
- Diseases of glomeruli or small blood vessels: glomerulonephritis, hemolytic-uremic syndrome
- Major blood vessel disease: renal artery thrombosis or embolism, renal artery stenosis
- Interstitial nephritis: medications, infection, crystals

Obstructive renal failure (postrenal)
- Congenital: ureteropelvic junction obstruction, posterior urethral valves
- Acquired: stones, abdominal/retroperitoneal tumors

TABLE 20.18 Causes of Chronic Renal Failure in Children

Congenital
Renal dysplasia or hypoplasia, cystic disease, obstructive uropathy

Hereditary
Alport syndrome, juvenile nephronophthisis, congenital nephrotic syndrome

Acquired
Focal segmental glomerulosclerosis, hemolytic-uremic syndrome, pyelonephritis or interstitial nephritis, renal venous thrombosis, polyarteritis nodosa, hypertensive glomerulosclerosis
Renal tumor

Metabolic
Diabetes, cystinosis, oxalosis

ponatremia, hyperkalemia, hypocalcemia, hyperphosphatemia, and hypermagnesemia. A reasonable approach to fluid management is to restrict fluids to insensible losses (35–45 ml/kg/day) plus replacement of any output the patient might have (urine, vomiting, diarrhea, nasogastric tube drainage). Monitoring of serum electrolytes should occur at least daily. It is important to maintain an appropriate caloric and protein intake. Protein restriction (1 g/kg/day) may be indicated to slow the development of azotemia.

In addition, the use of diuretics such as furosemide, either intermittently or by continuous infusion, may be useful in an attempt to convert oliguric ARF to nonoliguric ARF, which is associated with a better prognosis. **Dialysis** may be necessary to maintain an adequate fluid and electrolyte balance and to keep the patient hemodynamically stable (Table 20.19).

Children with CRF usually do not require hospitalization except for acute complications or for the initiation of dialysis. Patients are followed periodically for the side effects of uremia. A protein-restricted diet may be indicated to decrease the rate of progression of CRF but should be sufficient to provide the child's nutritional needs. Sodium restriction may be appropriate in patients with edema or hypertension, but supplements are necessary in individuals with salt-losing nephropathies. Potassium restriction should be the primary approach to prevention of hyperkalemia. Calcium gluconate, glucose and insulin, sodium bicarbonate, or potassium-binding exchange resins (e.g., Kayexalate) may be needed to

TABLE 20.19 Indications for Dialysis in Children

Acute renal failure (ARF)

- Symptomatic fluid overload unresponsive to conservative management
- Serious, life-threatening, or medically uncontrollable metabolic disturbances (hyperkalemia, intractable acidosis)
- Acute tubular necrosis associated with poisoning due to dialyzable or hemofilterable compound

Chronic renal failure (CRF)

- Early enough to prevent the development of severe malnutrition and uremic symptoms
- Decline in creatinine clearance to about 5–10 ml/min/1.73 m^2
- Fluid overload resulting in systemic hypertension or cardiovascular instability
- Severe restriction in fluid intake so that adequate nutrition cannot be provided
- Uncontrolled hyperkalemia, hyperphosphatemia, or acidosis
- Uremic signs or symptoms (e.g., changes in mental status, pericardial effusion)

treat hyperkalemia. Initial management of hypertension involves sodium restriction, weight loss, and exercise. Pharmacologic treatment of hypertension is indicated if patients are symptomatic or if end-organ damage is evident. Renal osteodystrophy can be prevented with the use of calcitriol and phosphate binders.

Use of **recombinant human erythropoietin** completely prevents anemia. Significant improvement in growth velocity in the growth-delayed child with CRF is possible with the use of **recombinant human growth hormone.** The optimal treatment for the pediatric patient with ESRD is **renal transplantation,** because it offers the greatest potential for complete rehabilitation. Dialysis is an important tool to maintain life until a successful transplantation can be accomplished (see Table 20.19).

SUGGESTED READINGS

Evaluation of Kidney Function

Greenberg A: *Primer on Kidney Diseases,* 2nd ed. San Diego, National Kidney Foundation, 1998.

Pennington DJ, Zerin JM: Imaging of the urinary tract in children. *Pediatr Ann* 28:678–686, 1999.

Proteinuria and Nephrotic Syndrome

Bargman JM: Management of minimal lesion glomerulonephritis: Evidence-based recommendations. *Kidney Int* 55:S3–S16, 1999.

Eddy AA, Schnaper HW: The nephrotic syndrome: from simple to the complex. *Semin Nephrol* 18:304–316, 1998.

Hogg RJ, Portman RJ, Milliner D, et al: Evaluation and management of proteinuria and nephrotic syndrome in children: Recommendations from a pediatric nephrology panel established at the National Kidney Foundation conference on proteinuria, albuminuria, risk, assessment, detection, and elimination. *Pediatrics* 105:1242–1249, 2000.

Keane WF, Eknoyan G: Proteinuria, albuminuria, risk. Assessment, detection, elimination (PARADE): A position paper of the National Kidney Foundation. *Am J Kidney Dis* 33:1004–1010, 1999.

Hematuria and Glomerulonephritis

Cilento BG Jr, Stock JA, Kaplan GW: Hematuria in children. A practical approach. *Urol Clin North Am* 22(1):43–55, 1995.

Diven SC, Travis LB: A practical primary care approach to hematuria in children. *Pediatr Nephrol* 14:65–72, 2000.

Feld LG, Waz WR, Perez LM, et al: Hematuria. An integrated medical and surgical approach. *Pediatr Clin North Am* 44(5):1191–1210, 1997.

Pan CG: Glomerulonephritis in children. *Curr Opin Pediatr* 9(2):154–159, 1997.

Rodriguez-Iturbe B: Postinfectious glomerulonephritis. *Am J Kidney Dis* 35(1):xlvi–xlviii, 2000.

Henoch-Schönlein Purpura

Rai A, Nast C, Adler S: Henoch-Schönlein purpura nephritis. *J Am Soc Nephrol* 10:2637–2644, 1999.

Saulsbury FT: Henoch-Schönlein purpura in children. *Medicine* 78:395–409, 1999.

Scharer K, Krmar R, Querfeld U, et al: Clinical outcome of Schönlein-Henoch purpura nephritis in children. *Pediatr Nephrol* 13:816–823, 1999.

Tizard EJ: Henoch-Schönlein purpura. *Arch Dis Child* 80: 380–383, 1999.

Urinary Tract Infection

American Academy of Pediatrics. Committee on Quality Improvement. Subcommittee on Urinary Tract Infection: Practice Parameter: The diagnosis, treatment, and evaluation of the initial urinary tract infection in febrile infants and young children. *Pediatrics* 1999; 103:843–852, 1999.

Downs SM: Diagnostic testing strategies in childhood urinary tract infections. *Pediatr Ann* 28:670–676, 1999.

Hellerstein S: Urinary tract infections in children: Why they occur and how to prevent them. *Am Fam Phys* 57:2440–2446, 1998.

Hoberman A, Wald ER: Treatment of urinary tract infections. *Pediatr Ann* 18:688–692, 1999.

Pennington DJ, Zerrin JM: Imaging of the urinary tract in children. *Pediatr Ann* 29(11):678–686, 1999.

Hypertension

Adelman RD, Coppo R, Dillon MJ: The emergency management of severe hypertension. *Pediatr Nephrol* 14: 422–427, 2000.

Bartosh SM, Aronson AJ: Childhood hypertension. An update on etiology, diagnosis, and treatment. *Pediatr Clin North Am* 46(2):235–252, 1999.

Drugs for hypertension. *Med Lett Drugs Ther* 41:23, 1999.

Feld LG, Springate JE, Waz WR: Special topics in pediatric hypertension. *Semin Nephrol* 18(3):295–303, 1998.

Flynn JT: What's new in pediatric hypertension? *Curr Hypertens Rep* 3(6):503–510, 2001.

National High Blood Pressure Education Program Working Group on Hypertension Control in Children and Adolescents: Update on the 1987 Task Force Report on High Blood Pressure in Children and Adolescents: A Working Group Report from the National High Blood Pressure Education Program. *Pediatrics* 98(4 Pt 1):649–658, 1996.

Sorof JM, Portman RJ: Ambulatory blood pressure monitoring in the pediatric patient. *J Pediatr* 136: 578–586, 2000.

Renal Tubular Acidosis

Halperin ML, Goldstein MB: Renal tubular acidosis. In *Fluid, Electrolyte and Acid–Base Physiology*, 3rd ed. Philadelphia, WB Saunders, 1999.

Johnson V, Perelstein E: Tubular diseases. In *Pediatric Nephrology*. Edited by Trachtman H, Gauthier B. Amsterdam, the Netherlands, Harwood Academic, 1998.

Rodriguez-Soriano J: New insight into the pathogenesis of renal tubular acidosis from functional to molecular studies. *Pediatr Nephrol* 14:1121–1136, 2000.

Acute and Chronic Renal Failure

Stewart CL, Barnett R: Acute renal failure in infants, children and adults. *Crit Care Clin* 133:575–590, 1997.

Warady BA, Alexander SR, Watkins S, et al: Optimal care of the pediatric end-stage renal disease patient on dialysis. *Am J Kidney Dis* 33:567–583, 1999.

Chapter 21

Rheumatology

Christy Sandborg

Juvenile rheumatic diseases are a family of inflammatory diseases that variably involve the musculoskeletal system, connective tissue, and vascular system. **Juvenile arthritis (JA)** is the most common type of rheumatic disease that affects children, followed by **systemic lupus erythematosus (SLE), juvenile dermatomyositis, vasculitis,** and **scleroderma.** Experts currently believe that autoimmunity is a key pathophysiologic feature. Although the precise precipitating events for these diseases are not known, many of them appear to be complex genetic traits with 6–12 genes contributing to the expression of disease. Some of these genes are in the human leukocyte antigen (HLA) region of chromosome 6; however, many non-HLA genes also appear to be contributors, including cytokines, apoptosis regulatory proteins, complement components, and immunoglobulin receptors. Other contributing factors to disease expression include age, pubertal stage, and environmental triggers (e.g., sun exposure, infectious agents). Some genes probably confer susceptibility to autoimmune diseases, as indicated by families affected by multiple autoimmune diseases.

JUVENILE ARTHRITIS

Juvenile arthritis (JA) is the most common rheumatic disease in children in the United States, affecting approximately 140/100,000–180/100,000 children. Arthritis (swelling or effusion, limitation of motion, tenderness or pain on motion, or increased heat) for longer than 6 weeks in one or more joints is a key feature. The onset of JA may occur at any time before 16 years of age.

Pathophysiology

The four main types of onset of JA, based on clinical features during the first 6 months of disease, are **pauciarticular JA, polyarticular JA, systemic JA,** and **juvenile spondyloarthropathies** (Table 21.1). It is important to classify patients into a type for prognostic reasons; some forms of disease may be relatively benign, whereas others may lead to significant functional disability or even death (Table 21.2).

Clinical and Laboratory Evaluation

History

Age and developmental level are important factors to consider in the history, because arthritis in children can begin at any age from 8 months through adolescence. Young children with significant joint swelling and inflammation may not complain directly of pain, so careful questioning of parents regarding the presence of morning stiffness, limp, or decreased use of an extremity may be helpful. As children grow older, their perception of pain or lack of function improves but fear, anxiety, or denial continue to affect their expression of pain. Parental observation continues to be a key element in the history, in addition to the clinical features that are characteristic of each type of JA (Table 21.3).

Physical Examination

Careful examination of the musculoskeletal system is necessary to document the presence of true **synovitis,** which is defined as either joint swelling or joint pain and limitation of motion. References that show the normal ranges of motion for all joints and the approach to the musculoskeletal examination in children are available. The number of joints involved and the severity of involvement are important to assess for both diagnostic and management purposes (see Table 21.3).

Careful general examination is required to detect evidence of nonarticular pathology in JA. Fever and rash are characteristic of the systemic form of JA, and the presence of these findings either by history or physical examination should prompt careful evaluation for other associated findings such as pneumonitis, pericarditis, hepatosplenomegaly, lymphadenopathy, and coagulopathies. Tachycardia, tachypnea, and irritability may be indications of serious systemic disease.

A potentially fatal condition known as **macrophage activation syndrome** occurs in a minority of children with systemic JA. This syndrome, which is often triggered by drugs or intercurrent viral illnesses, is manifested by disseminated intravascular coagulation as well as hepatic, pulmonary, and central nervous system (CNS) in-

TABLE 21.1 Types of Juvenile Arthritis (JA)				
Characteristic	**Pauciarticular**	**Polyarticular**	**Systemic**	**Spondyloarthropathy**
Percent of patients	30%–45%	30%–35%	10%–15%	10%–20%
Number of inflamed joints	< 5	≥ 5	Variable	Variable
Peak age of onset	1–3 years	Variable	Variable	7–16 years
Female–male ratio	4–5:1	3:1	1:1	1:3–4

volvement. Rapid recognition of this complication facilitates prompt, aggressive treatment to prevent severe morbidity or mortality.

Ophthalmologic inflammatory changes such as **subacute anterior uveitis** may occur, but physical findings are subtle. Neither conjunctival irritation nor significant complaints of eye pain usually are present. **Synechia** (irregular pupillary margins), cloudy anterior chambers, and cataracts may be seen in advanced cases, but in mild or early involvement, ophthalmologic slit lamp examination may be the only way to detect inflammatory changes in the anterior chamber.

Pediatric Pearl

The uveitis associated with JA, which is most commonly seen with the pauciarticular type of disease, is asymptomatic. Serial slit lamp examinations, performed as many as four times per year in high-risk patients, have successfully decreased the incidence of permanent eye damage from uveitis.

Laboratory Evaluation

No specific diagnostic test for the confirmation of JA is available. The presence of autoantibodies, especially antinuclear antibody (ANA) and rheumatoid factor, are not specific to any particular type of JA, although some trends are evident (see Table 21.3). In children with systemic JA who have very high fevers or appear toxic, presence of the coagulopathy associated with macrophage activation syndrome should be rapidly assessed.

Synovial fluid analysis is important when joint infection is being considered as a possible diagnosis. Typically, synovial fluid in JA is an inflammatory exudate with a white blood cell (WBC) count of 10,000–50,000 cells/μl, primarily neutrophils, and few red blood cells (RBCs). In contrast, septic arthritis is usually associated with higher WBC count (from 50,000 to more than 100,000 cells/μl). Because crystal arthropathies such as gout are exceedingly rare in children and adolescents, synovial fluid analysis to look for crystals is rarely necessary. Synovial biopsy, which is infrequently performed for diagnostic purposes, usually shows marked lymphocytic infiltration.

Imaging studies may be helpful in determining the severity of synovitis in JA. Plain radiographs usually are normal in early or mild disease, but cartilage loss, periarticular osteoporosis, erosions, sclerosis, subchondral lucency, and deformity may be visible in long-standing or severe disease. Radiographic evidence of sacroiliitis with sclerosis and erosions of the sacroiliac joints is di-

TABLE 21.2 Prognosis in Juvenile Arthritis (JA)

Pauciarticular onset

Generally good, with a minority of patients progressing to destructive arthritis; 30% of patients become blind if the disease is unrecognized and untreated

Polyarticular onset

40%–50% of patients progress to destructive arthritis; after 15 years, 50% are significantly disabled

Systemic onset

After 15 years, 50% of patients are significantly disabled

Spondyloarthropathy

Variable; may develop into classical ankylosing spondylitis

TABLE 21.3 Clinical Features of Juvenile Arthritis (JA)

	Type of JA			
	Pauciarticular	Polyarticular	Systemic	Spondylo-arthropathy
Pattern of joint involvement	Large joints; asymmetrical; often lower extremity, except hips	Both small and large joints; symmetrical	Polyarticular or oligoarticular pattern	Large joints; lower extremity (sacroiliac, hips, knees, ankles); frequent enthesitis
Other extra-articular features	Otherwise healthy	Possible low-grade constitutional symptoms; nodules if RF-positive	High, spiking fevers; eva-nescent, salmon-pink, macular rash; hepato-splenomegaly; adenopathy; anemia; pericardi-tis; macrophage activation syndrome	Psoriasis; acute anterior uveitis; urethritis; keratoderma blenorrhagica; inflammatory bowel disease
Subacute anterior uveitis	19% (ANA+) 7%–10% (ANA−)	7%–10% (ANA+) 3%–4% (ANA−)	Rare	Acute sympto-matic anterior uveitis
ANA	60%	40%–50%	< 10%	< 10%
RF	Negative	20%, usually in older children	Negative	Rare
WBC count (cells/μl)	Normal	8,000–15,000	15,000–30,000	8,000–15,000
Hgb (g/dl)	Normal	10–12	6–10	Normal
ESR (mm/hr)	5–40	20–80	50–150	5–60

ANA = antinuclear antibody; ESR = erythrocyte sedimentation rate; Hgb = hemoglobin; RF = rheumatoid factor; WBC = white blood cell.

agnostic for juvenile ankylosing spondylitis. Magnetic resonance imaging (MRI) is becoming a very useful modality to determine the extent of synovitis and cartilage involvement and to exclude other diagnoses such as trauma.

Differential Diagnosis

Three major conditions should be considered in the differential diagnosis of JA: trauma, infection, and neoplasm. Trauma is usually excluded based on history, clinical, and laboratory findings.

It is essential to rule out a bone or joint infection in pauciarticular JA, which often manifests initially in one joint, most frequently the knee or ankle. The high fevers, leukocytosis, and elevated acute phase reactants seen in systemic JA should prompt comprehensive evaluation to exclude infection. **Acute rheumatic fever** may account for a recent onset of arthritis and fever (see Chapter 13).

Lyme arthritis, which usually presents 1–2 years after exposure to the tick-borne *Borrelia burgdorferi,* is generally oligoarticular (see Chapter 9). Diagnosis depends on potential exposure. Laboratory evaluation for Lyme disease includes confirmation of a positive enzyme-linked immunosorbent assay (ELISA) test with a Western blot or similar test for multiple *B. burgdorferi* proteins.

Leukemia is another possibility. Twenty percent of children with acute leukemia present with bone pain, and in many cases this is so early in the course of disease that no abnormal cells may be seen in the peripheral smear. Rarely are there large synovial swellings in leukemia, but periarticular swelling and pain or point tenderness may be evident. Other juvenile rheumatic diseases may present initially with arthritis, including SLE, sarcoidosis, and vasculitis. Clinical and laboratory features help distinguish these diseases from JA (see the following sections).

Pediatric Pearl

Bone pain is a common presentation of childhood leukemia. Thus, when evaluating arthritis in children with an unusual clinical presentation (e.g., low-grade fever, weight loss, bone pain out of proportion to physical findings) and a low or low-normal total WBC count with lymphocyte predominance or atypical lymphocytes, or thrombocytopenia, bone marrow examination is necessary.

Management

Treatment of JA begins with nonsteroidal anti-inflammatory drugs (NSAIDs) [Table 21.4]. The major complications of low-dose methotrexate therapy are hepatic toxicity, allergies, mild bone marrow suppression, and rarely pneumonitis. It is rare for permanent or serious complications to occur in children with methotrexate. Currently, the tumor necrosis factor (TNF) receptor immunoglobulin G (IgG) fusion protein, etanercept, is approved for use in children. Etanercept is effective in as many as 70% of children who are resistant or intolerant to methotrexate. Other cytokine inhibitors such as a humanized monoclonal antibody to TNF and an interleukin-1 (IL-1) receptor antagonist are additional options.

Systemic or local corticosteroids are used in JA for selected indications only (Table 21.5). If corticosteroids are required, every effort should be made to decrease the dose to prevent the severe side effects of this family of medications.

SYSTEMIC LUPUS ERYTHEMATOSUS

The childhood form of **systemic lupus erythematosus (SLE),** the second most common rheumatic disease in children, is similar in many ways to the adult form except that organ system involvement is more frequent and more severe in children. This complex, multisystem disease, is rare before the age of 4 years, and females are more commonly affected than males. Prior to puberty, the female:male ratio is 3–4:1; after puberty, it is 7–8:1. The incidence increases until it peaks at the age of 20–30 years.

Pathophysiology

Many of the manifestations of SLE are caused by deposition of immune complexes along basement membranes of multiple tissues. Table 21.6 shows the common autoantibodies seen in SLE as well as those in other childhood rheumatic diseases. Without appropriate treatment, 30% of children with SLE progress to end-stage renal disease; however, with current medical management, overall survival at 15 years is estimated to be 90%.

Clinical and Laboratory Evaluation

History

The onset of SLE may be insidious or acute. Acute onset of fever in patients who are receiving treatment for SLE may indicate infection, a side effect of the commonly used corticosteroids and immunosuppressive agents.

TABLE 21.4 Management of Juvenile Arthritis

Standard First-Line and Second-Line Therapy

Start with nonsteroidal anti-inflammatory drugs (NSAIDs).
Consider initiation of low-dose methotrexate (0.3–0.6 mg/kg/week) if significant synovitis involving multiple joints persists for 3–6 months or radiologic evidence of destructive disease is present.
Consider intra-articular corticosteroid injection(s) if significant synovitis persists in ≤ 2 joints for 3–6 months.
Use sulfasalazine in spondyloarthropathy.

Lack of Response to Standard First-Line and Second-Line Therapy*

Consider parenteral methotrexate weekly (up to 1 mg/kg/week).
Consider systemic corticosteroid therapy in appropriate cases (see Table 21.5)
Use tumor necrosis factor (TNF) inhibitors (etanercept and infliximab).
Consider immunosuppressive agents (azathioprine, cyclosporin A, cyclophosphamide).
Consider intravenous immune globulin (IVIG) for systemic manifestations (efficacy not proven).
Consider surgery in cases in which medical treatment has been unable to control joint damage. In severe cases of JA, joint replacement may be performed during adolescence when growth is completed.

---

*IL-1 inhibitors and anti–T-cell antibodies are possible therapeutic agents now undergoing trials.

TABLE 21.5 Use of Corticosteroids in Juvenile Arthritis (JA)

Indications for high-dose systemic corticosteroid therapy (prednisone 2 mg/kg/day or pulse methylprednisolone 30 mg/kg/day for 3 days)
Symptomatic pericarditis, pneumonitis, cerebritis, coagulopathy, macrophage activation syndrome in systemic JA
Severe uveitis unresponsive to topical therapy

Indications for low-dose systemic corticosteroid therapy (prednisone < 0.5 mg/kg/day)
Significant anorexia
Failure to thrive
Pain, joint limitations significantly limiting quality of life

Indications for local corticosteroid therapy
Uveitis (ophthalmologic corticosteroids; subtenons injections for severe disease)
Persistent synovitis in ≤ 3 joints [intra-articular corticosteroid injections (triamcinolone hexacetonide)]

Physical Examination

The presentation of SLE in children is diverse, and a comprehensive examination is essential. The most common signs and symptoms are rash, arthritis, fatigue, weight loss, and fever (Table 21.7).

Laboratory Evaluation

Many laboratory findings are abnormal in children with active SLE (Table 21.8). Depressed complement levels are a reflection of immune complex formation and deposition; in fact, regular checking of complement components C3 and C4 is an excellent way of monitoring disease activity. Screening for **antiphospholipid antibodies,** the most common antibodies associated with hypercoagulability in SLE, should include anticardiolipin antibodies and lupus anticoagulant.

MRI, computed tomography (CT), magnetic resonance angiography, and conventional angiography may be helpful in assessing for cerebral vascular accidents and arterial thromboses. However, MRI and CT scans may be normal in patients with generalized **cerebritis,** and spinal fluid studies may also be entirely normal in these individuals. Metabolic scans such as positron emission spectroscopy (PET) or spectamine scanning may be useful but are often unable to distinguish between new or old disease, or mild or severe disease.

Evaluation of the extent of renal disease is often the most important diagnostic consideration in SLE, because renal involvement is the most

---

TABLE 21.6 Autoantibodies and Associated Diseases

Autoantibody	Disease
Antinuclear antibody (ANA)	SLE (98% of patients), JA, scleroderma, dermatomyositis, MCTD, Sjögren disease; positive in 10% of healthy children
Anti–double-stranded DNA	SLE (highly specific)
Anti-Smith	SLE (highly specific)
Antiribonucleoprotein	SLE, MCTD
Anti-Ro (SSA)	SLE, neonatal lupus syndrome, Sjögren syndrome
Anti-La (SSB)	SLE, neonatal lupus syndrome, Sjögren syndrome
Antihistone	SLE, drug-induced lupus
Anti–scleroderma 70	Systemic sclerosis
Anticentromere	Limited diffuse scleroderma
Antiphospholipid	SLE, antiphospholipid syndrome, MCTD, viral infections
Anticardiolipin	SLE, antiphospholipid syndrome, MCTD, viral infections
Antineutrophil cytoplasmic antibody	Vasculitis, inflammatory bowel disease
Antiplatelet, antierythrocyte, anti-WBC	SLE, antiphospholipid syndrome, MCTD
Anti–smooth muscle	Autoimmune hepatitis
Rheumatoid factor (RF)	JA, MCTD

JA = juvenile arthritis; MCTD = mixed connective tissue disease; SLE = systemic lupus erythematosus; WBC = white blood cell.

TABLE 21.7 Signs and Symptoms of Systemic Lupus Erythematosus (SLE) in Children*

Arthritis
Rash (malar, purpuric, vasculitic)
Alopecia
Constitutional symptoms (fever, weight loss, fatigue)
Oral and nasal ulcers
Cardiac disease (pericarditis, myocarditis)
Pulmonary disease (pneumonitis, pleural effusions, pulmonary hemorrhage, pulmonary hypertension)
Renal disease (glomerulonephritis, nephrosis, hypertension, renal insufficiency)
Hematologic abnormalities (anemia, bleeding, hypercoagulability)
Raynaud phenomenon
Central nervous system disease (cerebritis, seizures, cerebral vascular accidents, peripheral neuropathy, movement disorders)
Gastrointestinal (pancreatitis, vasculitis, microperforation, exudative ascites)

*Clinical manifestations listed in order of frequency of occurrence (from most common to least common.

powerful predictor of morbidity. It is now possible to classify patients according to risk of renal failure, which helps guide therapy (Table 21.9).

Differential Diagnosis

The most common infections that may mimic SLE are **infectious mononucleosis** and streptococcal infections (see Chapter 9). Lymphoid neoplasms can also resemble SLE, especially B-cell lymphoma, which may have associated positive ANAs. Drug-induced lupus occurs infrequently in children on anticonvulsants, minocycline, and methylphenidate (Ritalin). In addition, other rheumatic diseases of children must be distinguished from SLE, most notably systemic JA, dermatomyositis, scleroderma, mixed connective tissue disease, and vasculitis.

Management

Once the diagnosis of SLE is made, the key management principle is matching the intensity of the treatment to the severity of the disease—whether the manifestations are mild, moderate, or severe (Table 21.10). In general, corticosteroids are required to control disease in the majority of pa-

TABLE 21.8 Laboratory Abnormalities in Systemic Lupus Erythematosus (SLE)

Laboratory Test	Finding in SLE
CBC	
WBC count	2,000–4,000/μl (leukopenia)
Platelet count	100,000–150,000/μl (common)
	< 10,000/μl (infrequent)
Hgb	9–10 g/dl (common)
	< 8 g/dl (severe hemolytic anemia; infrequent)
ESR	Elevated
Complement levels	Low
Autoantibody screening	Antiphospholipid (50% of patients), ANA, among others
ANA	High titer in ≥ 98% of patients
Anti-DNA	Present in ≥ 60% of patients
Antiphospholipid antibodies	Present in 50% of patients
VDRL test for syphilis	False-positive
Circulating immune complexes	Immune complexes
Serum albumin	Hypoalbuminemia
Urinalysis	Proteinuria
	Presence of RBCs
Serum creatinine and BUN	Elevated in renal insufficiency

ANA = antinuclear antibody; BUN = blood-urea nitrogen; CBC = complete blood count; ESR = erythrocyte sedimentation rate; Hgb = hemoglobin; RBC = red blood cell; VDRL = Venereal Disease Research Laboratory; WBC = white blood cell.

TABLE 21.9 Renal Disease in Systemic Lupus Erythematosus (SLE)

WHO Classification	Pathologic Description	Associated Laboratory Findings	Prognosis
Type 1	Normal	Normal	No renal dysfunction
Type 2	Mesangial proliferation	Hematuria, mild proteinuria	No renal dysfunction
Type 3	Focal segmental Glomerulonephritis	Hematuria, proteinuria, hypoalbuminemia	Mild renal dysfunction
Type 4	Diffuse lupus nephritis	Hematuria, proteinuria, hypoalbuminemia, elevated serum creatinine	Significant risk of renal failure
Type 5	Membranous	Proteinuria, hypoalbuminemia	Risk of slow progression to renal failure

WHO = World Health Organization.

tients, but once disease is controlled, corticosteroids should be tapered to a minimal dose. Hydroxychloroquine and very low dose corticosteroids have been shown to be effective in preventing relapses of disease. When SLE is well controlled, many of the once-abnormal laboratory values return to normal, and in remission, almost all laboratory values are normal except perhaps for a positive ANA.

The use of intravenous cyclophosphamide has dramatically improved the outcome of severe lupus and lupus nephritis in children and adults. The major complications of cyclophosphamide are bone marrow suppression, infection, hemorrhagic cystitis, infertility, and increased future risk of neoplastic disease. Currently, infectious complications are the major cause of significant morbidity and mortality in children with SLE. Physicians should pay meticulous attention to any signs of potential infection, because even low-grade fevers may be significant in patients who take high-dose steroids and immunosuppressive agents. In addition, opportunistic infections are also found in SLE. All patients who take cyclophosphamide should receive prophylaxis for *Pneumocystis carinii*.

TABLE 21.10 Treatment of Childhood Systemic Lupus Erythematosus (SLE) Based on Disease Severity

Severity of SLE	Treatment
Mild	
Rashes, arthralgias, leukopenia, anemia, arthritis, fever, fatigue	NSAIDs Low-dose prednisone (< 0.5 mg/kg/day) Hydroxychloroquine Prednisone (1–2 mg/kg/day)
Moderate	
Mild disease + mild organ system involvement (mild pericarditis, pneumonitis, hemolytic anemia, thrombocytopenia, mild renal disease, mild CNS disease)	NSAIDs Hydroxychloroquine Low-dose methotrexate (0.5–1.0 mg/kg/wk) Mycophenolate mofetil, azathioprine, cyclosporine
Severe	
Severe, life-threatening organ system involvement (CNS disease, diffuse lupus nephritis, pulmonary hemorrhage)	High-dose corticosteroids (2–3 mg/kg/day or pulse methylprednisolone (30 mg/kg/day × 3 days) Intravenous cyclophosphamide (1000 mg/m^2 every 1–3 months) Plasma exchange

CNS = central nervous system; NSAID = nonsteroidal anti-inflammatory drug.

Pediatric Pearl

Infection is common in children with rheumatic disease who are receiving corticosteroids and immunosuppressive medications. Fever should prompt obtaining blood and other cultures. When faced with potential serious infections in immunosuppressed patients, it is appropriate and safe to start broad-spectrum antibiotics before culture results become available.

JUVENILE DERMATOMYOSITIS

Juvenile dermatomyositis is characterized by inflammation of the skeletal muscles and skin. The illness, which may occur any time during childhood, is slightly more common in girls.

Pathophysiology

Although juvenile dermatomyositis is outwardly clinically similar to adult dermatomyositis, it is distinct from the adult form of disease in several important ways. The juvenile disease is primarily a **vasculitis** with small vessel and capillary involvement, with no associated neoplasms, as in adult dermatomyositis. If the inflammatory process is well controlled, most children enter a permanent remission after 2–5 years of therapy.

Clinical and Laboratory Evaluation

History

The onset of juvenile dermatomyositis may be acute, with rapidly progressive weakness and rash over a few weeks, or insidious, with slow progression of signs and symptoms over years. In some cases, the weakness can be profound. Muscle pain is usually mild. Constitutional symptoms, such as fever, weight loss, or anorexia, may occur.

Physical Examination

Key clinical features of juvenile dermatomyositis are evident on physical examination (Table 21.11). Careful muscle strength testing is important to perform to monitor disease activity and response to treatment (Table 21.12).

Laboratory Evaluation

Abnormal muscle enzymes are detected in the vast majority of patients with juvenile dermatomyositis, including elevated creatine kinase, lactate dehydrogenase (LDH), aspartate aminotransferase (AST), and aldolase. Diagnostic procedures such as electromyography (EMG), MRI, and muscle biopsy may be helpful in ambiguous cases.

Differential Diagnosis

The major diagnoses that should be considered in children with muscle weakness are **muscular dystrophy** and neurologic disease. Other rheumatic diseases in children may have elements of inflammatory myopathy, including **SLE** and **scleroderma.**

Management

The mainstay of therapy in juvenile dermatomyositis is corticosteroids in dosages adequate to control inflammation, usually 1–2 mg/kg/day of prednisone. Normalization of muscle enzymes,

---

TABLE 21.11 **Clinical Features of Juvenile Dermatomyositis**

Organ/System	Symptoms and Signs
Skin	Heliotrope (purplish) rash over eyelids
	Erythematous thickened lesions over MCP and PIP joints (Gottron papules)
	Erythematous thickened lesions over elbows, knees, and malleoli, with malar rash
	Vasculitis lesions
	Calcinosis, soft tissue deposition of calcium
Muscle	Proximal and symmetric weakness
	Poor head and trunk control
	Gower sign
	Trendelenburg sway
Gastrointestinal	Vasculitis
	Microperforation
Pulmonary	Recurrent pneumothoraces
Cardiac	Rare myocardial involvement

MCP = metacarpophalangeal; PIP = proximal interphalangeal.

TABLE 21.12	Muscle Strength Testing	
Grades	% Function	Activity Level
5 Normal	100	Complete range of motion against gravity with full resistance
4 Good	75	Complete range of motion against gravity with some resistance
3 Fair	50	Full range of motion against gravity
2 Poor	25	Full range of motion without gravity
1 Trace	15	Evidence of slight contractility; no effective joint motion
0 No contraction	0	No evidence of muscle contractility

which occurs with treatment, are a good measure of adequate suppression of inflammation. One of the longer term complications of the disorder is subcutaneous calcifications or **calcinosis.** When early inflammation is well controlled, this complication is much less frequent. If the disease continues to be active, the addition of low-dose methotrexate to the corticosteroid regimen is appropriate. In cases of severe vasculitis involving the gastrointestinal (GI) tract, cyclophosphamide or cyclosporine may be helpful. Physical and occupational therapy is essential to improve strength and prevent muscle tightening.

SCLERODERMA

Scleroderma assumes two major forms in children: **localized scleroderma,** which is limited to focal areas of skin and subcutaneous tissues, is the most common form, and **diffuse scleroderma** (also called systemic sclerosis), which is very similar to the adult disease. Diffuse scleroderma is extremely rare in children.

Pathophysiology

Both forms of scleroderma are characterized by progressive fibrosis of affected tissues due to immune stimulation of fibroblast activity. Each form of scleroderma has different characteristics (Table 21.13).

Clinical and Laboratory Evaluation

History
Both types of scleroderma are typically of slow onset and have a gradually progressive course (over several years). However, further progression of localized scleroderma tends to stop after 5–7 years. Localized disease is first noticeable as a painless, nonpruritic skin lesion anywhere on the body. Diffuse scleroderma usually begins as **sclerodactyly** and **Raynaud syndrome.**

Physical Examination
Skin changes and other associated findings are evident in scleroderma (see Table 21.13). In diffuse disease, organ system involvement is the major morbidity in diffuse scleroderma. In the linear form of localized scleroderma, underlying bony involvement can impair growth of the facial bones or involved extremity and is seriously disfiguring. Sclerotic lesions crossing a joint may lead to decreased range of motion.

Laboratory Evaluation
ANAs are commonly positive in both localized and diffuse scleroderma, especially anti–scleroderma 70 and anticentromere antibodies (see Table 21.6). General laboratory tests are usually normal in both forms of the disease. Because there is little stimulation of the acute phase response, the erythrocyte sedimentation rate or C-reactive protein are unremarkable.

Imaging studies are very helpful in assessing the presence and severity of pulmonary disease. High-resolution CT of the chest may reveal alveolitis and fibrosis, which may eventually lead to severe pulmonary fibrosis, pulmonary hypertension, and cor pulmonale. Chest radiography may be normal. Pulmonary function tests, echocardiography (for pulmonary artery pressure estimates), and GI barium studies may be used to delineate the extent of disease.

Differential Diagnosis

The slow onset and progression of scleroderma in childhood makes diagnosis difficult; symptoms appear slowly. One of the earliest features in diffuse scleroderma is **Raynaud syndrome.** However, **Raynaud phenomenon** may occur in otherwise healthy individuals and never lead to significant disease. Scleroderma-like syndromes are associated with long-standing insulin-dependent diabetes mellitus, and skin and autoimmune changes are seen with allogeneic bone

TABLE 21.13	Characteristics of Diffuse and Localized Scleroderma		
Type	**Subtype**	**Skin Involvement**	**Associated Findings**
Diffuse scleroderma	Systemic sclerosis	Sclerosis proximal to MCP joints	Raynaud syndrome, esophageal dysmotility, atrophy and dilatation of small and large bowel, pulmonary fibrosis, pulmonary hypertension, cor pulmonale, nephrosclerosis, myocardial fibrosis
	Subacute diffuse scleroderma (CREST syndrome)	Sclerodactyly, telangiectasia	Esophageal dysmotility, Raynaud syndrome, calcinosis, milder pulmonary and renal disease compared to systemic sclerosis
Localized scleroderma	Morphea	One or more plaque-like atrophic hypopigmented lesions with lilac border	No associated organ system involvement No progression to diffuse scleroderma
	Linear scleroderma	One or more band-like sclerotic lesions extending along dermatomes, hypo- and hyperpigmentation	Local growth abnormalities underlying lesions on face, skull, and extremities Joint tightness and arthralgias No organ system involvement No progression to diffuse scleroderma
	Eosinophilic fasciitis	Thickened skin and subcutaneous tissues, "peau d'orange" appearance	Eosinophilia sometimes seen No organ system involvement

CREST = **c**alcinosis, **R**aynaud phenomenon, **e**sophageal involvement, **s**clerodactyly, **t**elangiectasia; MCP = metacarpophalangeal.

marrow transplantation. The lesions of localized scleroderma, which may appear very similar to a scar, may be confused with lichen sclerosis et atrophica or fungal infections.

Management

In localized scleroderma when symptoms are mild, emollients or creams are most useful. In cases of linear scleroderma in which patients are at risk for development of disability or significant cosmetic defect, low-dose methotrexate should be considered.

In diffuse scleroderma, the severity of involvement dictates the aggressiveness of treatment. Cyclophosphamide may be effective with significant pulmonary alveolitis and early fibrosis, and low-dose methotrexate, d-penicillamine, or low-dose corticosteroids may control milder forms of these conditions. Symptomatic treatment with H_2 blockers, proton pump inhibitors, and GI motility agents may be useful for GI problems, and calcium channel blockers may be helpful for Raynaud syndrome.

Systemic sclerosis progresses slowly, and cardiopulmonary manifestations currently account for the major life-threatening morbidity associated with the disorder. Early detection is required because late states of cardiopulmonary disease are often resistant to treatment. Angiotensin-converting enzyme inhibitors are an effective treatment for renal disease and malignant hypertension.

VASCULITIS

Many of the major forms of chronic vasculitis that affect adults also rarely affect children. The chronic forms of childhood vasculitis are discussed in this section. Two common forms of "transient" vasculitis, **Kawasaki disease** and **Henoch-Schönlein purpura,** will not be discussed here (see Chapters 13 and 20).

Pathophysiology

The most common forms of vasculitis in children may be differentiated according to their major clinical and pathologic manifestations (Table 21.14).

Clinical and Laboratory Evaluation

History

The history obtained in vasculitis reflects the type and extent of organ system involvement. Wegener granulomatosis is characterized by recurrent sinusitis and pulmonary disease. In contrast, polyarteritis may be characterized by constitutional symptoms such as fever and fatigue, as well as features of mesenteric vasculitis such as abdominal pain.

TABLE 21.14 | **Classification of Vasculitis in Children**

Vasculitis	Vessel Involvement	Associated Autoantibodies	Clinical Manifestations
Leukocytoclastic vasculitis	Small vessel perivascular polymorphonuclear cell infiltration		Urticarial vasculitis, palpable purpura
Henoch-Schönlein purpura	Small vessel perivascular polymorphonuclear cell infiltration, IgA immune complex deposition		Palpable purpura, GI vasculitis, glomerulonephritis, arthritis
Wegener granulomatosis	Small and medium vessel granulomatous vasculitis	c-ANCA, especially antiproteinase 3	Upper and lower respiratory tract involvement, glomerulonephritis
Crescentic (pauciimmune) glomerulonephritis	Focal or diffuse glomerulonephritis with crescents, rare immunoglobulin deposition	p- and c-ANCA	Glomerulonephritis
Churg-Strauss allergic granulomatosis	Small and medium vessel granulomatous vasculitis with eosinophils	p-ANCA	Pulmonary infiltrates with asthma syndrome
Polyarteritis nodosa	Small and medium necrotizing arteritis	p-ANCA, especially antimyeloperoxidase	GI and renal arteritis with microaneurysms; skin, CNS, hepatic, and muscle vasculitis
Microscopic polyangiitis	Small vessel necrotizing vasculitis	p-ANCA, especially antimyeloperoxidase	Pulmonary vasculitis, glomerulonephritis
Kawasaki disease	Medium and small vessel necrotizing arteritis		Fever, rash, mucocutaneous lesions, coronary aneurysms
Behçet syndrome	Small and medium vessel vasculitis		Anterior and posterior uveitis, aphthous ulcers, genital ulcers, small and large bowel colitis, thrombotic phenomenon
Giant cell (temporal) arteritis (not seen in childhood)	Large vessel granulomatous vasculitis		Temporal and cranial vasculitis, ocular involvement
Takayasu arteritis	Granulomatous vasculitis of the aorta and major branches		Hypertension, vascular insufficiency, aneurysms

ANCA = antineutrophil cytoplasmic antibody; CNS = central nervous system; GI = gastrointestinal.

Physical Examination

The key features of the physical examination reflect the type of organ system involvement in the various types of vasculitis (see Table 21.14). Hypertension suggests renal involvement, as in polyarteritis or Wegener granulomatosis. Altered peripheral pulses suggest large-artery involvement, as in Takayasu arteritis.

Laboratory Evaluation

One of the most helpful tests for diagnosis and monitoring of disease activity in vasculitis is antineutrophil cytoplasmic antibodies (ANCA), which are associated with the major forms of vasculitis (see Table 21.14). Inflammatory changes, including leukocytosis, thrombocytosis, and elevated acute phase reactants, are seen in active disease. **Glomerulonephritis,** with active urinary sediments and decreased creatinine clearance, leading to renal failure is a major complication of **Wegener granulomatosis**.

Imaging studies are helpful in understanding the extent of vasculitis. MRI and CT of the sinuses and chest are indicated in Wegener granulomatosis, and magnetic resonance angiography and conventional angiography are required in the evaluation of **Takayasu arteritis.**

Differential Diagnosis

It is essential to distinguish among the major types of vasculitis in children, because the extent and type of organ system involvement characterizes distinct clinical syndromes. However, when symptoms are vague, the major nonrheumatic diseases that should be considered are infectious (e.g., infectious mononucleosis) and neoplastic (e.g., lymphoma).

Management

The approach to management depends on both the type of vasculitis and the severity of involvement. Corticosteroids are the mainstay of treatment, but in certain types of vasculitis, corticosteroids alone may not be adequate. For example, cyclophosphamide is almost always indicated in Wegener granulomatosis and frequently in polyarteritis with organ system involvement. Other drugs that may be useful in milder forms of vasculitis such as microscopic polyangiitis include other immunosuppressive agents such as methotrexate.

PAIN SYNDROMES IN CHILDREN

Although rarely leading to permanent dysfunction or organ system damage, severe chronic pain may be extremely disabling unless recognized and treated. Pain syndromes in children may be frequently confused with rheumatic diseases. However, distinct features are helpful in distinguishing the major pain syndromes in children from rheumatic diseases (Table 21.15).

Pathophysiology

The etiology of pain syndromes may in part be developmental or mechanical. Familial associations are seen in benign limb pains and fibromyalgia. Psychologic causes are not associated except in conversion reactions, however, secondary depression due to chronic pain and disability is frequent.

Clinical and Laboratory Evaluation

History

The typical historical features of pain syndromes are a long onset period, as well as variable intensity and frequency (see Table 21.15). Females are more commonly affected than males, and onset occurs during puberty. Patients describe the pain as intolerable and unrelenting; as described, the severity of pain is greater than it is in other disease such as JA. The pain causes affected children to be unable to participate in normal activities.

Physical Examination

The physical examination is usually the basis for the diagnosis, with the major symptoms and signs as noted in Table 21.15. Typically, there is no evidence of joint swelling, skin rash, or other signs of inflammatory diseases. Muscle or diffuse extremity pain and tenderness are more common than joint tenderness.

Laboratory Evaluation

No laboratory abnormalities are evident with the pain syndromes. Severe disuse in reflex sympathetic dystrophy can be associated with osteopenia and changes detected by technetium bone scan.

Differential Diagnosis

The key conditions that must be distinguished from pain syndromes are trauma, other rheumatic diseases, neoplastic, and neurologic diseases. In some cases, **fibromyalgia** may be secondary to musculoskeletal disease due to SLE, JA, and trauma. Although psychological diseases (e.g., conversion reactions) may sometimes be confused with pain syndromes, the presenting symptoms and pain manifestations are frequently bizarre in these conditions.

TABLE 21.15	Characteristics of Common Pain Syndromes In Children				
Syndrome	Age at Onset (years)	F:M Ratio	Physical Findings	Description of Pain	Associated Features
Benign limb pains of childhood	4–13	F > M	None	Intermittent nocturnal pain in calves, thighs and shins	No pattern of recurrence
Patello-femoral pain	11–13	F > M	Crepitance, positive patellar apprehensive and compression tests, mild swelling	Grating, catching pain at edges of patella; instability	Increased with descending stairs, squatting kneeling, running; inability to sit for long periods without extending knee (theater sign)
Benign hypermobility syndrome	3+ (10% of population)	F > M	Hyperextensibility of elbows > 5°, genu recurvatum > 5°, hyperextension of MCP joints and thumbs	Aching in joints common	Familial occurrence, dislocation of joints, mitral prolapse; NO Ehlers-Danlos or Marfan syndromes
Juvenile fibromyalgia	10 through adolescence	F >>> M	> 13 tender areas at discrete anatomic locations	Aching, burning, pain at tender areas, palpation sometimes causing radiation; generalized, chronic, diffuse musculoskeletal pain	Fatigue, headaches, sleep disturbances, paresthesias, depression, anxiety
Reflex sympathetic dystrophy	8 through adolescence	F > M	Painful extremity with swelling; changes in temperature, color, perspiration pattern; occasionally > 1 extremity affected	Exquisite pain to light touch; chronic pain without touch	Disconnected affect from pain, "la belle indifference"
Psychogenic pain	7 through adolescence	F = M	None, unless induced injury	Unusual patterns of pain, unusual functional use of extremity or abnormal gait, intermittent severe pain, continuous severe pain	Psychologic disturbance (possible)

F = female; M = male; MCP = metacarpophalangeal.

Management

Accurate diagnosis is the key to management of pain syndromes. The families of many children are extremely concerned about the potential seriousness of symptoms and will continue to "doctor shop" until they find a physician who they believe has made a reliable diagnosis. Reassurance, often the first step, is very effective in the majority of milder pain syndromes. Intensive physical therapy, sometimes requiring inpatient therapy, is helpful in severe cases of **fibromyalgia** and **reflex sympathetic dystrophy.** In addition, psychological counseling for stress management, depression, and school dysfunction is often necessary in cases where significant disability and lack of normal functioning have occurred.

SUGGESTED READINGS

Burgos-Vargas R, Pacheco-Tena C, Vazquez-Mellado J: Juvenile-onset spondyloarthropathies. *Rheum Dis Clin North Am* 23:569, 1997.

Cabral DA, Tucker LB: Malignancies in children who initially present with rheumatic complaints. *J Pediatr* 134:53, 1999.

Cassidy JT, Petty RE: *Textbook of Pediatric Rheumatology.* New York, W.B. Saunders, 1995.

Gare BA: Juvenile arthritis—Who gets it, where and when? *Clin Exp Rheumatol* 17:367, 1999.

Glass DN, Giannini EH: Juvenile rheumatoid arthritis as a complex genetic trait. *Arthritis Rheum* 42:2261, 1999.

Lovell DJ, Giannini EH, Reiff A, et al: Etanercept in children with polyarticular juvenile rheumatoid arthritis. Pediatric Rheumatology Collaborative Study Group [see comments]. *N Engl J Med* 342:763, 2000.

Sandborg CI, Nepom B, Mellins E: Juvenile arthritis. In *Clinical Immunology*, 2nd ed. London, Mosby, 2001.

Sherry DD: Pain syndromes. In Isenkey DA, Miller JJI, eds. *Adolescent Rheumatology*. London, Martin Dunitz, Ltd., 1999.

Stephan JL, Zeller J, Hubert P, et al: Macrophage activation syndrome and rheumatic disease in childhood: A report of four new cases. *Clin Exp Rheumatol* 11:451, 1993.

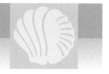

Chapter 22

Dermatology

Kimberly A. Horii and Alfred T. Lane

DEFINITIONS

To best understand the response of the skin to disease processes, it is first important to understand the structure of the skin (Figure 22.1). The skin can be divided into two layers, the epidermis and the dermis. The **epidermis** is the outer layer of skin that protects the body from the outside environment and maintains internal homeostasis. The epidermis contains **keratinocytes,** which divide and undergo a process of maturation called keratinization. This process results in the formation of the **stratum corneum,** an outer skin later that is less than 0.1 mm thick yet provides the majority of the barrier function of the skin. The **dermis,** the deeper layer of the skin, provides the blood supply, flexibility, and sensory innervation necessary for cutaneous function.

Before this discussion of skin disease in infants and children begins, it is also essential to understand the language of dermatology. Skin examination is necessary for identification of **primary lesions,** the first lesion to appear, and any secondary changes. The clinician should also be aware of the color, arrangement, and distribution of lesions. Often, only **secondary lesions** are apparent, and the correct diagnosis depends on finding less obvious primary lesions or attempts to correlate patient history with the appearance of secondary lesions. There are various types of primary and secondary lesions (Table 22.1).

DERMATOPHARMACOLOGY

Several principles of skin care are important in caring for infants and children. The epidermis, with its combination of cells surrounded by a lipid layer, provide a hydrophobic barrier that can be injured by the outside environment as well as by genetic abnormalities in production of the barrier. Recognized abnormalities in the barrier are **dry skin** and **dermatitis** (inflamed or irritated skin). Dry skin may be associated with scaling, roughened texture, and possible erythema (redness), and treatment often involves **topical creams, moisturizing lotions, or ointments** (Table 22.2). These **lubricants** smooth the skin and replace lipid in the stratum corneum.

Ointments are more greasy and occlusive than creams or lotions. The higher the humidity in the environment, the less occlusive the cream or lotion should be; in a drier environment, a greasier ointment or cream may feel better.

Care should be a consideration when applying any products to the skin, recognizing the potential for absorption of the product and systemic toxicity. **Topical steroids** are commonly used to treat inflamed skin conditions, irrespective of the cause. The strength of topical steroids ranges in potency from low to high (Table 22.3).

> ### Pediatric Pearl
> Only low- or moderate-potency topical steroids should be used in infants and children.

Dangerous and unwanted side effects may result from the use of high-potency topical steroids in young individuals.

SKIN LESIONS COMMON IN THE NEONATAL PERIOD

NEONATAL PUSTULES

Term infants may suffer from several common dermatologic conditions, including **erythema toxicum,** which develops 1–14 days after birth (Figure 22.2). The lesions appear as erythematous papules or pustules associated with multiple erythematous macules. The macules may be at the site of the pustules or elsewhere on the body. Typical sites of involvement include the face, trunk, and proximal extremities. Examination of a scraping of the pustule with Wright stain indicates that the pustule contains mainly eosinophils. The lesions resolve over several days to weeks, leaving no residua.

Infants born with pustules may have a condition called **transient neonatal pustular melanosis.** These pustules can be seen anywhere on the body but appear to be most common on the face and, occasionally, on the palms and soles. Wright stain of the pustule contents usually reveals predominance of polymorphonuclear leukocytes.

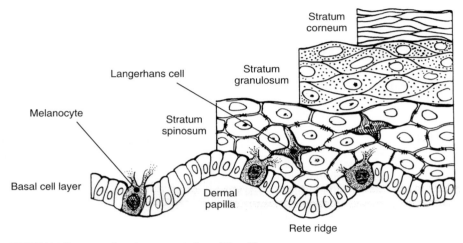

FIGURE 22.1 Cross sectional representation of the skin.

Cultures of both erythema toxicum and neonatal pustular melanosis should be sterile, and Gram stains should not show bacteria. These two common conditions should be distinguished from potentially serious infections such as herpes simplex, cutaneous candidiasis, and *Staphylococcus aureus* infection. Although both lesions appear to be of no consequence, because of their ap-

pearance at birth, they may be of great parental concern.

BIRTHMARKS

Vascular birthmarks are very common in children. Flat vascular lesions occur on the nape of the neck, where they are often called "stork bite,"

TABLE 22.1 **Definitions of Primary and Secondary Skin Lesions in Infants and Children**

PRIMARY SKIN LESIONS
- **Macule**—color change in the skin that is flat to the surface of the skin and not palpable.
- **Papule**—a solid, raised lesion 1 cm or less in diameter.
- **Plaque**—a solid, raised, flat-topped lesion larger than 1 cm in diameter.
- **Nodule**—a raised, solid lesion with indistinct borders and a deep palpable portion. If the skin moves over the nodule, it is subcutaneous in location; if the skin moves with the nodule, the nodule is intradermal.
- **Wheal**—an area of tense edema in the upper dermis, producing a flat-topped slightly raised lesion.
- **Vesicle**—a raised lesion less than 1 cm in diameter, filled with clear fluid.
- **Bulla**—a lesion larger than 1 cm in diameter, filled with clear fluid.
- **Cyst**—a raised lesion that contains a palpable sac filled with liquid or semisolid material.
- **Pustule**—a raised lesion filled with purulent exudate, giving it a yellow appearance.

SECONDARY SKIN CHANGES
- **Scaling**—small flakes on the skin surface, secondary to abnormal shedding or accumulation of stratum corneum cells.
- **Erosions**—moist, circumscribed, slightly depressed area representing a blister base with the roof of the blister removed.
- **Excoriations**—oval to linear depressions in the skin with removal of the epidermis, exposing a broad section of red dermis. Excoriations are the result of traumatic removal of the epidermis and upper dermis.
- **Crusting**—dried exudate of plasma combined with the blister roof, which sits on the surface of skin following acute dermatitis.
- **Atrophy**—the skin surface is depressed because of thinning or absence of the epidermis or subcutaneous fat.
- **Lichenification**—thickened plaques with accentuated skin markings secondary to chronic rubbing of the skin.
- **Fissures**—characterized by linear wedge-shaped cracks in the epidermis, extending down to the dermis and narrowing at the base.

TABLE 22.2 Examples of Common Over-the-Counter Emollients/Moisturizers

Petroleum jelly
Aquaphor ointment
Eucerin creme
Cetaphil cream
Moisturel cream
Mineral oil

---

or over the midnose or eyelid region, where they are called "salmon patch." About 0.3% of infants have **port-wine stains,** which are darker, red-blue, flat vascular lesions. Port-wine stains may be associated with either underlying brain or eye involvement or overgrowth of a limb when they are on an extremity.

Raised vascular birthmarks usually represent **hemangiomas** (Figure 22.3), which result from a proliferation of endothelial cells. Hemangiomas usually enlarge for the first 6–9 months of life and then start to flatten. Most of these lesions have flattened to skin level by the time children reach 10 years of age. Large hemangiomas can cause problems when they obstruct vision, obstruct the airway, or break down and ulcerate. Occasionally, lesions may trap platelets **(Kasabach-Merritt syndrome).** Affected infants present with profound thrombocytopenia and multiple areas of bruising. Ulcerated hemangiomas may require antibiotic therapy, as they are usually secondarily infected, most commonly with *S. aureus.* New advances in laser surgery have made early nonscarring therapy for both flat and raised vascular lesions possible.

TABLE 22.3 Topical Steroids Listed by Level of Potency*

Low potency
 Hydrocortisone 1%, 2.5%
 Desonide 0.05%

Moderate potency
 Fluocinolone acetonide 0.01%
 Hydrocortisone valerate 0.2%
 Mometasone furoate 0.1%
 Triamcinolone acetonide 0.1%

High potency
 Fluocinonide 0.05%
 Desoximetasone 0.25%

---

*Only low- or moderate-potency topical steroids should be used in pediatric dermatology.

SKIN LESIONS COMMON IN INFANTS AND OLDER CHILDREN

DIAPER DERMATITIS

Pathophysiology

Diaper dermatitis, a common condition seen in infants wearing diapers, is caused by a combination of skin wetness, pH elevation of the diaper-covered skin, and friction of the diaper against the skin. The elevated pH is secondary to urease activation, which breaks down the urea in the urine to ammonia and raises the pH. The elevated pH activates proteolytic enzymes that may injure the skin. In addition, secondary infection with *Candida albicans* may increase the severity and pain associated with diaper dermatitis (Figure 22.4). When diaper dermatitis is associated with erythematous red papules on the periphery of the central lesions, *C. albicans* may be the cause.

Management

Mild diaper dermatitis is easily treated with an application of a lubricant cream or ointment such as zinc oxide or petroleum jelly.

Pediatric Pearl

Superabsorbent gel disposable diapers have proved effective in preventing diaper dermatitis by absorbing wetness away from the skin and by buffering the pH back toward normal.

The addition of 1% hydrocortisone may be effective in decreasing the inflammation and tenderness. Hydrocortisone treatment is usually only necessary for several days.

Infants with *C. albicans* diaper dermatitis require a topical antifungal agent such as nystatin, miconazole, or clotrimazole. Many children who have *C. albicans* may have recurrences of diaper dermatitis and may need intermittent reapplication of the antifungal medication until they are out of diapers. These infants may also require the continuous application of lubricants or moisturizers in the diaper area with each diaper change.

ACNE

Acne vulgaris is a common skin condition that occurs in the pediatric age group. Although it may be seen in infants between 2 weeks and 6 months of age, it more commonly develops several years prior to the onset of adolescence. The lesions of acne are often apparent on areas of the face, upper chest, and the upper back.

Pathophysiology

The early lesions are the **blackhead,** which is also called an **open comedo,** and the **whitehead** which is also called a **closed comedo** (Figure 22.5). Both lesions represent obstruction of the sebaceous follicle just beneath the follicular opening in the neck of the follicle. The stratum corneum accumulates in this area, obstructing the orifice. Over time, with the accumulation of sebum and *Propionibacterium acnes* (bacterial overgrowth), the closed comedones may eventually become inflammatory papules and possibly pustules. Larger lesions may become nodules or cysts. With the formation of cysts, pitted scars may develop secondary to fibrosis in the dermis, which then pulls the overlying epidermis downward.

Pediatric Pearl

Acne is not caused by diet or dirty skin.

Many patients believe that acne is caused by dirty skin and aggressively scrub their skin in an effort to eliminate the acne. There are no data to support that facial scrubbing improves acne, and it definitely increases the irritative side effects. Keeping the face clean with only water or a mild, noncomedogenic cleanser is usually adequate. Patients in occupations where there skin is exposed to large quantities of grease may require avoidance of the greases or a more effective method of skin cleansing.

Management

Treatment of acne varies depending on severity (Table 22.4). For patients who present primarily with open and closed comedones or a few inflammatory papules and pustules, benzoyl peroxide, either as a 5%–10% over-the-counter lotion or as a 2.5%–10% prescription gel, may be adequate. Physicians should warn patients that the benzoyl peroxide may cause staining of clothes. Retinoic acid (tretinoin) is another excellent preparation that helps prevent the formation of comedones, the primary lesions of acne. This agent causes skin dryness and irritation and is also a photosensitizing drug that may increase the risk of developing a sunburn. Retinoic acid is available as a cream (0.025%, 0.05%, 0.1%); gel (0.01%, 0.025%); and micronized gel (0.1%). The creams tend to be less irritating and less drying than the gels, whereas the gels are more effective for those patients who believe that their skin is oily and greasy despite treatment with the cream. Adapalene gel (0.1%), a new synthetic product with retinoid activity, is not photosensitizing and causes less skin irritation.

Benzoyl peroxide and retinoic acid can also be used in combination. Usually, benzoyl peroxide is applied in the morning and retinoic acid is applied at night. It is important that retinoic acid be applied to skin without any other products and to skin that has not been washed in the previous 30 minutes. Washing the skin prior to the application hydrates the skin and increases the incidence of irritation from retinoic acid.

Patients who continue to have inflammatory papules and pustules despite therapy with topical benzoyl peroxide and retinoic acid may require additional treatment with antibiotics. Effective topical antibiotics include clindamycin phosphate

TABLE 22.4	Basic Treatment Guidelines for Acne Vulgaris

For few comedones, inflammatory papules, and pustules:
    Benzoyl peroxide gel or lotion
    Retinoic acid cream or gel

For many comedones, inflammatory papules, and pustules:
    Benzoyl peroxide gel or lotion
    Retinoic acid cream or gel
    Topical antibiotics
    Oral antibiotics

For many comedones, inflammatory papules, pustules, nodules, and cysts:
    Retinoic acid cream or gel
    Oral antibiotics
    Referral to dermatologist; patient may require systemic retinoids

1%, erythromycin 1%–2%, or sodium sulfacetamide 5%–10%. Oral antibiotics can be used for those patients who do not respond to topical antibiotic therapy or those patients for whom the application of multiple different products to their face becomes confusing. Tetracycline, doxycycline, or erythromycin are the most frequently prescribed oral antibiotics for acne and are usually taken in two divided doses per day.

All acne therapies require several weeks to months before a response is seen. Patient motivation is thus an important component of successful therapy. Initially, it is necessary to follow acne patients at 4–8-week intervals to evaluate response to therapy, to modify therapy as necessary, and to motivate the patient to continue therapy.

ATOPIC DERMATITIS

Atopic dermatitis, also known as eczema, is a common skin disorder, affecting 10%–15% of children. It has been described as the "itch that rashes," which emphasizes that the primary pathology is associated with **pruritus** (itching) and the results seen on the skin are lesions secondary to **excoriation.** Patients present with a history of pruritus and areas of excoriation on their face or other body sites (Figure 22.6). Atopic dermatitis can cause severe disability for children and their families secondary to the severity of pruritus and the intensity of the itching. For a discussion of the pathogenesis, clinical manifestations, and management of this disease, see Chapter 17, ATOPIC DERMATITIS.

Differential Diagnosis

Two conditions that must be differentiated from atopic dermatitis are **allergic contact dermatitis** and **scabies**. Usually, patients with allergic contact dermatitis have a history of exposure to poison ivy or poison oak. Often, the lesions in allergic contact dermatitis appear initially as vesicles that then become excoriated. Occasionally, linear vesicles can be seen where the leaf or stem of the plant has come in contact with the skin. Scabies is caused by a mite and is often associated with pruritus in other family members. This condition often appears to be worse on the hands and feet of infants and children (see SCABIES).

SEBORRHEIC DERMATITIS

Seborrheic dermatitis is common before 6 months of age and after puberty. It occurs as an accumulation of greasy scale on a base of erythema. When the condition involves the scalp of infants, it is known as **"cradle cap."**

Pathophysiology

Seborrheic dermatitis is thought to occur from a physiologic overproduction of sebum. In infants younger than 6 months of age, it is often difficult to distinguish this condition from atopic dermatitis.

Management

For those infants who have a thick accumulation of scale, application of mineral oil 30 minutes prior to washing the hair may help remove the scale. Treatment may involve low-potency topical steroids such as hydrocortisone cream in infants or fluocinolone solution in adolescents and young adults, applied once or twice a day to the area of dermatitis. Adolescents may require topical hydrocortisone applied to the areas of dermatitis on the face and fluocinolone applied to the areas of dermatitis on the scalp.

PSORIASIS

Although psoriasis is a common condition in adults, it is rather uncommon in children. Affected patients often present with **guttate lesions,** which are small papules 2–4 mm in size that suddenly appear on the central trunk with extension to the proximal and then distal extremities. Occasionally, 10–100 lesions may appear over several days.

Pathophysiology

Guttate psoriasis may follow a sore throat, particularly streptococcal pharyngitis, or a perianal streptococcal infection. More typical psoriasis can also occur in children, who have 1–20-cm erythematous plaques with overlying fine scale or thicker, silver-like scale. Often, children have genital involvement with dermatitis on the perineal area, inguinal folds, and labia or penis. Psoriasis is a condition associated with rapid proliferation of keratinocytes.

Management

Psoriasis can be a very difficult to treat and may require variation of therapy from time to time. Therapy often includes topical steroids, a topical tar preparation, a topical vitamin D analog (calcipotriene), or possibly ultraviolet light. For those patients who present with guttate lesions, evaluation for streptococcal disease may document a preceding infection. Often, therapy with antistreptococcal antibiotics may be beneficial as an adjunct to psoriasis therapy in these children.

PITYRIASIS ROSEA

Pityriasis rosea is a common condition of unclear etiology seen in children and adolescents. Children may present with an erythematous papule or plaque with scale. The lesion may resemble **psoriasis** or **tinea corporis** initially. Over 1–30 days, multiple new lesions may appear, usually on the central trunk. These lesions are often oval, with the long axis of the oval lesions parallel to the lines of skin stress. The configuration of these lesions on the back may result in a "pine tree" appearance (Figure 22.7). The lesions of pityriasis rosea often resolve in 6–10 weeks. If the lesions are symptomatic, a low-potency topical steroid or moisturizers may help relieve the pruritus.

URTICARIA

Urticarial lesions often present as individual lesions with a central **wheal** and a surrounding **flare** of erythema. These lesions can be seen with insect bites (**papular urticaria**) or associated with infection, drugs, food, cold, trauma, heat, or exercise. Often, the cause of urticaria is not identifiable, and the lesions will resolve over time. Individual lesions usually last several minutes to several hours, but episodes of recurring lesions may last for days to weeks. While investigating the cause of the urticaria, symptomatic therapy with oral antihistamines such as hydroxyzine or diphenhydramine may be useful.

PALPABLE PURPURA

Children who present with erythematous papules that do not totally lose their color when the overlying skin is stretched may have palpable purpura. These lesions are usually associated with bleeding from small vessels within the skin, usually caused by an inflammatory infiltrate injuring the vessels. A specific type of palpable purpura seen in children is called **Henoch-Schönlein purpura** (see Chapter 20). Purpura may also be associated with viral or bacterial infections. The presence of palpable purpura should alert the physician to the possibility of underlying severe disease and the need for more comprehensive evaluation.

VITILIGO

Occasionally, children may present with localized areas of total absence of pigment (Figure 22.8). In this condition the melanocytes are injured and absent from the area of the decreased pigment. Vitiligo is usually symmetrical, involving both arms, both legs, or both sides of the body. Affected areas do not tan and easily burn, even in darkly pigmented patients. The diagnosis is confirmed by sharp demarcation between areas where the pigment is normal. Vitiligo can be extremely difficult to treat, and response to therapy is often poor. Treatment options include potent topical steroids and ultraviolet therapy. The condition may result in major cosmetic deformity in darkly pigmented patients.

ALOPECIA AREATA

Alopecia areata, or acute hair loss, is often a very distressing condition for infants and children. Usually, complete hair regrowth eventually occurs in children, but a potential for long-term absence of hair or total body hair loss exists.

Alopecia areata is characterized by complete or almost complete hair loss in a local area, usually on the scalp (Figure 22.9). The lesions may be 1 cm or less in size or may involve all the hair on the entire body. Often, the lesion is noticed suddenly and may be identified to expand in involved surface area over time. **"Exclamation point"** hairs may occur at the periphery of the lesion; these tapered hairs become very thin at the skin site of hair growth. They eventually break off and fall out. Alopecia areata is usually not associated with scaling dermatitis of the scalp, but it does need to be identified and distinguished from **tinea capitis,** which usually manifests with broken-off hairs and dermatitis of the involved skin. Tinea capitis can be identified by a positive fungal culture of the involved area.

Spontaneous regrowth of hair occurs in 95% of cases. However, local treatment options include topical steroids, intralesional steroids, and allergic contact sensitization.

NEVI

Infants and children can be born with nevi **(congenital nevi)** or can develop nevi over time. Nevi are identified as brown to tan macules and papules that are sharply circumscribed. Recent data indicate that nevi appear to be sun induced. The number of nevi may be greater in children who experience more sun exposure during the first 10 years of life. Although malignant change is very uncommon in infants and children, the amount of sun exposure that children receive may increase their risk of developing **melanoma** as adults. Basic sun protection for infants, children, and adolescents may help prevent the development of skin cancer (Table 22.5). Education of children and parents about daily solar protection and sunscreen use is essential.

Nevi may develop on any area of the body but are most frequent on areas exposed to sun. Prior to and during puberty, many new lesions may evolve and old lesions may grow in elevation and width. Lesions that appear asymmetrical, have borders that are irregular, and have changing color or rapid changes in diameter are a greater concern. Although melanoma is uncommon in children, nevi that are undergoing changes may require evaluation over a period of time in order to identify the possibility of their being abnormal. Abnormal nevi should be biopsied to obtain a histologic diagnosis. If a melanoma develops, early excision of that melanoma may be curative. The longer and deeper the melanoma develops, the greater its risk of metastasis.

Pediatric Pearl

The ABCDs of skin cancer refer to the important clues to look for in a changing nevus: **a**symmetry (changes in shape), **b**orders (changes in edges), **c**olor (variation in color), and **d**iameter (> 6 mm).

INFECTIONS OF THE SKIN

BACTERIAL INFECTIONS

Infants and children are chronically exposed to minor cuts and injuries. Usually, these injuries heal without consequence and do not become infected. When infants do develop cutaneous infections, they are usually due to *S. aureus* or *Streptococcus pyogenes*. Superficial infections are called **impetigo,** and deeper-appearing lesions are known as **ecthyma.** These lesions may manifest as small fluid-filled vesicles that rupture easily or, more likely, as

---

TABLE 22.5 **Guidelines for Basic Sun Protection**

Keep infants < 6 months of age out of direct sunlight (sunscreen may be used on limited body surface areas that are not covered by clothing)
Use sunscreen with a minimum skin protection factor (SPF) of 15 for infants and children > 6 months of age with frequent reapplication every 2–4 hours
Wear protective clothing
Avoid sun exposure between 10 A.M. and 4 P.M.

---

erosions, which develop a honey-colored thick crust. The erosions occur on multiple sites of the skin distant to each other (Figure 22.10). Affected children sometimes have a prior history of injury or insect bite. Treatment is usually necessary with topical mupirocin or an oral antistaphylococcal antibiotic such as dicloxacillin, a first-generation cephalosporin, or erythromycin.

FUNGAL INFECTIONS

Fungal infections of the skin (**tinea corporis**) may appear as localized erythematous plaques with scale (Figure 22.11). Often, there is increased scale in the periphery of the lesion. Fungal infections of the scalp (**tinea capitis**) may develop as localized areas of dermatitis, usually with hair loss. Confirmation of the differential diagnosis of fungal infection of the skin necessitates scraping the periphery of the lesion and identifying hyphae in tissue partially dissolved in 10%–20% potassium hydroxide (KOH). Scalp infections usually require a culture to confirm the diagnosis. The best culture technique involves a brush, toothbrush, or swab rubbed against the skin and reapplied multiple times from the skin to the culture media.

Topical therapy with antifungal creams such as miconazole, clotrimazole, or terbinafine is usually effective for tinea corporis in children. Those infections involving the scalp require oral griseofulvin 10–20 mg/kg/day for a minimum of 6 weeks. It is necessary to follow children with scalp infections closely at 4–6-week intervals and treat them until cultures are negative. To maximize absorption of griseofulvin, children should take it with a meal that includes 4–8 ounces of fresh whole milk.

SCABIES

In infants and children, the infestation known as scabies often presents with increased irritability secondary to the severity of the pruritus. Older children and adults complain of pruritus, most marked on the hands and feet, although excoriations are frequently seen on other sites of the body. Often, several family members have pruritus and excoriations at the same time. The infestation is caused by the eight-legged mite *Sarcoptes scabiei*. The mite grows in the epidermis, where it lays its eggs.

Diagnosis

Confirmation of the diagnosis involves scraping the skin and finding the mite, which may be difficult, because infected patients may have only

10–20 mites. Often, only eggs or stool are apparent after scraping. It is important to check patients who have multiple family members with pruritus or individual patients who, on examination, have 2–10-mm linear burrows for scabies. Scraping involves lightly covering the site of the burrow as well as small papules with mineral oil and then using a number 15 blade scalpel for the actual scraping. The mite lives in the epidermis, and the upper layer of the epidermis is all that is necessary to obtain. In uncooperative infants and children, the potential for bleeding at the site of the scraping is real, and clinicians should warn parents about this. Occasionally, confirmation of the diagnosis may be possible by scraping lesions on a cooperative parent rather than an uncooperative child. The scraped skin is collected in a single mound on a slide and examined under magnification of 40–100x. Identification of the live mite, who may be moving about on the slide, or individual eggs or stool may be possible.

Management

Often, it is difficult to identify the mite's stool or eggs, and therapy is indicated when the diagnosis is suspected and multiple family members appear to be infested. Current recommended therapy is permethrin cream 5%. Application of the cream to the entire body from the neck down is necessary. Clinicians should be certain that the genital folds, the area between the toes and fingers, and the umbilical area are well treated. Often, therapy is applied at bedtime and washed off in the morning. Infants with involvement of their scalp and face require treatment of their entire body. It is essential to take care to prevent the topical therapy application from entering the eyes and causing irritation.

Pruritus may continue for several weeks after treatment because the mite and mite parts may still remain in the skin. The physician should reevaluate patients in 2–3 weeks to be certain that the therapy has effectively removed the infestation and that new lesions are not appearing. Because the mite can live as long as 3 days off the host, it is important to wash all bedding and recently worn clothing and not use them for at least 3 days. All family members and close household contacts should receive treatment at the same time, because family members may be infested and contagious, although they may not have symptoms. They can then reinfect the entire family, even after effective therapy of the symptomatic members.

HEAD LICE

The cause of head lice is the six-legged insect *Pediculosis capitis,* which lives in the scalp and usually passes from child to child. Often, the **nits** (lice eggs) are seen attached to the hair in the occipital regions. Under microscopic examination, the characteristic appearance of the nit can be confirmed. Occasionally, live lice are seen moving about the scalp. Usually, this is associated with pruritus, but many children are totally asymptomatic. All infested members of the family should be treated at the same time. Therapies for head lice include permethrin rinse 1% or malathion lotion 0.5%. Recently, there have been many reports of head lice that are resistant to common pediculicides.

VIRAL INFECTIONS (SEE CHAPTER 9, INFECTIOUS DISEASES)

Viral exanthems are commonly seen in children, who may present with fever and lymphadenopathy and then develop multiple erythematous macules and papules **(morbilliform eruption)** that involve the trunk, face, and extremities. However, often the eruptions are not diagnostic of a specific viral etiology, although in some cases, important clues obtained from the history and physical examination may be helpful in identifying a specific viral pathogen. When evaluating children for what appears to be a viral eruption, it is always necessary to obtain an adequate immunization history. **Measles** may be identified by its association with high fever, cough, rhinitis, and conjunctivitis. **Rubella (German measles)** is often less erythematous with faint, pink macules that appear first on the face and then spread to the proximal extremities. However, many other viruses may produce a similar eruption.

Varicella (chickenpox) has a more characteristic morphology. The lesions appear as tiny urticarial, edematous papules that rapidly become vesicles that often appear very translucent, as if they are a drop of water on the skin. The individual lesions rupture and become crusted while new lesions continue to evolve over a 5–7-day period. Often, lesions are apparent within the oral cavity and on the tongue. The advent of the varicella vaccine should mean that the incidence of the disease will decrease over time.

Herpes simplex may appear as grouped vesicles on an erythematous base, usually on the lip or face in children. The initial infection may be seen as multiple punched-out-appearing mouth ulcerations. Occasionally, herpes simplex lesions may occur on the hand or other body sites, where they

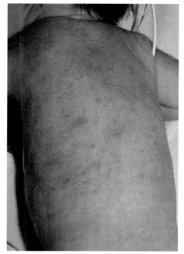

Figure 22.2

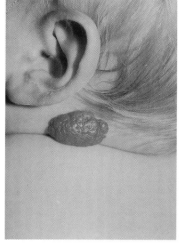

Figure 22.3

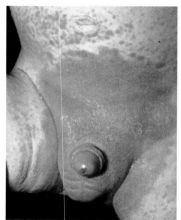

Figure 22.4

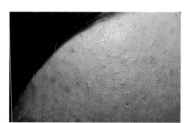

Figure 22.5

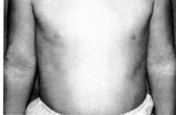

Figure 22.6

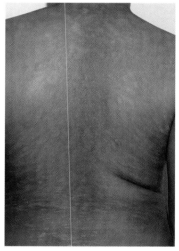

Figure 22.7

FIGURE 22.2 This 3-day-old healthy newborn has developed multiple erythematous macules and papules on the trunk, a classic sign of erythema toxicum.

FIGURE 22.3 This strawberry hemangioma is a proliferation of blood vessels that involute over time.

FIGURE 22.4 This infant has severe diaper dermatitis infected with *Candida albicans*. The periphery of the rash has multiple red papules and pustules that extend out of the area usually covered by the diaper.

FIGURE 22.5 Open and closed comedones, as well as inflammatory papules, are present on the forehead of an adolescent with acne vulgaris.

FIGURE 22.6 Atopic dermatitis is seen in this child as bilateral excoriations of the antecubital fossa with associated hypopigmentation.

FIGURE 22.7 The distribution of lesions in pityriasis rosea follows skin tension lines and resembles a pine tree in appearance.

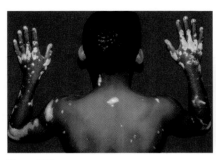
Figure 22.8

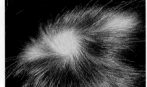
Figure 22.9

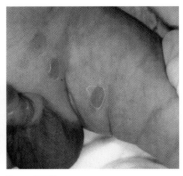
Figure 22.10

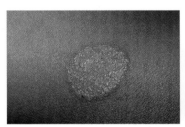
Figure 22.11

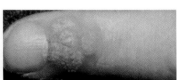
Figure 22.12

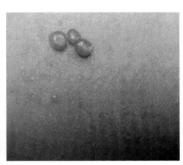
Figure 22.13

FIGURE 22.8 This child's vitiligo is somewhat symmetrical. It is very disfiguring and difficult to hide.

FIGURE 22.9 These three patches of alopecia without scale or erythema are an example of alopecia areata.

FIGURE 22.10 The bullous impetigo in the diaper area in this infant results from infection by *Staphylococcus aureus*. The stratum corneum has eroded centrally but remains on the edge, giving an appearance of a white collar around the lesion.

FIGURE 22.11 Patients with tinea corporis typically present with erythematous annular plaques with scale on the body.

FIGURE 22.12 The common wart at the end of this child's finger has a rough surface on a base of slightly inflamed skin. Note the grouping of several papules together.

FIGURE 22.13 Patients with molluscum contagiosum often present with groups of papules of different sizes. In this child, three papules of similar size are grouped together close to a much smaller, isolated papule.

may be extremely painful. It is possible to mistake them for a severe deep cellulitis. Presence of grouped vesicles on an erythematous base should prompt the examiner to be suspicious of herpes simplex or possibly of an allergic contact dermatitis. Therapy for the individual viral eruptions is dependent on the specific eruption and the stage of the eruption when the diagnosis is made.

Warts are common infections caused by the **human papilloma virus** (HPV) [Figure 22.12]. Different types of HPV are associated with different infections on different body sites. Therapy for the individual warts is dependent on body site location. Most warts eventually resolve over a 2–3-year period. Treatment usually involves trying to destroy infected tissue while limiting the damage to surrounding normal-appearing tissue. Therapy may be difficult and may require multiple attempts. Treatment methods include cryotherapy with liquid nitrogen, topical salicylic acid preparations, cantharidin, or immunotherapy.

Molluscum contagiosum presents as skin-colored dome-shaped papules that may have a central depressed area, giving the appearance of **umbilication** (Figure 22.13). This usually a benign condition is caused by a pox virus. The lesions are often different sizes ranging from 0.5 to 8 mm. These lesions can be sexually transmitted in adolescents and adults but are usually non-sexually transmitted in infants and children. Occasionally, the skin surrounding the lesions may show marked erythema and scaling. Treatment of the lesions consists of physical destruction of the overlying skin or removal of the lesions. This involves a sharp curette, and in young children, such a procedure may be painful and cause great resistance. Cure is often difficult; treatment of these lesions does not guarantee removal, because many lesions may recur. Over months to years, these lesions eventually resolve.

DRUG ERUPTIONS

Drug eruptions often appear as urticarial papules and areas of erythematous macules or large patches. The lesions may be pruritic. The onset of drug eruptions is usually between 3 and 14 days after the initial exposure to the drug. Antibiotics and antiseizure medications are common causes of drug eruptions in infants and children.

Occasionally, drug eruptions can be severe and associated with **exfoliation** of large areas of skin **(Stevens-Johnson syndrome)**. This exfoliation can also involve the mucous membranes, conjunctiva, and possibly the trachea. It is often difficult to separate a drug eruption from the eruption associated with a viral or bacterial infection.

SUGGESTED READINGS

American Academy of Pediatrics Committee on Environmental Health: Ultraviolet light: A hazard to children. *Pediatrics* 104:328–333, 1999.

Bakos L, Brito AC, Castro LC, et al: Open clinical study of the efficacy and safety of terbinafine cream 1% in children with tinea corporis and tinea cruris. *Pediatr Infect Dis J* 16:545–548, 1997.

Boiko S: Making rash decisions in the diaper area. *Pediatr Ann* 29(1):50–56, 2000.

Drolet BA, Esterly NG, Frieden IJ: Hemangiomas in children. *N Engl J Med* 341:173–181, 1999.

Eichenfield LF, Colon-Fontanez F: Treatment of head lice. *Pediatr Infect Dis J* 17(5):419–420, 1998.

Frieden IJ, Eichenfield LF, Esterly NB, et al: Guidelines of care for hemangiomas of infancy. American Academy of Dermatology Guidelines/Outcomes Committee. *J Am Acad Dermatol* 37:631–637, 1997.

Hartley AH: Pityriasis rosea. *Pediatr Rev* 1999;20(8):266–269.

Herbst RA, Hoch O, Kapp A, et al: Guttate psoriasis triggered by perianal streptococcal dermatitis in a 4-year-old boy. *J Am Acad Dermatol* 2000;42:885–887.

Hurwitz S: *Clinical Pediatric Dermatology*, 2nd ed. Philadelphia, WB Saunders, 1993.

Kazaks EL, Lane AT: Diaper dermatitis. *Pediatr Clin North Am* 47(4):909–919, 2000.

Knoell KA, Greer KE: Atopic dermatitis. *Pediatr Rev* 20(2):46–51, 1999.

Lookingbill DP, Marks JG: *Principles of Dermatology*, 2nd ed. Philadelphia, WB Saunders, 2000.

Nghiem P, Pearson G, Langley RG: Tacrolimus and pimecrolimus: From clever prokaryotes to inhibiting calcineurin and treating atopic dermatitis. *J Am Acad Dermatol* 46:228–241, 2002.

Pickering LK (ed): *2000 Red Book: Report of the Committee on Infectious Diseases*, 25th ed. Elk Grove Village, IL, American Academy of Pediatrics, 2000.

Raimer SS: New and emerging therapies in pediatric dermatology. *Dermatol Clin* 18(1):73–78,2000.

Resnick SD: Principles of topical therapy. *Pediatr Ann* 27(3):171–176, 1998.

Sidbury R, Paller AS: The diagnosis and management of acne. *Pediatr Ann* 29(1):17–24, 2000.

Silverberg NB, Lim JK, Paller AS, et al: Squaric acid immunotherapy for warts in children. *J Am Acad Dermatol* 42:803–808, 2000.

Silverberg NB, Sidbury R, Mancini AJ: Childhood molluscum contagiosum: Experience with cantharidin therapy in 300 patients. *J Am Acad Dermatol* 43:503–507, 2000.

Suarez S, Friedlander SF: Antifungal therapy in children: An update. *Pediatr Ann* 27(3):177–184, 1998.

Weston WL, Lane AT, Morelli JG: *Color Textbook of Pediatric Dermatology*, 3rd ed. St Louis, Mosby-Year Book, 2002.

Chapter 23

Trauma, Ingestions, and Burns

Jeffrey R. Avner and Young-Jin Sue

TRAUMA AND SHOCK

Trauma is the leading cause of death in children older than 1 year of age in the United States. Every year, almost 22 million children are injured, resulting in 13 million emergency department visits, 18,000 deaths, and more than $457 billion in health-related costs. Almost 50% of these injuries are the result of motor vehicle accidents; other major causes are drownings, fires, burns, and firearms. Blunt trauma, as opposed to penetrating trauma, is the predominant mechanism for the majority of injuries in children. However, the rate of penetrating trauma is increasing, especially in the inner cities. This section deals with the management of major trauma. It is important to realize that the best approach to trauma involves prevention. Prevention of unintentional injuries should be the primary goal of clinicians. To this end, pediatricians have made major strides by supporting regulations involving mandatory infant car seats, bicycle helmets, and fencing around pools.

Pathophysiology

The principles of trauma care are the same in all patients, but there are important anatomic and physiologic differences between children and adults. Children have a much greater total body surface area per weight and relatively less subcutaneous fat than adults, and stress to the body at the time of the trauma or undressing during the resuscitation can lead to increased evaporative losses and hypothermia. The resultant pathophysiologic cascade then increases peripheral vasoconstriction and causes metabolic acidosis and shock. Remember that children have a high metabolic rate with an oxygen consumption almost twice that of adults. Thus, even small physiologic changes can lead to significant effects.

In injured children, shock is primarily hypovolemic. (See DIFFERENTIAL DIAGNOSIS for a discussion of the types of shock.) Both blunt and penetrating trauma may cause lacerations of internal organs or extremities, which may account for a significant amount of acute blood loss. Injuries to the liver, spleen, pelvis, or femur can result in loss of 20%–40% of the circulating blood volume within an hour. There, it is imperative that the physician understands how children respond to such a blood loss. The early physiologic changes in response to hypovolemia are subtle. At first, blood loss leads to tachycardia as the body attempts to maintain cardiac output and thereby preserve organ perfusion. As the blood loss increases, children exhibit evidence of increased tachycardia, slowed capillary refill, lethargy or confusion, and decreased urinary output.

Pediatric Pearl

The ability of the child to maintain cardiac output is quite impressive. Only when acute blood loss approaches 30%–40% does blood pressure fall. Therefore, the physician should not rely solely on a child's blood pressure when evaluating the degree of blood loss.

Unique anatomic characteristics of children's shape and skeleton affect the type and severity of injuries. Children have a small oral cavity, a relatively large tongue, and a larynx that is more cephalad and anterior than that of adults. These factors, combined with lower respiratory reserve, often cause early respiratory compromise leading to hypoxia and hypercarbia. The head of children is also relatively large, especially in infancy, when it accounts for over 15% of the total body surface area. Therefore, the head is particularly vulnerable and bears the brunt of injury in blunt trauma. In fact, severe head injury occurs in 80%–90% of fatal pediatric trauma from motor vehicle crashes.

In addition, the skeleton of children is particularly compliant and very resilient. Because the chest wall is elastic, blunt chest trauma may cause serious lung injury in the absence of rib fractures. The liver and spleen are also poorly protected, and there is sparse perinephric fat surrounding the kidneys. Thus, children are predisposed to significant internal injury, regardless of the amount of external signs of trauma.

Clinical and Laboratory Evaluation

History
The history should be concise and should focus on the mechanism of the injury and the surrounding events. The paramedics or emergency medical technicians called to the scene report a child's initial vital signs, state of consciousness, any procedures they perform (e.g., intravenous line placement), and medications given. The timing of the injury, the timing of ancillary personnel arriving on the scene, and the timing of arrival of the patient to the emergency department are also important to estimate the amount of blood loss and the extent of injury. Past medical history should include current medical illnesses, current medications, allergies, and immunization status.

Physical Examination
The physical examination is closely tied to management. Trauma evaluation and management involve a "primary survey," the so- called ABCs of acute care stabilization and assessment (Table 23.1), for immediate life-threatening conditions, followed by a "secondary survey" for other types of injuries.

The primary survey begins with stabilization of the cervical spine in a hard collar and assessment of the **airway (A)** for signs of upper airway obstruction (e.g., stridor, gasping, no respirations). Inspection of the neck for jugular venous distention, tracheal deviation, or subcutaneous emphysema is part of airway management. The next step is auscultation of **breath sounds (B)** to check if they are present, and if so, evaluation of their quality and symmetry. Assessment of **circulation (C)** involves palpating the presence and quality of peripheral and femoral pulses and estimating peripheral perfusion with capillary refill time (normal: < 2 seconds). A quick neurologic examination to check for **disability (D)** is based on whether the child is awake, responds to verbal or painful stimulus, or is unresponsive. **Exposure (E)** involves complete undress of the child to check for other injuries. The primary survey should take less than 1 minute to perform.

The secondary survey includes a comprehensive physical examination from head to toe to identify all other injuries. It is important that this examination be orderly and include a rectal examination to determine the anal sphincter tone and the presence of occult blood. To assess the child's back and buttocks, it is necessary to "roll" the child to the side. This procedure usually requires two or three people to keep the child's neck in a neutral position; one person maintains

---

TABLE 23.1 Immediate Management of the Injured Child (ABCs)

Airway and cervical spine ("C" spine)
    Protect neck with rigid cervical collar
    Assess for airway obstruction
        Chin lift/Jaw thrust maneuver, if needed
        Prepare for endotracheal intubation, if needed
Breathing
    Administer 100% oxygen
    Place on continuous pulse oximetry monitoring
    Assess for quality and asymmetry of breath sounds
    Assess for work of breathing
Circulation
    Attach cardiac monitor leads
    Obtain intravenous access with two large-bore catheters
    Assess for signs of peripheral perfusion (pulses, capillary refill)
    Control hemorrhage
Disability
    Brief neurologic examination
    Level of consciousness (AVPU; **A**lert, responds to **V**erbal commands, responds to **P**ain, **U**nresponsive)
    Pupillary size and response to light
Exposure
    Completely undress child

the head and neck in line with the body while the others roll and inspect for injury.

Laboratory Evaluation

What laboratory studies are performed depends on several factors, including the mechanism of the trauma, the ability to assess the child, and the nature of the injuries. Radiographic studies (cervical spine, chest, and pelvic radiographs) and blood tests [complete blood count (CBC), spun hematocrit, type and cross- match, arterial blood gas] are warranted in children with multiple injuries. A urinalysis looking for hematuria may identify a urinary tract injury. Additional studies such as computed tomography (CT) scanning of the head or abdomen may be obtained after the resuscitation and reevaluation.

Differential Diagnosis

Children with major trauma are often in shock. Therefore, the physician must be able to recognize shock and identify its cause.

Hypovolemic Shock

The majority of children with major trauma present with some degree of hypovolemia. Deep or multiple lacerations, amputations, and obvious fractures are clear causes of the blood loss. However, it is essential to be acutely aware of occult injuries, especially in children who do not respond to initial fluid therapy. A large amount of unrecognized bleeding may accompany fractures of the pelvis or femur. Despite a seemingly soft, non-tender abdomen, severe intra-abdominal injuries such as lacerations or rupture of the liver or spleen may be present. In addition, young infants with head trauma can become hypotensive from blood loss into an epidural or subdural hematoma.

Estimates of the degree of hypovolemia due to the acute loss of blood often make use of several clinical parameters. With acute blood loss of up to 15% of the total blood volume, there is little if any change in the pulse, blood pressure, respiratory rate, mental status, or urinary output. However, as the blood loss exceeds 15%, the heart rate and respiratory rate begin to rise, and children become more anxious. The decline in blood pressure and noticeable decline in urine output does not become apparent until about 30%–40% of the blood volume is lost. This is a crucial point for management; blood pressure changes are a late finding in hypovolemic shock, whereas tachycardia and tachypnea occur earlier.

Obstructive Shock

Obstructive shock occurs when there is restriction of blood flow either to or from the heart. Children with severe injuries to the chest wall or penetrating chest wounds may have **pericardial tamponade,** which may lead to obstructive shock. Failing vital signs are associated with tachypnea, clear and equal breath sounds, neck vein distention, and distant heart sounds. Other causes of obstructive shock include **tension pneumothorax, flail chest, and hemothorax or pneumothorax.**

Cardiogenic Shock

Cardiogenic shock resulting from a **myocardial contusion or arrhythmia** may follow a direct, powerful blow to the sternum. In children, this may occur as an isolated injury (e.g., when a Little League player is hit in the chest with a fastball). Rapid deceleration injury can be seen with motor vehicle accidents. Fortunately, the hearts of children have a great degree of compliance and resiliency, so that myocardial infarctions and tearing of major vessels are rare.

Neurogenic Shock

A spinal cord injury may result in the loss of tone of the blood vessels with accumulation of fluid in the peripheral circulation. Thus, the classic picture of neurogenic shock is hypovolemia without tachycardia. The absence of tachycardia differentiates neurogenic shock from the more common hypovolemic shock. Concurrent chest or abdominal trauma is often present in neurogenic shock.

Septic Shock

Septic shock is uncommon in acutely injured children. However, children who are evaluated a long time after their injury or those who have penetrating abdominal injury are at risk for the development of sepsis. In isolated septic shock, tachycardia and normal or slightly decreased blood pressure occurs. Peripheral perfusion may be increased, leading to warm pink skin (warm shock, or decreased, leading to cool, clammy skin.

Management

In most cases, emergency medical workers notify the emergency department that they are transporting an injured child from the scene of the trauma to the hospital. At this time, the trauma team (pediatrician, emergency department physicians, surgeons, nurses, radiology technician) is assembled. The leader of the trauma resuscitation team is usually the trauma surgeon or the emergency department physician. It should be noted that optimal management of pediatric trauma involves a pediatrician, preferably a pediatric emergency medicine physician. The pediatrician should ensure that the unique characteristics of a child's anatomy and physiology are addressed.

The initial management of children with multiple trauma begins in conjunction with the primary survey [see Table 23.1]. Management proceeds in the standard sequence of the ABCs [**A**irway and cervical spine immobilization, **B**reathing, **C**irculation, **D**isability (neurologic), and **E**xposure]. Immediate correction of any abnormality noted during the primary survey is necessary.

It is necessary to immobilize the cervical spine in a rigid collar, if prehospital care providers have not already performed this. A clinician should talk to the child and see whether he can talk, hear, and understand. This clinician–patient interaction helps assess airway patency and central nervous system (CNS) function. If there is difficulty maintaining a patent airway, a chin-lift and jaw-thrust maneuver are necessary; these measures should help move the mandibular block of tissue forward and away from obstructing the airway. If these simple maneuvers are not effective, manual bag–valve–mask ventilation or endotracheal intubation may be warranted.

If there are signs of inadequate breathing, it is essential to look for evidence of a tension pneumothorax (asymmetric breath sounds, hyperresonant percussion note, tracheal deviation). To relieve a tension pneumothorax , a physician should insert a 16-gauge needle above the third rib into the second intercostal space in the midclavicular line.

To secure vascular access, it is necessary to insert two large-bore intravenous lines peripherally (usually in the antecubital fossa) or centrally (femoral vein). These large intravenous lines are essential because the hypovolemia is often profound. If immediate intravenous access is not secured in a young child, an intraosseous line can be used. Placement of an intraosseous line involves insertion of a 14- or 16-gauge intraosseous needle (e.g., bone marrow needle or any other large-bore needle with a stylet) into the flat surface of the anterior, proximal tibia, angling slightly away from the growth plate. Rapid fluid resuscitation requires administration of Ringer's lactate or normal saline in repeated increments of 20 ml/kg until adequate perfusion is restored. If blood loss continues or there is no response to the fluid boluses, rapid infusion of type-specific packed red blood cells (RBCs) is necessary. Control of any obvious source of bleeding entails the use of direct pressure or pneumatic splints.

A rapid neurologic assessment should include pupillary size and response to light, as well as a score on the Glasgow Coma Scale (Table 23.2). A score of 8 or less may be a sign of intracranial hypertension. In that case, it is important to elevate the head to 30° and implement hyperventilation in an attempt to reduce the intracranial pressure.

It is necessary to undress the child and perform a complete, detailed physical examination, including the buttocks and back. At this time, a Foley catheter is placed unless there is evidence of urethral disruption (blood at the urethral meatus or a scrotal hematoma). Certain management options are warranted in life- threatening conditions (Table 23.3). Further treatment is based on the specific injuries identified in the secondary survey.

During this first stage of trauma management, the physician should immediately consult appropriate specialists based on the child's most serious injuries. Specialists involved in the care of the injured child often include neurosurgeons, orthopedic surgeons, anesthesiologists, and radiologists. Because specialists usually focus on their area of expertise, the pediatrician must coordinate these services. In addition, the pediatrician should provide counseling to the parents, addressing their concerns and keeping them informed of further plans for the child.

TABLE 23.2 Glasgow Coma Scale*

Physical Feature	Score
Eyes	
Open spontaneously	4
Open to speech	3
Open to pain	2
No response	1
Best verbal response	
Oriented (coos and babbles)	5
Confused (irritable cries)	4
Inappropriate words (cries to pain)	3
Incomprehensible sounds (moans to pain)	2
No response	1
Best motor response	
Obeys (normal spontaneous movements)	6
Localizes (withdraws to touch)	5
Withdraws (withdraws to pain)	4
Abnormal flexion	3
Abnormal extension	2
No response	1
TOTAL SCORE†	3–15

*Parentheses indicate findings in preverbal children.
†Total score is sum of three parts.

TABLE 23.3	Management Options for Life-Threatening Conditions	
Finding	**Problem**	**Management**
Noisy breathing Stridor	Upper airway obstruction	Chin lift/jaw thrust Intubation
Neck pain or tenderness Head trauma Multiple trauma	Possible cervical spine fracture	Immobilize neck (hard collar) Lateral cervical spine radiograph
Asymmetric breath sounds and hyperresonant percussion note	Possible tension pneumothorax	Insert 16-gauge needle into second intercostal space in midclavicular line
Penetrating chest wound	Possible sucking chest wound	Loosely apply occlusive dressing Insert chest tube
Penetrating chest wound with muffled heart sounds or distended neck veins	Possible cardiac tamponade	Pericardiocentesis
Paradoxical chest wall movement	Flail chest	Positive pressure ventilation for respiratory distress

Orthostasis; pale, cool skin	Hypotension or shock	Establish two large-bore IV lines
		Give crystalloid boluses 20 ml/kg
		Transfusion
		    Emergent: type O, Rh-negative
		    Urgent: type-specific

IV = intravenous.

HEAD TRAUMA

Head trauma, a major cause of morbidity and mortality in children, accounts for 70%–80% of childhood deaths from trauma. Head trauma is very common, but fortunately, most cases are minor and do not require hospitalization. As with other types of trauma, prevention remains the best method to reduce the effects of these injuries. To this end, the enactment of legislative policies (national speed limit, mandatory child restraints, bicycle helmets) in recent decades have led to a decrease in the incidence of accidents that may cause head trauma.

Pathophysiology

At the exact moment of head trauma, there is direct impact of the brain against the skull, causing neuronal damage. Depending on the mechanism involved, this "primary injury" may cause cerebral contusion, laceration, hematoma, diffuse axonal injury, or diffuse brain swelling. The transient brain dysfunction that accompanies such injury may be associated with disruption of normal respiration and circulation. Nothing can change the immediate effects of the primary injury, because the damage occurs on impact.

Management of head trauma is centered on prevention of the "secondary injury" caused by the hypoxia, ischemia, and mechanical distortion that the primary injury sets in motion. Neuronal damage affects the autoregulation of cerebral blood flow and can lead to ischemic brain injury. At first, diffuse brain swelling causes displacement of cerebral buffering mechanisms (spinal fluid and vascular spaces) in an attempt to preserve the intracranial pressure. However, as the swelling increases, the intracranial pressure necessarily rises and causes further ischemia and hypoxia. If uncorrected, secondary brain injury leads to irreversible brain damage or death.

Clinical and Laboratory Evaluation

History
It is always important to ascertain the time and mechanism of injury as well as the initial manifestations at the scene of the event. The clinician should ask about the occurrence of loss of consciousness, seizures, vomiting, headache, and dizziness.

Physical Examination
To look for other injuries, the physician should perform a detailed neurologic examination as well as a complete physical examination. Signs of increased intracranial pressure include hypertension, abnormal respirations, irritability, visual change, papilledema, cranial nerve palsies,

and posturing. It is important to palpate the head and neck for hematoma, depression, and tenderness. Hemotympanum and clear rhinorrhea are signs of basilar skull fracture. Check the pupils for asymmetry, size, and reaction to light and record an initial score on the Glasgow Coma Scale (see Table 23.2). Unexplained skin bruising or retinal hemorrhages on funduscopic examination suggest child abuse.

Laboratory Evaluation

The need for blood tests is based on the severity of injury. If the injury appears minor and the child is awake and responsive with normal vital signs, no blood tests are necessary.

Skull films are rarely helpful because they are not predictive of intracranial injury, and most skull fractures do not require treatment. Indications for skull radiographs include a penetrating injury or suspicion of a depressed skull fracture.

CT scanning is the best method to look for the presence of intracranial injury. A CT scan is indicated for prolonged loss of consciousness (> 15 minutes), seizures, abnormal neurologic examination, abnormal mental status, or significant associated injury requiring an operation.

Differential Diagnosis

Usually, it is apparent from the history or the physical examination that a child has suffered head trauma. However, the physician should always consider head trauma in the differential diagnosis if there is a change in mental status or an altered level of consciousness. Children with significant head trauma from child abuse may present with only a history of apnea, cyanosis, poor feeding, or lethargy.

- A **concussion,** the most frequent type of head injury, is an immediate, transient interruption of normal neurologic function. Affected children often experience a period of loss of consciousness and may have posttraumatic amnesia.
- A **cerebral contusion** is an area of focal hemorrhage in the brain. This injury may occur at the point of impact between the brain and the skull or at the site directly opposite the impact (coup and contrecoup injury). There is often associated concussion.
- An **epidural hematoma** is a collection of blood just outside the dura. There is arterial bleeding, usually from a tear of the middle meningeal artery. The classic presentation is concussion, followed by a "lucid interval" when the child appears well, and then neurologic deterioration. However, no lucid interval or period of loss of consciousness is apparent in many cases.

- A **subdural hematoma** is a collection of blood just beneath the dura. This occurs as the result of tearing of the dural sinuses or bridging veins. The presenting symptoms may range from nonspecific neurologic findings to coma.

Pediatric Pearl

Unlike epidural hematoma, the mechanism that causes a subdural hematoma usually also results in underlying brain injury. This explains why subdural hematomas carry a worse prognosis than epidural hematomas.

Management

As with any trauma, management begins with stabilization of the cervical spine, airway, breathing, and circulation. If abnormal respirations, loss of protective airway reflexes, or signs of increased intracranial pressure (Glasgow coma score of < 8) are present, then endotracheal intubation followed by manual hyperventilation is warranted. Because endotracheal intubation is difficult and necessitates adequate sedation and muscle relaxation, only experienced personnel should perform it. If hypovolemia is present, Ringer's lactate or normal saline solution should be given in boluses of 20 ml/kg. Because cerebral perfusion pressure depends on the mean arterial pressure, restoration of the intravascular space is essential. Once euvolemia has been achieved, then fluid restriction to limit cerebral edema can begin. Immediate neurosurgical consultation is necessary. The head should be elevated to 30° and placed midline so there is no obstruction to venous outflow from the head. Increased intracranial pressure, if present, necessitates aggressive management (see Chapters 19 and 24).

In general, it is helpful to classify children into three categories based on their initial manifestations, Glasgow coma score, and the mechanism of injury. Children with **low-risk injuries** are asymptomatic with a normal neurologic examination. Management at home with observation by a parent is sufficient. Children with **moderate-risk injuries** have a history of altered consciousness, progressive headache, persistent vomiting, seizures, amnesia, or an associated injury. Neurosurgical consultation and a CT scan are warranted. The duration of observation in the emergency department and the need for hospitalization depend on the resolution or progression of symptoms. Children with **high-risk injuries** present with a depressed level of consciousness, focal neurologic examination, signs of increased intracranial pressure, or penetrating injury. Emergent management and neurosurgical consultation are necessary. Children with epidural hematomas and penetrating injuries require immediate operative intervention. Young patients with other severe injuries may require placement of intracranial pressure monitors.

Abuse should be suspected in infants with subdural hematomas or cerebral injury out of proportion to the degree of trauma sustained (see Chapter 24). In "shaken baby syndrome," rapid acceleration–deceleration injuries cause diffuse shearing of the gray and white matter, leading to diffuse cerebral edema. Retinal hemorrhages are often seen in the fundus of these children. Unfortunately, prognosis for this type of injury is very poor.

MINOR TRAUMA

This section concentrates on the management of **lacerations, abrasions, and puncture wounds,** which represent approximately 35% of all injuries seen in a pediatric emergency department. These injuries are common in the summer months when children spend more time engaging in outdoor activities such as bicycling, baseball, and basketball. As with other types of injuries, toddlers are at high risk because they often lack the experience and motor coordination of older children. Most lacerations occur on the face, mouth, and scalp; the head of children represents a large part of the total body surface area and is, therefore, easily subject to injury.

Pathophysiology

Two types of lacerations—those caused by glass and those caused by animal bites—deserve special consideration, because they are more common in children than adults. Injuries involving glass are responsible for as many as 20% of lacerations. Because these lacerations are caused by very sharp edges, the wounds tend to be deep and are often associated with injuries to nerves and tendons. In addition, many of these wounds contain fragments of glass, which, if undetected, may cause delayed healing, increased scarring, neurapraxia, and increased risk of infection.

Mammalian bites are another common source of injury in children. According to estimates, dog bites account for almost 90% of bite injuries, cats bites 5%, and human bites 3%. There are distinct differences in the type of injuries caused by dogs and cats. **Dog bites** can be very powerful, generating 150–450 pounds per square inch of pressure.

They cause lacerations, avulsions, and crush injury to soft tissue. Although **cat bites** are less forceful, they usually result in deep puncture wounds, because cats have very sharp teeth. Deep puncture wounds are associated with a high inoculum of bacteria into a small space, making irrigation and debridement difficult. Therefore, the infection rate is 20%–50% for cat bites compared with 5% for dog bites. The organisms responsible for infection also vary with the type of bite. Although *Staphylococcus aureus* and streptococcal bacteria are common in all bites, dog and cat bites often carry *Pasteurella multocida,* and human bites carry *Eikenella corrodens.*

Clinical and Laboratory Evaluation

History

The history should include when and where the injury occurred and the mechanism involved. (In wounds that are less than 12 hours old, primary closure is appropriate and does not increase the risk of infection.) The clinician should ask whether fragments of glass were present (e.g., with falls onto a shattered glass bottle). For bite wounds, it is important to identify the animal involved so that the risk of **rabies** can be better ascertained. Past medical history should include the child's immunization status and whether the child has allergies to antibiotics or local anesthetics.

With a **"closed fist injury,"** it is often difficult to obtain the correct history. This injury usually occurs when an adolescent punches someone in the mouth and sustains a small laceration over the metacarpophalangeal joint. The adolescent may not want to reveal that she was in a fight and often does not seek immediate attention. This injury can force a high inoculum of virulent oral bacterium deep into the fascial planes of the hand and is associated with a high risk of infection. The patient then presents 2 or 3 days after the injury with a serious hand infection. Thus, the presence of a laceration over the metacarpophalangeal joint in an adolescent should lead to the assumption of a closed fist injury.

Physical Examination

It is important to document the wound size, depth, and location by using pictures or diagrams if necessary; record whether the bottom of the wound is visible and whether glass or other foreign material is present in the wound. The physician should check the sensation, vascular supply, and motor function distal to the injury, as well as carefully inspect the wound and identify any nerve, muscle, tendon, or vascular injury. It is also necessary to perform a complete physical examination to look for other lacerations or trauma away from the site of the injury.

Laboratory Evaluation

Unless there is an unusual amount of blood loss or a history of a bleeding disorder, no blood tests are necessary. A radiograph of the involved area is warranted if there might be an associated fracture or if the wound was caused by glass. Most glass in use today is radiopaque, so a radiograph may show a retained glass fragment not seen on visual inspection of the wound.

Differential Diagnosis

Usually, the diagnosis of a laceration is evident, and the mechanism and causative agent are readily obtained. However, if the injury is not compatible with the history or the developmental age of the child, the physician should be concerned about the possibility of child abuse.

Management

It is necessary to clean all wounds of obvious debris and clotted blood by gentle washing or soaking in saline solution. With wounds less than 12 hours old and facial wounds less than 18 hours old, primary closure is allowable. The shaving of a small amount of hair from the surrounding area may be appropriate, but it is important to **leave eyebrows intact.** A dilute povidone solution is used to clean the area around the wound. The infiltration of 1% lidocaine usually provides local anesthesia. The physician should be aware that the **maximum dose of lidocaine is 4 mg/kg.** For better hemostasis, a combination of lidocaine with epinephrine may be used, **except when suturing end organs such as the fingers, ears, or nose.**

Pediatric Pearl

In an effort to reduce a child's pain, anxiety, and fear of needles, which is often associated with laceration repair, topical anesthesia may sometimes replace a lidocaine injection. A solution such as lidocaine–epinephrine–tetracaine (LET) applied directly to the wound via a solution-soaked gauze for 15–20 minutes may be effective.

Additional washing of the wound and irrigation with at least 200 ml normal saline, which should involve high-pressure irrigation with a sy-

ringe and a 20-gauge catheter, is appropriate. The clinician should extract any visible foreign body, excise necrotic skin, and debride free subcutaneous tissue. Exploration and repair of deep structures, if necessary, should occur. Deep lacerations require subcutaneous sutures (absorbable) to better oppose the skin. The clinician everts the skin edges and approximates them using the smallest nonabsorbable sutures that will do the job. **Staples,** which can be applied quickly, have a lower rate of tissue reactivity compared to sutures but do not allow as meticulous a closure. They are particularly useful for wound closure in noncosmetic areas (e.g., scalp, extremities) or in children with multiple trauma, when speed of repair is essential. Application of a sterile dressing completes the treatment process. Follow-up arrangement should be made for removal of nonabsorbable sutures.

Recently, tissue adhesives such as the glue-like substances cyanoacrylates have become a popular method for faster wound closure with less need for sedation and local anesthesia. Wound closure involves approximation of the wound edges with fingers or forceps and painting the tissue adhesive over the apposed wound edges; it is necessary to hold these together for 30 seconds to allow complete polymerization of the glue. There is no need for a dressing; the adhesive sloughs off in 7–10 days. Lacerations of toddlers' foreheads or chins are particularly amenable to this type of repair.

Vigorous soaking and irrigation of abrasions is necessary, because embedded debris is often present. A thin layer of antibiotic ointment and a sterile dressing are necessary.

High-risk wounds (Table 23.4) require consultation with a plastic surgeon. Because of the high risk of infection, primary closure of these wounds should be avoided unless a cosmetically important area is involved. **Prophylactic antibiotics** are necessary for wounds more than 18 hours old and for **all animal and human bites.** However, it is important to realize that **antibiotics are no substitute for thorough wound cleaning and judicious debridement.**

TABLE 23.4 **Wounds at High Risk for Infection**
Cat bites
Human bites
Hand wounds
Puncture wounds
Wounds more than 18 hours old
Wounds in an immunosuppressed child

Elevation of the injured area is required, and a splint may be necessary. Tetanus prophylaxis is based on the child's immunization status. For animal bites, the local health department can give advice regarding the need for rabies prophylaxis. Close follow-up is the rule for all children.

CARE OF TOXIC INGESTIONS AND FOREIGN BODIES

Toxic exposures are encountered frequently in children, in both exploring toddlers and experimenting adolescents. Successful management of poisonings requires a basic knowledge of toxicologic principles. Medical toxicology, the study of pathologic effects of exogenous substances on human physiology, is fundamental to the practice of therapeutic medicine, and a solid grounding in its principles is advantageous to the practitioner of any medical specialty. In addition, persistent history seeking, a meticulous physical examination, a few key diagnostics, and investigative curiosity are indispensable tools for the evaluation of poisoned children.

Pathophysiology

Pediatric poisonings fall into two important groups, which require distinctly different management approaches. **Accidental poisoning** occurs, for the most part, in **younger children** who have been left momentarily undersupervised. Usually, only **single agents** are ingested and, even then, in clinically **unimportant quantities.** Although the child's ability to communicate or the deductive abilities of adult witnesses may restrict the historical details, they are usually not purposeful attempts on the part of patients to mislead examiners.

In contrast, **intentional poisoning** largely occurs in **adolescents and adults**. Toxic substances may be used for recreational purposes or taken in overdose with the intent of self-harm. Often, **multiple substances** are involved in **significant quantities**. Consequently, these patients are at high risk for serious illness. For any of several reasons (e.g., avoidance of legal consequences, fear of parental reaction, seriousness of suicidal intent), patients may be unwilling to volunteer truthful information regarding the ingestion. Therefore, in the setting of an intentional poisoning, the examiner should be wary of potential inaccuracies in the patient's history.

The task of evaluating poisoned patients is simplified if the toxin can be determined with certainty. However, patients may be unable or unwilling to identify the toxic agent or agents, especially in the case of intentional overdose. In the latter case, the clinical skills of the examining physician are put to the test. Greater reliance is placed on the physical examination and diagnostic measures to offer critical clues to the identification of the toxin or toxins. In the absence of essential information, it is often necessary to prepare for the worst and enforce a period of observation.

Pediatric Pearl

If poisonings are intentional or occur in adolescents, the "worst case scenario" should be the basis of initial management, and selected standard diagnostic measures are warranted.

Clinical and Laboratory Evaluation

History

The primary goal when obtaining the history is to confirm that an ingestion has occurred and to determine the potential seriousness of the poisoning. Key questions in evaluating a poisoning are:

- What is the poison?
- When or over what period of time did the poisoning occur?
- How much poison was involved?
- By what route did the poisoning occur?
- Was the poisoning accidental or intentional?

One or more routes may result in poisoning. The most common is gut absorption following ingestion. Other routes of toxin absorption include inhalation, injection, and topical exposure. In children in particular, the dose of the toxin per body weight is often necessary for determination of the seriousness of the ingestion.

Occasionally, a patient comes to medical attention with signs and symptoms of an illness without a clear cause. Factors consistent with toxicologic causation include acute onset of illness, history of pica or previous ingestion, history of environmental stress or depression, past overdose attempts, at-risk age group (toddlers, adolescents), and a story that "just doesn't make sense." For the toddler who develops symptoms resembling a toxic exposure, knowing where the poisoning may have taken place is of help. For example, toxins found in a garage are distinct from the array of poisons available in the bathroom cabinet. Knowledge of past drug use patterns may help in the evaluation of an intoxicated adolescent. For the unknown overdose, it is necessary to conduct a dogged interrogation to identify all medications available in the home, including those belonging to other family members. If partially empty or unlabeled bottles are found, it is essential to make the correct product identification. References, pharmacists, prescribing physicians, and regional poison centers may be helpful.

Finally, the toxicologic management of a given patient must consider the patient's past medical problems, active medical conditions, current medications, and allergies. These not only may provide insight into the current clinical picture but also may alert the physician to potential contraindicated therapies or drug interactions.

Physical Examination

The physical examination provides critical clues to the severity and nature of the poisoning. It begins with the initial assessment of cardiorespiratory stability and vital signs and progresses to a rapid assessment of neurologic function and methodical head-to-toe examination. Equally important is the ongoing observation and repeated evaluation of the patient as the case unfolds. Absence of physical findings may be consistent with a nontoxic ingestion. However, early in the course of serious ingestions, children may also be free of symptoms. Countless toxins may result in nonspecific symptoms such as drowsiness, vomiting, or abdominal distress. Certain groupings of symptoms may suggest specific classes of toxins. These **"toxidromes,"** if present, are especially useful in the evaluation of the unknown poisoning (Table 23.5).

Certain compounds or class of compounds may consistently produce a specific sign or symptom following overdose. **Depressed level of consciousness** is a hallmark of CNS depressants such as alcohols, opioids, barbiturates, and benzodiazepines. CNS depression may be secondary, resulting, for example, from insulin-mediated hypoglycemia or cellular asphyxia due to carbon monoxide. Respiratory depression is a commonly seen complication of severe CNS depression. **Seizures** may result from a number of sympathomimetic agents such as theophylline, cocaine, and amphetamines as well as phenylpropanolamine and pseudoephedrine, two common ingredients of over-the-counter cold preparations. Antidepressants, antihistamines, and isoniazid are therapeutic drugs that may also cause seizures in overdose. Camphor and pesticides, which are commonly found in the home, are two epileptogenic poisons.

Some substances that are commonly involved in poisonings result in certain signs and symptoms (Table 23.6). **Hypotension** may result from bradycardia as seen with parasympathomimetic agents such as organophosphate pesticides or with sympatholytic antihypertensives such as β

| TABLE 23.5 | Common Toxidromes |

Anticholinergic poisoning
  Hot as Hades
  Blind as a bat
  Red as a beet
  Dry as a bone
  Mad as a hatter

Cholinergic poisoning (DUMBBELS)
  Diarrhea
  Urination
  Miosis
  Bronchorrhea
  Bradycardia
  Emesis
  Lacrimation
  Salivation

Narcotic poisoning
  Pinpoint pupils
  Coma
  Respiratory depression

Sympathomimetic poisoning
  Tachycardia
  Hypertension
  Mydriasis
  Excitation
  Diaphoresis
  Delirium, psychosis
  Seizures

| TABLE 23.6 | Major Signs and Symptoms of Some Common Poisonings |

Agent	Signs and Symptoms
Acetaminophen	No symptoms (early)
	Hepatic failure (late)
Iron	Vomiting, abdominal pain
	Hypotension
Salicylates	Hyperpnea, vomiting
	Metabolic acidosis
Albuterol	Tachycardia, excitation
Diphenhydramine	Lethargy, tachycardia, seizures
"Superwarfarins"	No symptoms (early)
	Bleeding (late)
Ethanol	Lethargy, ataxia
	Hypoglycemia
Isoniazid	Seizures

blockers. Hypotension with tachycardia occurs in the setting of hypovolemia resulting from severe vomiting, diarrhea, and third-space redistribution that is seen with many heavy metals and plant toxins. **Dysrhythmias** commonly occur following overdose of tricyclic antidepressants and cardiac medications such as digitalis and quinidine. In children with hyperthermia, sympathomimetic drugs, salicylates, and anticholinergic agents warrant consideration.

In addition, characteristic **odors** may also provide clues to the intoxicant. Most people are familiar with the odors of ethanol and mothballs. Methyl salicylate smells of wintergreen, and organophosphate pesticides smell of garlic. **Burns** of the oral mucosa or skin are an important physical finding following ingestion of caustic compounds.

Laboratory Evaluation

The diagnostic measures selected depend on the history, clinical appearance, and intentionality. For most accidental childhood ingestions of a single agent such as bleach, a cold preparation, or detergents, observation alone is sufficient if children have no symptoms. After small ingestions of acetaminophen, salicylates, or ethanol, drug levels are not required if the amount ingested does not approach toxic doses. For unclear reasons, ethanol is associated with hypoglycemia in young children. Therefore, it is good to offer something sweet while observing the small child who has ingested an unknown quantity of ethanol. If the amount ingested cannot be calculated with reasonable certainty, symptoms are present, the amount consumed is great, or there is doubt concerning the verity of the history, diagnostic and therapeutic measures are indicated.

The intentional overdose requires an entirely different approach. A very low threshold for diagnostics and decontamination is essential despite the apparent triviality of the poisoning. In all adolescent or intentional ingestions where the history may be inaccurate, assays for commonly available drugs such as acetaminophen and an electrocardiogram (ECG) are routinely indicated.

For many toxins, blood levels are not useful because they do not correlate with clinical toxicity. For several commonly ingested agents (i.e., salicylates, acetaminophen, ethanol, theophylline), blood levels are rapidly performed in most clinical laboratories and provide useful information about prognosis and guide therapeutic interventions. For other drugs, the mere qualitative presence in blood or urine has important implications for patient disposition. For example, finding cocaine or opioids in a small child should prompt a child welfare investigation.

Pediatric Pearl

It is impossible to screen for all agents, and the specific panels of drugs screened vary between laboratories. The toxicology screen should only be used as an adjunct to clinical suspicion regarding a specific drug or drugs, and the clinician should be familiar with the drugs included in a given screen.

Aside from drug levels, other routine laboratory evaluations may help assess the unknown intoxication. Both hypoglycemia and electrolyte disturbances may result from and contribute to toxic syndromes. Immediate determination of blood glucose is warranted in every lethargic or comatose child. Likewise, a therapeutic trial of naloxone in an obtunded child may diagnose opioid intoxication by producing abrupt arousal. It is important to use caution with naloxone in patients who are known to be habitual users of opioids, because sudden administration of the antagonist may precipitate withdrawal. For toxins known to cause bleeding, coagulopathy, hepatic toxicity, renal compromise, rhabdomyolysis, or respiratory failure, the selective use of the CBC, prothrombin time (PT), partial thromboplastin time (PTT), serum chemistries, and blood gas values are indicated both to determine baseline values and to monitor the evolution of the illness.

Radiographs have selective utility in poisonings. Aside from demonstrating pneumonitis or pulmonary edema, radiographs may be of help in diagnosing ingestion of certain drugs that are radiopaque in large enough quantities. The mnemonic "CHIPSS" can be used to remember the radiopaque compounds (Table 23.7). Absence of radiopacity on the abdominal radiograph does not rule out ingestion of these substances.

The presence of an elevated anion gap metabolic acidosis [sodium − (chloride + bicarbonate)] of greater than 12–16 mEq/L suggests several toxins. The mnemonic "AT MUDPILES" can be used to remember the substances that cause metabolic acidosis (Table 23.8). Similarly, an elevated osmol gap (range: $-5 - +15$ mOsm), calculated by the equation

$$\frac{2(sodium) + glucose}{18} +$$

$$\frac{blood\ urea\ nitrogen\ (BUN)}{2.8}$$

TABLE 23.7	**Radiopaque Compounds**

Chlorinated compounds (chloral hydrate, carbon tetrachloride, *p*-dichlorobenzene)
Heavy metals (iron, mercury, lead)
Iodine
Phenothiazines
Slow-release preparations (enteric-coated analgesics)
Stuffers (cocaine- or heroin-filled packets)

may be associated with the toxic alcohols or diuretics. However, a nonspecific elevation of the osmol gap is seen in many other disease states (e.g., liver disease, sepsis).

Assessment and Differential Diagnosis

After the history, physical examination, and selected diagnostics have been initiated, the clinician must assess the nature and seriousness of the poisoning.

- Given the identity and quantity of the toxin involved, has a poisoning occurred?
- Is the patient ill now, or is the patient likely to become ill?
- Are there nontoxicologic disease processes that may be taking place instead of or in addition to the poisoning (e.g., traumatic and infectious causes, which should always be considered in the evaluation of the altered or febrile child)?
- To minimize the morbidity that may result from the poisoning, what treatment does the patient need?
- How soon is intervention warranted?

Management

As with any emergency, attention to life-threatening processes is the initial priority. The basic life support sequence of **airway (A), breathing (B),** and **circulation (C)** is critical to the success-

ful management of toxicologic emergencies (see Table 23.1).

After immediate stabilization, the cornerstone of toxicologic management is **decontamination.** The objective of decontamination is to minimize systemic absorption of the toxin. For skin or mucous membrane exposure, this consists of washing or irrigation of the contaminated surfaces. In the case of intoxication by inhalation, removal from the source of toxic vapors to fresh air or the administration of humidified oxygen is indicated. For ingested toxins, gut decontamination consists of one or more of the following: gastric emptying by emesis or lavage, the administration of a sorbent such as activated charcoal, and the addition of a cathartic.

In considering **gastric emptying,** the clinician must consider the safety of the procedure and the likelihood of removing substantial amounts of toxin. In general, both emesis and gastric lavage may predispose individuals to aspiration if performed in patients who are lethargic, comatose, or seizing. The ingestion of corrosive agents and hydrocarbons are contraindications because both procedures may exacerbate gut mucosal damage, increase the risk of perforation, or lead to aspiration. Emesis with syrup of ipecac, used strictly with medical supervision, is useful for initiation of decontamination at home. Although gastric lavage is the preferred method of gastric emptying in the hospital setting, its use is increasingly controversial.

TABLE 23.8	**Substances Causing Anion Gap Acidosis**

Alcohols
Toluene
Methanol
Uremia
Diabetic ketoacidosis or other ketoacidosis (alcoholism, starvation)
Paraldehyde or **P**henformin
Iron or **I**soniazid
Lactic acidosis
Ethylene glycol
Salicylates or **S**trychnine

Pediatric Pearl

Most toxicologists accept that gastric lavage still has a place in the treatment of massive, life-threatening ingestions for which alternative treatments are insufficient (e.g., sustained-release calcium channel blockers). If gastric lavage is used in an obtunded individual, measures to secure a safer airway (i.e., endotracheal intubation) must be taken beforehand.

Activated charcoal avidly adsorbs to a large variety of toxins and may be safely administered in most patients. However, it does not adsorb heavy metals, hydrocarbons, and alcohols well. Potential adverse effects of charcoal include (1) aspiration, particularly when administered forcibly to obtunded individuals, and (2) charcoal inspissation in the gut with potential for perforation in the patient with ileus.

Cathartics theoretically decrease absorption by decreasing transit time. In repeated doses, they may result in dehydration and electrolyte imbalance. Whole bowel irrigation with an iso-osmotic solution such as polyethylene glycol is sometimes useful for hastening elimination of pills or particles that have passed beyond the stomach, especially those that are not adsorbed by charcoal. Gut decontamination is most effective when instituted early, before significant absorption has occurred.

Several measures may hasten postabsorptive elimination of a substance. Examples include hemodialysis, charcoal hemoperfusion, ionized diuresis, and multiple doses of activated charcoal. For dialysis to be useful, a toxin should be small enough to traverse the dialysis membrane, possess a small volume of distribution (i.e., largely limited to the intravascular space), and have a low degree of protein binding. Lithium and methanol are examples of such compounds. Ionized diuresis works for weak acids such as salicylates by trapping the charged form of the drug in alkaline urine and thereby enhancing renal elimination of the drug. Multiple doses of charcoal are effective in enhancing elimination of drugs such as theophylline by adsorbing drug, which backdiffuses into the gut, or by interrupting enterohepatic cycling of other drugs (e.g., carbamazepine).

A nationwide network of regional poison information centers is available 24 hours a day to medical practitioners to provide assistance in management of specific poisonings. Several resources are available: **POISINDEX,** a computerized data bank of medicinal, industrial, and environmental toxins that is regularly updated; a library of toxicologic reference texts; and a staff of medical toxicologists. In addition, the centers also may be able to supply telephone numbers for other area experts such as the local botanical gardeners or herpetologists. They may help predict the symptoms that may occur with a given toxin and are instrumental in directing the clinician toward the safest course of therapy.

Foreign body ingestion is often included in the discussion of childhood poisonings, although it is not necessarily a toxicologic problem. Most ingested foreign bodies pass through the gut with no absorption and, consequently, do not result in systemic illness. Occasionally, the size or shape of the ingested object causes it to lodge in the gut. If arrested in the lower esophagus, it should be removed endoscopically to avoid the potential for regurgitation and aspiration into the airway. Once beyond the lower esophageal sphincter, round objects such as coins rarely cause problems. Larger objects may result in obstruction and require surgical removal. Button batteries rarely fragment in the gut and usually do not require removal. However, patients who ingest button batteries warrant careful observation for signs that caustic contents have leaked, resulting in gut mucosal ulceration and abdominal pain. Although elevated blood and urine mercury levels may occur following the fragmentation of mercuric oxide button batteries, no reports of resulting systemic mercury toxicity have appeared. In contrast, the sudden absorption of the contents of a ruptured cocaine bag has nearly uniformly lethal consequences.

Several antidotes protect against or reverse the toxicity of specific toxic agents by a multitude of mechanisms (Table 23.9). The antagonism of opioids by naloxone is well known.

After stabilization and treatment of poisoned patients, meticulous supportive care is of paramount importance for the eventual recovery. Monitoring of vital signs and serial examinations, vigorous respiratory support and toilet, maintenance of fluid and electrolyte homeostasis, and management of infectious complications are critical early in the course of the severely poisoned patient. As recovery proceeds, psychiatric intervention and preventive education is appropriate. Acute awareness of potential drug interactions, both of ingested toxins and of drugs administered therapeutically, is important throughout the treatment period.

OFFICE OR EMERGENCY DEPARTMENT CARE OF BURNS

Burns are a common cause of injury in children. Each year more than 200,000 children receive treatment for burn injuries. In addition, signifi-

TABLE 23.9	Some Toxins and Their Antidotes
Toxin	**Antidote and Mechanism of Action**
Acetaminophen	N-acetylcysteine; prevents formation of toxic metabolite
Warfarin	Vitamin K; acts as cofactor for synthesis of coagulation factors
Organophosphates	Atropine; acts as muscarinic antagonist
	Pralidoxime; reactivates cholinesterase
Digoxin	Digoxin-specific antibodies; effect immunoneutralization
Lead	Dimercaprol; effects chelation
Methanol	Ethanol; competitively inhibits alcohol dehydrogenase
Nitrites	Methylene blue; helps reduce methemoglobin

cant morbidity and mortality often occur; only motor vehicle accidents cause more accidental deaths in children. The peak incidence of burn injury occurs in toddlers (1–5 years), and the injuries usually occur as the result of scalding from hot liquids. Although burns from house fires are less common, they account for almost half of all burn-related deaths. This higher mortality is probably related to associated smoke inhalation.

Pathophysiology

Direct thermal injury causes cell death at the time of the burn. Immediate release of local mediators, especially histamine, which causes a transient increase in vascular permeability, then occurs. After a short lag period, release of additional vasoactive substances such as serotonin and prostaglandins further increases permeability. Altogether, these factors result in marked tissue edema, accentuating the ischemic damage of the injured cells.

The severity of the direct tissue injury is related to the temperature of the causative substance and the duration of contact.

☀ Pediatric Pearl

Because the ischemic injury may extend 3–7 times more deeply than the level of the direct injury, the final depth of the burn may be delayed for 4–5 days.

Usually, the severity can be estimated by the depth of the burn. **First-degree burns** such as sunburn involve only the epidermis. These red and painful burns do not blister and resolve without scaring in 3–5 days. **Second-degree burns** are partial-thickness burns that involve the entire epidermis and varying degrees of dermis. Superficial second-degree burns (involving the top one-half of the dermis) are usually red or mottled with blisters, swelling, and intense pain. Healing occurs in

1–2 weeks without scarring. Deep second-degree burns appear mottled with a broken epidermis and a wet or weeping surface. Depending on the amount of nerve destruction, these burns may or may not be painful. Healing occurs slowly, often resulting in a scar. **Third-degree burns** are full-thickness burns involving damage to all layers of the skin and subcutaneous tissue. The skin is broken with a white or leathery appearance. The burn surface is usually dry and painless, because the nerve endings are destroyed. At this level there is no functional barrier to bacterial infection. Healing is prolonged and may necessitate skin grafting. **Fourth-degree burns** extend from the skin through the subcutaneous tissue and fascia to the bone. Tissue necrosis, edema, and coagulopathy are extensive and may cause systemic toxicity. These burns usually require skin grafting.

Clinical and Laboratory Evaluation

History

The history-taking process should involve learning more about the circumstances that resulting in the burn injury. It is essential to ascertain whether the mechanism of the injury (explosion, thrown from vehicle, house fire) may have caused internal injuries or fractures. Determination of the circumstances of the injury, the nature of the agent involved, and the duration of exposure is important. Flash burns from fires or scalding from boiling water usually causes second-degree burns, whereas fires, explosions, hot grease, or hot oil often cause third-degree burns. Questions about the nature and duration of smoke inhalation and fire are warranted. Exposure to combustion of carbon-containing products such as wood (with house fires), methane with clogged heating vents), or gasoline (with blocked automobile exhaust) should prompt concerns about carbon monoxide poisoning. Any conflict between the circumstances of the injury and the severity or appearance of the burn as well as the degree of supervision may lead the physician to suspect child abuse or neglect. The child's tetanus immunization status is important to determine; it may be necessary to administer a booster.

Physical Examination

It is appropriate to consider the physical examination in terms of the ABCs for burns.

- **Airway:** Signs of upper airway obstruction (stridor), which may occur as a result of thermal injury to the pharynx, and clinical signs that may indicate the presence of inhalation injury (Table 23.10) may be evident.
- **Breathing:** Signs of respiratory distress (retractions, wheezing, tachypnea, cyanosis) may result either from direct inhalation injury to the lung or from the effects of smoke inhalation and carbon monoxide production. In addition, significant burns to the chest wall, especially if they are circumferential, may impede chest wall excursion and cause hypoxia.
- **Circulation:** Increased vascular permeability and edema formation around the injured tissue can cause significant fluid loss. This may be worsened by associated internal injuries. Assessment of circulation includes examination of pulse rate, capillary refill, skin color, skin temperature, quality of peripheral pulses, and mental status.
- **Depth:** Estimates of the depth (degree) of the burn are based on clinical appearance, as previously described (see PATHOPHYSIOLOGY).
- **Extent:** Estimates of the total extent of the burns may involve use of the "rule of 9s" (Table 23.11) or the system that dictates that one surface of the child's hand represents 1% of body surface area. It is important to note any circumferential burns of the chest and extremities.
- **Fractures:** This includes identification of fractures and internal injuries.
- **Globes:** In the presence of facial burns, it is necessary to inspect the eyes for burns, abrasions, and foreign material.

TABLE 23.10 Clinical Signs Associated With Inhalation Injury

Singing of nasal hair
Carbon deposits in the oropharynx
Oropharyngeal edema
Facial burns
Carbonaceous sputum
Altered mental status

TABLE 23.11 Rule of 9s for Estimating the Extent of Burns

	Child (%)	Adolescent (%)
Head	18	9
Each arm	9	9
Trunk	18	18
Back	18	18
Each leg	14	18

Laboratory Evaluation

For minor burns, no laboratory tests are indicated. If exposure to smoke or other combustible gases occurred, an arterial blood gas and co-oximetry for determination of carboxyhemoglobin levels are appropriate. If there are major burns (> 10%–15% second-degree burns) or associated injury, then baseline blood tests (CBC, electrolytes, PT, PTT, type and cross-match) and urinalysis (for hemoglobin and myoglobin) should be obtained. In children with respiratory distress, inhalation injury, or significant chest wall burns, an arterial blood gas is warranted.

Differential Diagnosis

Burn injury is usually apparent from the history and physical examination. Two specific types of burns—chemical and electrical—require special mention. Chemical burns often have prolonged exposure and penetrate deep into the dermal layers. Electrical burns are usually very serious, despite their initial minor appearance, because the electrical current can destroy muscles and blood vessels deep to the contact site. Affected patients may develop cardiac ischemia or dysrhythmia (if the current passed through the heart) as well as complications from muscle breakdown (myoglobinemia).

The physician should also be aware of burns that are characteristic of child abuse: patterned or small circular burns (from an iron, lighter, or cigarette), sharply demarcated burns of the extremities or buttocks (from intentional immersion in scalding bath water), or other burns not consistent with the history.

Management

Management should proceed based on the evaluation of the "ABCs" (see Table 23.1). If signs of airway compromise (e.g., stridor) or signs associated with the development of upper airway obstruction following inhalation injury are present (see

Table 23.10), endotracheal intubation should be used to secure the airway. Direct laryngoscopy with a flexible endoscope, by an experienced emergency medicine or ear, nose, and throat physician, may help assess the degree of pharyngeal edema. It is important to provide 100% oxygen to all patients with suspected smoke inhalation or signs of respiratory distress. Nebulized β_2-agonists (albuterol) are indicated for signs of bronchospasm (e.g., wheezing). For children with cardiovascular compromise or more than 10% second-degree burns, intravenous fluid resuscitation with normal saline or lactated Ringer's solution is appropriate. As already noted, there is significant fluid loss at the site of the burn. The amount of intravenous fluids required is the child's maintenance fluid requirement plus additional fluids to compensate for the loss through the burned tissue (2–3 ml/kg body weight/ % body surface area burned). One-half of the calculated fluid deficit should be administered in the first 8 hours. Placement of a Foley catheter to monitor urine output is appropriate, and insertion of a nasogastric tube to decompress the stomach is also warranted. Circumferential burns of the extremities may cause vascular compromise and a compartment syndrome. Significant burns to the chest may cause respiratory compromise. These types of burns may necessitate an immediate surgical intervention such as an escharotomy. In this procedure, an incision is made for the entire length of the eschar in order to allow the skin edges to separate and relieve the tension.

Once the child is stabilized, the physician should focus on wound care. Burns can be extremely painful, so prompt sedation and analgesia is essential. Unlike adults who can express their pain with complaints, children's cries are often not appreciated by the providers as a sign of pain, thereby delaying the administration of pain medications. Thus, as soon as the ABCs are secured, children should receive sedation. The method of sedation depends on the experience of the physicians and existing emergency department protocols. A dose of morphine (0.1 mg/kg given IV, IM, or SQ) is usually effective and has the advantage of being readily reversed with naloxone if needed.

Room temperature, saline-soaked gauze pads can be used initially to cover the burned areas. Do *not* apply ice or cold dressings because of the risk of developing hypothermia. Notify the hospital's burn service (plastic or general surgeon) for any significant burns. To dress the burns, remove the saline gauze and clean the burns gently with saline solution, using aseptic technique. It is ap-

TABLE 23.12 Burns That Require Hospitalization
Second-degree burns over > 10% BSA
Third-degree burns over > 2% BSA
Significant smoke inhalation
Associated injuries (e.g., fracture, head trauma)
Perineal burns
Second-degree burns involving face, ears, hands, or feet
Second-degree burns that are circumferential or cross a joint
Electrical burns
Deep chemical burns
Suspected child abuse

BSA = body surface area.

propriate to remove devitalized tissue, but intact blisters (which themselves provide a sterile dressing) should remain. The application of topical antimicrobial agents to all second- and third-degree burns is warranted. A *thin* layer of Silvadene can be applied to the burns, but because the silver can leave a hyperpigmented scar, bacitracin is preferred for cosmetically important areas such as the face. A single layer of fine-mesh gauze followed by two or three layers of fluffed absorbent gauze is used to provide a closed dressing. If needed, give a tetanus booster. Certain types of burns require hospitalization are (Table 23.12). The use of hyperbaric oxygen for burn management and carbon monoxide poisoning is controversial.

SUGGESTED READINGS

Avner JR, Baker MD: Dog bites in urban children. *Pediatrics* 88:55–57, 1991.

Avner JR, Baker MD: Lacerations involving glass: The role of routine x-rays. *Am J Dis Child* 146:600–602, 1992.

Baker MD, Selbst SM, Lanuti M: Lacerations in urban children. *Am J Dis Child* 144:87–92, 1990.

Deitch EA: The management of burns. *N Engl J Med* 323:1249–1253, 1990.

Goldfrank LR, Flomenbaum NE, Lewin NA, et al (eds): *Toxicologic Emergencies*, 6th ed. Stamford, CT, Appleton & Lange, 1998.

Hansbrough JF: Pediatric burns. *Pediatr Rev* 20(4):117–123, 1999.

Haydel MJ, Preston CA, Mills TJ, et al: Indications for computed tomography in patients with minor head injury. *N Engl J Med* 343:100–105, 2000.

Kulig K, Bar-Or D, Cantrill SV, et al: Management of acutely poisoned patients without gastric emptying. *Ann Emerg Med* 14:562–567, 1985.

Marx JA (ed): *Rosen's Emergency Medicine: Concepts and Clinical Practice*, 5th ed. St. Louis, Mosby, 2002.

Mlcak R, Cortiella J, Desai MH: Emergency management of pediatric burn victims. *Pediatr Emerg Care* 14:51–54, 1998.

Olson KR, Pentel PR, Kelley MT: Physical assessment and differential diagnosis of the poisoned patient. *Med Toxicol* 2:52–81, 1987.

Pond SM, Lewis-Driver DJ, Williams GM, et al: Gastric emptying in acute overdose: A prospective randomized controlled trial. *Med J Aust* 163:345–349, 1995.

Quinn J, Wells G, Sutcliffe T, et al: Tissue adhesive versus suture wound repair at 1 year: Randomized clinical trial correlating early, 3-month, and 1-year cosmetic outcome. *Ann Emerg Med* 32:645–649, 1998.

Resh K, Schilling C, Borchert BD, et al: Topical anesthesia for pediatric lacerations: A randomized trial of lidocaine-epinephrine-tetracaine solution vs. gel. *Ann Emerg Med* 32:693–697, 1998.

Sanchez JI: Childhood trauma: Now and in the new millennium. *Surg Clin North Am* 79(6):1503–1535, 1999.

Schiller WR: Burn management in children. *Pediatr Ann* 25(8):434–438, 1996.

Schutzman SA, Barnes P, Duhaime A, et al: Evaluation and management of children younger than two years old with apparently minor head trauma: Proposed guidelines. *Pediatrics* 107:983–993, 2001.

Singer A, Hollander J, Quinn JV: Evaluation and management of traumatic lacerations. *N Engl J Med* 337:1142–1148, 1997.

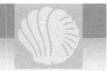

Chapter 24

Pediatric Intensive Care

Lorry R. Frankel and Joseph V. DiCarlo

A clerkship rotation in the pediatric intensive care unit (PICU) is too brief to allow a complete understanding of the therapeutic regimens used in the unit. Students might best benefit by focusing on (1) the common manifestations of organ dysfunction and failure experienced by children and (2) the largely supportive role the critical care team plays in their recovery. It is necessary to seek out unifying features in the various manifestations of the **systemic inflammatory response syndrome** that are always present in a multidisciplinary PICU, whether in a child recovering from extensive spinal fusion surgery who now is flushed and tachycardic, with a widened pulse pressure and rising oxygen requirement; in a 2-year-old with profound septic shock induced by *Streptococcus pneumoniae;* in a newborn with severe cardiac dysfunction after prolonged corrective heart surgery; or in an immunosuppressed adolescent whose pneumonia insidiously blossomed into total lung consolidation. Each of these situations represents different manifestations and severity of the systemic inflammatory response syndrome.

The PICU functions in two ways: (1) primarily, to support critically ill children and give them time to heal, and (2) to provide a safe and efficient environment for the multidisciplinary team working with children and their families. The vast majority of children admitted to the PICU survive the experience. Occasionally, admission is prolonged, and in a few cases, children succumb to their disease. Pediatricians should be aware of the psychosocial dynamics encountered among children, parents, and relatives, and the teams of health professionals who provide the care.

In most active academic PICUs, the patient "mix" is evenly divided between medical and surgical patients. Most patients are admitted emergently, and 20%–30% of these may be admitted via a critical care transport service. The remainder of admissions are scheduled—usually postoperative patients requiring a high level of monitoring and nursing care not available on general care units. These children may need mechanical ventilation, invasive intravascular monitoring, and frequent attention by both the nursing and medical staff.

ORGANIZATION OF PEDIATRIC INTENSIVE CARE UNITS

PICUs are usually directed by a physician certified in pediatric critical care medicine and staffed by other subspecialists (anesthesiologists, cardiologists, pulmonologists, cardiovascular surgeons). A hospital critical care committee helps formulate policy for the PICU (e.g., admission and discharge criteria for PICU patients) and a **quality assurance program**. Admission and discharge criteria must be specific and clearly define which patients are to be admitted to the PICU or, if available, an intermediate care unit (Table 24.1).

The quality assurance program offers the opportunity to examine clinical practice patterns and their influence on patient outcomes. An example of a quality assurance project might include surveys of extubation criteria, reintubation rates for failed extubations, and evidence of airway injury following intubations performed by different techniques. Another quality assurance issue, especially in the era of managed care, is the overutilization of PICU beds.

TECHNIQUES FOR MONITORING CRITICALLY ILL INFANTS AND CHILDREN

Most PICU patients require some type of respiratory support, and many also need cardiovascular support. Frequent (**noninvasive**) or continuous (**invasive**) monitoring of vital signs and arterial blood gases is usually an integral part of PICU care (Table 24.2). It is important that age-specific criteria be used for setting monitor alarms. Normal values for heart rate, blood pressure, and respiratory rate vary with a child's development.

Continuous **pulse oximetry**, developed in the mid-1980s, has revolutionized respiratory monitoring in the PICU and is now the standard for bedside oxygenation monitoring. The advantage of pulse oximetry is that it can be used in patients of all ages. Its accuracy is somewhat dependent on tissue perfusion; therefore, its utility may be limited in patients with significant vasoconstriction and poor perfusion. **Transcutaneous moni-**

| TABLE 24.1 | Admission and Discharge Criteria in Pediatric Intensive Care Units |

Pediatric Intensive Care Unit (PICU)

ADMISSION CRITERIA

Patients with the following conditions who require invasive monitoring (e.g., arterial lines, central venous pressure lines, pulmonary arterial lines, intracranial pressure monitoring devices):
- Evidence of respiratory impairment or failure
- Cardiovascular compromise, including shock and hypotension (hypertensive crisis may be managed in the ICU)
- Acute neurologic deterioration, which includes status epilepticus, coma, or evidence of increased intracranial pressure
- Acute renal failure requiring dialysis
- Bleeding disorders that require massive transfusions

DISCHARGE CRITERIA

When the following discharge criteria are met, the PICU attending physician will arrange the transfer of the patient to an appropriate setting within the hospital or to a referring hospital. The primary attending physician will be notified of such discharge from the PICU. Discharge from the PICU may take place when the patient's disease process reverses itself to the point that the patient
- Requires no invasive monitoring
- Requires no airway protection (intact cough and gag reflexes)
- Is hemodynamically stable

Pediatric Intermediate Intensive Care Unit (PIICU)

ADMISSION CRITERIA
- Patients who do not require respiratory assistance for acute respiratory failure but require continuous monitoring of vital signs, noninvasive blood gas analysis (e.g., O_2 saturations, transcutaneous PO_2 and PCO_2), including those patients who require chronic ventilatory assistance with tracheostomies in place
- Patients who are in **early** cardiovascular failure and require continuous monitoring of vital signs and noninvasive monitoring
- Patients with a patent airway who require observation for acute neurologic deterioration (e.g., status epilepticus)
- Patients who have multiple organ failure but require nursing care not available in other parts of the hospital (e.g., acute renal failure, diabetic ketoacidosis, trauma victims)

DISCHARGE CRITERIA
- Patients who no longer require level of skilled nursing care provided in PICU
- Patients whose disease process has reversed itself to the point that they can be safely managed in other parts of the hospital

---

toring of oxygen (PO_2) or carbon dioxide (PCO_2) tension is of limited use in the PICU.

Capnography measures the end-tidal CO_2 concentration in exhaled gas and is more commonly used in intubated patients. The highest concentration of CO_2 sampled in the respirator circuit represents the alveolar CO_2 concentration, which should be very close to the arterial ($PaCO_2$) concentration. In patients with acute pulmonary disease where intrapulmonary shunting exists, the end-tidal CO_2 reading may not be accurate. Furthermore, neither pulse oximetry nor end-tidal CO_2 devices can provide data about arterial pH, which is usually a critically important part of the patient's assessment. Thus, these noninvasive modalities are usually supplemented by **arterial blood gas** sampling. Other noninvasive moni-

toring techniques used in the PICU are detailed in Table 24.2.

Invasive monitoring is often utilized in patients who are in shock or in need of infusions of vasoactive agents. Central venous access is used for the administration of vasoactive drugs as well as for the determination of **central venous pressure (CVP). Pulmonary artery thermodilution (e.g., Swan-Ganz) catheters** are occasionally used for more sophisticated monitoring, although these catheters are more difficult to insert in children than in adults. A pulmonary thermodilution catheter can measure central venous pressure, pulmonary capillary wedge pressure (which reflects left atrial and usually left ventricular filling pressures), cardiac output, and mixed venous oxygen saturation. These data allow the

TABLE 24.2 Pediatric Intensive Care Unit (PICU) Monitoring Devices

Monitoring Device	Site	What is Measured	Monitoring Limitations/Concerns
Noninvasive Monitoring			
Cardiorespiratory	Chest leads	Heart rate, rhythm, respiratory rate	Only provides a lead 2 recording; may have difficulty with dys-rhythmia recognition
Transcutaneous	Chest	PaO_2 $PaCO_2$	Surface electrodes that warm the skin to 43°C can cause thermal injuries; must be changed every 3–4 hours; useful in neonates only
Pulse oximetry	Digits/nasal bridge	Continuous O_2 saturation values	Very useful in well-perfused patients
Capnography	End of endotracheal tube	Breath-by-breath analysis of CO_2 in intubated patients' end-tidal CO_2	Need graphic picture to determine end-tidal plateaus
Blood pressure	Arm cuff	"Dinamap" can cycle blood pressure every 1–5 minutes	Similar to cuff pressure (cuff size important)
EEG	Scalp surface	Provides for continuous monitoring of cranial electrical activity	Requires specialized technician for placement
Invasive Monitoring			
Arterial	Dorsalis pedis, radial, posterior tibial axillary, femoral	Continuous blood pressure monitor; able to draw frequent blood gases and other labs	Expertise in placement and monitoring; may require cut-down technique; loss of distal perfusion
Central venous access	Femoral, subclavian, external/internal jugular, antecubital	Central venous pressure monitoring useful in shock states and for administration of vasoactive agents	Requires expertise in placement, especially in young infants; multilumen catheter for multiple drips
Pulmonary artery ("Swan-Ganz") catheter	Placed through sheath in internal jugular, femoral, or subclavian vein	Cardiac output, pulmonary capillary wedge pressure Indications Septic shock Cardiogenic shock High PEEP Barbiturate coma	Less commonly used in children; helpful in titration of therapy
Intracranial pressure monitoring	Subdural bolts; epidural fiberoptic devices; intraventricular catheter	Intracranial pressure when CNS pathology is associated with significant cerebral edema (e.g., severe head injury), Reye syndrome, Glasgow Coma Scale score ≤ 8	Neurosurgeon usually inserts device; requires expertise in monitoring; may be used for therapeutic intervention if required

CNS = central nervous system; EEG = electroencephalogram; PEEP = positive end-expiratory pressure.

calculation of both systemic and pulmonary vascular resistances, oxygen consumption, and intrapulmonary shunt fractions.

Intracranial pressure monitoring devices assist in the management of intracranial pathology commonly encountered with severe head injuries, severe central nervous system (CNS) infections, or Reye syndrome (see NEUROLOGIC INTENSIVE CARE). The specific monitoring device used depends on the clinical indications, the neurosurgeon's familiarity with different types of devices, and the location in the cranium where it can be most safely inserted. The monitor may be placed on top of the dura (epidural device), under the dura (subdural device), or directly into the ventricular system (intraventricular monitor). Intraventricular devices have the added advantage of being useful for therapeutic removal of cerebrospinal fluid (CSF). Each of these devices may be associated with a variety of complications including infection, bleeding, injury to brain tissue, and monitor malfunction. The more invasive devices (i.e., subdural and intraventricular monitors) are associated with a greater risk of infection and thus are usually removed after 5–7 days.

BASICS OF ASSISTED VENTILATION

Mechanical ventilation is utilized in children with either pulmonary or nonpulmonary causes of **respiratory failure**. Pulmonary pathologies that result in the need for mechanical ventilation include airway obstruction, severe pneumonias that result in respiratory failure (increase in $PaCO_2$ and respiratory acidosis), accumulation of significant amounts of fluid in the pleural space, and injuries to the chest wall that produce an unstable thoracic cage. Nonpulmonary indications for ventilatory support include CNS pathologies that produce either ineffective respiratory efforts (e.g., Cheyne-Stokes respirations) or none at all (apnea), severe cardiac failure with the development of pulmonary edema, multisystem organ failure as seen in sepsis, massive gastrointestinal (GI) hemorrhage, intra-abdominal masses or ascites that produce pressure on the diaphragm and result in decreased lung volumes, and severe forms of trauma.

The usual physiologic indications for mechanical ventilation include one or more of the following: **hypoxia** (i.e., $PaO_2 < 60$ mm Hg, or $SaO_2 < 90\%$ in an $FIO_2 > 0.50$–0.60), **hypercarbia** (i.e., $PaCO_2 > 55$–60 mm Hg), or **respiratory acidosis** (pH < 7.25).

Once the decision has been made to begin mechanical ventilation, equipment and pharmaco-

logic agents appropriate for the patient's age and weight must be readied. Necessary adjuncts include oxygen (in tanks or via a central system), proper-sized face masks, ventilation bags, laryngoscopes (blades vary in size from 00 for neonates to 3 for older children and can be either straight or curved), and endotracheal tubes (2.5–8.0 mm in diameter). The size of the tube selected depends on age and the underlying disease process (e.g., patients with croup may require a smaller tube).

Pediatric Pearl

A useful formula to determine size of endotracheal tubes is: **Tube size = [Age (in years) + 16] ÷ 4**

Appropriate doses of medications should be calculated and drawn up before intubation. If children are apneic or comatose and have virtually no airway protective mechanisms, an endotracheal tube can be placed emergently with little resistance. However, it is more common for patients to be alert; therefore, pharmacologic agents are used to sedate and relax children so that the intubation can be performed safely and efficiently. Commonly used agents include narcotics (morphine or fentanyl), benzodiazepines (diazepam or midazolam) and muscle relaxants (either a depolarizing agent such as succinylcholine or a nondepolarizing agent such as pancuronium). Other agents that may be used include short-acting barbiturates (thiopental) and dissociative anesthetics such as ketamine.

During intubation, patients should be monitored for heart rate and oxygen saturation and should receive the highest concentration of oxygen possible. Positioning patients on their back with some neck extension and chin lift facilitates the insertion of the laryngoscope blade and the endotracheal tube (Figure 24.1). Once the tube has been inserted, the accuracy of the tube location is determined by auscultation of both lung fields, evidence of condensation of gas in the tube, and a postintubation chest radiograph. Choice of nasotracheal versus oral intubation depends on the preference of the individual physician. Although technically more difficult, nasal tubes offer more stability and are better tolerated. Complications from endotracheal tubes include injury to the glottis and subglottic areas, right mainstem intubation, pneumonias, and esophageal intubations. Uncuffed tubes are used more often in pediatrics, because they are associated with less airway injury than cuffed tubes.

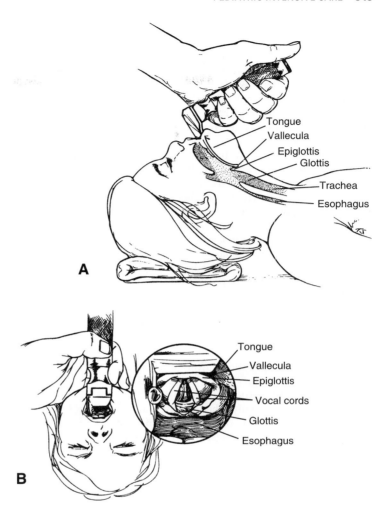

FIGURE 24.1 A. Position of the head for direct laryngoscopy. Note the laryngoscope is held in the left hand. The endotracheal tube is advanced with the right hand. **B.** Visualization of the glottic area at the time of intubation.

After the endotracheal tube is stabilized, the ventilator circuit is connected. Conventional mechanical ventilators can be divided into **time cycled, pressure-limited,** and **volume-cycled** ventilators. Time-cycled ventilators terminate an inspiratory breath after a preselected inspiratory time elapses. Pressure- limited ventilators are commonly used in the care of critically ill neonates with hyaline membrane disease. In these ventilators, the desired **peak inspiratory pressure** is delivered until the pressure limit is reached and until the ventilator time cycles "OFF." Volume-cycled ventilators are designed to deliver a preset **tidal volume** with each breath. Volume ventilation has become the mainstay of ventilatory support for children. Nonconventional ventilators (jet ventilators, oscillators, or flow interrupters) are used to deliver **high-frequency ventilation,** which has

been used to reduce barotrauma in very severe forms of lung injury.

After selecting the type of ventilator to be used, the mode of ventilation required is determined based on the pathophysiology and patient age. Most common is **intermittent mandatory ventilation,** which allows the patient to breathe spontaneously with a mechanical inflation provided at preset intervals—the intermittent mandatory ventilation rate. Other common forms of mechanical ventilation include **assist control, synchronized intermittent mandatory ventilation,** and **pressure support ventilation**. For these modes, patients must be able to breathe spontaneously in order to trigger the ventilator; muscle relaxants cannot be used. In pressure support ventilation, the ventilator supplements each breath with additional pressure in order to increase the inspired tidal volume to achieve appropriate gas exchange. Pressure support has been shown to be useful in patients with neurologic disease who cannot generate a large enough tidal volume on their own (e.g., severe forms of Guillain-Barré syndrome).

Mechanical ventilation has several potential complications. Critically ill children often need sedation and possibly muscle paralysis in order to ensure a safe course of mechanical ventilation. If patients are not comfortable with the therapy, the risk of complications increases. In addition, mechanical ventilation may affect other organ systems, most notably the cardiac and renal systems. The increased pressure in the alveolar spaces may be transmitted to the pulmonary vascular bed, resulting in increased pulmonary artery resistance, increased workload on the right heart, displacement of the interventricular septum to the left, and decreased cardiac output. Urine output may be reduced as a result of redistribution of organ blood flow. By carefully selecting ventilator settings, these effects of positive pressure ventilation can be minimized.

Pulmonary complications from mechanical ventilation include injury to the airway and the development of subglottic stenosis. Positive pressure ventilation, especially when the mechanical preset pressure or airways resistance is high, may exert **barotrauma** on the lungs, which can result in air leaks (pneumothorax, subcutaneous emphysema, pneumoperitoneum, or pneumopericardium). Although rare, chest tube drainage is indicated when pulmonary status is compromised secondary to an air leak. Because mechanical ventilation is associated with many complications, it is necessary to assess a child's ventilatory status frequently so that weaning and extubation are not unnecessarily delayed.

RESPIRATORY DISEASES THAT REQUIRE PEDIATRIC INTENSIVE CARE

Impending respiratory failure must be recognized and stabilized on a timely basis. Failing to do so can subject children to prolonged periods of hypoxemia and acidosis. Such conditions can cause neurologic damage or death. The primary respiratory pathologies that lead to PICU admission can be categorized according to several criteria: the specific anatomic sites that are affected; the specific age groups that are at risk; the specific symptoms (e.g., stridor, wheezing, tachy-

pnea, or dyspnea) they produce; or specific etiologies. Understanding the anatomic relationships in the airways of children and how they differ from those of adults leads to a recognition of how they predispose children to a unique array of airway diseases.

UPPER AIRWAY OBSTRUCTION
Pathophysiology

Upper airway obstruction can be a life-threatening event, especially because the severity of the situation may be overlooked by individuals unfamiliar with children. Disorders of the upper airway are far more common in children because of structural factors that make the child more vulnerable to infectious agents, allergens, foreign body aspiration (small objects or foods such as peanuts, popcorn, and grapes), toxins, and traumatic injuries (Table 24.3).

The radius of the airway is smaller in children than in adults. As a result, there is an exponential increase in the resistance to airflow in clinical situations that result in airway narrowing, such

TABLE 24.3 Common Causes of Airway Obstruction

Infections
  Viral croup
  Epiglottitis
  Supraglottitis
  Tracheitis
  Pharyngeal/peritonsillar abscess
  Severe hypertrophy of tonsils or adenoids

Congenital
  Webs
  Vocal cord paralysis
  Tracheomalacia or laryngomalacia
  Subglottic stenosis
  Vascular abnormalities (hemangiomas, vascular rings)

Acquired (other than infectious)
  Trauma, either external or internal (e.g., subglottic stenosis)
  Foreign body aspirations

Central nervous system (CNS) disorders
  Head trauma
  CNS infections
  Status epilepticus
  Neuromuscular disorders
  Drug-induced dysfunction (e.g., narcotics, anesthetics, tranquilizers)

as occurs during the inflammation produced by croup or epiglottitis. In addition to the smaller airway, other factors that may predispose the child to airway obstruction are the presence of the cricoid membrane, mucosal tissue that swells when irritated, and the potential loss of upper airway muscle tone during sleep. This last factor is important when managing a child who has received anesthetic or narcotic agents for pain relief in the postoperative period. The most common presenting symptom in a child with airway obstruction is **stridor,** and this may be accompanied by alterations in respiratory rate and effort.

Differential Diagnosis

The most commonly encountered forms of severe upper airway obstruction are caused by infections. Acute croup syndromes may be caused by viruses or bacteria. Classically, **croup** (also known as **acute laryngotracheitis**) is caused by viral agents such as parainfluenza, influenza, or respiratory syncytial virus (RSV). Bacterial infections may produce either **epiglottitis** (*Haemophilus influenzae*) or **bacterial tracheitis** (*Staphylococcus aureus*). A syndrome of acute **supraglottitis** has also been described and is associated with viral illness. The viral croup syndromes are usually self-limiting and require very little in the way of PICU care. However, children with epiglottitis, tracheitis, or supraglottitis may require instrumentation of the airway in order to overcome the obstruction. Other serious causes of upper airway obstruction include severe tonsillar and adenoidal hypertrophy, acute tonsillitis, or a retropharyngeal abscess.

Foreign body aspiration is another major cause of upper airway obstruction in children, especially in young toddlers. Other common causes of airway obstruction include congenital anomalies of the airway, congenital defects of the tracheobronchial tree, vascular anomalies that produce extrinsic compression on the trachea or bronchi, and acquired problems such as neoplasm. Sometimes, these conditions produce only mild symptoms until an upper respiratory tract infection occurs, at which time severe obstruction may result.

PICU Management

Children who present with acute airway obstruction should have cardiorespiratory monitoring and pulse oximetry and should be observed continuously. They should be maintained in a position of comfort; if stable and not in impending respiratory failure, this may be on the parent's lap. An anesthesiologist and a pediatric surgeon or otolaryngologist should be notified, and equipment for emergency airway access should be at the bedside. Oxygen or racemic epinephrine may be administered, and patients reassessed for signs of improvement.

Careful history-taking is warranted, and if the history is appropriate for the aspiration of a foreign body (e.g., a toddler who eats peanuts and then coughs), the diagnostic and therapeutic procedure of choice is **rigid bronchoscopy**. This is usually performed under general anesthesia in the operating room. However, if the history is not definitive for foreign body aspiration or the symptoms are unusual, the clinician may wish to examine the airway at the bedside. **Flexible fiberoptic bronchoscopy** is ideal for this purpose and can help identify congenital airway anomalies such as **hemangioma, subglottic stenosis** (either acquired or congenital), **tracheomalacia,** or **laryngomalacia** or may demonstrate a pulsatile mass resulting from a **vascular ring** producing extrinsic compression of the airway.

A lateral radiograph of the neck region may assist in identifying a swollen epiglottis; however, it is important to minimize diagnostic procedures (e.g., blood drawing for arterial blood gases, intravenous injections, radiographs) until the patient's airway is secured. A careful examination by an experienced physician should be performed so that the obstruction is not worsened. In children with suspected **epiglottitis,** attempting to visualize the obstruction by direct laryngoscopy may lead to acute total airway obstruction. Such patients are usually taken to the operating room with either a pediatric surgeon or an otolaryngologist and an anesthesiologist present in case intubation is not possible and a tracheostomy is required. Once they are intubated, such patients are brought to the PICU. Additional problems that need to be addressed in caring for these patients are the need for sedation and the possibility of associated pulmonary disease (e.g., pneumonia or pulmonary edema) or a systemic disease that may accompany infection. Chapter 9, Infectious Diseases, provides more complete details on the clinical and laboratory findings in children with croup and epiglottitis.

So by the time many children with upper airway obstruction reach the PICU, a diagnosis has usually been made and the airway has been secured. These children usually benefit from positive pressure ventilation because of associated pulmonary disease. Patients with epiglottitis are usually intubated the shortest period of time (1–3 days). Those with viral croup and tracheitis may require 5–8 days of airway support. The bacterial infections require antibiotics directed against specific pathogens. The use of steroids for treatment of croup syndromes remains controversial. Once patients are extubated, racemic epinephrine is effective in reducing the airway swelling that often accompanies the postextubation period.

In children with a **peritonsillar** or **retropharyngeal abscess,** surgical drainage of the abscess is required in addition to aggressive medical management with antibiotics. Some centers place an endotracheal tube prophylactically to maintain the airway and prevent aspiration of infected contents.

SMALL AIRWAYS AND PARENCHYMAL LUNG DISEASE

Pathophysiology

In this broad category of lung pathologies, the most common conditions are **bronchiolitis, asthma,** and **pneumonia,** each of which can produce significant respiratory compromise (Table 24.4). Most infectious diseases of the airway are viral in nature, and most of the care required for these patients is supportive. When the clinician is able to diagnose a bacterial agent or a specific virus for which antiviral therapy is available (e.g., cytomegalovirus), specific therapy can be added to supportive measures.

Bronchiolitis is probably one of the more complicated acute pulmonary diseases encountered in the young child (see Chapter 9, Infectious Diseases). Bronchiolitis is an acute inflammation of the small airways that results in bronchoconstriction via chemical mediators such as the leukotrienes (L4), increased mucous secretion, epithelial cell destruction, and edema of the airways. Bronchiolitis can produce small airway disease accompanied with severe wheezing similar to that in asthma. In addition, significant parenchymal injury associated with the infection may exist; on chest radiography, this may be interpreted as pneumonia or atelectasis.

Differential Diagnosis

Bronchiolitis is predominantly a disease of infancy and is usually caused by viruses. Young infants are particularly susceptible because of small airway diameter, an unstable chest wall, the potential for fatigue of the respiratory muscles, and a very reactive pulmonary vascular bed. **RSV, parainfluenza, influenza,** and **adeno-**

TABLE 24.4 Types of Lower Airways Disease in Children

Infections
    Bronchiolitis (RSV, parainfluenza, influenza)
    Pneumonia (viral or bacterial)
Allergic
    Status asthmaticus
Foreign body
    Usually food, but may be plastic toys
Vascular anomalies
    Usually produce stridor, but may result in collapse of bronchus and produce atelectasis
Pulmonary edema
    Cardiogenic pulmonary edema secondary to congestive heart failure
    In children with either congenital or acquired heart disease
    Secondary to upper airway obstruction
    Noncardiogenic pulmonary edema (ARDS)
    After severe pulmonary injury or systemic illness
    Neurogenic pulmonary edema following severe neurologic insult
Chronic disorders
    Bronchopulmonary dysplasia
    Cystic fibrosis
Aspiration
    Swallowing disorders
    Gastroesophageal reflux
    Esophageal abnormalities
    Brainstem injury that results in poor cough and gag reflexes

---

ARDS = adult (or acute) respiratory distress syndrome; RSV = respiratory syncytial virus.

virus have been associated with this disease. RSV is probably the most common and usually produces epidemics of severe bronchiolitis, typically in the winter months. Those infants who are most at risk are those with underlying cardiopulmonary diseases (e.g., congenital heart disease, bronchopulmonary dysplasia that is seen in graduates of neonatal intensive care units who have had severe lung disease) and immunocompromised children. Infants with bronchiolitis infrequently require hospitalization, and only a small percentage (3%—7%) of those admitted to the hospital with bronchiolitis require intensive care.

Asthma is another severe form of reversible airways disease that may require admission to the PICU. Acute deterioration in asthmatic patients is often secondary to an allergen in the environment that produces a cascade of inflammatory reactions resulting in increased mucus production, bronchiolar edema, and bronchoconstriction (see Chapter 18, Pulmonology). These patients present with wheezing and dyspnea that are similar to the symptoms of bronchiolitis, but the patients are usually beyond infancy.

Other acute lung injuries that may necessitate care in the PICU are bacterial and other types of pneumonias; inhalation injuries (hydrocarbon, smoke); severe aspirations; and lung injuries following trauma. These events can produce a very complex and severe inflammatory response that results in a lung injury called the **adult (or acute) respiratory distress syndrome,** which is the end product of a series of chemical reactions that produce severe necrosis and both alveolar and interstitial disease. The mortality rate may be as high as 50%—60%. Unlike the respiratory distress syndrome seen in neonates where hyaline membranes form as a result of an inability to manufacture surfactant, hyaline membrane formation occurs despite adequate surfactant production in adult respiratory distress syndrome. Further details on the clinical and laboratory evaluation of patients with small airway disease can be found in Chapter 18.

PICU Management

Supportive measures in children with small airway disease include adequate hydration, oxygen therapy to maintain an arterial oxygen saturation of more than 90%, and bronchodilators to decrease airway resistance. The $PaCO_2$ and pH must be monitored for evidence of impending respiratory failure. Those patients who are retaining CO_2 out of proportion to their ventilatory rate and effort may require endotracheal intubation (Table 24.5). The ventilatory requirements for these patients can be problematic, because they may have both increased airways resistance secondary to severe small airway disease and decreased lung compliance secondary to alveolar disease. One of the strategies commonly used in the ventilation of these patients is to prolong the inspiratory and expiratory times in order to facilitate lung emptying. Generous tidal volumes are required to adequately inflate the lungs and maintain adequate minute ventilation, while the patient is ventilated with slow rates to provide for the long inspiratory/expiratory times. Children may require sedation and possibly muscle relaxants in order to tolerate these ventilator settings.

For infants with severe bronchiolitis resulting from RSV, antiviral therapy with the drug ribavirin is available, although its efficacy is still controversial. Ribavirin is administered via an aerosolized apparatus, so that the drug is delivered directly into the airways.

TABLE 24.5 Treatment of Respiratory Failure

Goals
- Avoidance of hypoxemia
- Avoidance of acidosis
- Avoidance of carbon dioxide retention

Basic Interventions
- Oxygen by mask, tent, or nasal prongs: maintain oxygen saturation of $> 90\%$
- Hydration: if the patient is in respiratory distress, keep status of nothing by mouth (NPO)
- Mechanical ventilation: indicated if the patient is apneic or has evidence of significant respiratory distress or failure
  $PaCO_2 > 60\text{–}65$ mm Hg
  $pH < 7.25$
  $PaO_2 < 60$ mm Hg in an $FIO_2 > 0.5$

Adjuncts to the previously described treatments include the use of aerosolized bronchodilators and the maintenance of fluid and electrolyte balance. Albuterol, administered in both intermittent and continuous treatment regimens, provides some benefit by decreasing small airway disease. The nutritional status of these children may also require careful attention. If infants do not tolerate enteral feeding, **total parenteral nutrition** is indicated.

Few children admitted to the PICU with **status asthmaticus** require mechanical ventilation, although they may still need aggressive respiratory treatment, including aerosolized bronchodilators and continuous administration of intravenous aminophylline or isoproterenol, in order to avoid mechanical ventilation. A careful search should be performed for causes of acute exacerbation in these patients (e.g., presence of intercurrent infections such as *Mycoplasma pneumoniae*). Because inspissated, tenacious mucus often contributes to the need for mechanical ventilation in asthmatic children, fiberoptic bronchoscopy may bring about dramatic improvement. Less invasively, DNAase may enhance the clearance of mucus.

Recovery from adult respiratory distress syndrome is more likely if the triggering event can be reversed or removed, and if the cascading immune response can be turned off. Thus, one might expect total recovery from adult respiratory distress syndrome triggered by massive transfusion (e.g., after trauma or surgery) in a host with a normal immune system. However, in children with severe immune deficiency (e.g., severe combined immune deficiency or early in the process of bone marrow transplantation), recovery is far more problematic even if the triggering event (e.g., bacterial pneumonia) can be controlled. In these children, it is likely that the remaining intact immune components function in the absence of the normal checks and balances; the inflammatory process in this scenario is often insidious and unrelenting.

The respiratory support for adult respiratory distress syndrome has evolved over the past two decades in favor of a gentler approach. At the peak of the illness, when pulmonary compliance is greatly reduced, normal levels of arterial oxygenation can be obtained only by applying high levels of **positive end-expiratory pressure,** large tidal volumes, and high fractional inspired oxygen concentrations. Such aggressive therapy puts children at great risk for barotrauma, including pneumothoraces and dramatic amounts of subcutaneous emphysema. Severe barotrauma often heralds a patient's demise, from superinfection, cardiovascular compromise, or pulmonary parenchymal failure (i.e., fibrosis).

Conversely, using a strategy that embraces the concept of "permissive hypercapnia," the lungs of children with adult respiratory distress syndrome may be protected. This strategy allows for marginal oxygenation and a moderate respiratory acidosis. Smaller tidal volumes and lower levels of positive end-expiratory pressure are used. Volume-cycled ventilation is often abandoned in favor of time-cycled, pressure-limited techniques. In the latter, a high gas flow rate brings the airway pressure to the desired level nearly instantaneously, which is then held for the prescribed inspiratory time. Flow actually decreases over the duration of inspiration. The area under this "square-wave" represents the same tidal volume achieved by volume-cycled ventilation at the expense of a higher peak pressure. The latest generation of microprocessor-controlled ventilators can mimic the square-wave pattern in volume mode (Figure 24.2). These changes may reduce the likelihood or severity of barotrauma, and children may then have more time to eliminate the trigger and turn off the immune cascade.

Arterial and central venous catheters are often utilized for physiologic monitoring, and rarely a pulmonary artery catheter is placed to assist in the determination of the optimal positive end-expiratory pressure and to calculate pulmonary shunt fractions. Therapy for adult respiratory distress syndrome may also include the use of bronchoscopy to retrieve inspissated mucus, bronchoscopic washing to look for evidence of infection, aggressive respiratory therapy treatments to clear secretions, and generous nutritional support. Less common therapies include **high-frequency venti-**

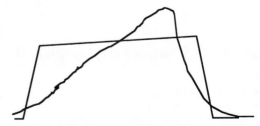

FIGURE 24.2 Graphic comparison of tracings from volume-cycled ventilation (peaked wave form) versus time-cycled ventilation (square wave form). In this example, the patient is administered the same tidal volume with both techniques. However, this is achieved with a lower airway pressure using the time-cycled, pressure-limited technique, which allows for a reduction of airway injury from barotrauma.

lation when there is evidence of significant barotrauma. **Extracorporeal membrane oxygenation (ECMO)** has also been used in an attempt to rescue some of these patients; however, its effectiveness in patients with advanced lung injury is not encouraging. Finally, **inhaled nitric oxide** has been shown to relax both the bronchial and pulmonary vascular smooth muscle and improve oxygenation.

SHOCK

Pathophysiology

In children, cardiovascular compromise may have many causes (Table 24.6) that share the common denominator of decreased cardiac output with a resultant decrease in oxygen and substrate delivery to the tissues. **Hypovolemia** is probably the most common cause of shock in the pediatric age group. The next most common cause of shock is **septic or distributive shock** and, finally, **cardiogenic shock.**

Clinical signs and symptoms of shock vary depending on the degree of compensation. **Compensated shock** occurs when patients have been able to maintain adequate cardiac output through compensatory mechanisms that maintain the blood pressure within a normal range. **Decompensated shock** is said to occur when patients are hypotensive and acidotic. If allowed to progress, hypotension, poor peripheral perfusion, altered level of consciousness, and multisystem organ failure may develop. This is classically labeled the "shock state." Therapy for shock is most effective when instituted in the early phases. The mortality rate in shock states increases as the patient progresses from a compensated to a decompensated shock state. Irreversible shock results in multisystem organ failure in which cardiopulmonary failure may be profound. These patients develop subsequent cardiac arrest leading to death.

PICU Management

The keys to successful treatment of shock are rapid recognition, assessment for multiorgan involvement, and the institution of aggressive measures to avoid irreversible shock. Vascular access must be obtained rapidly (Figures 24.3 and 24.4). This may involve an **intraosseous catheter** for initial fluid administration until it is possible to insert a large-bore intravenous line. All patients should be placed on a cardiorespiratory monitor as well as a pulse oximeter, and oxygen should be administered. If patients do not respond to these initial measures, a fluid bolus, vasoactive drugs, or both, should be administered. All of these efforts are directed to support vital organ perfusion. Appropriate laboratory studies are sent to determine the underlying cause, and specific therapy should be started as soon as an etiology is identified. Evaluation of the pulmonary system with arterial blood gases is performed to provide appropriate therapy to correct hypoxemia and hypercapnia. Assessment should be performed for liver dysfunction and bleeding problems that can accompany shock. Coagulation parameters that are abnormal should be corrected with appropriate blood products. If renal failure has been significant, the use of dialysis may be indicated.

HYPOVOLEMIC SHOCK

Hypovolemic shock is the most common cause of shock in children. Loss of circulating blood volume is followed by a series of cardiac and peripheral compensatory adjustments that attempt to restore blood pressure and perfusion to critical organs. The most common causes of hypovolemia in children are vomiting and diarrhea. Patients usually present with a history of fluid

---

TABLE 24.6   Common Causes of Shock in Children

Hypovolemic shock
- Vomiting
- Diarrhea
- Blood loss
- Osmotic diuresis (e.g., diabetes)
- Nephrotic states
- Increased insensible loss (e.g., burns, heat stroke)

Distributive or septic shock
- Sepsis (bacterial or viral)
- Spinal cord injury
- Anaphylaxis
- Drug toxicity

Cardiogenic shock
- Congenital heart disease (especially left-sided obstructive lesions)
- Cardiomyopathies
- After open heart surgery with bypass
- Myocardial ischemia
- Sepsis
- Barbiturate-induced coma
- Mechanical ventilation effects on the myocardium
- Tamponade
- Trauma

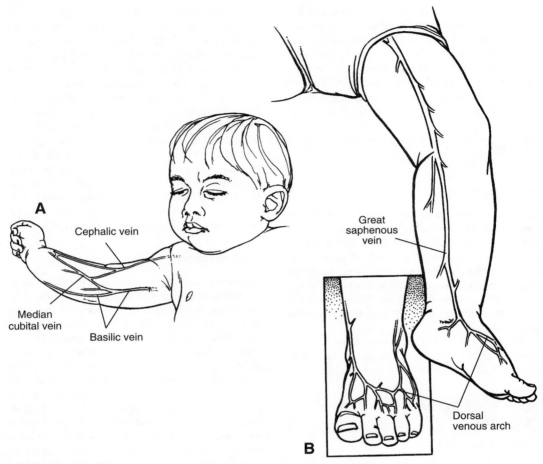

FIGURE 24.3 The various sites commonly used for vascular access in the infant. **A.** Veins of the upper extremity: the cephalic, basilic, and the median cubital veins. **B.** Saphenous veins of the foot. **C** and **D.** Femoral vein and its landmarks as well as the technique commonly used to insert a catheter. **E.** Intraosseous catheter inserted in the tibia.

loss (e.g., severe diarrhea). However, hypovolemic shock may also be a component of **capillary leak injuries,** such as those seen with severe trauma or overwhelming sepsis. Hypotension is a late finding in hypovolemic shock, as blood pressure can usually be maintained during rapid volume loss by an increase in systemic vascular resistance; however, this compensation is at the expense of normal cardiac output. It is not until an approximately 50% loss of circulatory volume that blood pressure decreases below acceptable standards.

Patients with compensated hypovolemic shock usually respond to a rapid bolus (20 ml/kg) of isotonic fluids (normal saline or lactated Ringer's solution). If a patient shows improvement, appropriate fluid replacement is warranted (see Chapter 4, Principles of Pediatric Nutrition, Fluids, and Electrolytes). On occasion, children may require 40–80 ml/kg within the first 4 hours of PICU admission to restore vascular filling pressures and to maintain cardiac output.

If the fluid losses surpass the compensatory ability of the body, the decompensated form of shock occurs, and children develop hypotension, tachycardia, and signs of organ hypoperfusion (decreased urine output, altered state of consciousness). This form of shock requires very aggressive support, which usually surpasses simple fluid administration. Other therapeutic maneuvers include oxygen, correction of the acidosis, and the use of inotropic agents (e.g., catecholamine drips). Central venous access is used for measurement of CVP to assist in fluid management.

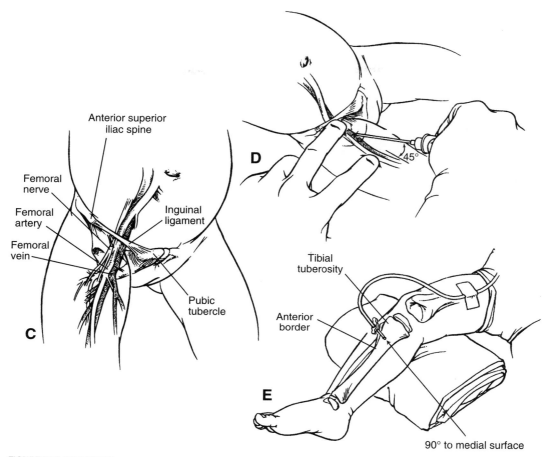

Anterior superior
iliac spine

Femoral
nerve

Femoral
artery

Femoral
vein

Inguinal
ligament

Pubic
tubercle

C

D

45°

Tibial
tuberosity

Anterior
border

E

90° to medial surface

FIGURE 24.3 *(CONTINUED)*

DISTRIBUTIVE SHOCK

Distributive shock results in inadequate tissue perfusion secondary to abnormalities in the distribution of blood flow to various organs. Distributive shock occurs following vasomotor paralysis, with increased venous capacitance, and when physiologic shunts redistribute blood past capillary beds. Chemical mediators play an important role in the pathogenesis of this complex phenomenon. Distributive forms of shock are seen in anaphylaxis, sepsis, and CNS injury. The alterations in hemodynamics in distributive shock are similarly complex. For example, life-threatening infections may be accompanied by depletion of intravascular volume secondary to a capillary leak phenomenon, combined with a marked decrease in cardiac contractility resulting from circulating toxins. Unlike other forms of decreased cardiac output where mixed venous oxygen saturation is decreased, in distributive shock mixed venous oxygen saturation may actually increase reflect-

ing the body's inability to extract oxygen from the capillary bed.

> ### Pediatric Pearl
>
> The mixed venous oxygen saturation is generally a good index of the ratio of systemic oxygen supply and demand. However, in distributive shock, the mixed venous saturation may increase due to the decreased ability of the tissues to extract oxygen.

The basic goals of treatment for distributive shock are the same as in the other forms of shock (i.e., to improve hemodynamics and avoid irreversible shock). Because patients may have both intravascular hypovolemia and alterations in cardiac output, the clinician must focus on these alterations in developing a therapeutic plan. Hypovolemia secondary to capillary leak and the third spacing of fluid requires volume replacement,

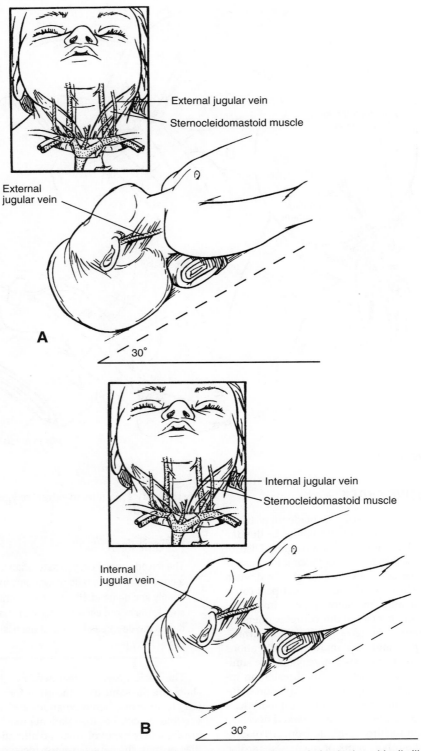

External jugular vein

Sternocleidomastoid muscle

External
jugular vein

30°

A

Internal jugular vein

Sternocleidomastoid muscle

Internal
jugular vein

30°

B

FIGURE 24.4 A and **B.** Some sites used for central venous cannulation in the critically ill child. The veins of the neck include the internal jugular, subclavian, and external jugular. **C** and **D.** Techniques for the cannulation of some of these vessels.

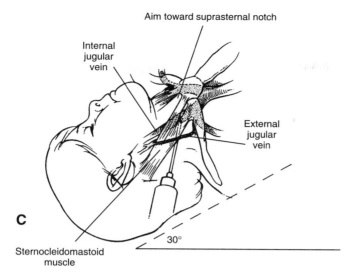

Aim toward suprasternal notch

Internal
jugular
vein

External
jugular
vein

C

Sternocleidomastoid
muscle

30°

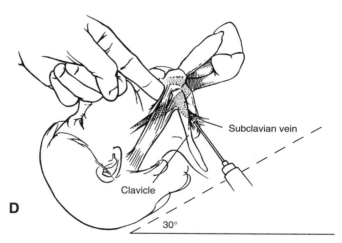

Subclavian vein

Clavicle

D

30°

FIGURE 24.4 *(CONTINUED)*

usually in the form of colloid. The decrease in cardiac output can be reversed with adrenergic inotropic agents such as dopamine, epinephrine, or dobutamine. However, if the systemic vascular resistance is very low, an α-adrenergic agent such as norepinephrine may help.

In the early 1990s, studies in adults with severe septic shock suggested that outcome may be enhanced by increasing cardiac output and oxygen delivery to supranormal values, which implies that pulmonary artery catheters should be widely used. In fact, these catheters are rarely inserted in PICUs. Extensive research has sought agents that can short-circuit various points along the inflammatory cascade. None of these agents have come

into general use. Global suppression of immune function (e.g., with corticosteroids) has been shown to be ineffective. Yet in the past 20 years, survival rates for septic shock and for adult respiratory distress syndrome have improved substantially, most likely benefiting from the maturation of critical care as a medical and nursing discipline.

CARDIOGENIC SHOCK

Cardiogenic shock usually results from a disease process that decreases cardiac function (**contractility**), leading to poor cardiac output. The cause may be a dysrhythmia, a pericardial effusion, a congenital heart defect, an acute infection that affects the myocardium (myocarditis), or one of the cardiomyopathies. Patients who have undergone open heart surgery using cardiopulmonary bypass may also develop transient cardiac dysfunction. This primary pump failure results in an inability to deliver oxygen and substrates to meet the metabolic demands of the body. These patients have tachycardia, a metabolic acidosis, and cool extremities, as systemic vascular resistance is elevated. The mixed venous oxygen saturation (< 65%) and the index of oxygen extraction obtained from a pulmonary artery catheter are below normal.

The treatment for cardiogenic shock is directed toward increasing cardiac contractility. Oxygen should be administered to correct systemic hypoxemia. Acidosis should be corrected, and although usually predominantly metabolic in nature, mechanical ventilation may be of help, particularly because it also reduces the oxygen demands of breathing. Pharmacologic agents that increase cardiac contractility and reduce afterload are used to improve cardiac output (Table 24.7). Finally, temporary mechanical support of the circulation may be instituted. A "cardiac" ECMO circuit can provide partial bypass via a veno-venous route if oxygenation is not at issue. **Left ventricular assist devices,** which are external pumps whose influx and efflux ports are implanted directly in one or both ventricles, greatly augment cardiac output. Some devices are portable enough to allow easy ambulation. These mechanical devices should only be used if there exists a reasonable chance for recovery (e.g., ECMO for "cardiac stun" after heart surgery) or transplantation (e.g., left ventricular assist devices for dilated cardiomyopathy).

TABLE 24.7 | **Therapy for Shock**

Volume Replacement

Crystalloids: Ringer's lactate or normal saline
- Are used to replace external fluid losses (vomiting, diarrhea) or third spacing due to burns, injury, and sepsis
- 20–60 ml/kg may be required in the first 1–2 hours
- Are relatively inefficient volume expanders when compared with others with a higher oncotic pressure
- May move outside the vascular space within 30 minutes

Colloids: albumin 5%, fresh frozen plasma (FFP), blood, or limit dextrans
- 10–20 ml/kg
- Help to restore the vascular compartment faster, may provide for clotting factors and increased oxygen-carrying capacity when blood is used

Inotropic and Afterload Reduction Therapy

- Oxygen, calcium, and correction of the acidosis
- Inotropic agents shift to a new position on the Frank-Starling curve

Drug	Dose (μg/kg/min)	Effects
Dopamine	2–5	Vasodilator, especially in splanchnic and renal vessels, promotes diuresis
	5–10	Increases inotropic state of heart; causes moderate tachycardia and peripheral vasoconstriction
	10–30	Produces both inotropic and chronotropic effects plus strong vasoconstriction
Dobutamine	1–15	Mostly inotropic activity; potent vasodilator
Epinephrine	0.05–0.2	Chronotropic and inotropic; reserved for when patient has very low systemic vascular resistance
	> 0.2	Vasoconstrictor
Norepinephrine	0.01–1.0	Potent vasoconstrictor
Nitroprusside	0.05–4.0	Potent vasodilator used in hypertensive crises or as an afterload reducer in cardiogenic shock
Nitroglycerin	0.05–4.0	Potent vasodilator; used in pulmonary hypertensive crises
PGE_1	0.05–0.1	Potent arterial dilator used in newborns to maintain patency of the ductus arteriosus in ductal-dependent cardiac defects; may be used as a pulmonary vasodilator

PGE_1 = prostaglandin E_1.

NEUROLOGIC INTENSIVE CARE

Examples of neurologic injury requiring intensive care include asphyxial injuries such as **near-drowning** or **near-miss sudden infant death syndrome (SIDS), CNS trauma,** conditions resulting from **status epilepticus,** and **coma** after **drug ingestions** or from metabolic disorders such as **Reye syndrome**. Neurologic intensive care differs considerably from other forms of PICU management, not only because failure may result in death, but because survivors may persist in a vegetative coma state or have severe neurologic dysfunction either due to the primary etiologic event or a secondary brain injury.

The major focus of neurologic intensive care is to minimize the effects of the primary injury and to avoid secondary injury. In the initial assessment and management of children with neurologic injury, the focus is on the ABCs of resuscitation (**airway, breathing,** and **circulation**). After appropriate interventions have taken place to avoid hypoxemia and hypotension, a quick yet thorough neurologic examination is performed. For this purpose of rapid neurologic assessment, the **Glasgow Coma Scale** is a simple, reproducible tool that also has some prognostic value. A score of less than 9 is suggestive of severe injury; these patients may require further imaging tests [computed tomography (CT) or magnetic resonance imaging (MRI)], airway support and respiratory monitoring, and possibly intracranial pressure monitoring. The Glasgow Coma Scale can be used as a tool for repeated patient evaluations, both in the emergency room and in the PICU. The Glasgow Coma Scale is usually modified when used for assessing infants and toddlers. It is important to note that pharmacologic agents such as anticonvulsants, analgesics, or muscle relaxants used to facilitate intubation modify the neurologic assessment.

HEAD TRAUMA

Once patients have been stabilized and an initial neurologic assessment performed, further evaluation is made to determine if a life-threatening situation requiring surgical intervention, such as an intracranial hemorrhage, exists. This evaluation is usually performed in collaboration with both a general surgeon and a neurosurgeon. The general surgeon is responsible for ensuring that intra-abdominal or intrathoracic lesions are not responsible for the patient's altered mental condition. This evaluation is often aided by the use of head and body CT imaging. However, before patients are moved to the scanner, it is the pediatric intensivist's responsibility to ensure that they are adequately oxygenated and ventilated as well as hemodynamically stable. While in the scanner, patients should be monitored to avoid the potential for secondary injury.

In children, most serious head injuries are nonpenetrating. These result most often from falls, although "**shaken baby syndrome,**" a form of child abuse, can also produce significant intracranial injury. Less than 25% of these traumatic injuries produce significant intracranial hematomas that necessitate neurosurgical intervention. However, injuries may be so severe that small deep intracerebral hemorrhages occur secondary to the tearing of small blood vessels deep in the brain parenchyma. Rapid movement of the brain can also result in the shearing of axons, leading to diffuse brain swelling. This injury is more common in children and may result in increased intracranial pressure and secondary brain injury.

INCREASED INTRACRANIAL PRESSURE

Depending on the cause of acute neurologic deterioration, different approaches to PICU management may be indicated. If **increased intracranial pressure** is a potential problem, then an intracranial pressure monitoring device should be placed by a neurosurgeon. Children may be placed in a drug-induced coma to facilitate ventilatory management and to help reduce intracranial pressure. In this situation, continuous electroencephalogram (EEG) monitoring may be performed, allowing titration of medication to an electrical therapeutic end point.

Other specific neurologic management techniques to decrease intracranial pressure include hyperventilation, fluid restriction, altering patient position in the bed, diuresis, and appropriate use of analgesics. Hyperventilation has been used to decrease the $PaCO_2$ from a normal of 40 mm Hg to 25–30 mm Hg, resulting in vasoconstriction of the cerebral vasculature and a reduction of cerebral blood flow to about 50% of normal. This level of cerebral blood flow is sufficient to avoid ischemia, yet diminishes the contribution that increased blood flow may have to the total volume in the intracranial vault and the increased intracranial pressure. After 24–48 hours of hyperventilation, intracranial blood flow may normalize. There is evidence that profound hyperventilation has little effect beyond this time. For this reason, hyperventilation is usually reserved for acute and abrupt elevations in intracranial pressure.

The use of pharmacologic agents such as barbiturates, calcium channel blockers, and lidocaine to lower intracranial pressure are often necessary adjuncts to the care of these critically ill children. When using these agents, the clinician must have a clear understanding of their significant side effects, especially on the cardiovascular system. Although the results of various clinical and experimental studies do not demonstrate a clear neurologic benefit from these agents, they do decrease intracranial pressure and are useful for that purpose.

Fluid management and diuretics are another important component in the treatment of increased intracranial pressure. The injured brain may develop a capillary leak syndrome and a propensity to retain fluid, resulting in increased cerebral edema and significant secondary injury. By decreasing total body water content and increasing serum osmolarity, a gradient is established between the intracellular compartment and the extracellular compartment that draws fluid out of the cells and thereby reduces the potential for cerebral edema formation. Thus, patients should be fluid restricted to 50%—60% of maintenance if hemodynamically stable. Some patients may require inotropic support in order to maintain blood pressure in an appropriate range. Diuretic therapy may be of help in keeping the CVP between 0 and 2 mm Hg and the serum osmolarity between 295 and 320 mOsm. Aggressive treatment for patients with increased intracranial pressure is continued until the pressure returns to the normal range for at least 24 hours. The clinician can then begin weaning patients off diuretics, hyperventilation, and barbiturates. The intracranial pressure monitoring device is removed once patients no longer require it.

STATUS EPILEPTICUS

Status epilepticus (or "status") refers to the severest form of seizure activity lasting more than 30 minutes. Before a detailed workup, the intensivist must ensure that the ABCs of resuscitation are addressed. Children with severe status are at risk for losing patency of their airways and developing aspiration pneumonia or apnea. Other systemic complications of status epilepticus include blood pressure instability (early hypertension, late hypotension), hypoxia, hypercarbia, acidosis, hyperthermia, electrolyte abnormalities, and an increase in cerebral blood flow and cerebral oxygen consumption.

Once the emergency ABC assessments have been made, the intensivist then focuses on trying to stop the seizure activity. This is most commonly accomplished with intravenous anticonvulsants such as diazepam or lorazepam. If the seizure continues, a longer acting anticonvulsant such as phenytoin or phenobarbital can be used. Phenytoin is very effective in controlling tonic–clonic seizures in children. However, it has a relatively low lipid solubility and therefore may take 10–30 minutes before an effect is seen. Recently fosphenytoin, which is claimed to be gentler on veins during administration, has begun to replace phenytoin. However, rapid administration of either can induce severe cardiac depression. Phenobarbital is the least lipid soluble of these agents and therefore has the slowest onset of action, although in status epilepticus its activity may be enhanced as a result of changes in blood pH and blood pressure.

If the seizure activity persists despite the use of these agents, a more aggressive approach is indicated. In this situation, the goal of therapy is not only stopping the seizures but also preventing secondary brain injury. Therapeutic maneuvers are designed to enhance cerebral protection by reducing cerebral metabolism. Pharmacologic agents including a general inhalational anesthetic or a short-acting barbiturate may be useful. Therapy at this level usually requires the combined expertise of a pediatric neurologist, an intensivist, and possibly a neurosurgeon. These patients may require an intracranial pressure monitoring device if increased pressure is implicated in causing the seizures. Continuous EEG monitoring is also useful in regulating cerebral protective therapy. These pharmacologic agents also have adverse effects on cardiovascular dynamics, and thus cardiac output needs to be monitored. Other agents that may be useful include intravenous lidocaine (1–2 mg/kg/hr) or rectal paraldehyde (0.15 ml/kg of a 4% solution; however, paraldehyde is no longer available in the United States).

METABOLIC ENCEPHALOPATHIES

Metabolic encephalopathies and **Reye syndrome** represent a third group of neurologic emergencies that often require PICU admission. Although there are many causes of toxic–metabolic encephalopathies in childhood (Table 24.8), Reye syndrome is the one that has had the most significant impact on pediatric neurologic intensive care. Reye syndrome is an acute hepatoencephalopathy that is usually preceded by a viral infection (usually varicella or influenza) and is more common in children who are receiving salicylates. It results in

TABLE 24.8 Causes of Encephalopathies in Childhood

Congenital or inherited conditions

Perinatal asphyxia
Hypoglycemia
Inborn errors of metabolism
Aminoacidurias
Organic acidemias
Hyperammonemia
Storage diseases
Degenerative neurologic diseases

Infections

Meningitis (bacterial and viral)
Brain abscess

Trauma

Cerebral vascular injuries

Organ failure

Hepatic failure (Reye syndrome)
Uremia

Disorders of electrolytes and minerals

Hypercalcemia
Hypernatremia
Water intoxication
Vitamin A toxicity

Ingestions

Mushrooms
Lead poisoning

acute hepatic dysfunction with marked elevations in serum transaminases, serum ammonia, and abnormalities of coagulation studies. Signs of increased intracranial pressure develop, although if the increased intracranial pressure is managed aggressively, the chances for full recovery are excellent. As with trauma and status epilepticus, if the clinician focuses on the ABCs, guarantees adequate substrate delivery to the brain, and intervenes to decrease intracranial pressure, secondary brain injury can be minimized.

SUGGESTED READINGS

Bardella IJ: Pediatric advanced life support: A review of the AHA recommendations. American Heart Association. *Am Fam Physician* 60(6):1743–1750, 1999. (n.b. erratum in *Am Fam Physician* 1:61(9):2614, 2000.)

Derish MT: Unconventional forms of respiratory support. In *Nelson Textbook of Pediatrics,* 16th ed. Edited by Behrman RE, Kleigman RM, Jenson HB. Philadelphia, WB Saunders, 2000, pp 275–276.

DiCarlo JV, Frankel LR: Neurologic stabilization. In *Nelson Textbook of Pediatrics,* 16th ed. Edited by Behrman RE, Kleigman RM, Jenson HB. Philadelphia, WB Saunders, 2000, pp 272–273.

Frankel LR, Mathers LH: Shock. In *Nelson Textbook of Pediatrics,* 16th ed. Edited by Behrman RE, Kleigman RM, Jenson HB. Philadelphia, WB Saunders, 2000, pp 262–266.

McIntyre RC Jr, Pulido EJ, Bensard DD, et al: Thirty years of clinical trials in acute respiratory distress syndrome. *Crit Care Med* 28(9):3314–3331, 2000.

Ostermann ME, Keenan SP, Seiferling RA, et al: Sedation in the intensive care unit: A systematic review. *JAMA* 283(11):1451–1459 2000.

Rogers M, Nichols DG (eds): *Textbook of Pediatric Intensive Care,* 3rd ed. Baltimore, Williams & Wilkins, 1996.

Chapter 25

Pediatric Surgery

Gary E. Hartman and
Rebecca Evangelista

PREOPERATIVE MANAGEMENT

The principles of preoperative evaluation and management of children are similar to those of adults. Important differences are dictated by the age of the child, the condition prompting the operation, whether the operation is elective or emergent, and the presence of coexisting congenital anomalies or physiologic derangement.

ELECTIVE SURGERY

The most common elective surgical procedures in children are repair of **inguinal hernia, orchiopexy,** and **myringotomy** (placement of ear tubes) for chronic or recurrent otitis media. More than 70% of these procedures are currently performed on an outpatient basis. General anesthesia is used in all major and most minor procedures on children, unlike in adults. It is essential that preoperative evaluation focus on detecting conditions that increase the risk of general anesthesia.

Clinical and Laboratory Evaluation

History
The clinician should obtain a complete history of previous problems with general anesthesia for both the patient and patient's family members. Prematurity, especially with a history of apnea, presents a special concern because of the increased risk of **postanesthetic apnea**. The incidence of life-threatening apnea is greatest during the first 24 hours following general anesthesia and mandates in-hospital respiratory monitoring for patients at high risk. Most authorities consider infants to be high risk if they are (1) currently on home apnea monitors or (2) less than 52–60 weeks total conceptual age (gestational age at birth plus postnatal age). Recent or current upper respiratory infection also increases the risk of general anesthesia and should prompt delay of an elective procedure until the infection is clearly resolved.

Knowledge of a **congenital cardiac defect** is important for proper physiologic management as well as the opportunity to administer preoperative prophylactic antibiotics to prevent bacterial endocarditis. Obtaining a complete history of **drug allergy** or sensitivity is always extremely important. Specific inquiries of inpatients with myelodysplasia and congenital urinary tract malformation regarding sensitivity to latex is essential. Severe, potentially fatal allergic reactions, or anaphylaxis, associated with latex are common in these patients.

Physical Examination
It is necessary to perform a careful, complete physical examination in an attempt to detect anomalies not yet clinically apparent that may compromise the performance of or recovery from the proposed operation. In addition to concentrating on the area of surgical interest, the physical examination should focus on cardiorespiratory function. In most cases, clinical evidence of **upper respiratory tract infection** (rhinorrhea, cough), particularly **lower respiratory tract involvement** (abnormal breath sounds, wheezing), should result in postponement of the procedure. Presence of a **cardiac murmur** discovered during a preoperative evaluation warrants a full cardiac evaluation (see Chapter 13). As previously mentioned, prophylaxis against bacterial endocarditis (penicillin, ampicillin plus gentamicin) should be instituted based on the organisms likely to be encountered in the specific operative field involved.

Laboratory Evaluation
The need for routine laboratory studies is usually quite limited. In the past, most hospitals required every patient entering the operating room to have a minimum of a complete blood count (CBC), urinalysis, and chest radiograph. A routine preoperative chest radiograph, in the absence of pulmonary or cardiac symptoms, is no longer recommended because of the extremely low incidence of anomaly detection. Most centers no longer require mandatory laboratory examinations for elective operative procedures unless there is clinical suspicion of an abnormality. However, it is necessary to obtain a hematocrit if the patient appears anemic and a type and cross-match if blood loss is possible. Preoper-

ative autologous or directed blood donation may be appropriate if significant blood loss is anticipated.

General Management

On the day of surgery, all centers require that patients refrain from ingesting solids or liquids for some time prior to the operation. This helps reduce acidity and volume of gastric contents in an effort to decrease the risk of aspiration during induction of anesthesia. In children, this time has been shortened to 6–8 hours for solids and 2 hours for clear liquids. If major gastrointestinal (GI) procedures are planned, most surgeons restrict oral intake for 8–12 hours prior to the operation. A bath with antibacterial soap the evening before the operation significantly reduces bacterial colonization and the risk of infection. Shaving is rarely necessary in children; if necessary, it should be performed in the operating room.

EMERGENCY SURGERY

If the surgical condition is such that an elective operation is not possible, any physiologic derangement that increases the risk of general anesthesia or of the procedure itself should be corrected provided that the procedure is not unduly delayed. In patients requiring emergency surgery, attention must be directed at correcting hemodynamic, respiratory, GI, and metabolic derangements.

Hemodynamic Abnormalities

Hemodynamic abnormalities are usually the result of hypovolemia, primarily from loss of fluid and occasionally from loss of blood. Correction of hypovolemia with isotonic fluid or blood is critical to prevent cardiovascular collapse from the vasodilation that accompanies the administration of anesthesia. It is necessary to replace fluids, as in dehydration (see Chapter 4).

Respiratory Conditions

Newborns and young children are more dependent on diaphragmatic function for adequate ventilation than older children and adults. Support with supplemental oxygen may be warranted in patients with hemodynamic instability. Severe abdominal distention resulting from intestinal obstruction, ileus, or intraperitoneal fluid may compromise respiratory status. Children may require intubation and assisted ventilation prior to surgery.

Pediatric Pearl

It is necessary to maintain a low threshold for assisted ventilation, particularly in young infants.

Gastrointestinal Dysfunction

GI dysfunction is nearly universal in seriously ill children regardless of whether the pathology is intra-abdominal. It is necessary to institute nasogastric tube placement and suction early during resuscitation to reduce the risk of aspiration and respiratory embarrassment caused by intestinal distention. If the distention or condition is not severe enough to warrant a nasogastric tube, children should at least be given nothing by mouth (NPO) if the need for urgent operation is a possibility.

Metabolic Abnormalities

Metabolic abnormalities are primarily related to fluid losses that result in hypokalemic alkalosis after repeated vomiting or metabolic acidosis secondary to hypovolemia. Fever can trigger seizure activity in young children and may rise precipitously with general anesthesia. It is necessary to attempt to control temperatures higher than 38.5°C during the preparation for operation using either rectal acetaminophen or a tepid sponge bath. Other metabolic abnormalities may be due to associated medical conditions and may require substantial effort to correct without causing excessive delay of the operation.

POSTOPERATIVE MANAGEMENT: RESPONSES TO SURGERY

Stress Response

The considerations in managing children following an operation are similar to those in preoperative management with the caveat that they are superimposed on the background of a different physiologic state (i.e., that of the **stress response**) [Figure 25.1]. The concept of the stress response refers to the physiologic alterations that follow significant injury (accidental or operative) or severe infection. Studies over many decades have documented the existence of the stress response in adults. Physiologic studies in newborns and young children have only recently confirmed the occurrence of a similar response in young individuals, although it is clinically apparent. The magnitude of this response is related to the magnitude of the injury and the severity of any accompanying infection.

A constellation of events, including **fever, pituitary and stress hormone elaboration,** and **increased acute phase protein synthesis,** characterize the stress response (see Figure 25.1). Patients are "hyperdynamic" and catabolic. Increases in heart rate and blood pressure are due to increased core temperature and elevated levels of catecholamines. Sodium conservation and water conservation are driving priorities that result in elevated levels of **antidiuretic hormone, renin–angiotensin,** and **aldosterone**. Increasing amounts of available fuel meet the increased metabolic demands, with elevation of **corticosteroids** and **glucagon** and decreased levels of and sensitivity to **insulin**.

Recognizing the stress response is important because the definition of "normal" parameters for **heart rate, blood pressure, serum glucose,** and **urine volume** must be interpreted based on the phase of the stress response. Modest elevations of blood pressure are likely due to a catecholamine surge–induced increase in peripheral vascular resistance and should not be considered abnormal or a requirement for antihypertensive therapy. Similarly, serum glucose immediately after a major operation is commonly in the range of 250–300 mg/dl and falls naturally within 6–8 hours.

Hemodynamic Abnormalities

Hypovolemia, the most common hemodynamic abnormality in children following an operation, continues for some time following the procedure. Fluid loss, which occurs during surgery from exposure of the peritoneal or pleural surfaces, is usually of extracellular fluid. Replacement with isotonic solutions is necessary. Urine volume, which is decreased as a result of elevated antidiuretic hormone, is no longer an adequate single monitor of intravascular volume status. It is necessary to monitor heart rate, peripheral perfusion, acid–base status, serial hematocrit, and mental status all for proper volume assessment. Frequent physical examinations are crucial.

Pediatric Pearl

Reliance on hemodynamic parameters such as central venous pressure or pulmonary artery wedge pressure should never replace physical examination.

In the setting of severe sepsis or myocardial dysfunction, the use of inotropic drugs such as dopamine or dobutamine may improve hemodynamic performance. Clinicians should neither use these agents instead of or before adequate volume replacement nor should they use them solely to achieve a normal blood pressure. Adequate tissue perfusion, not mean arterial blood pressure, is the major barometer of resuscitation.

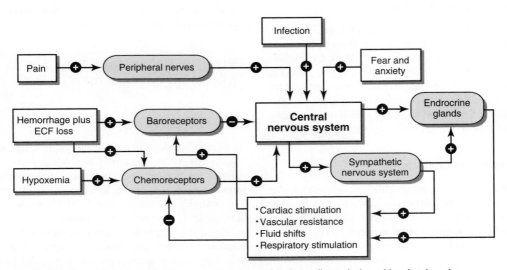

FIGURE 25.1. Stress response. Overview of the neuroendocrine reflexes induced by shock and trauma. ECF = extracellular fluid.

Respiratory Response

In addition to any respiratory compromise imposed by the condition requiring operation, both general anesthesia and an abdominal or thoracic incision can further exacerbate respiratory dysfunction. General anesthesia produces **respiratory ciliary paralysis** lasting 24 hours or more. This ciliary dysfunction combined with airway dehydration and decreased cough and respiratory excursion due to discomfort impairs clearance of airway secretions leading to atelectasis and mucous plugging. Adequate analgesia, humidified oxygen, respiratory effort, and mobilization minimize these problems. Prolonged effects of anesthesia, aspiration pneumonia, and hemodynamic instability are the primary reasons for assisted ventilation in postoperative children.

In neonates, the primary indications for ventilatory support are (1) excessive abdominal wall tension resulting from closure of abdominal wall defects and (2) risk of pulmonary hypertension associated with congenital diaphragmatic hernia. After repair of abdominal wall defects, the decreased compliance resulting from the tight abdominal wall requires ventilatory pressures significantly higher than would normally be necessary. As the abdominal wall gradually relaxes, the inflation pressures can be returned to more standard levels to prevent hyperinflation or barotrauma.

Gastrointestinal Response

Paralytic ileus accompanies nearly every major operation in children. The duration of the ileus depends on the magnitude of intestinal dysfunction present preoperatively, the magnitude and type of operative procedure, and the presence of any intervening complications. The ileus characteristically resolves in the small bowel first, then stomach, and then colon. Although return of bowel sounds is an encouraging sign, the passage of flatus and stool herald true resolution of the ileus.

Nasogastric decompression remains an important tool in postoperative management of children, especially young children who may swallow large amounts of air while crying or sucking on a thumb or pacifier. Single-lumen tubes offer the advantage of a large lumen but can become obstructed by mucus or gastric mucosa when placed on continuous suction. For this reason, intermittent suction is preferred and patency can be maintained by frequent irrigation with a small volume of saline. Double-lumen or sump tubes are specifically designed for continuous suction but the suction lumen size is limited because of the additional sump lumen, and

they are particularly prone to obstruction. Any tube placed across the gastroesophageal junction increases the risk of gastroesophageal reflux and aspiration. Therefore, the tubes should remain in place only as long as necessary and should be kept maximally functional.

Metabolic or Nutritional Response

The postoperative neuroendocrine milieu produces predictable alterations in the metabolism of electrolytes and energy sources. **Serum sodium** falls as a result of increased antidiuretic hormone levels and sodium losses through the GI tract. This tendency is aggravated if excessive amounts of hypotonic fluid are used for resuscitation or maintenance fluid. **Serum glucose** is predictably elevated immediately following an operation but should fall within 6–8 hours. Normal amounts of glucose, 4–6 mg/kg/min, can be infused on return from the operating room in all but extreme cases. Insulin administration in nondiabetic children causes a precipitous fall in serum glucose and is dangerous in the immediate postoperative period.

The stress response is characterized by increased secretion of catabolic hormones. Presumably, this provides glucose and amino acids to the area of injury in adequate amounts. The body's ability to induce **positive nitrogen balance** during the early recovery phase has commanded great attention. It is now well documented that adults and older children can be driven into positive nitrogen balance within 24 hours after surgery. What is not clear is whether this is desirable. Available studies in adults suggest that in previously well-nourished patients, the infectious complications of parenteral nutrition equal or outweigh any metabolic benefits. However, patients with significant acute weight loss (20%–25%) may benefit from early nutrition. In previously well-nourished patients who are expected to ingest near-normal enteral calories by 7 days after the operation, the risks of parenteral nutrition are probably not justified.

COMMON PEDIATRIC SURGICAL CONDITIONS

ACUTE ABDOMINAL PAIN

Pathophysiology

Abdominal pain is classified as **visceral, somatic,** or **referred**. Visceral pain fibers are located in the muscular wall of the hollow viscera and in the capsule of solid organs. They respond to changes in geometry, primarily stretch, and their threshold is lowered by inflammation and ischemia. Visceral pain is transported via the autonomic nervous system and is perceived as dull, aching, or cramping. Because this pain is transmitted via bilateral fibers of the sympathetic system, it is perceived in the midline. The location of the pain is related to the embryologic origin of the involved viscera. Structures of foregut origin produce epigastric pain, structures of midgut origin produce periumbilical pain, and structures of hindgut origin produce lower abdominal visceral pain.

Visceral pain from the hollow viscera is due to distention or disordered motility caused by intestinal obstruction, gastroenteritis, or ureteral or biliary calculi. Visceral capsules of the solid organs may be stretched by passive congestion or hemorrhage. Although visceral pain is usually the earliest sign of an intra-abdominal process, it is nonspecific and frequently associated with nonbilious reflex vomiting.

Somatic pain is the type of pain that arises from the abdominal wall and parietal peritoneum. It is mediated by the spinal nerves that innervate the abdominal wall and enter the spinal cord through the dorsal root ganglia. Somatic pain, which is stimulated by changes in pH or temperature that may accompany chemical or bacterial inflammation, is sharp or pricking and generally constant. More localized than visceral pain, somatic pain is usually perceived in one of the four abdominal quadrants: right lower and upper and left lower and upper. To determine its cause, the clinician must be familiar with the organs located in each of the quadrants and their pathologic processes.

Referred pain is the term used when pain is perceived in an area of the body other than the site of its origin. It occurs because afferent neurons arising from different sites have shared central pathways. Irritation of the left hemidiaphragm (levels C3, C4, and C5) by blood from a ruptured spleen may be associated with pain in the left shoulder because of the somatic innervation of the shoulder by the same nerve roots. Knowledge of the patterns of referred pain can assist in diagnosis in cases with equivocal or confusing abdominal findings.

In children, the most common cause of acute abdominal pain requiring surgical intervention is **appendicitis** (see Chapter 15). Obstruction of the appendiceal lumen by inspissated stool is the initial pathophysiologic event. This is associated with visceral pain perceived in the periumbilical region because of the midgut origin of the appendix. As the intraluminal pressure increases, the blood supply to the wall of the appendix is compromised, producing necrosis and eventual perforation. Inflammation of the appendix progresses to involve the parietal peritoneum, which produces somatic pain in the right lower quadrant. Perforation with spillage of fecal material and bacteria results in generalized peritonitis with diffuse abdominal pain and toxemia.

Clinical and Laboratory Evaluation (Figure 25.2)

History

The duration, location, and intensity of abdominal pain are essential features of the history. Colicky pain is usually due to hyperperistalsis (e.g., in intestinal obstruction or attempted passage of ureteral or biliary calculi). Constant pain is usually visceral in origin. Location of the pain is helpful in narrowing the diagnostic possibilities, particularly with somatic pain. If pain is localized to one quadrant of the abdomen, the organs in that quadrant and their disease processes determine the likely diagnosis. Vomiting preceding the pain, especially in association with diarrhea, favors gastroenteritis over appendicitis. Vomiting associated with early appendicitis is reflex in nature and usually follows the onset of pain. Appendicitis proceeds to perforation within 72 hours of onset of symptoms; therefore, visceral pain lasting longer than 3 days is rarely due to appendicitis. Progression of the pain from a periumbilical to a right lower quadrant location is classic for appendicitis. It represents the progression from visceral to somatic pain, a progression highly suggestive of a surgical condition.

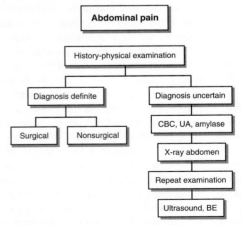

FIGURE 25.2. Flow diagram for diagnostic evaluation of children with acute abdominal pain. BE = barium enema; CBC = complete blood count; UA = urinalysis.

In evaluating children with abdominal pain, it is important to question patients or parents specifically about symptoms related to other abdominal organ systems (genitourinary, hepatobiliary, pancreatic). Flank pain, dysuria, urethral discharge, menstrual cycle, or menstrual abnormalities are important historical points.

Diarrhea may be a symptom of **viral gastroenteritis; inflammatory bowel disease;** or, occasionally, **appendicitis.** In gastroenteritis or infectious enterocolitis, diarrhea is frequent, large in volume, and foul smelling. Children with appendicitis may have frequent, small-volume loose stools as a result of irritation of the sigmoid colon from the inflamed appendix.

Knowledge of preexisting conditions is also important because other nonsurgical conditions such as **sickle cell disease** and **porphyria** can cause abdominal pain. **Nephrotic syndrome** is associated with a significant incidence of abdominal pain from **primary bacterial peritonitis** requiring antibiotics but not surgery.

Physical Examination

Inspection of the patient and the abdomen reveals important diagnostic clues. Appendicitis with local or generalized peritonitis causes the child to lie still, frequently with the thighs flexed and the knees elevated. Movement increases the pain because of the inflamed peritoneum and abdominal wall. Colicky pain associated with intestinal hyperperistalsis or ureteral or biliary obstruction causes the child to writhe in agony and frequently assume a knee–chest position in an attempt to minimize the discomfort. It is essential to interpret the results of auscultation, an important part of the abdominal examination, in light of the clinical context. Bowel sounds are categorized according to frequency and pitch. Hyperactive bowel sounds are related to hyperperistalsis as seen in gastroenteritis or the early stages of appendicitis. Hypoactive bowel sounds indicate decreased peristalsis, which is typical for paralytic ileus associated with sepsis or the peritonitis resulting from a perforated appendix.

Palpation is frequently the most important portion of the abdominal examination. The goal of palpation is to detect direct tenderness associated with inflammation of the abdominal wall and peritoneum. It is important to gain the child's confidence with a slow, cautious manner. Distraction of the child with conversation while the examining hand is gently palpating each quadrant is a useful strategy. Resistance of the abdominal wall muscles to palpation signifies irritation of the parietal peritoneum from underlying inflammation.

Rebound tenderness refers to pain elicited by induced movement of the abdominal wall. The most sensitive method of detecting rebound tenderness is by gentle percussion in each quadrant.

Pediatric Pearl

The combination of direct and rebound tenderness is a powerful indication of an underlying inflammatory process, usually one that requires surgical intervention.

Rectal or pelvic examination is necessary to complete the physical evaluation of abdominal pain. The information gained by rectal examination includes the presence or absence of fecal impaction or constipation, rectal wall tenderness, and a palpable mass in the right perirectal fossa or adnexal regions. In sexually active girls, the pelvic examination is directed at detecting adnexal masses or evidence of sexually transmitted diseases (STDs) that cause **pelvic inflammatory disease.** Prepubertal girls may have an imperforate hymen, producing abdominal pain when the initial menses accumulates in the vaginal and endometrial canals. This condition manifests as a bulging hymen with blood behind it.

Laboratory Evaluation

Laboratory studies often are not helpful in establishing the diagnosis of appendicitis. However, they are important in excluding other conditions that may mimic appendicitis or other acute surgical conditions. A CBC is routine. An elevated white blood cell (WBC) count with a left shift neither confirms nor excludes appendicitis. In fact, appendicitis commonly occurs in the face of a normal WBC count. Anemia, especially microangiopathic anemia with thrombocytopenia, is highly suggestive of **hemolytic-uremic syndrome,** which may manifest as severe abdominal pain (see Chapter 20, ACUTE AND CHRONIC RENAL FAILURE). Similarly, sickle cell anemia is associated with abdominal pain resulting from visceral infarctions or abdominal pain crises. Thrombocytosis may be a sign of **Henoch-Schönlein purpura** (see Chapter 20).

Urinalysis is crucial if urinary symptoms are present or if the pain is lateral or flank in location. Appendicitis may be associated with a mild pyuria or hematuria of 20–30 cells/high power field but should not be associated with bacteriuria. Proteinuria and microscopic hematuria are found frequently in hemolytic-uremic syndrome and Henoch-Schönlein purpura. Serum amylase and liver function tests are appropriate in children with abdominal trauma or if the pain is epigastric or radiates to the back.

Radiography is not necessary if a diagnosis is secure on the basis of the history and clinical examination. If the diagnosis is in doubt, plain abdominal radiographs, ultrasound, computed tomography (CT), or occasionally barium enema may be helpful. It is appropriate to evaluate supine and upright films of the abdomen for severe constipation, fecalith, ileus or small bowel obstruction pattern, and pneumoperitoneum. Calcified fecaliths are present in 20% of children with appendicitis. Pneumoperitoneum is rare. Ultrasound has been used to augment clinical examination with good reliability. However, because the results must be interpreted with clinical suspicion, false-positive and false-negative rates are approximately 10%. Ultrasound is particularly helpful in girls in whom tubo-ovarian anomalies may simulate appendicitis and in young children with perforated appendicitis. Rapid CT with "triple contrast" (enteral, intravenous, rectal) has accuracy rates equal to skilled ultrasonography and is used in many centers in preference to ultrasound. With the improvements in ultrasonography and CT, barium enema is rarely needed in diagnosing appendicitis but is helpful, particularly in cases of inflammatory bowel disease.

☀ Pediatric Pearl

It is necessary to obtain plain radiographs of the chest if children have a history of cough or significant upper respiratory infection. **Right lower lobe pneumonia** is a well-known cause of abdominal pain that is sometimes strikingly similar to appendicitis.

Differential Diagnosis

The differential diagnosis of acute abdominal pain includes a number of conditions (Table 25.1). It is critical to distinguish between conditions that require a surgical solution and those that resolve spontaneously or with nonoperative measures. Most children with acute abdominal pain are ultimately labeled as suffering from gastroenteritis or abdominal pain of unknown origin. Appendicitis is the most common surgical condition producing abdominal pain in children.

Occasionally, after the initial examination, and laboratory and imaging studies, diagnosis of the abdominal pain is still uncertain (see Figure 25.2). In such cases, the most reliable method of excluding a surgical condition involves admission for intravenous hydration and serial examination by the same observers. Progression of pain, especially with the development of direct abdominal tenderness and muscular rigidity, is the most reliable indicator of a process requiring operative treatment. Resolution of pain and resumption of oral intake while under observation are the most reliable signs that the child is not in need of surgery.

Management

Conditions that require operative therapy include **appendicitis, Meckel diverticulitis,** and **torsion of the ovary or omentum**. Removal of a nonperforated appendix may involve conventional laparotomy or laparoscopic techniques. Perioperative antibiotics are usually warranted, although there is some controversy as to their necessity. Recovery from the associated ileus is usually prompt, and in most children, discharge follows 2–4 days after the operation. Perforated appendicitis is much more complicated, requiring 7–10 days of broad-spectrum antibiotics. A prolonged ileus requiring nasogastric suction and intravenous hydration may be necessary. Drains are used for well-formed abscesses and in some centers for all children with perforated appendicitis.

Meckel diverticulitis, which is clinically indistinguishable from appendicitis, requires resection of the involved intestine followed by anastomosis. Again, nasogastric suction and intravenous hydration are necessary for 2–5 days along with antibiotics. Recovery from resection of an infarcted ovary or segment of omentum is

TABLE 25.1	Most Frequent Causes of Abdominal Pain in Children by Age Group
Preschool	**School Age**
Gastroenteritis	Gastroenteritis
Appendicitis	Appendicitis
Intussusception	Ovarian cyst/torsion
Hemolytic-uremic syndrome	Henoch-Schönlein purpura
Pneumonia	Inflammatory bowel disease

similar to that seen after surgery for nonperforated appendicitis.

INTESTINAL OBSTRUCTION

Pathophysiology

Propulsion of food and liquids through the GI tract requires coordinated peristalsis and adequate lumen size. Disordered peristalsis and intrinsic or extrinsic narrowing of the lumen may produce similar symptoms, specifically vomiting, abdominal distention, pain, and absence of flatus or stool. Disordered peristalsis, as in paralytic ileus or intestinal dysmotility, is considered a functional obstruction, whereas narrowing of the lumen from any cause is considered a mechanical obstruction. Intraluminal obstruction may result from abnormally thick meconium in newborns, enteric contents in patients with cystic fibrosis, or a bezoar of organic or inorganic objects ingested by patients with severe neurologic abnormalities.

Intestinal obstruction is classified as complete or incomplete; the distinction is based on a combination of clinical and radiographic criteria. **Complete obstruction** is evident by the lack of flatus or stool and radiographic absence of intestinal gas beyond the point of obstruction. **Incomplete obstruction** is marked by continued passage of flatus or stool and by radiographic evidence of gas beyond the obstruction. Intestinal obstruction is also classified according to location (small bowel versus colonic) and etiology (i.e., adhesive, intussusceptive, malignant). Symptoms relate to the level of obstruction and its completeness. Patients with obstructions of the stomach, duodenum, and upper jejunum present with vomiting early after the obstruction occurs with little, if any, abdominal distention. Patients with obstruction of the lower small bowel and colon present with delayed onset of vomiting and prominent distention.

Once established, intestinal obstruction results in pooling of secretions and fluid in the intestinal lumen, intestinal wall, and peritoneal cavity. Fluid loss may be dramatic and consists of losses from the extracellular compartment. In many types of intestinal obstruction, especially if the obstruction is complete, vascular supply to the intestine is compromised. Initially this is due to venous congestion but can proceed to arterial insufficiency with intestinal necrosis and perforation if not relieved within a few hours. In the absence of vascular compromise, untreated intestinal obstruction produces progressive intestinal dilation and fluid loss.

Clinical and Laboratory Evaluation

History

In evaluating children with possible intestinal obstruction, specific attention should be focused on the GI system. Specific aspects of vomiting are important, including onset, frequency, and whether the vomitus is bilious or nonbilious. Obstruction of the stomach or duodenum proximal to the ampulla of Vater results in nonbilious vomiting, whereas all obstructions distal to the ampulla are accompanied by bile-stained emesis. Bile staining, which frequently signifies a mechanical obstruction or severe paralytic ileus, is generally considered to suggest a surgical condition until proven otherwise. Pain from intestinal obstruction is crampy and midline as a result of the distention and increased peristalsis. The progression of pain in severity and frequency, especially if it is localized, is suggestive of intestinal ischemia.

A history of stooling pattern is helpful particularly in newborns. **Meconium** is first passed within 24 hours of birth in 95% of normal infants. Failure to pass meconium in the first 24 hours is highly suggestive of an obstruction, in particular **Hirschsprung disease**.

☀ Pediatric Pearl

Even after an intestinal obstruction becomes complete, stool and flatus may continue to pass as a result of evacuation of the bowel distal to the obstruction. Therefore, the passage of stool or flatus cannot be used to date the onset of obstruction or to exclude obstruction.

Fever is unusual in the absence of intestinal perforation and may suggest an alternate diagnosis such as gastroenteritis or urinary tract sepsis. Other non-GI symptoms can help identify the abdominal symptoms as secondary findings resulting from a paralytic ileus. History of previous abdominal surgery is extremely important. The illness that prompted the initial procedure may recur or **adhesions** that form after the initial procedure can cause obstruction.

With possible obstruction in neonates, it is necessary to explore the maternal history for evidence of **polyhydramnios** (increased amniotic fluid volume), which is associated with obstruction of the upper jejunum and proximal GI tract. A history of anomalies such as **cystic fibrosis** or **Hirschsprung disease** in siblings should alert the clinician to the possibility of these or associated conditions.

Physical Examination

General inspection yields important information regarding hydration status and systemic toxicity. In newborns, evidence of genetic or developmental anomalies should be specifically sought. Infants with Down syndrome have an increased incidence of Hirschsprung disease and duodenal atresia, and those with other syndromes may also have an increased risk of GI anomalies.

Inspection of the abdomen should focus on the presence or absence of distention, visible discoloration, or evidence of previous operations. Abdominal distention in intestinal obstruction is due to multiple dilated loops of small bowel or colon and generally signifies obstruction of the mid-small bowel or beyond. In small children in whom the abdominal wall is thin, erythema frequently heralds the presence of underlying peritoneal inflammation; this condition is seen earliest in the midline and lateral to the rectus muscles where the abdominal wall is thinnest.

Auscultation of bowel sounds is an essential part of the examination. High-pitched sounds of increased frequency are the classic findings of intestinal obstruction. Decreased frequency of bowel sounds or a silent abdomen is found in children with paralytic ileus or obstruction complicated by intestinal ischemia.

Palpation of the abdomen should focus on detection of abdominal wall tension or resistance, presence of palpable loops of bowel, or abdominal masses. A sausage-shaped mass in the right upper quadrant or epigastrium may be palpable in early cases of **intussusception** before marked distention of the small bowel occurs. In infants with suspected **pyloric stenosis,** careful palpation of the upper abdomen should reveal a palpable olive-sized mass in 80% of patients with this condition. The infant must be relaxed, which can be facilitated by a pacifier and flexing the thighs.

☀ Pediatric Pearl

The technique of sham feeding is especially effective in allowing deep palpation. After placement of a nasogastric tube the infant is allowed to take Pedialyte or glucose water from a bottle while an assistant aspirates the stomach with a syringe. This technique quiets the infant, relaxes the abdominal wall, and keeps the stomach from distending.

The characteristic "olive" is transverse in orientation, mobile, 1–2 cm in length, and located in the epigastrium or right upper quadrant. If an olive is palpable, no further diagnostic studies are necessary.

Examination of the groin is essential; **inguinal hernia** is the single leading cause of intestinal obstruction in children. It is necessary to examine children for hernias from the side, with the testis grasped in the examiner's dominant hand, unlike in adults. The fingers of the nondominant hand are used to palpate the spermatic cord at the level of the pubis. The presence of bowel or fluid in the hernia sac produces a thickened spermatic cord. The distinction between fluid and intestine is usually straightforward, but difficult cases may be aided by transillumination of the scrotum or, in small infants, bimanual examination of the internal ring with a digit in the rectum.

Rectal examination itself may be diagnostic, as in the case of **imperforate anus,** where the absence of a communication or presence of a dimple makes the diagnosis. Typical rectal examination findings in Hirschsprung disease are absence of a rectal vault and a snug feel to the examining digit. Large pelvic masses may produce rectal obstruction and be easily palpated by rectal examination. Occasionally, the intussusceptum (invaginated bowel) of an intussusception is palpable as a rectal mass; these rarely prolapse through the anus.

Laboratory Evaluation

Laboratory studies in children with intestinal obstruction should focus on detecting complications such as dehydration and sepsis. A CBC with a differential and platelet count is usually warranted to exclude complicating anemia or a left shift that raises the suspicion of intestinal ischemia or associated sepsis. A right shift producing lymphocytosis may suggest severe gastroenteritis, simulating obstruction. Serum electrolytes and renal function are important in identifying electrolyte abnormalities such as hypokalemic alkalosis from recurrent vomiting. Azotemia and acidosis from intravascular volume depletion are common complications of intestinal obstruction.

Radiographic studies help identify the cause of obstruction. Workup should begin with plain radiographs of the abdomen obtained in two or three views. In addition to a supine film, a film in the upright or lateral decubitus position is necessary to identify air-fluid levels and to detect a small pneumoperitoneum from possible perforation. In newborns, a lateral view with the patient prone or held upside down may help demonstrate air in the rectum in cases of imperforate anus or suspected Hirschsprung disease.

In most instances, the diagnosis is not obvious from plain radiographs, and a contrast study, usually a contrast enema, is necessary. If meconium ileus or its postneonatal equivalent is suspected, the enema should be performed with a water-soluble contrast agent. The contrast material can break up the thickened enteric contents due to its hyperosmolarity, which causes movement of water into the intestinal lumen. In cases of gastric outlet or duodenal obstruction, injection of air through the nasogastric tube may be as helpful as injection of radiopaque contrast. Ultrasound has been very helpful in confirming the diagnosis of pyloric stenosis in infants without palpable masses. More complex imaging studies are rarely, if ever, necessary in the evaluation of intestinal obstruction.

Differential Diagnosis

The differential diagnosis of intestinal obstruction in children is highly dependent on age and symptoms (Table 25.2). In newborns, the combination of history, physical examination, and plain radiographs of the chest and abdomen can make the diagnosis quite certain. A contrast enema is usually performed to confirm the diagnosis or to exclude additional atresias or anomalies.

Management

Diagnosis and treatment should proceed simultaneously. Systemic derangements of hydration, electrolytes, and sepsis are urgent priorities. Both nasogastric suction and intravenous resuscitation with isotonic solution such as normal saline or lactated Ringer's solution should begin promptly. Clinical evidence of dehydration and hypovolemia after evaluation of skin turgor, peripheral perfusion, mental status, and urine volume may warrant bolus infusions of 10 ml/kg. It is necessary to initiate broad-spectrum antibiotics because of the risk of translocation of bacteria and systemic sepsis, even in the absence of intestinal infarction.

The diagnosis and degree of obstruction determine the definitive therapy. Most obstructions from postoperative adhesions resolve with

nasogastric suction, fluid replacement, and nutritional therapy. This is especially true if the obstruction is incomplete and it is early in the postoperative period. Complete obstructions from postoperative adhesions usually require operative treatment.

Initial treatment of obstructions from **incarcerated inguinal hernias** involves manual reduction of the hernia in addition to general resuscitative measures. It is rare that incarcerated hernias are truly irreducible in children. After reduction of the hernia, monitoring of infants for evidence of intestinal injury and continued obstruction is necessary. Hernia repair is appropriate when patients have stabilized and intestinal and scrotal injuries have resolved.

Pyloric stenosis is frequently associated with significant hypokalemic alkalosis. Preoperative preparation should concentrate on adequate potassium replacement, which is determined by serum concentrations of potassium and chloride. A low serum chloride with an elevated bicarbonate level indicates persistent potassium depletion regardless of the serum potassium level. Division of the hypertrophied muscle (pyloromyotomy) is all that is required to relieve the obstruction; it produces excellent results. Entry into the lumen of the pylorus is infrequent but can be disastrous if not recognized and repaired at the time of surgery.

The usual treatment for **imperforate anus** and **Hirschsprung disease** is a temporary colostomy followed by definitive reconstruction at the age of 12–18 months. **Intestinal atresias and malformations** such as duplication require limited intestinal resection with primary anastomosis. **Malrotation and adhesive obstructions** require lysis of adhesive bands and resection only if segments are nonviable.

Meconium ileus is a special circumstance. If it is not complicated by intestinal ischemia and is recognized on contrast enema, nonoperative relief with enemas of hyperosmolar contrast agents may be appropriate. Refluxing these agents into the dilated segment of intestine allows mixing of

TABLE 25.2	Causes of Intestinal Obstruction in Children by Age Group	
Newborn	**Infants**	**Children**
Inguinal hernia	Inguinal hernia	Inguinal hernia
Hirschsprung disease	Intussusception	Adhesions
Atresia	Malrotation	Meconium ileus equivalent
Malrotation	Duplication	Appendicitis
Meconium ileus	Appendicitis	
Imperforate anus	Pyloric stenosis	

the agent with the abnormally thick meconium; this can result in a change in the consistency of the meconium so that it can pass through the colon and resolve the obstruction. It is not unusual for repeat administrations of the agent to be necessary. If these attempts are unsuccessful, operative therapy should consist of attempts to milk the material into the colon by injecting Gastrografin or *N*-acetylcysteine into the lumen. Resection is appropriate only if the bowel is nonviable. Because these patients (who most likely have cystic fibrosis) will have difficulty with absorption in the future, limited resection is necessary.

Pediatric Pearl

Meconium ileus in newborns is strongly suggestive of cystic fibrosis.

Meconium ileus equivalent is the term applied to the same type of obstruction occurring in older children with cystic fibrosis. It is very common in these patients. Relief usually involves nonoperative methods. However, other conditions that require operation (adhesions, intussusception) may also occur and warrant consideration in the differential diagnosis.

ABDOMINAL MASS

Pathophysiology

Most abdominal masses in children produce few, if any, symptoms other than the presence of the mass itself. The exceptions are unusually large tumors that produce respiratory compromise if they are located in the upper abdomen or produce rectal or bladder obstruction if they are located in the pelvis. **Vascular tumors** that trap platelets or produce congestive heart failure are usually confined to the liver. Some tumors may produce symptoms as a result of secretion of hormones: **neuroblastomas** may produce vasoactive intestinal peptide, resulting in watery diarrhea; **Wilms tumors** may be associated with hypertension caused by renin production; and **pheochromocytomas** cause episodic hypertension and diaphoresis as a result of catecholamine excess. The GI masses associated with pyloric stenosis, intussusception, or intestinal duplication are usually overshadowed by the GI obstructive symptoms (see INTESTINAL OBSTRUCTION).

Clinical and Laboratory Evaluation (Figure 25.3)

History

Maternal history and careful questioning regarding GI function are important in evaluating newborns with an abdominal mass. **Polyhydramnios** (increased amniotic fluid volume) is often associated with high-level intestinal obstruction, and **oligohydramnios** (decreased amniotic fluid volume) is associated with impaired renal function. In older children, abdominal pain and vomiting usually indicate that the mass is GI in origin, whereas hematuria obviously direct attention toward a renal lesion. A history of unusual eye movements (**opsoclonus–myoclonus**) suggests the presence of a neuroblastoma.

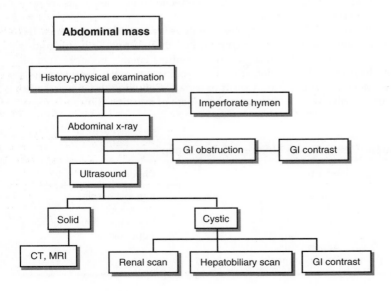

FIGURE 25.3. Flow diagram for the diagnostic evaluation of children with an abdominal mass. CT = computed tomography; GI = gastrointestinal; MRI = magnetic resonance imaging.

Physical Examination

Location of the mass is the most important piece of information obtained from a careful abdominal and rectal examination (Figure 25.4). Upper abdominal masses are related to the liver, spleen, adrenals, or kidneys. Bilateral flank masses are almost always renal (e.g., those seen in polycystic disease). Midline lower abdominal masses are likely to be related to the bladder, vagina, ovary, or retroperitoneum. In small children with palpable masses, transillumination may offer quick reassurance that the lesion is cystic.

General examination should specifically look for subcutaneous nodules, periorbital ecchymosis, superficial hemangiomas, and jaundice. Pallor and weakness suggest systemic disease and tachypnea, rales, and wheezing suggest congestive heart failure associated with a vascular malformation. Congenital aniridia, hemihypertrophy, and Beckwith-Wiedemann syndrome are associated with an increased incidence of Wilms tumor.

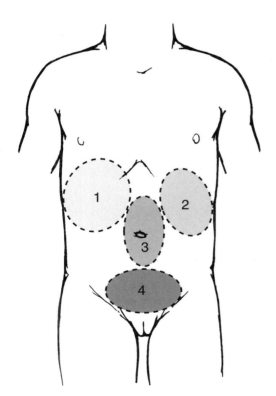

FIGURE 25.4. Likely organ of origin of abdominal mass by location. *1* = liver, gallbladder, kidney, adrenal; *2* = spleen, stomach, kidney, adrenal; *3* = pancreas, retroperitoneum, mesentery, bowel; and *4* = bladder, uterus, ovary.

Laboratory Evaluation

A CBC may reveal evidence of marrow involvement with anemia or thrombocytopenia, leukemia with elevated WBC, or thrombocytosis in some solid tumors. Serum determinations of α-fetoprotein and β-human chorionic gonadotropin (β-HCG) and of urine vanillylmandelic acid and homovanillic acid are warranted in children with solid tumors.

Plain radiographs of the abdomen may be helpful if calcification suggestive of neuroblastoma or teratoma is identified. Contrast study of the GI tract is indicated if evidence of intestinal obstruction is apparent on plain films. Ultrasonography to distinguish cystic from solid masses and the likely organ of origin should be next. Further cross-sectional imaging such as CT or magnetic resonance imaging (MRI) for evaluation of solid tumors is generally necessary. In the case of solid renal masses, ultrasonographic evaluation of the inferior vena cava and right atrium to detect tumor thrombus prior to any attempts at resection is also warranted.

Differential Diagnosis

The differential diagnosis of an abdominal mass in children depends on age, the cystic or solid nature of the mass, and the presence of associated symptoms (Table 25.3). In newborns, most lesions are cystic, although neuroblastoma and teratoma occur with some frequency. In older children, most lesions are solid, with neuroblastoma and Wilms tumor being the most common. It is necessary to refer children with solid tumors to a pediatric oncology center early in the evaluation to facilitate diagnostic studies and to ensure a multidisciplinary approach to treatment.

Management

After careful diagnostic evaluation, patients with solid tumors need either diagnostic biopsy or tumor resection. The method of confirming the diagnosis and the decision whether to attempt resection depend on the type of tumor and the presence of distant or local spread. This decision is usually made in consultation with a pediatric oncologist, a pediatric surgeon, and a radiotherapist. Malignant tumors usually require additional chemotherapy or radiotherapy. If dissemination is widespread or if complete resection cannot be performed, chemotherapy may be warranted before resection is attempted.

Cystic lesions may require operative therapy, medical management, or observation. **Adrenal**

TABLE 25.3 Types of Abdominal Masses in Children	
Cystic	**Solid**
Hydronephrosis	Neuroblastoma
Multicystic dysplastic kidney	Wilms tumor
Adrenal hemorrhage	Teratoma
Ovarian cyst	Hepatoblastoma
Choledochal cyst	Mesoblastic nephroma
Hydrometrocolpos	Hemangioendothelioma
Mesenteric cyst	Infantile polycystic kidneys
Intestinal duplication	Rhabdomyosarcoma

hemorrhage is a neonatal condition that resolves spontaneously, although it must be distinguished from a **cystic neuroblastoma** by measuring urinary catecholamines. Serial ultrasound examinations are used to monitor its resolution. **Ovarian cysts** are common in newborns, resulting from stimulation from maternal hormones. Recent studies using prenatal ultrasonography have shown that many of these cysts resolve spontaneously, particularly if they are 3 cm or less in diameter. **Ovarian cysts with torsion** require operative therapy in an attempt to preserve the ovary and the fallopian tube.

Obstructive uropathy requires further investigation, including voiding cystourography, renal nuclear scan, and possible cystoscopy. Chronic suppressive antibiotic therapy is used in children with severe **vesicoureteral reflux** and partially obstructing uropathy.

Cysts of the mesentery, bowel wall, or **extrahepatic biliary tree** require excision with reconstruction. **Hydrometrocolpos,** which presents in the neonatal period or at the onset of menses, warrants excision of the imperforate hymen or, in cases of distal vaginal atresia, vaginal reconstruction.

SUGGESTED READINGS

Ashcraft KW: *Pediatric Surgery,* 3rd ed. Philadelphia, WB Saunders, 2000.

Burd RS, Whalen TV: Evaluation of the child with suspected appendicitis. *Pediatr Ann* 30:720–725, 2001.

D'Agostino J: Common abdominal emergencies in children. *Emerg Med Clin North Am* 20:139–153, 2002.

Dehner LP: *Pediatric Surgical Pathology,* 2nd ed. Baltimore, Williams & Wilkins, 1987.

Harrison MR: Surgically correctable fetal disease. *Am J Surg* 180:335–342, 2000.

Hartman GE, Shochat SJ: Abdominal mass lesions in the newborn: Diagnosis and treatment. *Clin Perinatol* 16:123–135, 1989.

O'Neill JA: *Pediatric Surgery,* 5th ed. St. Louis, Mosby-Year Book, 1998.

Pearl RH, Irish MS, Caty MG, et al: The approach to common abdominal diagnoses in infants and children. *Pediatr Clin North Am* 45:1287–1326, 1998.

Schmeling DJ, Coran AG: Hormonal and metabolic response to operative stress in the neonate. *J Parenter Enteral Nutr* 15:215–238, 1991.

Chapter 26

Pediatric Surgical Subspecialties

Rebecca Evangelista, Paul Harris,
David M. Merer, Marijean M. Miller,
Lane S. Palmer, Lisa Menasse-Palmer,
and Gary E. Hartman

LIMP AND DEVELOPMENTAL GAIT DISTURBANCES*

One of the most important characteristics that distinguishes human beings from lower animal species is that humans walk erect on two legs. Therefore, it is not surprising that humans have an inherent interest in the development of normal gait and in the disturbances of gait or limp. Perhaps the most celebrated event of early childhood is when a child first walks; therefore, it is not surprising that some of the most frequent concerns of parents and pediatricians involve questions about gait. At the time a toddler is beginning to walk and even in preparation for this event, attention focuses on the lower extremities and feet. Similarly, limp is an extremely common complaint in pediatric practice, which invariably generates concern and should never be dismissed without thorough investigation to determine the cause. Loss of function or diminished function of the lower extremities is often more disabling than that of the upper extremities. Therefore, it is important to correctly evaluate and manage conditions arising in children that interfere with the normal functions of standing, walking, running, skipping, and jumping.

Unlike disturbances involving the upper extremities, where localization of pain or dysfunction is likely to indicate the specific anatomic site of involvement, the symptom of limp or painful gait is a complex summation of functions of the entire lower extremity and even of the lower abdomen. A limp can result from conditions arising in the toe, foot, ankle, leg, knee, thigh, hip, inguinal region, abdomen, or back. Furthermore, conditions affecting the nervous system, skeleton, muscles, joints, skin, soft tissues, and even

the psyche may precipitate limping as the major or sole presenting symptom. With the most severe form of limp, children may refuse to walk, making localization of the problem even more difficult. To add to the complexity, the etiology of conditions resulting in a limp may be developmental, traumatic, neoplastic, infectious, metabolic, or psychologic, as in mimetic limp or conversion reaction.

Because gait is a complex function comprised of both static or structural components as well as active or dynamic movements at different levels, it is necessary to understand normal patterns of development and variations of normal to advise parents about the ultimate outcome of their child's condition. Gait represents a summation of many factors at different levels (i.e., hips, femora, tibiae, feet) that may result in a single observation by parents or the pediatrician that a child's gait is abnormal.

The approach to a child with a limp is important. Topics of discussion in this section include diagnostic considerations, evaluation, causal conditions, and management, as well as issues relating to normal and abnormal development of gait.

Pathophysiology

For the purposes of this discussion, a **limp** is any **disturbance in gait**. The most severe form of limp is refusal to walk or inability to walk at all. Mild forms of limp according to this definition even include such entities as **genu varum (bowleg)** and **genu valgum (knock-knee),** because they involve altered symmetry and form of gait. Normal gait is comprised of symmetrical, alternating, rhythmical motions involving two phases, the stance phase and the swing phase. In contrast to running, one foot is always in contact with the ground at all times. There is no upper body swaying or lurching, but normally there is loose arm swinging bi-

---

*"Limp and Developmental Gait Disturbances" was written by Paul Harris, M.D.

laterally. If the stance phase is shortened because of pain on weight-bearing, an antalgic limp results. If the swing phase is shortened, some abnormality in the hip joint should be suspected.

Limps may be categorized in several ways to develop a differential diagnosis:

- **Function versus pain** (Table 26.1). Some limps are purely functional in nature and do not usually cause pain (e.g., **Trendelenburg or glu-teus medius limp**), some limps combine pain and dysfunction (e.g., **antalgic gait**), and some result in painful extremity without dysfunction (e.g., **osteoid osteoma**). There is a wide spectrum of disease and overlap within these three categories, but it is quite useful to assess the patient accordingly. In addition, patients' symptoms and signs may change over time, moving them from one category to another.

- **Level** (Table 26.2). Disturbances may occur at any level in the lower extremity or even abdomen or back and still result in limp. They may be unilateral or bilateral. Therefore, efforts to localize the level and laterality of the disturbance are most helpful. Occasionally, symptoms attributed to one level may actually represent pathology at a different level; knee pain may actually be due to disease in the hip joint, as in **slipped capital femoral epiphysis (SCFE)**. Symptoms referable to one side may actually represent pathology of the contralateral extremity (e.g., unequal leg lengths) or be a predictor of bilateral involvement (**Legg-Calvé-Perthes disease**).

- **Etiology** (Table 26.3). Localization alone or the presence or absence of pain may be insufficient to identify and properly manage the condition in all cases, because there are multiple causes of limp. A complete differential diagnostic consideration by etiology is essential. For example, SCFE, Legg-Calvé-Perthes disease, transient synovitis, and septic arthritis all affect the developing hip joint but their different etiologies mandate radically different management.

TABLE 26.1 **Types of Limp and Conditions Causing Gait Disturbance**

Functional (No Pain)
Trendelenburg (gluteus medius)
Quadriceps femoris
Steppage
Unequal leg lengths (PFFD)
Mimetic limp
Posttraumatic limp
Genu varum/genu valgum
Femoral torsion
Tibial torsion
Pes planus (flexible)
Metatarsus varus

Pain and Dysfunction
Antalgic gait
Short swing (back pain)
Enigmatic limp
Traumatic limp
    Toddler's fracture
    Foreign body
Joint infections
Perthes disease
Transient synovitis
SCFE
JRA
Patellofemoral malalignment syndrome
Osteochondritis dissecans
Pes planus (rigid)
Pes cavus (rigid)
Tight shoes

Painful Extremity (Normal Function)
Tumors of bone
    Osteoid osteoma
    Osteogenic sarcoma
Osgood-Schlatter disease
Kohler disease
Trauma
Osteomyelitis
Growing pains (shin splints)
Leukemia

JRA = juvenile rheumatoid arthritis; PFFD = proximal focal femoral dysplasia; SCFE = slipped capital femoral epiphysis.

Clinical and Laboratory Evaluation

Whether the differential diagnostic considerations are evaluated on the basis of presence or absence of pain, level of dysfunction, or specific etiology, the systematic approach remains the same. The integration of a careful and complete history; complete physical examination, including a neurologic examination; and appropriate use of laboratory and imaging studies should lead to a properly constructed list of diagnostic considerations that can then be pursued and properly managed.

History

At birth, the practitioner should observe infants for two major factors: (1) congenital **malformations,** which are usually genetic in origin, and (2) congenital **deformations,** which are secondary to intrauterine position and forces. Specific commonly occurring conditions in the second category are considered here. In addition, as children grow, develop, and learn to walk, certain changes

TABLE 26.2	**Causes of Limp by Level and Etiology**	
Level	**Disease**	**Etiology**
Hip	CHD	Developmental
	Femoral torsion	Developmental
	PFFD	Developmental
	SCFE	Developmental/traumatic
	Perthes disease	Traumatic?
	Septic arthritis	Infectious
	Transient synovitis	Traumatic/viral/inflammatory
	Femoral neck fracture	Traumatic
	Arthritis	RA: inflammatory
Knee	Genu recurvatum	Congenital
	Genu varum–genu valgum	Developmental
	Blount disease	Developmental
	Rickets	Metabolic
	Osgood-Schlatter disease	Traumatic
	Septic arthritis	Infectious
	Patella fracture, subluxation	Traumatic
	Osteochondritis dissecans	Developmental/traumatic
	Chondromalacia patella	Developmental/traumatic
	Menisci and ligament tears	Traumatic
Tibia	Tibial torsion	Developmental
	Toddler's fracture	Traumatic
	Growing pains/shin splints	Developmental/traumatic
Foot	Metatarsus adductus	Developmental
	Clubfoot	Developmental
	Pes planus, pes cavus	Developmental
	Foreign body/tight shoes	Traumatic
Other	Tumors	Neoplastic
	Leukemia	Neoplastic
	JRA	Inflammatory
	Neurologic	Cerebral palsy
	Psychiatric	Mimetic (conversion)

CHD = congenital hip dislocation; JRA = juvenile rheumatoid arthritis; PFFD = proximal focal femoral dysplasia; RA = rheumatoid arthritis; SCFE = slipped capital femoral epiphysis.

normally take place as fetal positional effects diminish and other familial patterns emerge in the ultimate attainment of a normal neutral gait.

Information about intrauterine position or observations made by parents or staff soon after birth are useful because most conditions have their onset at that time. For example, a history of breech delivery is significant in the evaluation for the presence of congenital hip dislocation (CHD). Age of onset or when first observed helps place the condition within its natural historical background.

With the exception of some of the developmental disorders in which intrauterine position determines the condition, and physical examination is the mainstay of diagnosis, both a history and a complete physical examination are necessary. Age, sex, race, onset, character, localization, systemic symptomatology, function and limitations, relief of symptoms, and family history all are important elements of a complete history of the child presenting with limp or gait disturbance.

AGE. Certain conditions occur more often at specific ages; SCFE at 10–17 years (adolescence), Legg-Calvé-Perthes disease at 4–9 years, and osteogenic sarcoma and Ewing sarcoma in the second decade of life.

For developmental conditions in younger children and infants, it is important to determine the natural history of each condition producing gait disturbance in the individual child whether or not a particular condition is abnormal. For example, mild to moderate bowing is not abnormal in an 8-month-old infant but may be a sign of progressive disease in a 3-year-old child. Similarly, genu valgum in a 4-year-old child is not as bothersome to the pediatrician as this same finding in a 1-year-old toddler. In addition, flatfoot in a toddler does

| TABLE 26.3 | Characteristics on Physical Examination of Various Disorders of the Lower Extremity | |

Part of Body	Abnormal Physical Findings	Etiology to be Considered
Hip	Abduction, external rotation on flexion	SCFE
	Obesity, limp, external rotation, decreased hip rotation	SCFE
	Trendelenburg gait/sign, decreased abduction	CHD
	Limp, limitation of internal rotation, abduction, may be thigh atrophy	Transient synovitis
	Antalgic gait, limitation of range of joint motion, decreased internal rotation and abduction, flexion contracture, atrophy, and tenderness of thigh muscle	Legg-Calvé-Perthes disease
	Swelling of thigh, pain on movement of joint, systemic findings, fever, increased WBC count	Septic hip
Knee	Tenderness and swelling over anterior tibial tuberosity	Osgood-Schlatter disease
	Tenderness of patella articular surface, painful crepitance	Chondromalacia patella
	Tenderness of medial condyle, limp, swelling, decreased range of motion	Osteochondritis dissecans
	Mass in popliteal fossa, painless	Baker cyst
	Joint effusion, localized tenderness over lateral or medial joint, positive McMurray test, atrophy of quadriceps	Menisci injuries
Leg	Painless limp, compensatory scoliosis, unequal leg lengths	CHD, congenital neurofibromatosis
	Persistent pain, limp, tender or nontender mass	Tumor Osteoid osteoma Osteochondroma Osteogenic sarcoma Ewing sarcoma
Foot	Rigidity of foot, deep arch versus absent arch	Pes cavus, pes planus

CHD = congenital hip dysplasia; SCFE = slipped capital femoral epiphysis; WBC = white blood cell.

not warrant great concern or require therapeutic intervention.

SEX. Note that CHD is associated with a female: male sex ratio of 6:1. There is an increased incidence of CHD in Lapps, southern Tyrolean Italians, and certain Navajo Indian peoples, and a significant preponderance of excessive bowing and Blount disease in West Indian blacks.

RACE. Although some conditions are rare in certain ethnic groups (e.g., Ewing sarcoma in blacks), too much significance should not be placed on race as a differential point in the history.

ONSET. When was the limp or pain first noted? Was it sudden, gradual, or insidious? These questions help clarify the duration or chronicity of the disorder. It is most important to determine whether a condition is of recent onset or of long standing. Conditions of sudden or recent onset are more likely to be secondary to trauma or to require more aggressive, prompt intervention. The limp or pain associated with Legg-Calvé-Perthes dis-

ease, SCFE, or juvenile rheumatoid arthritis may well be intermittent, whereas persisting pain of recent onset may be associated with toxic synovitis or septic arthritis.

CHARACTER OF PAIN. Is the pain or limp intermittent or constant? Is it severe, mild, or only present at certain times? Is it worse during the day or night? Does the pain interfere with normal activities such as running or walking? Symptoms in conditions involving bones such as osteoid osteoma are likely to be more severe at night, whereas conditions involving joints or weight-bearing surfaces become symptomatic with daytime activities.

LOCATION OF PAIN. Where is the pain experienced most acutely? It may be extremely helpful if the child or parent can localize the pain to a particular region of the lower extremity such as the toes, foot, ankle, or knee. One significant exception to this rule involves knee pain. A history of pain in the knee may indicate a local problem such as arthritis, osteomalacia of the patella, or a problem with ligaments or cartilage of the joint. Knee pain is also a frequent complaint in conditions affecting the hip joint such as Legg-Calvé-Perthes disease or SCFE. Children with either of these conditions may have no symptoms referable to the hip but may present only with referred intermittent knee pain.

Similarly, back pain in children may be a symptom of problems with the lower extremities such as the fairly common condition of unequal lengths of the legs, which may produce an almost unrecognizable disturbance in gait. Even intra-abdominal conditions such as acute appendicitis and inguinal adenitis may cause an abnormal gait and lower extremity pain on the affected side.

Although a history of trauma may help distinguish between the two broad entities of traumatic and atraumatic limp, the presence or absence of such a history may be of no aid or may be misleading. Active children, who sustain multiple episodes of minor trauma daily, may be unable to recall a specific significant event even after serious injury. Conversely, parents or children frequently associate the onset of limp or pain with a specific traumatic event that may bear no causal relationship to it. Because the management and the prognosis of traumatic limp differ in such important ways, it is essential to consider the possible unreliability of a history of a very specific traumatic event.

Is there a history of trauma? What are the circumstances surrounding the incident? As previously mentioned, a history of trauma may be exceedingly helpful in elucidating the problem, but it may also be misleading. The absence of a definitive history of trauma does not rule it out as the precipitating event.

SYSTEMIC SYMPTOMS. Does the ill child have any more generalized symptoms or signs? Is there a history of fever or rash? Are joints other than those of the lower extremity involved? Is weight loss, fatigue, or anorexia present?

Pediatric Pearl

A history of fever associated with joint pain should alert the clinician to such conditions as septic arthritis, toxic synovitis, juvenile rheumatoid arthritis, and acute rheumatic fever.

The absence of fever or other systemic symptoms is more likely to implicate trauma, developmental conditions, or tumor. Leg pain may be the presenting complaint of a child with acute leukemia who subsequently is noted to have other manifestations of systemic illness.

FUNCTION AND LIMITATION OF MOTION OR ACTIVITIES. Does the presenting pain or discomfort interfere with, alter, or curtail daily activities such as school sports, climbing stairs, walking, and running? Osgood-Schlatter disease, which may be exacerbated by contact sports, may prevent active participation in these sports. However, it may cause relatively little discomfort during swimming or bicycling. Is there limitation of motion or pain involved in a particular joint? Where does the patient think the pain emanates from?

RELIEF OF SYMPTOMS. What treatment or home remedy seems to relieve the pain? Does rest help? Does using aspirin relieve symptoms? Is the condition more noticeable at the beginning of the day or in the evening? Joint pain associated with juvenile rheumatoid arthritis is classically more prominent in the morning but becomes less noticeable as things loosen up during daytime activities. The pain of osteoid osteoma is relieved by aspirin.

FAMILY HISTORY. Do other family members have or have they ever had similar symptoms? Children are great imitators and may at times mimic a favorite relative or other household member for attention or other secondary gain. Some conditions such as unequal leg lengths have a familial pattern that can be revealed by an accurate history. What do the family and the patient think is the cause of the pain or limp? This seemingly naive question frequently elicits pertinent historical data that the physician would not otherwise have gleaned by routine questioning. In addition, this question tells the practitioner what worries the family most and whether this concern is real or irrational. Of course, this question may also elicit a great deal of material that is or appears to be irrelevant, but the time it takes is usually well spent.

Family history often aids in the evaluation of gait disturbances, because tendencies toward torsional deformities, genu varum or genu valgum, and foot deformities often have repetitive familial patterns. This may help reassure anxious parents while alerting the physician to a predisposition toward physiologic excess.

Often, the pediatrician's role is simply to determine whether the condition is resolving or progressing. This is accomplished by obtaining accurate historical data and sequential evaluations. Many of the conditions discussed can be bilateral. Physiologic and minor positional variations tend to be symmetric, whereas more severe deformities are often unilateral or asymmetric.

Therefore, the parents' perception of which side is worse or abnormal is important.

Historical data should include information on the child's preferred sleeping position. Orthopedic gait disturbances are not necessarily caused by aberrant sleeping positions, but may be exacerbated or prevented from spontaneous resolution by continued fixation of an existing deformity. Most torsional deformities are exacerbated when the infant sleeps in the prone position, whereas supine slumbering allows natural resolution to occur more rapidly. Many parents are afraid to allow young infants to sleep on their backs for fear of regurgitation and aspiration. However, the supine position is the preferred sleeping position now recommended by the American Academy of Pediatrics (AAP) because of the association of prone sleeping position with sudden infant death syndrome (SIDS).

Can the older child sit cross-legged or does he prefer to sit in the reverse tailor position? Does he run with a flailing or eggbeater pattern? These characteristics are all compatible with the diagnosis of excessive femoral anteversion.

Many parental concerns focus on the gait of the toddler who is just beginning to stand or walk. Feet and legs turning in or out, bowing, stumbling, falling, and waddling may all be normal stages of development in the newly ambulatory child, but excessive clumsiness and frequent falling over her own feet in a toddler may imply internal tibial torsion with metatarsus adductus.

Physical Examination

It is always necessary to perform a complete and thorough physical examination. Certain physical findings are common in infants and children who present with gait disturbances (Table 26.4).

EXAMINATION OF THE HIP OF THE NEWBORN AND INFANT. Physical examination of the hip joints is performed at birth, at the time of discharge from the nursery, at 2–3 weeks, and again at 4–6 weeks.

Pediatric Pearl
Detection of hip abnormality is important in the immediate newborn period.

Frequent and complete range of motion tests are necessary to screen for the presence of hip dislocation and to confirm the absence of pathology in infants who have noticeable ligamentous laxity or ligamentous clicks.

TABLE 26.4	**Physical Findings in Gait Disturbances**
Conditions	**Physical Findings**
Congenital hip dislocation (CHD)	Positive Ortolani maneuver or Barlow test Shortening of leg Asymmetry of skin folds Limitation of abduction Trendelenburg gait
Excessive femoral anteversion	Characteristic sitting position Increased internal rotation Decreased external rotation Compensatory external tibial torsion Intoeing—negative angle of gait
Genu varum	Increased tibiofemoral angle 25°
Genu valgum	Negative tibiofemoral angle 15°
Blount disease	Severe progressive bowing—bilateral with radiographic findings
Internal tibial torsion	Intoeing gait Negative thigh-foot axis—10–15°
External tibial torsion	Positive thigh-foot axis Outtoeing gait
Metatarsus adductus	Wide space between first and second toes Prominence at base of fifth metatarsal convexity of lateral border of foot Concave crease on medial aspect of foot
Talipes equinovarus (clubfoot)	Forefoot adduction Supination heel varus Ankle equinus
Pes planus or pes cavus	Rigidity of arch or foot

A reduction test, or **Ortolani maneuver,** is performed with the infant lying comfortably supine on a firm surface by grasping the lower limb with the fingers extended over the greater trochanter and simultaneously lifting and abducting (see Figure 2.9A). The maneuver should be performed gently but firmly. If dislocation is present, a palpable clunk is appreciated as the head of the femur pops back into the acetabulum.

The reverse maneuver or dislocation test, known as the **Barlow maneuver,** is performed by grasping the leg in the same manner as for the Ortolani maneuver but pressing down and simultaneously adducting (see Figure 2.9B). If the femur pops out, it is felt and can be confirmed by the Ortolani maneuver. Small degrees of crepitance or slight sensations of clicking are usually due to ligaments, cartilage, or other soft tissue structures and do not indicate dislocation.

Shortening of one extremity or asymmetric skin folds may be suggestive of a problem but are difficult to assess and are unreliable in arriving at a diagnosis, especially since the condition may be bilateral and thus appear symmetric. Although it is desirable to make the diagnosis on physical grounds alone within the first month of life, examination of the hip joints should be repeated at all routine examinations during the first year (Figure 26.1).

In older infants (2–4 months), the previously described tests no longer yield positive results because a dislocated hip is not easily reduced by a simple manual maneuver. The most prominent and pathognomonic finding is severe limitation of abduction of the hip joint. Shortening and asymmetry with telescoping become more prominent and recognizable in unilateral disease. In children who have begun to walk, the development of Trendelenburg gait or sign is indicative of CHD until proven otherwise. The natural history of this condition is such that patients may learn to walk, run, and compensate without symptoms or obvious signs of gait disturbance such as waddling until their teens or even young adulthood. At this time, severe deformity of the acetabulum, femoral head, and false acetabulum has occurred.

EXAMINATION OF THE CHILD WITH A LIMP. The following sequence is helpful.

Evaluate the apparent site of pain or dysfunction, examining all adjacent structures, including abdomen, back, and inguinal region, before considering any further diagnostic procedures. Inspect the skin for any discoloration, rash, sites of trauma or puncture, and swelling over joints. It helps to ask a child to point with one finger to where there is pain or discomfort on walking.

Observe the child's stance when he is completely undressed; look for symmetry of both extremities. Avoidance of heel or toe walking indicates foot problems. Check for equal levels of the iliac crests, and measure leg lengths from the anterior–superior iliac spine to the medial malleolus. It is also useful to measure thigh and calf circumference to detect muscle wasting or hemihypertrophy.

Next, observe the child in the sitting position, and again check the levels of the iliac crests from behind. Unequal leg lengths cause asymmetry of the iliac crest heights while standing but not while sitting. Inspect the feet and toes for plantar lesions or lesions such as ingrown toenails.

Then examine the child in the supine position for passive range of motion and stability of all joints. Examine the knee for stability by the anterior—posterior and lateral–medial stressing maneuvers as well as for crepitance and pain on flexion. Inspect the patient's shoes to determine excessive or uneven wear. Local knee joint tenderness, joint effusion, atrophy of the quadriceps muscles, and a positive **McMurray test** (flexion and extension of the knee with the tibia externally rotated and internally rotated, producing a palpable and painful clunking) are indications of traumatic knee injury, especially to a meniscus.

Passively flex the hip joint fully in the supine position. If the thigh abducts and externally rotates, it is almost pathognomonic for SCFE. Palpate the feet for flexibility and suppleness and the entire region of suspected pain or dysfunction for tenderness. Table 26.3 indicates the diagnoses that are associated with certain physical findings.

If developmental gait abnormalities are suspected, it is essential to examine the child in several positions on the examining table and perform the various maneuvers described below. Ask the child to walk and then run, with and without shoes. The act of running may accentuate the limp and provide further evidence of the degree of disability. It may also help to observe the child ascend and descend stairs. Because gait is the summation of many factors at different levels affecting the lower extremities, physical examination helps answer the following questions:

- At what level (hips, femur, knees, tibia, foot) does the problem exist?
- Is the condition within range of normal for a developing infant or child, or does it represent an aberration of severe degree?
- Is the condition bilateral or asymmetric?

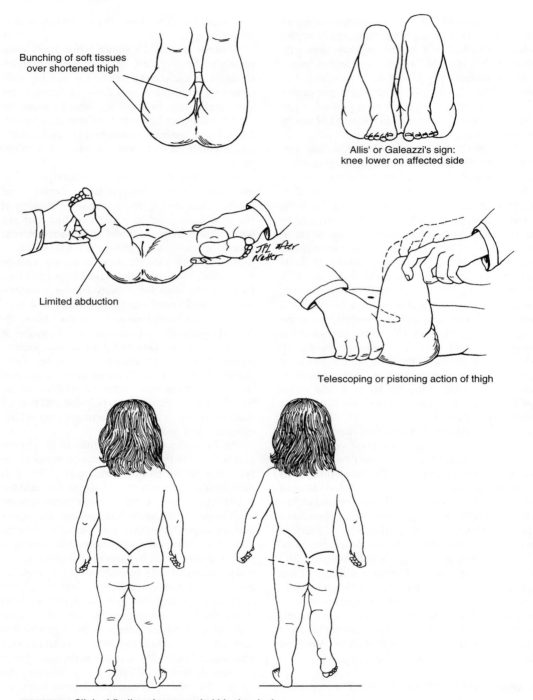

Bunching of soft tissues over shortened thigh

Allis' or Galeazzi's sign: knee lower on affected side

Limited abduction

Telescoping or pistoning action of thigh

FIGURE 26.1 Clinical findings in congenital hip dysplasia.

- Is the gait disturbance made up of several components, compensatory or cumulative?
- What is the specific pathognomonic or diagnostic sign present to confirm or rule out the diagnosis being considered?

ASSESSMENT OF LEVEL OF INVOLVEMENT. The three components that must be evaluated are hip rotation, thigh–foot angle, and foot axis or shape. All three of these are most easily measured with the infant lying comfortably on her belly with someone playing with the child at the head of the examining table. With the knee flexed, the thigh and leg are allowed to fall laterally from the vertical position as far as they naturally go from the midline (Figure 26.2A, B). This rotates the thigh internally; the number of degrees of internal rotation is the angle made by the lower leg and the vertical midline position. Similarly, the leg is now folded in toward and across the midline, and the angle of external rotation of the femur is recorded on the other side of the midline. Normally, the sum of external and internal rotation is 100° or more. The limits of internal and external rotation vary with age. Infants have up to 90° of external rotation, and can easily bring the leg all the way down on the table, but they may only have 10°–20° of internal rotation. As the child becomes older, the external rotation diminishes and internal rotation increases. Evaluation of rotational components should be performed separately on each leg (see Figure 26.2A–C).

ANGLE OF GAIT. It is important to perform a physical examination of children who are being evaluated for a limp or abnormal gait related to a torsional deformity to determine the level and degree of deformity. The resultant components of femoral, tibial, and pedal contributions produce a neutral gait, outtoeing, or intoeing. The term **angle of gait** refers to the angle the foot makes with an imaginary line on the floor in the direction the child is walking (line of progression) [see Figure 26.2E].

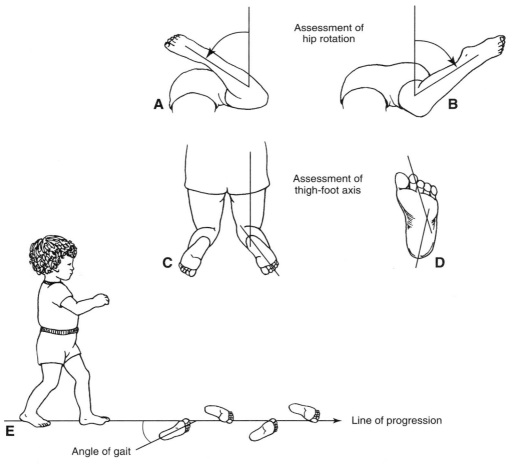

FIGURE 26.2 Evaluation for torsional deformity. *A* and *B:* assessment of hip rotation; *C* and *D:* assessment of thigh–foot axis; *E:* assessment of angle of gait, which is made by estimating the average angle of each step while watching the child walk.

Most toddlers learn to walk outtoe about 20° from this line and gradually approach 5°–10° by 2 years of age. Outtoeing is common in the general population and is not abnormal. Intoeing, which is expressed in negative degrees from the straight line, may represent components of internal tibial torsion, femoral torsion, or metatarsus adductus.

The angle of gait in children who are not yet walking obviously is not obtainable. Even children who are able to strut around the office are often self-conscious and will vary their gait tremendously. Casual observations and parental observations of children's gait are most helpful. Symmetric gait angles also help the pediatrician concentrate on which side is most affected.

THIGH–FOOT AXIS. The next measurement is the thigh–foot axis, which defines the degree of tibial torsion. The foot is dorsiflexed passively to 90° while the child continues to lie prone and while the examiner grasps the toes and distal foot (see Figure 26.2C). The angle observed between the axis of the thigh and the axis of the foot is approximated by observation and expressed positively for the outtoeing foot and negatively for the intoeing foot. It is also possible to evaluate the thigh–foot axis with the child sitting, flexing the knee and ankle joints to determine the relative axis of joint movements. However, this requires more interpretation by the examiner and more infantile cooperation than the prone thigh–foot axis measurement previously described.

EXAMINATION OF THE FOOT. With the infant prone, the shape of the bottom of the foot is observed and the axis of the hindfoot is compared with the axis of the forefoot. Normally, the two should make a straight line. In forefoot deformity such as metatarsus adductus, the forefoot axis makes an obtuse angle with the hindfoot axis toward the midline (see Figure 26.2D). At this point, it is essential to palpate the foot and determine its rigidity or suppleness. The degree to which the forefoot can be brought passively to the midline axis of the hindfoot largely determines the severity of the deformity and the treatment indicated. Other physical findings compatible with the diagnosis of metatarsus adductus or metatarsus varus are convexity on the lateral side of the foot and concavity with a crease on the medial side. Prominence or bulging at the base of the fifth metatarsal and a wide space between the first and second toes may also be noted but alone are not diagnostic. In metatarsus adductus, the deformity is limited to the forefoot, which is adducted and often supinated, whereas in clubfoot, there is an ad-

ditional heel varus and ankle equinas that is rigid.

Calcaneovalgus deformity may also be noted. This merely denotes a foot that is held naturally in dorsiflexion and eversion but that is usually supple and may be passively brought into normal position.

Another measure that we like to perform for the sake of both the pediatrician and the parents is to fold the baby back up into the most naturally occurring fetal position, which usually involves crossing the legs and folding in the feet. In this manner, it is easy to demonstrate the contribution of fetal intrauterine position to the various torsional components.

Physical examination of the lower extremities to evaluate **bowleg (genu varum)** and **knock-knee (genu valgum)** is largely a matter of observation. Visually inspect the child walking and, if of age, lying in the supine position. The degree of genu varum or genu valgum deformity is usually apparent as mild, moderate, or severe. It is subject to interpretation as physiologic or pathologic depending on the degree of deformity, the age of the child, and the presence or absence of symmetry. It is important to feel the knee and other joints for ligamentous laxity, and it may be helpful to measure the distance between the knees and ankles in the standing older child. However, these methods are only clinical approximations of the tibiofemoral angle, which must be determined radiographically if pathology is suspected.

Pes planus or flatfoot is mentioned here only because of its association with external tibial torsion and outtoeing. The hypermobile or everted foot may cause excessive positive angle of gait but rarely causes pain. Physical examination is synonymous with determining the relative degree of suppleness or rigidity. A supple foot may be considered normal in infants and toddlers. Ask older children to stand on tiptoes to demonstrate the functioning presence of an arch and ligaments. If the foot is rigid, whether flat or **deeply arched (pes cavus),** the examination is considered abnormal. Excessive eversion with bulging of the astragalus and concomitant outtoeing is the only significant criterion for abnormality.

Laboratory Evaluation

Laboratory studies of blood or serum are not very helpful in developmental disorders such as tibial torsion, developmental dysplasia (or displacement) of the hip (DDH), and Blount disease but are diagnostic in genu varum secondary to rickets. Newer imaging techniques are useful and have revolutionized the accuracy with which these diagnoses may be made. Plain-film radiography, fluoroscopy, arthrography, ultrasonography, computed tomography (CT), and magnetic resonance imaging (MRI) provide more accurate diagnostic information than was previously available. Detailed consideration of all these imaging techniques is beyond the scope of this discussion.

At least one striking example of progress should be noted; the use of real-time ultrasonography in identifying DDH in infants is most important because it shows the relationship of the nonossified structures not visualized on plain films. It may further help differentiate DDH from acetabular dysplasia and proximal focal femoral dysplasia. As Table 26.5 shows, certain radiologic findings in various developmental conditions are associated with specific gait disturbances.

Table 26.5 also indicates laboratory tests that are useful in the diagnosis of limp and pain and gait disturbances in children. In the presence of an elevated erythrocyte sedimentation rate (ESR) it becomes increasingly important for the pediatrician to obtain further diagnostic laboratory determinations, including rheumatoid factor, antinuclear antibody (ANA), HLA-B27, serum complement, antistreptolysin O titer, and viral titers. As discussed in Chapter 9 (Infectious Diseases), the diagnosis of septic arthritis ultimately rests on joint aspiration with demonstration of organisms on smear or culture and blood cultures.

An elevated white blood cell (WBC) count and ESR associated with fever and limb pain also suggest osteomyelitis (see Chapter 9). Blood cultures and radiographs should be obtained. In addition, a radionuclide bone scan is indicated for early detection of osteomyelitis because radiographic findings of the condition lag 10–14 days behind symptomatology.

Management

The pediatrician caring for children with limp or gait disturbances must be familiar with major trends in management and must also know when to seek orthopedic consultation. This discussion does not concentrate on management except as outlined in specific conditions.

Congenital Hip Dislocation

The new, preferred terminology for these conditions is **developmental dysplasia (or displacement) of the hip (DDH)**. This term includes CHD as well as subluxation and acetabular dysplasia. This term also recognizes that these problems may

arise in utero, at the time of birth, or even during infancy. DDH is an important developmental condition that ultimately results in gait disturbance if it is not recognized and treated during the first few months of life. Because DDH involves the hip joint and is thus not a static deformity, the clinician must administer a screening or diagnostic maneuver to detect its presence. Like most of the other conditions considered in this section, there is a definite relationship between the intrauterine position of the infant and subsequent development of the deformity.

DDH is six times more common in females than males. The left hip is four times more likely to be the involved joint but bilateral hip dislocation does occur in 25% of cases. More often, DDH is a congenital deformation rather than a congenital malformation of embryologic maldevelopment (i.e., a condition acquired shortly before or after birth). Between 30% and 50% of children with DDH are delivered by breech. Therefore, it has been recommended that all infants delivered by breech should be fully evaluated for the possibility of DDH.

In most instances, newborn infants have dislocatable hips with otherwise normal structural anatomy except for loose or stretched joint ligaments. In about 20% of cases the deformity is more severe and long-standing with resultant in utero deformity of the femoral head and acetabulum. The former cases respond to positional treatment, whereas the latter may require more aggressive intervention.

The diagnosis of DDH is made primarily by physical examination at the time of birth as previously described, and this represents one of the most important prescriptive newborn screening tests. In addition, the pediatrician must consider this condition when examining well children from birth to 6 months. Several case reports describe children found to have DDH at several months of age despite normal newborn examinations. Although radiographic studies at birth may be misleading, ultrasonography of the hip joint has become a very useful modality in making the diagnosis and may even be advocated as a screening technique.

The simplest method of treatment of uncomplicated DDH discovered at birth is the use of the Pavlik harness, which holds the relocated femoral head in position while allowing for rotation as well as diaper changes. The duration of treatment (usually several months) is determined by the progress of the individual infant.

Children older than 6 months of age with frank dislocation that does not reduce with the Ortolani

| TABLE 26.5 | **Laboratory Tests in the Differential Diagnosis of Limp** | | |

Part of Body	Common Diagnostic Considerations	Diagnostic Tests	Anticipated Results
Hip	SCFE	X-ray (AP frog leg) Technetium bone scan	Increased width of epiphysis, frank slip, increased uptake on the joint
	Transient synovitis	X-ray	Usually normal, occasional widening of joint spaces on traction
		Ultrasound-fluid	
		CBC	Normal
		ESR	Normal
	Legg-Calvé-Perthes disease	X-ray	Usually normal or slightly increased Widening of joint space
		MRI	Widening of epiphyseal line, increased density of femoral head, increased width of neck of femur
		Technetium bone scan	Decreased uptake in FC–epiphysis initially, later increased uptake
	Septic hip	CBC and blood culture	Increased WBC count with shift
		ESR	Increased
		X-ray	Increased soft tissue and capsular swelling with lateral displacement of the proximal femur
	Developmental dysplasia of the hip (DDH) [CHD]	Ultrasound (newborn)	Interpreted by ultrasonographer
		X-ray (older child)	Increase in acetabular angle Lateral displacement of femoral neck Discontinuous Shenton line
	Excessive femoral anteversion	X-ray	Anteversion of femoral neck > 50°
	Genu varum	X-ray	Tibiofemoral angle > 25° of varus
	Genu valgum	X-ray	Tibiofemoral angle > 15° of valgus Asymmetry Short stature
Knee	Osgood-Schlatter disease	None	Normal
	Chondromalacia patella	X-ray arthroscopy	Usually normal, rough articular surface
	Baker cyst	Transillumination needle aspiration	Positive gelatinous fluid
	Traumatic conditions	Radiography	Displacement of patella, bone fragments, degeneration of patella
	Dislocation of patella	Arthrography	Diagnostic
	Subluxation of patella	Arthroscopy	Diagnostic
	Injuries of the menisci	MRI	Diagnostic
	Fracture of anterior tibial spine	MRI	Diagnostic
Leg (femur or tibia)	Osteoid osteoma	X-ray	Radiolucent nidus surrounded by sclerotic bone
	Osteochondroma	X-ray	Ossification
	Osteogenic sarcoma	X-ray	Lytic and calcified areas of bone
	Ewing sarcoma	X-ray	Lytic lesions
	Trauma	X-ray	Various fractures
	Blount disease	X-ray	Abrupt medial angulation and fragmentation of proximal tibia
	Rickets	X-ray	Osteoporosis Bowing Widening of epiphyseal plate Fraying of metaphysis and cortical thinning
		Ca^{2+}, PO_4, alkaline phosphatase, PTH	Diagnostic
	Tibial torsion	—	Not helpful

TABLE 26.5	Laboratory Tests in the Differential Diagnosis of Limp *(Continued)*		
Part of Body	**Common Diagnostic Considerations**	**Diagnostic Tests**	**Anticipated Results**
Foot	Metatarsus adductus	—	Usually normal
	Equinovarus	X-ray	Complex
	Pes planus	—	Normal

AP = anteroposterior; CBC = complete blood count; CHD = congenital hip dislocation; ESR = erythrocyte sedimentation rate; FC = fluorocytosine; MRI = magnetic resonance imaging; PTH = parathyroid hormone; SCFE = slipped capital femoral epiphysis; WBC = white blood cell.

maneuver must be referred to a pediatric orthopedist for evaluation and treatment. During the first year of life, the developing acetabulum molds to the shape of a femoral head. Therefore, the goal of management is to maintain position of the femoral head within the acetabulum without compromising the vascular supply. At no time should clinicians use forceful maneuvers or apply devices that damage these delicate structures. In children between 1 and 5 years of age, various methods of treatment (molding, traction, casting, surgical reduction) may be necessary and warranted, but in children older than 5 years of age, the end result of attempting to bring the femur down into the acetabulum may be unsatisfactory. In these cases, where there is no chance of having a normally functioning hip joint, many orthopedists recommend leaving the dislocated femur in its false acetabulum rather than attempting complex heroic surgical procedures.

Management of affected children becomes a joint venture, and the pediatrician should not abandon the child or defer to all orthopedic opinion. Continued support, interpretation, evaluation of compliance, and advice to the family make the orthopedist's intervention more effective and sensitive to the family's needs and, in the long run, lead to a more successful outcome.

Septic Arthritis of the Hip

Septic arthritis is the most important diagnosis to make promptly in the differential diagnosis of hip joint disease. In its classic form, the findings are fairly straightforward, but atypical or early presentations may mimic other conditions. Subsequent morbidity resulting from destruction of the femoral head and neck is directly proportional to duration of delay in recognition and instituting treatment. Therefore, this condition must be considered whenever there is recent onset of limp associated with joint findings. The diagnosis must be made early and treatment instituted promptly.

Septic arthritis of the hip joint may arise at any age from the neonatal period through adolescence. It is usually bacterial in origin, with organisms entering the joint space via a hematogenous route from a distant site of infection or by direct skin portal of entry from recent trauma or puncture. Pneumonia, otitis media, pharyngitis, or skin infection have all been associated with subsequent septic arthritis. Organisms responsible for the infection include *Haemophilus influenzae* in neonates and young infants, pneumococcus, streptococci, gonococcus, and salmonella, with the latter occurring especially in children with sickle cell disease.

The history is that of a sudden onset of fever, hip pain, limp, or total failure to move the extremity, often associated with or following an infection. On examination, children appear seriously ill. Any movement of the affected joint elicits pain, and swelling and erythema overlie the proximal thigh. The joint is splinted in flexion, external rotation, and abduction. Tenderness to palpation of the overlying soft tissues is often present.

The diagnosis of septic arthritis is suspected clinically and then confirmed by appropriate laboratory tests. It is imperative to make this diagnosis as early as possible to avoid destruction of joint tissues. A markedly elevated WBC count with a left shift and an elevated ESR are characteristic. Although radiographs of the hip made very early in the course of the disease may be negative, they usually reveal soft tissue swelling, capsular swelling, and lateral and upward displacement of the femur. Ultrasonography may help demonstrate the presence of fluid and epiphyseal displacement. More advanced cases show subluxation and destruction of the femoral head. In neonates, whose ossification is incomplete, there may be displacement of the medial metaphysis from the acetabulum.

If the diagnosis of septic hip is suspected, needle aspiration of the joint must be performed promptly for both diagnosis and identification of the organism. Recovery of the organism from the hip joint may be unsuccessful, and a negative

Gram stain or culture does not exclude the diagnosis of septic arthritis. Frequently the organism is obtained by multiple blood cultures rather than by direct aspiration of the hip.

Transient Synovitis

This condition, which is also known as **toxic synovitis,** is the most common cause of nontraumatic limp in children. Although this condition is relatively benign, self-limited, and of short duration, it is very significant because of potential difficulties in distinguishing it from other more serious conditions.

Transient synovitis occurs in children of both sexes between the ages of 2 and 12 years, but it is most common in boys between 5 and 10 years of age. The etiology is unknown but many children have an antecedent history of a mild viral illness associated with intermittent fever.

The presenting complaint is usually the gradual onset of unilateral limp. Children may complain of knee or hip pain and often bend forward at the hip on the affected side as flexion of the joint relieves symptoms. They either refuse to walk or manifest a mildly painful gait with only moderate discomfort and occasionally have a low-grade fever.

Examination of the hip reveals no tenderness, warmth, or swelling, but discomfort is elicited on extension, internal rotation, and abduction of the hip. The gait and natural resting position of the affected side reflect flexion, external rotation, and adduction of the hip joint.

Laboratory examinations are helpful only because the complete blood count (CBC) and ESR are usually normal; therefore, the test results rule out other conditions. Radiographic examinations of the hip are usually completely normal but occasionally may show some widening of the joint space between the head of the femur and the acetabulum medially and, on traction views, superiorly. A bulge of the capsule is seen rarely on the lateral side, and on occasion, alternations of soft tissue shadows are seen laterally. Ultrasound may show small amounts of fluid in the joint.

Treatment involves bed rest and analgesics for 3–5 days. Although traction has been used by some orthopedists to relieve discomfort, this is rarely if ever necessary except as a means of keeping the child at rest. The condition is invariably self-limited and of short duration. There are usually no sequelae but the condition may recur.

Legg-Calvé-Perthes Disease

This disease is a potentially serious condition if not recognized early. Fortunately, it is not common, with an estimated annual incidence of 1:18,000. It occurs most often in Caucasian children between the ages of 4 and 9 years and has a sex predominance of boys over girls of 5:1.

Legg-Calvé-Perthes disease, an avascular necrosis of the femoral head, is usually considered to represent an osteochondrosis of the capital femoral epiphysis. The etiology is unknown but may be related to repeated trauma to an area known to have poor vascularization. Low-birth-weight children, children with constitutional delay of growth, and children with retarded bone age have a significantly higher incidence than the general population. Children with an antecedent history of transient synovitis are susceptible. The condition is bilateral in 10%–18% of cases, and there is an increased familial frequency.

Children with Legg-Calvé-Perthes disease most often present with an intermittent limp of insidious onset associated with knee pain. The gait is antalgic with pain in the groin, lateral hip, or inner aspect of the knee. However, no pain may be present, and often the history is so subtle that the diagnosis is delayed because the parents or the physician do not attribute sufficient significance to the symptoms.

On examination, shortening of the stance phase occurs in symptomatic children, along with limitation of internal rotation and abduction on passive manipulation of the hip joint. In long-standing cases, there may also be some flexion contraction and mild atrophy of the leg muscles on the affected side. These children are afebrile.

Laboratory studies reveal a normal CBC and ESR. The principal aid to diagnosis is radiography. There are four distinct stages: (1) widening of the distance between the femoral head and the acetabulum, (2) collapse of the femoral head with increased density and characteristic subcapsular semilunar lucencies, (3) increase in width of the femoral neck, and (4) reossification of the femoral head and metaphysis. In early stages before radiographic changes become obvious, a technetium scan will show decreased epiphyseal uptake in contrast to the diffuse increased uptake seen in transient synovitis. In addition, weighted MRI studies of the hip show early necrosis before radiographic changes are visible.

The pediatrician has an important role in diagnosing and caring for children with Legg-Calvé-Perthes disease. First, the diagnosis must be suspected and established, which requires an appropriate index of suspicion and a correct diagnostic approach, and second, the pediatrician must participate with the orthopedist and family in carrying out a plan of treatment.

The basic goals of treatment are reduction of weight-bearing on the affected side for a prolonged period of time while maintaining motion and containment to prevent deformity, alter growth disturbance, and joint diseases. This may involve 2–4 years of continued follow-up and planning. The range of treatment may include periods of bed rest and traction, braces, crutches, or surgical intervention. There are many different approaches to eliminating weight-bearing, and each affects the child's life to a variable degree. Therefore, the pediatrician is essential to help plan an acceptable therapeutic program.

Slipped Capital Femoral Epiphysis

SCFE is a serious, common condition of obese preadolescents and early adolescents. It occurs in boys between 10 and 17 years of age and in girls between 8 and 15 years of age and is bilateral in 20%–30% of patients. Before fusion of the epiphyseal plate has taken place, boys have the disorder two to four times more frequently than girls, and blacks are more predisposed than whites. About 80% of all cases fall into this category, with a slowly progressive chronic slip of the femoral shaft off the capital head through the epiphysis. The remaining 20% have a more acute process, usually associated with significant trauma. This latter group is comprised of younger children, including newborns, who have sustained shearing trauma, especially from automobile accidents or abuse.

Typical presentation of the larger group involves an antalgic gait with pain in the knee, groin, buttock, or lateral hip. Again, the limp may be subtle or intermittent, and the pain may not be particularly severe. Superimposed trauma may exacerbate a chronic low-grade slip. Symptoms may have been present for many months before being recognized, but the moment the diagnosis is suspected or confirmed, immediate hospitalization is indicated to prevent further slip.

To perform the physical examination, place the child in the supine position and passively flex the hip. If the patient has SCFE, the hip abducts and rotates externally instead of flexing in the same neutral plane as the knee. This maneuver should be part of the routine adolescent examination as well because the history of limp or pain can frequently appear later in the course of the disease.

In SCFE, laboratory findings are normal and the diagnosis is made on clinical and radiologic grounds alone. Posterior–anterior, frog-leg, and lateral views must be obtained to visualize subtle or early findings. Initially, there is an increase in the width of the epiphysis with irregular margins. As the condition progresses, there is a lat-

eral movement of the femur in relation to the head, which slips medially with shearing of the epiphyseal plate. Discontinuity of the medial border of the head of the femur at the level of the epiphysis demonstrates the degree of displacement or slippage.

Treatment of SCFE is prompt surgical pinning of the epiphysis to prevent further slippage. Immediate hospitalization and orthopedic consultation are indicated as soon as the diagnosis is established. The pediatrician should provide long-term follow-up and be aware of the possibility of contralateral involvement at a later date.

Torsional Deformities

The management of torsional deformities in children is largely medical; few surgical interventions are warranted. The pediatrician should know how to determine which conditions need treatment and how to use the few effective splints or devices available.

TIBIAL TORSION. Whether or not an infant presents with tibial torsion is largely due to three factors: heredity, intrauterine position, and sleeping position. Probably the most significant of these is intrauterine position, which determines the basic deformity. Sleeping position is never causative but may further exacerbate the condition or prevent spontaneous resolution by maintaining the abnormal position for many hours during the day and night. Although there may be familial trends in gait patterns and torsional deformities, no specific hereditary patterns have been documented.

The more common deformity is internal tibial torsion, which is frequently associated with varying degrees of metatarsus adductus. Although this condition usually resolves spontaneously with weight-bearing, progression without resolution prior to 18 months of age results in lifelong gait disturbance. External tibial torsion is usually of little significance unless it is extreme or asymmetric, with more than 20° variance between extremities.

The internal tibial torsion together with metatarsus adductus results in an abnormal gait, often noticed when the child begins to walk. In most mild to moderate situations, the condition resolves spontaneously without treatment before the age of 18 months. However, because the condition is positional in nature, sleeping posture may exacerbate or prevent spontaneous resolution. The pediatrician should advise parents to encourage sleeping in the supine position as early as possible. One helpful hint involves hanging a mobile above the crib; this attracts the child's attention and allows him to fall asleep on his back. After 18 months of age, spontaneous correction is unlikely, and many orthopedists recommend night splints. The Denis Browne bar, which maintains the feet in the desired position, supposedly exerts external rotational forces that correct the deformity. Unfortunately, compliance is usually marginal because children hate these contraptions, and the results are questionable because no researchers have performed prospective controlled trials. Late sequelae of unresolved external tibial torsion are largely cosmetic and not functional. If they are asymmetric, correction can be obtained surgically by derotational tibial osteotomy, but this is rarely indicated. External tibial torsion is not a problem. A slight outtoeing gait is quite common and tolerable.

EXCESSIVE FEMORAL ANTEVERSION. This torsional deformity occurs at the level of the hip and might better be termed "femoral torsion." Actually, all infants have femoral anteversion at birth, and it is not until 1–2 years of age that the femur begins to rotate externally in relation to the neck of the femur. Femoral anteversion represents a failure of progression and a persistence into childhood and adult life of the normally anteverted position.

A familial pattern may be partially responsible for failure to respond to normal weight-bearing forces in shaping the neck and head of the femur. There is still some debate as to whether an abnormal sitting position (reverse tailor position) is primary or secondary in this condition. Some experts believe that the condition arises because children with the deformity are able to sit comfortably in this position. We believe that the condition is secondary but do not encourage children to sit in the W position, because it may exacerbate or prolong a previously existing deformity.

There is no known preventive treatment for excessive femoral anteversion other than cautioning the parents not to allow the child to sit in the reverse tailor position. Sitting cross-legged (Indian style) prevents further progression of this deformity, but the ultimate outcome must await young adulthood. At that time, if the disability is judged to be severe, with a very abnormal gait, patellofemoral malalignment syndrome, and attendant chondromalacia patellae, femoral osteotomy may be indicated. There is no evidence that continued femoral anteversion leads to hip joint disease (arthritis) in later life; therefore, if signs and symptoms are tolerable, surgery should be avoided. Many children have compensatory external tibial torsion that corrects the angle of gait when walking and provides good cosmetic appearance. In these instances, only athletic activities (including running) are significantly altered, and the decision regarding surgery is elective.

GENU VARUM (BOWLEG) AND GENU VALGUM (KNOCK-KNEE). Most normal infants are born with mildly to moderately bowed legs (i.e., physiologic bowing). The bowing is clearly related to the intrauterine position, where the lower extremities are folded up cross-legged on one another. There is a gradual disappearance of the bowing during the first 2 years of life, by which time the tibiofemoral angle approaches 0°. The process does not stop here, because most normal children then go to a phase of physiologic valgus. This peaks at 3 years of age, after which it returns to about 5° of valgus by 7 years of age.

The etiology of excessive physiologic bowing or excessive genu valgum deformity is unknown, but it is thought that hereditary factors play more of a role than environmental factors (i.e., walking habits). As long as the development is symmetrical and not excessive, bowleg at younger than 2½ years of age and knock-knees between 2½ and 7 years of age should be considered variants of normal.

BLOUNT DISEASE (TIBIA VARA). This growth disturbance results in severe genu varum deformity. It is often associated with internal tibial torsion, which tends to exacerbate the condition. The etiology of this progressive disease, which represents a growth disturbance of the epiphyseal and metaphyseal region of the posterior-medial aspect of the proximal tibia, is disputed. One school of thought suggests that there is a disturbance in growth and ossification (dysplasia of bone) of the medial part of the proximal tibial epiphysis–metaphysis. The other school of thought attributes the problem to abnormal lines of force transmitted across the medial tibiofemoral compartment secondary to early walking patterns of obese children.

Blount disease is most common among blacks with many cases reported from the West Indies and West Africa. The condition has also been reported in Scandinavia. Initially, it may be impossible to differentiate excessive physiologic genu varum from early Blount disease, even with radiologic criteria. The spectrum of genu varum may include Blount disease at the extreme and that familial or genetic predisposition probably accounts for its occurrence in some families and not in others.

The management of physiologic symmetric genu valgum and genu varum requires no intervention whatsoever. No special shoes, exercises, or braces are indicated, and the use of a Denis Browne splint actually exacerbate bowed legs. Reassurance that the bowing noted in toddlers under 2 years of age and the knock-knees commonly observed between 2 and 7 years of age are within the normal range is the most important aspect of pediatric assessment and counseling.

On the other hand, the pediatrician must be able to recognize when either of these conditions is asymmetric or of extreme variation with a poor prognosis. Severe genu varum deformity with a tibiofemoral angle of more than 25°, which has not resolved by 2 years of age, is considered to have a poor prognosis for spontaneous resolution. Black infants with severe bowing should be evaluated carefully for progression and for the presence of Blount disease.

Knock-knees of moderate degree occurring up to 7 years of age may be considered within normal limits. Asymmetry or a tibiofemoral angle of more than 15° of valgus or association with short stature are indications for orthopedic intervention, because spontaneous resolution is unlikely. A distance of more than 3 inches between the medial malleoli in a 10-year-old child is not likely to correct spontaneously.

Severe genu varum deformity that requires intervention may be managed by either a long leg brace with lateral pull strap, a frame brace, or a Blount brace. Severe genu valgum deformity, on the other hand, may require surgical intervention with procedures designed to alter the medial distal femoral and medial proximal tibial epiphyses.

RICKETS. This condition should always be considered as a possible cause in the differential diagnosis of bowing, particularly in a breast-fed black child. Vitamin D–deficient rickets, as well as other less common types occurring in infancy while skeletal maturation is progressing, may be responsible for excessive bowing that easily is recognized on radiographic examination.

Foot Deformities

By far the most common cause of foot deformities resulting in a gait disturbance is intrauterine fetal position with subsequent molding. Metatarsus adductus, which is often associated with internal tibial torsion, is usually a flexible forefoot deformity that can be corrected passively by manual manipulation. On the other hand, rigid metatarsus with talipes equinovarus (clubfoot) probably represents deformity of longer intrauterine positioning and is not spontaneously correctable without surgical intervention.

Metatarsus adductus is a condition involving mild to moderate forefoot deformities that are flexible and handled by the pediatrician and the parent without orthopedic intervention. Because this condition most often resolves spontaneously, it is not clear whether passive stretching exercises with each diaper change and handling of the infant are truly contributory or are more for peace of mind. However, sleeping position is important in internal tibial torsion. If the infant can be encouraged to sleep in the supine position, the continuous pressure on the lateral aspect of the foot is removed allowing the forefoot to develop normally.

In severe, asymmetric or rigid forefoot abnormalities, the application of casts changed every 2 weeks is recommended. This may be followed with outflare shoes (to maintain position) and combined with a Denis Browne splint if the condition is associated with internal tibial torsion.

There is still some controversy concerning the management of flexible **flatfoot**, or **pes planus**. Although many podiatrists and orthopedists still recommend high-topped shoes with a Thomas heel and scaphoid pad, no special treatment for asymptomatic pes planus is necessary. Special shoes or arches may make the pronation and eversion less noticeable, but there is no evidence that any nonsurgical treatment alters the natural configuration of the foot. On the other hand, if there is any degree of rigidity, pes cavus, or pain associated with foot deformity, orthopedic intervention is warranted and may involve surgical procedures.

Worried parents can be reassured that all infants appear flatfooted until chubbiness has resolved, arch function develops with walking, and up to 50% of the population has some degree of flatfoot without disability.

Foot Pain

Limp in children can also be caused by pain in the foot. Several major causes of foot pain warrant consideration (Table 26.6). The causes of foot pain may be divided according to the frequency of the occurrence in various age groups. It is beyond the scope of this chapter to describe all the causes of foot pain individually. However, it may be noted that developmental conditions such as pes cavus and pes planus, stress fractures, and sprains, and certain tumors of bone are more likely to appear in older children, whereas infections, occult fractures, and inflammatory conditions are more prevalent in younger children. Conditions such as ill-fitting shoes, foreign body, plantar warts, and trauma may occur at any age.

The major function of shoes at any age, including infancy, is to protect the feet from trauma such

TABLE 26.6	Probable Causes of Foot Pain by Age	
0–6 Years	**6–12 Years**	**12–19 Years**
Ill-fitting shoes	Ill-fitting shoes	Ill-fitting shoes
Foreign body	Foreign body	Foreign body
Occult fracture	Accessory navicular	Ingrown toenail
Osteomyelitis	Occult fractures	Pes cavus
Juvenile rheumatoid arthritis	Tarsal coalition (peroneal spastic	Hypermobile flatfoot with tight
Rheumatic fever	flatfoot)	Achilles tendon
	Ingrown toenail	Ankle sprains
	Ewing sarcoma	Stress fractures
		Ewing sarcoma
		Synovial sarcoma

as puncture wounds. Children and infants who go without shoes (especially in summertime) are exposed to a greater variety of traumatic conditions than those who wear shoes or sneakers. A history of going barefoot is helpful in arriving at the diagnosis of local trauma.

OTORHINOLARYNGOLOGY*

Pediatric otolaryngology is a growing field. In the past 25 years, tremendous advances have been made in such diverse areas as laryngeal reconstruction, skull base surgery, audiology, and surgery for severe hearing impairment and craniofacial anomalies. The material included in this chapter is an overview of five medical problems that might be encountered in either an outpatient clinic or an inpatient setting. They are otitis media, adenotonsillectomy, epiglottitis, epistaxis, and sinusitis. For those interested in a more in-depth discussion on any of these or other topics in otolaryngology, a number of excellent texts exist (see SUGGESTED READINGS).

OTITIS MEDIA

Otitis media is a major health problem in infants and children. It is one of the most common reasons for "sick visits" in pediatric offices, with 50%–90% of children experiencing at least one episode within the first year of life. The pediatrician needs to be familiar with the various types of otitis media, their treatments, and possible complications. There are four classes of otitis media: acute, persistent, and recurrent otitis media, plus otitis media with effusion (OME).

"Otorhinolaryngology" was written by David M. Merer, M.D.

Acute Otitis Media

Acute otitis media (AOM) is characterized by the rapid onset of symptoms that may include otalgia, fever, or irritability. The most common causes are *Streptococcus pneumoniae, H. influenzae,* and *Moraxella catarrhalis.* History and pneumatic otoscopy are the basis for diagnosis of AOM. Bubbles, air-fluid levels, and otorrhea are obvious signs. Researchers who evaluated findings noted on otoscopy to establish which factor most consistently predicted infection found that color, mobility, and tympanic membrane position could be used most accurately.

Pediatric Pearl

The light reflex is an inconsistent finding in AOM, and it should not be the sole basis for diagnosis.

Treatment of AOM includes antipyretics and analgesics as well as appropriate antibiotics such as amoxicillin, erythromycin with sulfisoxazole, or trimethoprim–sulfamethoxazole. Cefaclor, loracarbef, and amoxicillin–clavulanate are appropriate in those children who fail to respond to initial therapy. A more in-depth approach to the topic of AOM can be found in Chapter 9 (Infectious Diseases).

Persistent Otitis Media

Middle ear effusions may persist for 2 months after the acute infection in 20% of children. Risk factors for persistent otitits media include atopic history, a previous history of recurrent otitis media, and enlarged adenoids. One researcher found that 31% of these effusions contained ampicillin-resistant *H. influenzae,* while 51% had ampicillin-susceptible *S. pneumoniae* or *H. influenzae.* Persistent middle ear effusions do not warrant any specific treatment except close observation to check for evidence of hearing loss. There has been no conclusive evidence that even with persistent effusion **without hearing loss,** the use of antibiotics or myringotomy with tympanostomy tube placement has any more efficacious outcome than just close observation and follow-up even if the effusion has not resolved within 3 months (Figure 26.3). However, the recommendation for intervention with myringotomy and tube placement should be accelerated if there is evidence of bilateral hearing loss.

Recurrent Otitis Media

Multiple bouts of AOM with complete resolution between episodes is called recurrent AOM. The bacteriology of these infections is identical with that of AOM, although recurrence soon after a course of antibiotics may signify the presence of a resistant organism. Children who have frequent bouts of AOM in rapid succession should be evaluated for underlying conditions that may give them a predilection for ear infections (e.g., poor

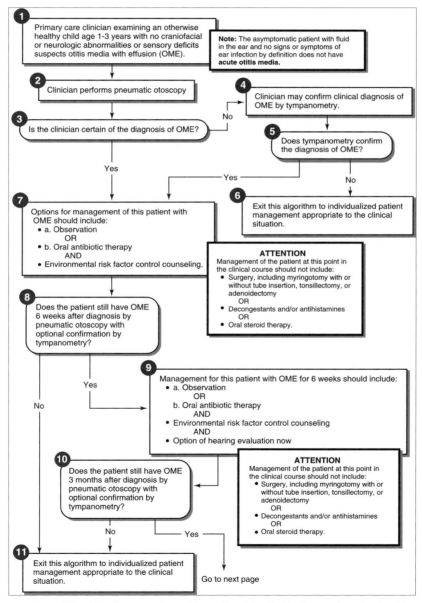

FIGURE 26.3 Algorithm for managing otitis media with effusion in an otherwise healthy child of 1–3 years of age. *(continued)*

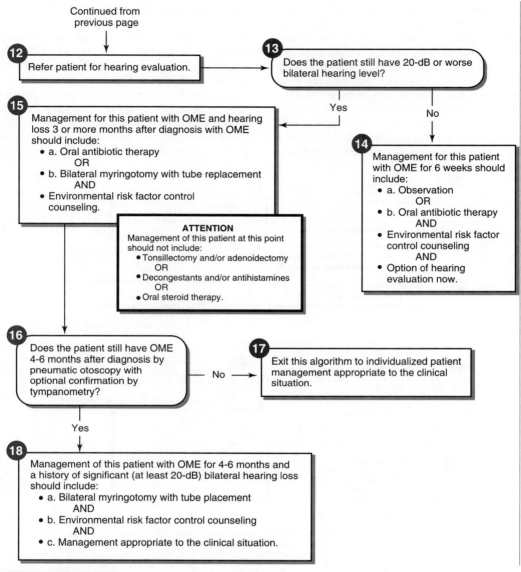

FIGURE 26.3 *(CONTINUED)*

immune function, sinusitis, respiratory allergies, submucous cleft palate, nasopharyngeal mass).

If there is no evidence of physical or physiologic abnormality, the physician must next decide how to treat the recurrent infections. Two common methods are (1) antibiotic prophylaxis and (2) myringotomy and tube placement with or without adenoidectomy.

Prophylaxis is a once-daily dose of antibiotics, usually given at bedtime. Current recommendations are amoxicillin 20 mg/kg or sulfisoxazole

75 mg/kg (trimethoprim–sulfamethoxazole is never used for prophylaxis). Antibiotics continue throughout the entire respiratory infection season (frequently 3 months). Evaluation every 6–8 weeks for new-onset effusion or "breakthrough" AOM is appropriate. If either condition occurs, the pediatrician should consider myringotomy and tube placement.

Myringotomy and insertion of tubes is the most common surgical procedure performed on children for which general anesthesia is required.

This procedure prevents the symptoms of AOM, although persistent otorrhea occurs in 5%–15% of patients. This can be treated with oral antibiotics and local antibiotic–cortisone drops. The overall complication rate is 11%. Other complications include persistent tympanic membrane perforation, atrophic tympanic membrane, granuloma formation, tympanosclerosis, cholesteatoma, and ossicular disruption.

Adenoidectomy performed concurrently with myringotomy and tube placement remains controversial. Some studies appear to show that adenoidectomy decreases the frequency of otitis media. Moreover, the effect is independent of adenoid size, which suggests that the location of the adenoid and its reservoir of pathogenic bacteria is as important in the pathogenesis of otitis media as physical obstruction of the eustachian tubes. Therefore, the decision for or against adenoidectomy should be individualized. Children with chronic upper airway obstruction or those with recurrent or chronic OME who have had one or more myringotomies with tube insertions may be good candidates for adenoidectomy.

Otitis Media With Effusion

Otitis media with effusion (OME) is the fourth type of otitis media (see Figure 26.3). Fifty percent of children with OME may be asymptomatic. Recent literature indicates that two-thirds of effusions contain bacteria, with one-half of these containing *H. influenzae, S. pneumoniae,* or *M. catarrhalis.* Physical examination may reveal a retracted or bulging tympanic membrane, which may be opacified or translucent, and fluid may be amber or bluish. There should be no history of ear pain, fever, or other symptoms suggesting an AOM.

OME is usually associated with an upper respiratory infection and resolves without treatment. Some physicians prefer not treating the effusion, knowing that it will resolve. The treatment of chronic OME is a subject of controversy. OME causes mild to moderate hearing loss, and recent studies have examined the effects of chronic OME on communication development. This research indicates that OME may be associated with learning disorders, attention and auditory processing deficits, and deficits of higher-order auditory processing (i.e., signal detection in background noise). However, opponents of these studies believe that while early deficits have been documented in some children, the long-term consequences are negligible.

Persistence of the effusion for longer than 2 months, frequent recurrences (i.e., OME for four of 6 months), changes in the tympanic membrane, or concurrent sensorineural hearing loss should be taken into account when making treatment decisions. **Most physicians begin with a trial of antibiotics.** Decongestants, antihistamines, and corticosteroids have not proven efficacious in children. Recent guidelines support close observation and monitoring if there is no evidence of bilateral hearing loss. Even with unilateral hearing loss, the recommendation is expectant observation. However, with an effusion for 3 months or more and evidence of bilateral hearing loss, intervention is recommended; the most well supported procedures are myringotomy and placement of tympanostomy tubes. Figure 26.3 delineates these recent guidelines.

Complications of Otitis Media

If treatment for AOM, chronic OM, and cholesteatoma is not adequate, complications may develop. The complications of otitis media may be divided into two types—aural and intracranial (Table 26.7). Causes of complications are spread of infection beyond the air cells of the temporal bone or bony destruction. Factors that influence the spread of infection include the type and virulence of the infecting organism, antibiotics, host response, anatomic barriers, and drainage.

Signs of complications range from headache, seizures, and spiking fevers to vertigo, sudden hearing loss, and anterior–inferior displacement of the pinna with postauricular swelling. The pediatrician who suspects that a child has a complication of either AOM or chronic otitis media should contact an otolaryngologist immediately. Complications related to AOM typically require drainage, surgical debridement if bony destruction is present, and high-dose intravenous antibiotics. A neurosurgical consult is indicated if intracranial complications are present. Complications from chronic otitis media require surgical intervention to debride granulation tissue and remove cholesteatoma. The surgery varies depending on the aural or intracranial structures involved.

ADENOTONSILLITIS

During the early twentieth century, adenotonsillectomy was a common treatment for adenotonsillitis. Physicians performed the procedure for various reasons, including enuresis, epistaxis, upset stomach, asthma, and stammering. Although modern otolaryngologists use more rigorous preoperative criteria, controversy surrounding management of adenotonsillar disease in children still exists.

The palatine tonsils are paired structures located along the lateral wall of the oropharynx, while the adenoids (pharyngeal tonsils) are found on the posterior–superior wall of the nasopharynx, in close proximity to the eustachian tubes and sinus ostia. Both are composed of large masses of lymphoid tissue that enlarge until puberty and then regress. Their immunologic function is complex; they appear to affect both local immunity (i.e., antibody production to specific bacteria) and systemic immune surveillance. However, there is no evidence that adenotonsillectomy adversely affects immune function.

The microbiology of the adenoids and tonsils is similar. Although group A beta-hemolytic streptococcus is the organism most physicians associate with adenotonsillitis, *S. pneumoniae, Staphylococcus aureus,* and *H. influenzae* as well as Epstein-Barr virus, herpes simplex virus, and various anaerobes may also play important roles.

The tonsils are easily visualized in the oropharynx. To evaluate their inferior extension, the clinician should use a tongue depressor. It is necessary to grade the tonsils on the basis of obstruction of the airway as 1+ ($< 25\%$), 2+ (25%–50%), 3+ (51%–75%), and 4+ ($> 75\%$). Erythema, exudate, tonsilloliths, or other abnormalities may also be present.

It is not possible to visualize the adenoids without the use of special equipment (nasopharyngeal mirror or fiberoptic nasopharyngoscope). Therefore, the best methods for diagnosis of adenoid hypertrophy are by clinical history (nasal obstruction, snoring, mouth-breathing) and physical examination (hyponasal speech; adenoid facies; openmouthed, dull appearance; elongated face; dark circles under the eyes).

The **drug of choice** for treating adenotonsillitis is **penicillin** (clindamycin or erythromycin for allergic children), although antibiotics effective against beta-lactamase-producing organisms may be warranted in resistant cases.

The indications and contraindications for **adenotonsillectomy** have been well documented (Table 26.8). The **most common indication is recurrent infection**. In one study, researchers demonstrated that tonsillectomy is effective in preventing recurrent tonsillitis–pharyngitis; however, this particular study required that children had at least seven episodes in 1 year, five epi-

---

TABLE 26.7 **Complications of Otitis Media**

Aural
  Hearing loss (conductive and sensorineural)
  Otorrhea
  Tympanosclerosis
  Acute and chronic tympanic membrane
    perforation
  Chronic otomastoiditis
  Cholesteatoma
  Acute mastoiditis with bony destruction
  Ossicular erosion
  Labyrinthine erosion/labyrinthitis
  Facial nerve paralysis

Intracranial
  Meningitis
  Lateral sinus thrombosis
  Extradural abscess
  Subdural abscess
  Brain abscess

---

sodes annually for 2 years, or three episodes annually for 3 years to be in the study. The pediatrician should not use these criteria dogmatically but should consider surgical intervention when the infections have a significant effect on the everyday functioning of the child (i.e., missing a significant amount of school or work because of illness). Guidelines shared by the American Medical Association and the American Academy of Pediatrics (AAP) recommend tonsillectomy for children with four or more documented episodes of pharyngitis annually.

Obstructive sleep apnea is also a common indication for surgery. This condition is characterized by loud snoring, periods of apnea, restlessness, coughing and choking during sleep, and daytime somnolence.

Pediatric Pearl

Children with obstructive sleep apnea may initially present with complaints of daytime sleepiness, lack of energy, and poor school performance. Careful questioning uncovers a history of loud snoring and restless sleeping.

Rare complications of sleep apnea include cor pulmonale and failure to thrive. The diagnosis may be made by recording the individual during sleep and listening for apneic episodes or by a sleep study that more accurately records the frequency of apneic and hypopneic episodes.

The most common complications of adenotonsillectomy are pain and bleeding. Bleeding may occur within the first 24 hours or between the fifth and tenth postoperative day (late postoperative bleeding). Less common complications include hypernasal speech (encountered in children with undiagnosed submucous cleft palate or after laceration of the soft palate), tongue or tooth trauma, neuropathies (lingual or hypoglossal), or pseudoaneurysm of the carotid artery.

EPIGLOTTITIS

Acute epiglottitis, also called supraglottitis, is an inflammatory condition affecting the supraglottic structures (epiglottis, aryepiglottic folds, false vocal cords). It affects children between 2 and 8 years of age (although cases in children as young as 7 months have been reported) and is seen more often during the winter and spring months. Children present with the sudden onset of stridor, drooling, odonotophagia, and high fever. Stridor, a harsh noise caused by the turbulent flow of air through a partially obstructed airway, is one of many physical signs diagnostic of airway compromise.

Pediatric Pearl

Epiglottitis is a medical emergency that requires prompt attention by a physician capable of securing the airway by either intubation or tracheotomy. If the diagnosis is suspected, direct visualization of the larynx is usually performed in the operating room.

A detailed history, careful physical examination, and appropriate radiographic and laboratory tests help identify the cause of stridor. The differential diagnosis of stridor is extensive (Table 26.9).

Epiglottitis results from infection with *H. influenzae* type b, although pneumococci and group A beta-hemolytic streptococcus have also been implicated. Inspiratory stridor results from obstruction in the supraglottic airway; biphasic stridor, by obstruction in the subglottis, glottis, or extrathoracic trachea; and expiratory stridor, by obstruction of the thoracic trachea or bronchopulmonary tree. Fortunately, the incidence of epiglottitis has substantially decreased with the introduction of routine *H. influenzae* vaccination.

In cases of suspected epiglottitis, **airway control** and administration of **intravenous antibiotics**

should not be delayed. It is necessary to complete the history and physical examination as quickly as possible. The clinician should avoid manipulating the pharynx, because this may cause acute worsening of the airway obstruction. A WBC count and blood cultures are warranted (bacteremia occurs in 50% of patients). A lateral neck film, if time permits, demonstrates swelling of the supraglottic structures.

After transfer to the operating room, the pharynx and larynx are visualized (the epiglottis is usually red and swollen) and intubation occurs. The otolaryngology team is available if a tracheotomy is required. Cultures are appropriate after intubation. Intravenous antibiotics are necessary (a second- or third-generation cephalosporin) until children are safely extubated. The criteria for extubation vary; it is usually performed when an air leak develops around the endotracheal tube or within 24 hours of the cessation of fever. After children begin taking oral antibiotics and their condition stabilizes, they may be discharged.

EPISTAXIS

Epistaxis is a common complaint in the pediatric population. This condition, which is typically a self-limited process caused by a mild mucosal abrasion, may be the first sign of a more serious underlying disease.

The nasal cavity receives blood from the internal and external carotid artery systems (Table 26.10). The most common bleeding site, called the Kiesselbach plexus or Little area, is located along the anterior septum and corresponds to the convergence and anastomosis of arteries from both systems. However, bleeding sites may be located in any part of the nasal cavity. Those sites located posteriorly or superiorly tend to be more difficult to control.

The **initial intervention for epistaxis** should consist of **digital pressure** applied to the nares for 10 minutes. In a majority of cases, this will be the only intervention necessary. Bleeding that cannot be controlled with pressure may require the application of topical vasoconstrictors (Neo-Synephrine 0.25%), evacuation of clot from the nasal cavity, cautery (silver nitrate), or packing with a self-expanding nasal tampon. An experienced physician may choose to place a Vaseline nasal pack or to pack the nasopharynx for improved hemostasis.

After the bleeding has been controlled, the physician should obtain a careful history, keeping in mind the differential diagnosis of epistaxis

TABLE 26.8 Traditional and Current Indications for and Contraindications to Tonsillectomy and Adenoidectomy

Definite indications for tonsillectomy

Recurrent acute or chronic tonsillitis
Tonsillitis resulting in febrile convulsions
Peritonsillar abscess
Tonsillar hypertrophy obstructing respiration or deglutition
Diphtheria carrier
Biopsy necessary to define tissue pathology

Definite indications for adenoidectomy

Recurrent middle ear disease secondary to eustachian tube obstruction
Adenoid hypertrophy obstructing respiration
Sinusitis or its complications secondary to adenoid obstruction of the posterior sinus ostia

Equivocal or relative indications for tonsillectomy and adenoidectomy

Recurrent sore throats
Recurrent otalgias
Recurrent or chronic rhinitis
Recurrent upper respiratory infections
Snoring or mouth breathing
Failure to thrive
Large tonsils or tonsillar debris
Cervical lymphadenopathy
Tuberculous adenitis
Systemic diseases secondary to β-hemolytic streptococcal infections (rheumatic fever, rheumatic heart disease, nephritis)

Relative contraindications to tonsillectomy and adenoidectomy

Cleft palate
Presence of tonsils or adenoids
Acute infections, including tonsillitis and respiratory infections
Younger than 3 years of age

Definite contraindications to tonsillectomy and adenoidectomy

Blood dyscrasias (leukemias, purpuras, aplastic anemias, hemophilia)
Uncontrolled systemic diseases (diabetes, heart disease, seizure disorders)

(Table 26.11). The duration of the epistaxis and previous episodes and their frequency of occurrence, as well as easy bruisability, any history of nasal trauma (including picking), nasal drug abuse, or recent upper respiratory infections are all pertinent, as is a family history of bleeding disorders.

In stable children who are ready for discharge, the clinician must address the underlying cause of the epistaxis. Humidification of the home environment is important. Normal saline sprays and Vaseline ointment help prevent crusting and moisten the mucosa. It is necessary to advise patients against nose picking, the use of nasal drugs, or other "habits" that might adversely affect the nasal cavity and cause further epistaxis.

Severe bleeding may rarely require surgical ligation of the internal maxillary, anterior eth-moid, or posterior ethmoid artery or embolization via selective artery catheterization. Children with severe epistaxis require hospitalization for observation. Those with severe or recurrent epistaxis require a more thorough medical workup to ensure that the epistaxis is not a sign of an underlying illness.

SINUSITIS

When evaluating children for sinusitis, the pediatrician tries to distinguish between a bacterial infection of the sinuses and allergies or an upper respiratory tract infection. This is complicated in young children who are, more often than not, poor historians and unable to describe the most important symptoms of an acute sinus infection.

TABLE 26.9 Differential Diagnosis of Stridor

Upper airway

Choanal atresia
Pharyngeal mass
Large tonsils and adenoids
Craniofacial anomalies

Larynx

Laryngomalacia
Vocal cord paralysis
Glottic hemangioma
Laryngeal mass/cyst
Subglottic stenosis
Papilloma
Infectious process (croup, epiglottitis)

Lower airway

Tracheomalacia
Vascular ring
Tracheal stenosis
Aspirated foreign body
Tracheoesophageal fistula
External compression

TABLE 26.10 Nasal Arterial Supply

Internal carotid system

Anterior ethmoid artery
Posterior ethmoid artery

External carotid system

Sphenopalatine artery
Greater palatine artery
Labial artery

The sinuses develop as outpouchings of the nasal chamber. The ethmoid and maxillary sinuses are clinically significant at birth and reach adult size by the ages of 12 and 18 years, respectively. The ethmoid sinuses are composed of multiple thin-walled cells located between the nasal cavity and the orbit. The anterior cells drain into the middle meatus, while the posterior cells drain into the superior meatus. The maxillary sinuses occupy the body of the maxilla. The roof corresponds to the floor of the orbit, the floor to the alveolar process of the maxilla, and the medial wall to the lateral wall of the nasal cavity. It drains into the middle meatus through a common ostium shared with the anterior ethmoid cell.

The frontal and sphenoid sinuses are not easily distinguished for several years. The frontal sinus, which is situated in the frontal bone adjacent to the anterior cranial fossa and drains into the middle meatus, becomes evident at the age of 6–8 and reaches adult size by the age of 18. The sphenoid sinuses, which are contained within the sphenoid bone and drain into the superior meatus, become evident at the age of 7 years and reach adult size by the age of 12–15. The optic nerve, pituitary gland, internal carotid artery, and cavernous sinus are all adjacent to the sphenoid sinus.

Three elements affect normal function of the sinuses: ciliary function, patency of the sinus ostia, and quality of the secretions. Factors that cause obstruction of the sinus ostia (allergies, viral upper respiratory infection, trauma, nasal polyps); impaired ciliary function (immotile cilia syndrome); or a change in the viscosity of secretions (viral upper respiratory infection, cystic fibrosis) may all cause retention of secretions in the sinuses.

The classic bacteria found in acute sinusitis include *S. pneumoniae, H. influenzae, M. catarrhalis,* and *Streptococcus pyogenes.* The results of cultures taken from the nose, nasopharynx, and throat do not accurately predict the bacteria in infected sinus secretions, and they are not currently recommended as a guide for therapy.

Common symptoms of acute sinusitis in adults and older children are headache, facial pain, and fever. Young children may not be able to describe their symptoms, which may lead to a delay in diagnosis. Signs and symptoms frequently associated with sinusitis include purulent rhinorrhea, sore throat, fever, cough (frequently at night), fetid breath, and irritability.

Physical examination may not be of help in diagnosing sinusitis in young children. The physician should attempt to elicit tenderness by percussing or palpating over the sinuses. Intranasal examination may reveal a mucopurulent discharge or foul odor. Shrinking the nasal mucosa with Neo-Synephrine 0.25% after initial evaluation allows better visualization of the middle meatus (over the inferior turbinates), the site of drainage of the frontal, maxillary, and anterior ethmoid sinuses.

Standard sinus radiographs may be of help in finalizing a diagnosis of sinusitis. An air-fluid level strongly correlates with an active disease process. Plain sinus films are notoriously nonspecific and inaccurate in the pediatric population, however, and the diagnostic modality of choice is the CT scan.

TABLE 26.11	Etiology of Epistaxis in Children

Common causes

Inflammation
    Upper respiratory tract infections
        Viral
        Bacterial
    Childhood exanthems
    Rheumatic fever
Trauma
    Dry air
    Injury, external, with or without fracture
    Patient induced (nose picking)
    Foreign body
Allergic rhinitis with or without accompanying inflammation

Uncommon causes

Alterations of intravascular factors of hemostasis
    Platelet abnormalities
        Idiopathic thrombocytopenic purpura (quantitative change in platelets)
        Thrombocytopathic purpuras (qualitative change in platelets, such as with von Willebrand disease or Glanzmann thrombasthenia)
    Coagulation defects
        Hemophilia A and B (Christmas disease)
        Bleeding caused by anticoagulant drugs such as warfarin
Hypertension
Idiopathic
    Polymorphic reticulosis
    Pyogenic granuloma
Neoplasms
    Benign
        Juvenile nasopharyngeal angiofibroma
        Polyps
        Meningocele and meningomyelocele
    Malignant leukemias
Parasite in nasal or nasopharyngeal space
Structural
    Deviation of the septum
    Adhesions between septum and lateral nasal wall
Trauma
    Postsurgical bleeding
    Chemical and caustic agents

Treatment includes antibiotics (amoxicillin, trimethoprim–sulfamethoxazole, erythromycin–sulfonamide), topical decongestants (Neo-Synephrine 0.25%), and systemic decongestants. Topical decongestants should be discontinued within 5 days to avoid a rebound phenomenon. If symptoms do not improve within 2–3 days, reevaluation is essential. Antibiotic coverage should be changed to include beta-lactamase–producing bacteria (cefuroxime, amoxicillin–clavulanate). If symptoms persist, an otolaryngology consult is warranted. A child with refrac-

tory sinusitis may require admission to the hospital for intravenous antibiotics. A CT scan of the sinuses should be obtained to evaluate the extent of the disease. Surgical options include maxillary sinus irrigation, frontal sinus trephination, and intranasal endoscopic sinus drainage.

Complications of acute sinusitis are infrequent but can be severe. Orbital complications range from periorbital cellulitis to orbital abscess and cavernous sinus thrombosis, and intracranial complications include meningitis, epidural abscess, and brain abscess. Children with suspected complications should have an otolaryngology and other relevant consult immediately.

UROLOGY*

TESTICULAR TORSION

Testicular torsion is the most common cause of acute scrotal pain and swelling in children and affects 1 in 4000 males. Torsion may occur prenatally and manifest itself as a nontender scrotal mass at birth or may present anytime through puberty as a surgical emergency.

Pathophysiology

Torsion may occur above the investment of the tunica vaginalis that surrounds the testicle (extravaginal torsion) and is more common in the perinatal period (Figure 26.4A). Intravaginal testicular torsion is more common in older children and adolescents and occurs when the testicle twists within the tunica vaginalis. The predisposing anatomic abnormality in this variant is the "bell-clapper deformity" where the tunica vaginalis has a high insertion onto the spermatic cord (see Figure 26.4B). In either type, twisting initially impedes venous return, resulting in venous thrombosis; subsequently, arterial blood flow is compromised, leading to ischemic necrosis. Unless spontaneous or surgical reduction occurs, infarction will lead to testicular atrophy.

The immediate inciting event leading to testicular torsion is poorly understood. Some factors that have been proposed include cremaster muscle hyperactivity, scrotal trauma, changes accompanying puberty including hormonal (rising testosterone) or anatomical (increased testicular volume) maturations, and vigorous exercise.

Clinical and Laboratory Evaluation

Testicular torsion typically presents as acute onset of pain that may gradually increase in intensity. The pain is usually localized to the affected testis and scrotum but may be referred to the inguinal region or lower abdomen. Previous episodes of transient pain with or without swelling of this type suggest intermittent testicular torsion. Nausea, vomiting, and anorexia often occur. Fever is a very uncommon sign and, if present, is usually low grade.

Physical examination reveals an exquisitely tender testicle. The testicle may ride high or lie transversely in the scrotum and the cremasteric reflex is reliably absent. Prehn sign, relief of pain by elevation of the testicle, is not dependable. Scrotal erythema and edema as well as a reactive hydrocele may be found as the ischemic process proceeds. "Knots" in the spermatic cord may be palpable above the testicle.

Laboratory data demonstrate a normal or only modestly elevated WBC count. Urinalysis is usually normal, although the presence of WBCs does not exclude the diagnosis of testicular torsion. If the clinical diagnosis remains in doubt, a technetium-99m pertechnetate scan to evaluate testicular blood flow can assist in making a diagnosis. Decreased blood flow to the testicle results in an area of decreased radioactive activity or "cold spot" on the scan. A long-standing torsion or missed torsion manifests as a hyperemic rim surrounding the cold spot. Scrotal ultrasonography with duplex Doppler, which also displays reduced flow to the twisted testicle, is often easier to obtain but is more operator dependent than a radionuclide study. If the diagnosis of testicular torsion is clinically in question, radiologic studies should be initiated only if they would not delay surgical intervention more than 6 hours after the onset of symptoms.

Differential Diagnosis

The acute pain and swelling found in testicular torsion can be attributed to several conditions, including testicular torsion, acute epididymitis or orchitis, incarcerated hernia, torsion of a testicular appendage, and acute hydrocele (Table 26.12). Briefly, an infectious process of the testicle or epididymis may be associated with dysuria, urinary frequency and urgency, urethral discharge, pyuria and bacteria on urinalysis, and increased flow on nuclear scan. Hernias are usually palpable, and incarceration may be associated with bilious vomiting and abdominal pain. The appendix testes and appendix epididymis, müllerian and wolffian duct remnants, respectively, may twist and are palpable as focally tender areas at the upper pole of the testis. An ischemic appendix testes may appear as a "blue dot" visible through the scrotal skin; radionuclide scans are normal or exhibit increased flow.

"Urology" was written by Lane S. Palmer, M.D., and Lisa Menasse-Palmer, M.D.

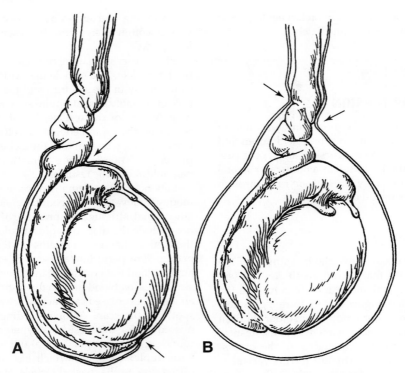

FIGURE 26.4 Anatomic relationship between the testis and tunica vaginalis in extravaginal (*A*) and intravaginal (*B*) torsion.

Management

Testicular torsion is a surgical emergency. Prompt, accurate diagnosis is imperative for surgical salvage of the testicle. The best testis survival is obtained when orchidopexy is performed within 6 hours of the onset of symptoms; only about 10% of twisted testicles are spared orchiectomy if surgery is performed after 24 hours. Irrespective of the fate of the twisted testicle, orchidopexy is performed on the contralateral testis to prevent its torsion. Manual detorsion with sedation as an emergent temporizing measure may be attempted; however, if it is successful, elective orchidopexy is indicated within 48 hours as acute retorsion is common.

PHIMOSIS

Problems related to the foreskin (prepuce) occur commonly in ambulatory pediatric settings. At birth, the prepuce normally obscures the glans and meatus and can be retracted in 4% of boys. By 6 months of age, 20% of boys have a fully retractable foreskin; the number increases to 50% by 1 year of age and to 90% by 3 years of age.

Pathophysiology

Phimosis is defined as nonretractability of a previously retractable foreskin. Smegma and skin oil production allow for the natural separation of the prepuce from the glans. Injury from forcible retraction of the prepuce and local infection from poor hygiene are the most common causes of true phimosis. These processes lead to scarring of the preputial ring and eventual fibrosis.

Clinical and Laboratory Evaluation

With phimosis, there may be ballooning of the prepuce during voiding. Infection associated with phimosis (**posthitis**) often presents as preputial edema, erythema, and tenderness.

Management

Management should include oral antibiotics to treat any infection. A dorsal slit (incision of the dorsal aspect of the prepuce) to assist with drainage is made if necessary. Circumcision can be performed electively after the inflammation has subsided. A foreskin that has never been retracted and is not in-

TABLE 26.12 Differential Diagnosis of Acute Scrotal Pain and Swelling

	Incarcerated Hernia	Torsion of the Testis	Acute Hydrocele	Inguinal Lymphadenitis	Torsion of the Appendix Testis	Acute Epididymitis
Age	Infancy	Preadolescence	Infancy	Any	Preadolescence; younger than torsion of testis	Adolescence; if infant, anatomic anomaly likely
Onset of pain	Sudden, severe; increases when testis lifted	Sudden, severe	Gradual; may be painless	Gradual, mild	Sudden, moderate; localized to one pole (blue dot)	Gradual, may become severe; early on, limited to epididymis and cord
Groin swelling	Yes	No	Maybe (hydrocele of cord)	Below inguinal ligament	No	No
Overlying redness	Yes	Yes	No	Yes	Yes	Yes
History	Prematurity; hernia noted on prior examinations	Trauma to scrotum; cryptorchidism	None	Lower extremity infection	Trauma to scrotum	Urologic instrumentation; catheterization
Mobility of mass	Fixed at groin	Movement increases pain	Yes, mobile	Fixed below inguinal ligament	Fixed on testis	Relief of pain when lifted
Transillumination	Sometimes	No	Yes	No	No	No
Associated features	Intestine palpable at internal ring on rectal examination; bowel obstruction; bilious vomiting	Testis lies transverse, high in scrotum; right lower quadrant pain, gastrointestinal symptoms, fever, leukocytosis may mimic appendicitis	Internal ring normal on rectal examination; canal empty above mass	Canal, testis, and scrotum normal	Canal normal; "blue dot" at superior pole	Associated urethritis leads to dysuria, pyuria, and urgency
Management	Early reduction, surgical repair in 1–2 days; immediate surgery if unable to reduce	Immediate surgery, including contralateral exploration and fixation	Nonoperative; hydrocelectomy if persists after 2 years of age	Antibiotics	Symptomatic; excision if scrotum is explored	Antibiotics

flamed, infected, or scarred requires no treatment. Although some physicians believe that forcible retraction of the foreskin is important for satisfactory hygiene, this often causes significant pain, fright, skin cracking, bleeding, and ultimately scarring. If the prepuce is completely nonretractile, it should be left alone unless problems occur.

PARAPHIMOSIS

Pathophysiology

Paraphimosis is the inability to place the foreskin in its natural position following retraction. A preputial ring can act as a tourniquet, resulting in venous congestion and edema of the glans and foreskin. Enlargement of the glans worsens the paraphimosis and may progress to arterial occlusion. Necrosis and gangrene may develop if the process continues.

Clinical and Laboratory Evaluation

Paraphimosis appears as a grossly edematous prepuce located proximal to the glans. A tight ring of skin is noticeable at the base of the edematous prepuce and glans. Impingement on the urethra may interfere with the urinary stream or cause urinary retention in the extreme case.

Management

Treatment of paraphimosis involves firmly grasping the glans to reduce the edema followed by manual replacement of the prepuce over the glans. If this fails, an incision of the constricting preputial ring is essential, if necessary, with a dorsal slit. After reduction, application of ice and the administration of oral antibiotics may be help. A secondary circumcision can be performed after the inflammation abates.

POSTHITIS/BALANITIS

Pathophysiology

Posthitis and **balanitis** refer to inflammation of the prepuce and glans, respectively; accompanying cellulitis may or may not be present. In uncircumcised boys, they may occur secondary to phimosis or may result in phimosis following the inflammatory process. In circumcised boys, contact dermatitis from urine or soap may induce balanitis.

Clinical and Laboratory Evaluation

The penis appears erythematous, swollen, warm, and tender at the glans (balanitis) or prepuce (posthitis). If the infection affects the urethral meatus, a secondary meatitis may result. Children may complain of dysuria and voluntarily refrain from voiding as the ammoniacal urine makes contact with the inflamed area. A purulent discharge may exude from under the prepuce.

Management

Medical management is appropriate. In the majority of cases, warm sitz baths and topical antibiotics are satisfactory. In some cases, oral antibiotics may be necessary.

HYPOSPADIAS

Hypospadias is the congenital displacement of the urethral meatus ventrally on the penis. The incidence of this common anomaly is 1 in 300 boys and is often associated with chordee (fibrous tissue that creates an abnormal ventral penile curvature). The urethral meatus may be located anywhere from the distal glans to the penoscrotal junction and perineum. Fifty to seventy percent of hypospadias are located anteriorly on the glans, corona, or distal penile shaft (Figure 26.5). The etiology of hypospadias is unknown but may be multifactorial; there is a familial risk of 8%–14% if fathers or brothers are affected.

Pathophysiology

A working knowledge of urethral embryology is essential for understanding the development of hypospadias. The male urethra forms between weeks 8 and 15 of gestation. The urethral folds, which line the two edges of the urethral plate, fuse in the midline and become tubular in a proximal to distal direction. The terminal urethra forms from an ectodermal plug that channels its way from the distal glans and meets the endodermally derived urethra at the subcoronal position. Anomalous fusion of the urethral folds or abnormal formation of the ectodermal plug results in hypospadias.

Clinical and Laboratory Evaluation

Thorough inspection of the external genitalia is warranted. The prepuce is generally deficient ventrally and may be redundant dorsally. The skin proximal to the meatus is usually thin. The location of the meatus may be anywhere: just below a dimple at the very distal glans or hidden between the halves of a bifid scrotum or in the perineum. Chordee may be present on inspection or may be elicited only by an "artificial erection" (intraoperative injection of saline into the corpora cavernosum). The urinary stream is generally unaffected but may be deflected downward by the location of the meatus. It is necessary to palpate the scrotum for the presence of both testes.

Differential Diagnosis

Hypospadias may be an isolated condition or associated with other anomalies including cryptorchidism and inguinal hernia. It may represent a form of intersex, particularly when located proximally or associated with unilateral or bilateral cryptorchidism. It is important to remember that when hypospadias is related to a possible intersex state, sex assignment should be delayed and may not correspond to the child's karyotype.

An impalpable testis may reflect a chromosomal abnormality (mixed gonadal dysgenesis), androgen insensitivity, or true hermaphroditism. If neither gonad is palpable, the pediatrician should consider a defect in steroidogenesis (congenital adrenal hyperplasia).

Management

Treatment involves surgical reconstruction, usually performed at 6–18 months of age. The surgical goal is to provide the child with a normal-appearing and functioning penis. All techniques involve reconstruction of the urethra so that the meatus is closer to its usual position and straightening of the chordee. The foreskin is frequently used in the repair; thus, circumcision should *not* be performed pending consultation with a pediatric urologist.

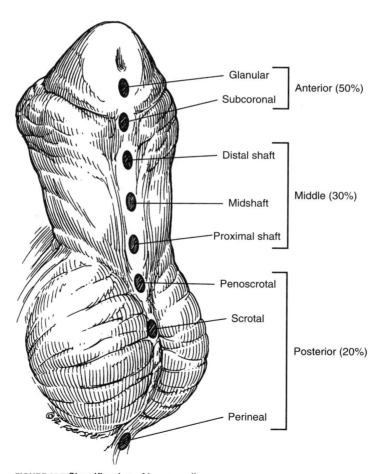

FIGURE 26.5 Classification of hypospadias.

Repair of distal hypospadias is generally an ambulatory procedure, while more proximal repairs may require brief hospitalization.

CRYPTORCHIDISM

Undescended testes, or cryptorchidism, is the most common urogenital congenital anomaly. It has an incidence of 3.4% at birth, which decreases to 0.8% by 1 year of age.

> ### Pediatric Pearl
>
> Low birth weight and prematurity are associated with higher rates of cryptorchidism.

Histologic changes in the cryptorchid testis are found by the second year of life and pose a risk for malignancy and infertility. Thus, undescended testes require treatment before a child's second birthday.

Pathophysiology

Although the mechanism of testicular descent is not well understood, postulated theories include traction on the gubernaculum, differential growth of the body wall, increased intra-abdominal pressure, and hormonal factors. Embryologically, testicular descent begins during the eighth week of gestation with attachment of the gubernaculum to the epididymis. The transabdominal phase of testicular descent from the abdomen to the internal inguinal ring is finished by week 12. A dormant period exists until week 28, after which the transinguinal phase begins leading the testis from the internal inguinal ring into the scrotum. Testicular descent may become arrested at any point in development.

Biopsy of cryptorchid testes, particularly intraabdominal testes, demonstrate histologic abnormalities. These include decreased number of germ cells, greater number of hormonally dormant Sertoli cells, increased collagen deposition, and fibrosis around the seminiferous tubules. The contralateral testis, even if normally descended, may also demonstrate abnormal histology. Fertility is generally reduced, and 20% of men may remain infertile despite surgical correction in childhood.

Testicular neoplasm is 20–45 times greater in undescended testes, with an overall incidence of 4%–11%. Seminoma is the most common malignancy. Although correction (hormonal or surgical) does not reduce malignant potential, it does allow for self-examination and earlier tumor detection.

Clinical and Laboratory Evaluation

Undescended testes may be classified according to location: truly cryptorchid (arrested in the normal path of descent), ectopic (arrested in an abnormal position), or retractile (able to be brought into the scrotum followed by retraction) [Figure 26.6]. The truly cryptorchid testis may be located anywhere along the normal pathway of descent, including the abdomen. Ectopic testes are found outside of the normal pathway. Testes that are found high in the scrotum and can be brought to the normal position, albeit temporarily, are **retractile** and are not at an increased risk of infertility or malignancy. Physical examination should also focus on the size and shape of the penis, because cryptorchidism in the presence of an abnormal phallus may reflect a hormonal aberration or an intersex condition.

In the case of bilateral impalpable cryptorchidism, it is necessary to evaluate serum hormone levels. Low testosterone and high gonadotropin levels suggest primary testicular failure or absent testes. If normal or low levels of gonadotropins and testosterone are present, a stimulation test with human chorionic gonadotropin (hCG) is indicated to assess the presence of functioning testicular tissue. An increase in serum testosterone implies functioning testicular tissue; it is necessary to determine the location.

Differential Diagnosis

The truly cryptorchid testes may be an isolated feature or associated with intersex (refer to the section on the differential diagnosis of hypospadias). Retractile and ectopic testes are generally isolated findings unrelated to an intersex condition.

Management

The following general principles apply to the management of undescended testes (Figure 26.7):

- Surgical correction (orchidopexy) is the primary treatment modality in the United States, while hormonal stimulation is the mainstay of treatment in Europe.
- Treatment should be instituted before 2 years of age.
- Radiographic studies are of limited value in searching for the undescended testis.

VESICOURETERAL REFLUX

The retrograde passage of urine from the bladder to the ureter, **vesicoureteral reflux (VUR),** is commonly found during the evaluation of urinary

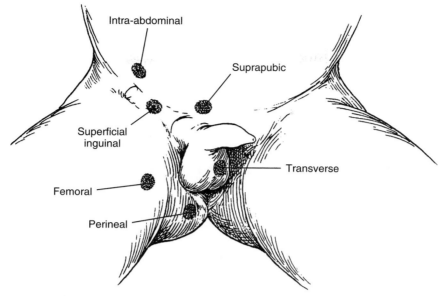

FIGURE 26.6 Location of undescended testes.

tract infections. Although the exact incidence is not known, a familial tendency is reported with approximately 30% of siblings having VUR. The importance of detecting VUR lies in the prevention of infection and subsequent impairment of renal function. VUR may be minimal or grossly deform the renal collecting system and ureter. The international classification system of VUR is depicted in Figure 26.8.

Pathophysiology

VUR can be divided into **primary** (abnormal mechanics at the vesicoureteral junction unrelated to obstruction or abnormal voiding) and **secondary** (related to obstruction or abnormal voiding). The ureter passes through the bladder at an oblique angle such that the roof of this tunnel compresses the ureter as the bladder fills with urine. The ratio of the tunnel length to ureteral diameter is supposedly important in maintaining competence of this mechanism (minimal ratio of 3:1). Any aberrancy in this valvular mechanism can lead to VUR. Similarly, any distortion of the ureteral orifice or displacement from its normal position can result in VUR. These abnormalities include ureteral duplication, ectopic ureteral location, and ureterocele (cystic dilatation at the ureteral orifice). Furthermore, high bladder pressures or obstruction to the flow of urine (posterior urethral valves, tumors, urethral strictures) may lead to disruption of the normal valvular mechanism.

VUR in the presence of infected urine poses a significant threat to renal function. Bacteria gain entry to the renal medulla through abnormal papilla, stimulating an immune response. Superoxide, released to kill the bacteria, damages the tubular cell wall and produces a renal scar. Scarring leads to contraction of the renal parenchyma overlying the affected papilla and loss of function (reflux nephropathy). At its worst, end-stage renal disease ensues with subsequent need for dialysis or renal transplantation.

Clinical and Laboratory Evaluation

The first febrile urinary tract infection or a history of VUR in a sibling or parent should prompt a search for VUR. Symptoms may reflect either the urinary tract infection (fever, vomiting, failure to thrive, dehydration, lethargy) or VUR (colicky-type back pain, hypertension). Accurate documentation of infected urine obtained from urethral catheterization, suprapubic aspiration, or a "clean-catch" in older children is acceptable; urine cultures from bagged specimens are valuable only if negative prior to administration of antibiotics and should be avoided.

After documentation of a urinary tract infection, the radiographic evaluation begins with a sonogram of the bladder and kidneys. The presence of hydronephrosis or dilated ureters raises the possibility of VUR, although low-grade VUR is not excluded by a normal sonogram. **Voiding**

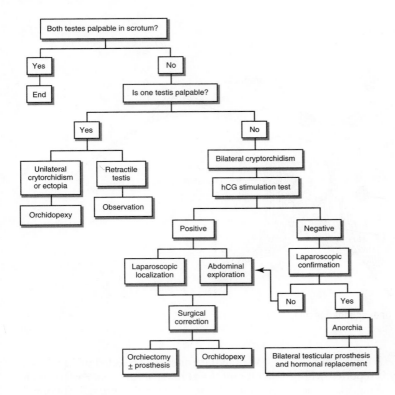

FIGURE 26.7 Algorithm for the evaluation and management of undescended testes. hCG = human chorionic gonadotropin.

cystourethrography is then performed by placing a urethral catheter and filling the bladder with iodinated contrast. Fluoroscopic or static images of the urinary tract looking for the presence of contrast in the ureter or renal collecting system confirm the diagnosis. Assessment of renal function by either nuclear renogram or intravenous pyelogram is performed in the presence of documented VUR. Cystoscopy is reserved for those children who require surgical correction or who have repeated episodes of cystitis.

Differential Diagnosis

VUR is one cause of hydronephrosis or hydroureter. Other conditions are possible (Table 26.13).

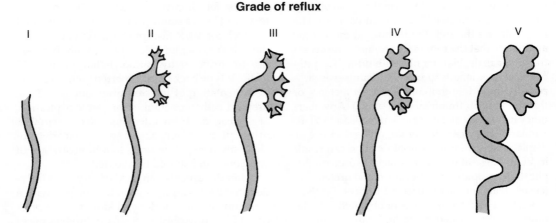

FIGURE 26.8 International classification of vesicoureteral reflux.

Management

The management of the different grades of VUR are predicated on their respective rates of spontaneous resolution and the prevention of urinary tract infections.

- **Grades I–II VUR** resolve in 80% of children. Antibiotic prophylaxis is the treatment of choice for lower grades of reflux. Affected children are followed with serial urine cultures, serum creatinine levels, and voiding cystourethrography.
- **Grade III VUR** resolves in 50% of children. The consensus on optimal management is divided between advocates for chemoprophylaxis and advocates for surgical intervention.
- **Grades IV–V VUR** are unlikely to resolve spontaneously. These cases require surgical correction (ureteral reimplantation into the bladder).

OPHTHALMOLOGY*

INJURIES TO THE EYE

Approximately one-third of childhood blindness results from trauma. Injury from sharp objects, explosives and strong chemicals are the most common. Symptoms of eye injury include pain, tearing, photophobia, redness, and bleeding, which all require immediate evaluation. Any lid or periorbital hemorrhage or swelling is of little consequence but should prompt a complete evaluation for more serious injuries such as intraocular hemorrhage or retinal detachment. **Lacerations of the lid,** especially those involving the lid margins or medial canthus, require evaluation and repair by an ophthalmologist.

Hyphema, blood in the anterior chamber, results from blunt or penetrating injury and presents as bright or dark red fluid between the cornea and iris. It usually resolves with bed rest and head elevation. However, elevation of intraocular pressure can cause blindness. Surgical evacuation of a clot or irrigation of the anterior chamber may reduce intraocular pressure and prevent staining of the cornea.

Perforating wounds of the eye necessitate immediate evaluation by an ophthalmologist. However, the pediatrician plays a key role in initial diagnosis and treatment. Signs of a perforating

---

*"Ophthalmology" was written by Rebecca Evangelista, M.D., and Marijean Miller, M.D.

TABLE 26.13 Differential Diagnosis of Hydronephrosis and Hydroureter
Vesicoureteral reflux (VUR)
Ureteropelvic junction obstruction
Megaureter
Prune belly syndrome
Posterior urethral valves
Neurogenic bladder
Diabetes insipidus
Urinary tract infection
Prior ureteral or renal pelvic surgery
Urethral stricture
Ureterocele

injury include collapse of the anterior chamber, distortion or displacement of the pupil, or protrusion of the dark uvea into the wound. Manipulation should be minimized. The clinician should place a sterile bandage and rigid shield over the injured eye for protection until further evaluation by the ophthalmologist occurs.

Presenting symptoms of **corneal abrasions** usually include pain, foreign body sensation, tearing, or redness, which are easily seen with fluorescein dye. A fluorescein dye–impregnated paper strip is applied to the conjunctiva, and the yellow dye "stains" the epithelial defect, making it visible under blue light. Treatment consists of antibiotic eye ointment to prevent infection and bandaging the eye. Examination of the eye, preferably by an ophthalmologist, should take place the following day. Contact lens wearers are susceptible to ulcers of the cornea with aggressive gram-negative organisms and should see an ophthalmologist as soon as possible.

Foreign body removal usually requires only irrigating or gently wiping the eye. Lid eversion is necessary if the object is lodged under the upper lid. An ophthalmologist should remove embedded foreign bodies and take care of follow-up after removal of a metallic foreign body.

Chemical injuries require immediate and copious irrigation until the eye pH normalizes. It is necessary to obtain a specific history about the chemical. Caustic alkaline products may continue to damage the tissue long after initial contact requiring continued close, long-term care.

Fracture of the orbit, which is possible to miss on plain radiography, warrants evaluation by CT scan if suspected. Fracture of the floor of the orbit can result in entrapment of the inferior rectus muscle and may require immediate surgical repair.

RETINOPATHY OF PREMATURITY
(SEE CHAPTER 10 [NEONATOLOGY])

Retinopathy of prematurity (ROP) refers to a spectrum of retinal angiopathy found in preterm infants. A retinal examination is necessary for all preterm infants born at or before 32 weeks' gestation, or a low birth weight (1500 g), or both. Continued examinations every 1–2 weeks until the retina matures are warranted. Major risk factors for ROP are prematurity, degree of retinal immaturity at birth, and hyperoxia. Respiratory distress, apnea, bradycardia, heart disease, infection, hypoxia, hypercarbia, acidosis, and anemia may be contributing factors.

The current international classification describes the zone in the eye affected and stages the severity of new anomalous blood vessel formation. Infants who develop threshold ROP undergo laser photocoagulation to the avascular retina to arrest progression. Despite this treatment, some infants eventually develop retinal detachments, necessitating surgical repair. Ultimately, significant visual impairment may still occur in infants with severe ROP.

GLAUCOMA

Glaucoma in children is usually the result of a developmental abnormality in the filtration angle of the anterior chamber or residual tissue impeding drainage. The condition may be congenital or develop secondary to several other disease processes, including ROP, trauma, intraocular tumor, Sturge-Weber syndrome, Marfan syndrome, congenital rubella, and a number of chromosomal syndromes. It may be inherited in what many experts believe to be a multifactorial fashion. The glaucoma is usually bilateral but asymmetric and generally sporadic. Symptoms include tearing, photophobia, corneal clouding, and progressive enlargement of the eye.

Initial treatment is surgery, which should be performed as soon as the patient's medical condition allows. Often several procedures are required before adequate results are obtained. Long-term medical therapy usually follows.

CATARACTS

Cataracts refer to any opacity of the lens. They may occur in children for several reasons, including trauma, metabolic disturbances, intrauterine infection, heredity, and as a part of several multisystem syndromes. Management of clinically significant cataracts involves removing the affected lens material to create a clear visual axis and then correcting the resulting visual defect. This is accomplished with glasses, contact lenses, or lens implants. Affected children may also have associated sensory deprivation **amblyopia** that needs correction.

CONJUNCTIVITIS

Inflammation of the conjunctivae, a common condition in children, may result from a wide range of insults. **Acute purulent conjunctivitis** is usually bacterial; the most frequent organisms are *Staphylococcus*, pneumococci, *H. influenzae*, and streptococci. These infections respond well to topical antibiotics. Newborn infants with conjunctivitis require careful consideration of gonococcal and chlamydial infections. Children may also develop **viral conjunctivitis**, often in conjunction with a viral upper respiratory infection.

Membranous and pseudomembranous conjunctivitis, which are potential sequelae of infectious conjunctivitis, may require surgical removal of the fibrin-rich exudate. **Allergic conjunctivitis** is best treated with cold compresses and over-the-counter drops. **Chemical conjunctivitis** results from several liquids and air-borne substances. Thorough, copious irrigation is often adequate treatment.

STABISMUS

Strabismus refers to misalignment or deviation of the eye. Conditions include **esotropia (inward)**, **exotropia (outward)**, vertical, and torsional deviation. The deviation may lead to reduced depth perception, transient diplopia, or suppression of central vision of the deviated eye. Children younger than 8 years of age suppress a deviated eye, resulting in **amblyopia**, or poor visual development in that eye. **Accommodative esotropia** occurs when the eyes overconverge during accommodation.

During a comprehensive ophthalmologic examination, the clinician may identify causative factors such as cataract or the need for unilateral glasses. The **Hirschberg test** involves a flashlight pointed at the eyes. The position of corneal reflection is normal when the light reflex is symmetric and well centered. The "cover-uncover" and "alternate-covers" tests look for eye deviation while moving an eye occluder. Normally a covered eye will not move while the other is fixed on a target. With strabismus, the eye under the occluder shifts and a refixation movement can be seen when the occluder is switched to the other eye.

Goals of treatment are to achieve the best possible vision and alignment. Patches and glasses are prescribed when needed. Amblyopia may be reversed with patching, and accommodative esotropia often can be corrected with glasses. Congenital esotropia and partially accommodative esotropia require surgery. Surgical correction of alignment should occur at the earliest possible time to allow for normal development.

RETINOBLASTOMA

Two-thirds of cases of this tumor of the retina are bilateral; they occur due to a dominantly inherited predisposition on chromosome 13. Diagnosis often takes place before 2 years of age. The sporadic cases that usually occur after 2 years of age are unilateral. The tumor usually develops on the posterior portion of the retina and rarely metastasizes.

The presenting sign is **leukokoria,** the typical yellowish white reflex. Some patients also present with loss of vision, pain, or pupillary irregularity. The diagnosis requires a complete, careful funduscopic examination, which often necessitates anesthesia in children. A CT scan to determine the extent of involvement in the surrounding structures and evaluate the pineal gland is also necessary. Staging is based on whether there are single or multiple lesions and the extent of the retina involved.

Pediatric Pearl

The presence of a yellowish white reflex (**leukokoria**) is highly suggestive of retinoblastoma.

Standard treatment of unilateral disease for large tumors is enucleation of the eye. In bilateral disease, chemotherapy with adjunct laser phototherapy can be successful in preserving vision. Children with retinoblastoma remain at risk of developing other tumors (e.g., sarcomas) into adulthood.

SUGGESTED READINGS

Limp and Developmental Gait Disturbances
Common orthopedic problems. *Pediatr Clin North Am* 33(6), 1986.

Harris P: Limp and gait disturbance. Norwalk, CT, Appleton-Century-Crofts, 1983.

Hensinger RN: Congenital dislocation of the hip. *Ciba Clin Symp* 31:5, 1979.

Morrisy RT: *Lovell and Winter's Pediatric Orthopaedics,* 3rd ed. Philadelphia, JB Lippincott, 1990.

Ozonoff MB: *Pediatric Orthopedic Radiology,* 2nd ed. Philadelphia, WB Saunders, 1992.

Shelov S, Mezey A, Edelmann C, et al: Pediatric primary care: A symptomatic approach. In *Major Problems in Clinical Pediatrics.* Edited by Shelov S, Mezey A, Edelmann C, et al. Philadelphia, WB Saunders, 1981;XXI.

Smith DM: Recognizable patterns of human deformation. In *Major Problems in Clinical Pediatrics.* Edited by Shelov S, Mezey A, Edelmann C, et al. Philadelphia, WB Saunders, 1981;XXI.

Tolo VT, Wood BL: *Pediatrics in Primary Care.* Baltimore: Williams & Wilkins, 1993.

Otorhinolaryngology
Bluestone CD, Stool SE: *Pediatric Otolaryngology,* 3rd ed. Philadelphia, WB Saunders, 1995.

Bluestone CD, Stool SE, Scheetz MD (eds): *Pediatric Otolaryngology,* 2nd ed. Philadelphia, WB Saunders, 1990.

Cumming CW (ed): *Otolaryngology—Head and Neck Surgery,* 2nd ed. St Louis, CV Mosby, 1993.

Gates GA (ed): *Current Therapy in Otolaryngology—Head and Neck Surgery,* 5th ed. Chicago, Mosby-Year Book, 1994.

Paradise JL, Bluestone CD, Bachman RZ, et al: Efficacy of tonsillectomy for recurrent throat infections in severely affected children: results of parallel randomized and nonrandomized clinical trials. *N Engl J Med* 310:674–683, 1984.

Schwartz R, Rodriguez W, Schwartz D: Office myringotomy for acute otitis media: Its value in preventing middle ear effusion. *Laryngoscope* 91:616–619, 1981.

Yankelowitz S, Gravel J, Wallace I, et al: A clinical research form for use in documentation of middle ear effusion. *Ear Hearing* 12:296–298, 1991.

Urology
Arant BS: Vesicoureteral reflux and renal injury. *Am J Kidney Dis* 17:491, 1991.

Avellan L: The incidence of hypospadias in Sweden. *Scand J Plast Reconstr Surg* 9:129, 1975.

Cass AS, Cass BP, Verraraghaven K: Immediate exploration of the unilateral acute scrotum in young male subjects. *J Urol* 124:829, 1980.

Duckett JW: Hypospadias. In *Adult and Pediatric Urology.* Edited by Gillenwater JY, Grayhack JT, Howards SS, et al. St Louis, Mosby-Year Book, 1991:2103–2140.

Edwards D, Normand ICS, Prescod N, et al: Disappearance of vesicoureteral reflux during long-term prophylaxis of urinary tract infection in children. *Br Med J* 2:285, 1977.

Hadziselimovic F: *Cryptorchidism. Management and Implications.* New York, Springer-Verlag, 1983.

Hadziselimovic F: Pathogenesis of cryptorchidism. *Clin Androl* 7:147–162, 1981.

Hadziselimovic F, Girard J, Herzog B: Lack of germ cells and endocrinology in cryptorchid boys from one to six years of life. In *Cryptorchidism.* Edited by Bierich JR, Giarola A. New York, Academic Press, 1979:129–134.

Kogan SJ: Fertility in cryptorchidism: An overview in 1987. *Eur J Pediatr* 146(suppl 2):s21, 1987.

Leape LL: Torsion of the testes: Invitation to error. *JAMA* 200:669, 1967.

Martin DC: Germinal cell tumors of the testis after orchidopexy. *J Urol* 121:422, 1979.

Noe HN: The long-term results of prospective sibling reflux screening. *J Urol* 148:1739,1992.

Ransley PG, Risdon RA: Reflux and renal scarring. *Br J Radiol Suppl* 14:1, 1978.

Redman AJ, Scribner LJ, Bissada NK: Postcircumcision of phimosis and its management. *Clin Pediatr* 14:407, 1975.

Rolleston GL, Maling TMJ, Hodson CJ: Intrarenal reflux and the scarred kidney. *Arch Dis Child* 49:531, 1974.

Scorer GC, Farrington GH: Congenital deformities of the testes and epididymis. London: Butterworth, 1971.

Skoglund RW Jr, Chapman WH: Reduction of paraphimosis. *J Urol* 104:137, 1970.

Stage KH, Schoenvogel R, Lewis S: Testicular scanning: Clinical experience with 72 patients. *J Urol* 1981;125:334.

Weiss R, Duckett J, Spitzer A: Results of a randomized clinical trial of medical vs. surgical management of infants and children with grades III and IV primary vesicoureteral reflux (United States). *J Urol* 148:1667, 1992.

Williamson RCN: Death in the scrotum: Testicular torsion. *N Engl J Med* 196:338, 1977.

Williamson RCN: Torsion of the testes and allied conditions. *Br J Surg* 63:465, 1976.

Ophthalmology

Isenberg SJ: *The Eye in Infancy*, 2nd ed. St. Louis, Mosby-Year Book, 1994.

MacCumber MW: *Management of Ocular Injuries and Emergencies*. Philadelphia, Lippincott-Raven, 1998.

Nelson, LB: *Harley's Pediatric Ophthalmology*, 4th ed. Philadelphia, WB Saunders, 1998.

Figure and Table Credits

FIGURES

2.1 From Frankenburg WK, Dodds J, Archer P, et al: The Denver II: A major revision and restandardization of the Denver Developmental Screening Test. *Pediatrics* 89:91–97, 1992.

2.2 Courtesy of Michael Jellinek, MD, Massachusetts General Hospital.

2.3 From Ogden CL, Kuczmarski RJ, Flegal KM, et al: Centers for Disease Control and Prevention 2000 growth charts for the United States: Improvements to the 1977 National Center on Health Statistics version. *Pediatrics* 109:48, 2002. http://www.cdc.gov/growthcharts

2.4 From Ogden CL, Kuczmarski RJ, Flegal KM, et al: Centers for Disease Control and Prevention 2000 growth charts for the United States: Improvements to the 1977 National Center on Health Statistics version. *Pediatrics* 109:52, 2002. http://www.cdc.gov/growthcharts

2.5 From Ogden CL, Kuczmarski RJ, Flegal KM, et al: Centers for Disease Control and Prevention 2000 growth charts for the United States: Improvements to the 1977 National Center on Health Statistics version. *Pediatrics* 109:47, 2002. http://www.cdc.gov/growthcharts

2.6 From Ogden CL, Kuczmarski RJ, Flegal KM, et al: Centers for Disease Control and Prevention 2000 growth charts for the United States: Improvements to the 1977 National Center on Health Statistics version. *Pediatrics* 109:51, 2002. http://www.cdc.gov/growthcharts

2.7 From Ogden CL, Kuczmarski RJ, Flegal KM, et al: Centers for Disease Control and Prevention 2000 growth charts for the United States: Improvements to the 1977 National Center on Health Statistics version. *Pediatrics* 109:49, 2002. http://www.cdc.gov/growthcharts

2.8 From Fleisher GR, Ludwig S (eds): *Textbook of Pediatric Emergency Medicine,* 4th ed. Philadelphia, Lippincott Williams & Wilkins, 2000, p 740.

2.9 From Algranati PS: *The Pediatric Patient: An Approach to History and Physical Examination.* Baltimore, Williams & Wilkins, 1992, p 39.

2.10 From the American Academy of Pediatrics. In Pickering L (ed): *2000 Red Book: Report of the Committee of Infectious Diseases,* 25th ed. Elk Grove Village, IL, American Academy of Pediatrics, 2000.

2.11 From Committee on Practice and Ambulatory Medicine, Recommendations for preventive pediatric health care, American Academy of Pediatrics (AAP): *Pediatrics* 105(3):645, 2000.

3.1 From Fleisher GR, Ludwig S: *Textbook of Pediatric Emergency Medicine,* 3rd ed. Baltimore, Williams & Wilkins, 1993, p 1506.

3.2 From Fleisher GR, Ludwig S: *Textbook of Pediatric Emergency Medicine,* 3rd ed. Baltimore, Williams & Wilkins, 1993, p 1506.

3.3 From Fleisher GR, Ludwig S: *Textbook of Pediatric Emergency Medicine,* 3rd ed. Baltimore, Williams & Wilkins, 1993, p 1506.

3.4 Adapted from Brookman RR, Rauh JL, Morrison JA, et al: The Princeton Maturation Study, 1976, unpublished data for adolescents in Cincinnati, Ohio. Used with permission of Ross Products Division Laboratories Inc., Columbus, OH 43215. From Assessment of Pubertal Development, 1986, Ross Product Division, Abbott Laboratories Inc.

3.5 Adapted from Brookman RR, Rauh JL, Morrison JA, et al: The Princeton Maturation Study, 1976, unpublished data for adolescents in Cincinnati, Ohio. Used with permission of Ross Products Division Laboratories Inc., Columbus, OH 43215. From Assessment of Pubertal Development, 1986, Ross Product Division, Abbott Laboratories Inc.

4.1 From *Caring for Your Baby and Young Child: Birth to Age 5* by Steven Shelov and Robert E. Hannemann, copyright © 1991 by American Academy of Pediatrics. Used by permission of Bantam Books, a division of Random House, Inc., pp 76, 77.

4.2 From *Caring for Your Baby and Young Child: Birth to Age 5* by Steven Shelov and Robert E. Hannemann, copyright ©1991 by American Academy of Pediatrics. Used by permission of Bantam Books, a division of Random House, Inc., p 74.

4.3 From Berry PL, Bel Sha CW: Hyponatremia. *Pediatr Clin North Am* 37(2):351–364, 1990.

4.4 From Kallen RJ: Diarrheal dehydration in infancy. *Pediatr Clin North Am* 37(2):265–286, 1990.

8.1 Based on Berk ML, Monheit AC: The concentration of health expenditures revisited. *Health Aff (Millwood)* 20(2):9–18, 2001.

8.3 Based on Levit K, Smith C, Cowan C, et al: Inflation spurs health spending in 2000. *Health Aff (Millwood)* 21(1):172–181, 2002, and National Health Care Expenditure Projections: 2001–2011, Personal Health Care Expenditures Aggregate and Per Capita amounts, Percent distribution and Average Annual Percent Change by Source of Funds: Selected Years 1980–2010. http://www.hcfa.gov/stats/NHE-Proj/proj2001/Proj2001.pdf

8.4 Based on Levit K, Smith C, Cowan C, et al: Inflation spurs health spending in 2000. *Health*

Aff (*Millwood*) 21(1), 2002, and National Health Care Expenditure Projections: 2001–2011, Personal Health Care Expenditures Aggregate and Per Capita amounts, Percent distribution and Average Annual Percent Change by Source of Funds: Selected Years 1980–2010. http://www.hcfa.gov/stats/NHE-Proj/proj2001/Proj2001.pdf

8.5 Based on data from Letsch SW, Lazenby HC, Levit KR, et al: National health expenditures, 1991. *Health Care Finance Rev* 14(2):1–30, 1992.

8.7 Managed care fact sheets. http://www.mcareol.com/factshts/factnati.htm

10.1 From OH W: Fluid and electrolyte management. In *Neonatology: Pathophysiology and Management of the Newborn.* Edited by Avery GB. Philadelphia, JB Lippincott, 1987, p 776.

10.2 From OH W: Fluid and electrolyte management. In *Neonatology: Pathophysiology and Management of the Newborn.* Edited by Avery GB. Philadelphia, JB Lippincott, 1987, p 776.

10.3 Courtesy of Richard Barth, M.D., Division of Pediatric Radiology, Stanford University.

10.4 Courtesy of Richard Barth, M.D., Division of Pediatric Radiology, Stanford University.

10.5 Courtesy of Richard Barth, M.D., Division of Pediatric Radiology, Stanford University.

10.7 Courtesy of Richard Barth, M.D., Division of Pediatric Radiology, Stanford University.

10.8 Courtesy of Richard Barth, M.D., Division of Pediatric Radiology, Stanford University.

10.9 From Martin RJ, Miller MJ, Carlo WA: Pathogenesis of apnea in preterm infants. *J Pediatr* 109:733, 1986.

10.11 Courtesy of Richard Barth, M.D., Division of Pediatric Radiology, Stanford University.

10.12 Courtesy of Richard Barth, M.D., Division of Pediatric Radiology, Stanford University.

11.2 From Gelehrter TD, Collins FS: *Principles of Medical Genetics.* Baltimore, Williams & Wilkins, 1990, p 173.

11.3 From Gelehrter TD, Collins FS: *Principles of Medical Genetics.* Baltimore, Williams & Wilkins, 1990, p 29.

11.4 From Gelehrter TD, Collins FS: *Principles of Medical Genetics.* Baltimore, Williams & Wilkins, 1990, p 36.

13.1A Repinted with permission from Rudolph AM: *Congenital Diseases of the Heart: Clinical Physiological Considerations,* 2nd ed. Armonk, NY: Blackwell Publishing, 2001.

13.1B Courtesy of Dr. Abraham M. Rudolph, University of California, San Francisco.

13.3 From Lilly LS: *Pathophysiology of Heart Disease.* Baltimore, Williams & Wilkins, 1993.

13.11 Adapted from Gillette PC, Garson A Jr: *Pediatric Arrhythmias: Electrophysiology and Pacing.* Philadelphia, WB Saunders, 1990.

13.12 Adapted from Gillette PC, Garson A Jr: *Pediatric Arrhythmias: Electrophysiology and Pacing.* Philadelphia, WB Saunders, 1990.

13.13 Adapted from Committee on Rheumatic Fever, Endocarditis, and Kawasaki Disease: Prevention of Bacterial Endodarditis: Recommendations by the American Heart Association. *JAMA* 277:1794–1801, 1997. *Circulation* 96:358–366, 1997. © 1997, American Medical Association.

14.3 From New MI, del Balzo P, Crawdford C, et al: The adrenal cortex. In *Clinical Pediatric Endocrinology,* 2nd ed. Edited by Kaplan SA. Philadelphia, WB Saunders, 1990, p 188, as adapted from New MI, Levine LS: Congenital adrenal hyperplasia. *Adv Hum Genet* 4:251–376, 1973.

14.6 From Sperling MA: Diabetes mellitus. In *Clinical Pediatric Endocrinology,* 2nd ed. Edited by Kaplan SA. Philadelphia, WB Saunders, 1990, p 128.

14.8 From Sperling MA: *Physician's Guide to Insulin-Dependent (type I) Diabetes. Diagnosis and Treatment.* Arlington, VA, American Diabetes Association, 1988.

14.10 From Bacon GE, Spencer ML, Hopwood NJ, et al: *A Practical Approach to Pediatric Endocrinology,* 3rd ed. Chicago, Year Book Medical Publishers, 1990, p 124.

18.6 From Taussig L, Landau L, Le Souef P, et al (eds): *Pediatric Respiratory Medicine,* St. Louis, Mosby, 1999.

20.1 From Hogg RJ et al: Evaluation and management of proteinuria. *Pediatrics* 105:1244, 2000.

20.3 Reproduced with permission from Greenberg A: *Primer on Kidney Diseases.* San Diego, National Kidney Foundation, 2nd ed. 1998, p 130.

20.4 Reproduced with permission from Diven SC et al: A practical primary care approach to hematuria. In *Pediatric Nephrology,* vol 14. Springer-Verlag, 2000, p 69.

20.5 Reproduced with permission from Hellerstein S: Urinary tract infections in children. *Am Fam Phys* 57:2445, 1998.

22.1 Reprinted with permission from Lookingbill DP, Mark JG: *Principles of Dermatology.* Philadelphia, WB Saunders, 1993, p. 6.

25.1 From Gann DS, Ameral JF: The pathophysiology of trauma and shock. In *The Management of Trauma,* 4th ed. Philadelphia, WB Saunders, 1984, p 38.

26.1 Modified after illustrations by Frank K. Netter, MD, from Hensinger RN: *Ciba Clin Symp* 31:1. 1979. Copright 1979, CIBA Pharmaceutical Company, Division of CIBA-GEIGY Corporation.

26.2E From Algranati PS: *The Pediatric Patient: An Approach to History and Physical Examination.* Baltimore, Williams & Wilkins, 1992, p 107.

26.3 From Stool SE, Berg AO, Berman S, et al: Managing otitis media with effusion in young children. Quick reference guide for clinicians. AHCPR publication no. 94–0623. Rockville, MD, Agency for Health Care Policy and Research, Public Health Service, US Department of Health and Human Services, July 1994.

26.4 Reproduced with permission from Gosalbez R Jr, Woodard JR: Testicular torsion calls for urgent intervention. *Contemp Urol* 4(8):76–84,

1992. Copyright Medical Economics Publishing.

26.5   Reproduced with permission from Duckett JW Jr: Successful hypospadias repair. *Contemp Urol* 4(4):42–55, 1992. Copyright Medical Economics Publishing.

26.6   Reproduced with permission from Freedman AL, Rajfer J: Cryptorchism: Reliable surgery amid uncertainties. *Contemp Urol* 4(1):59–70, 1992. Copyright Medical Economics Publishing.

26.8   Reproduced with permission from Freedman AL, Rajfer J: Cryptorchism: Reliable surgery amid uncertainties. *Contemp Urol* 4(1):59–70, 1992. Copyright Medical Economics Publishing.

TABLES

1.1   Adapted from Apgar V: Proposal for new method of evaluating the newborn infant. *Curr Res Anesth* 32:260, 1953.

2.1   From *Caring for Your Baby and Young Child: Birth to Age 5* by Steven Shelov and Robert E. Hannemann, copyright © 1991 by American Academy of Pediatrics. Used by permission of Bantam Books, a division of Random House, Inc., p 136.

2.2   Adapted from American Academy of Pediatrics. In Pickering L (ed): *2000 Red Book: Report of the Committee of Infectious Diseases,* 25th ed. Elk Grove Village, IL, American Academy of Pediatrics, 2000.

2.3   From American Academy of Pediatrics. In Pickering L (ed): *2000 Red Book: Report of the Committee of Infectious Diseases,* 25th ed. Elk Grove Village, IL, American Academy of Pediatrics, 2000.

2.4   From Centers for Disease Control and Prevention: Vaccine adverse event reporting system—United States: Requirements. *MMWR* 39, 1990.

3.3   Adapted from Drugs for sexually transmitted disease. *Med Lett* 33(860): 119–124, 1991.

3.4   Adapted from Hatcher RA, Trussell J, Stewart F, et al: *Contraceptive Technology,* 16th rev. ed. New York, Irvington Publishers, 1994.

3.5   Adapted from Hatcher RA, Trussell J, Stewart F, et al: *Contraceptive Technology 1900–1992,* 15th rev. ed. New York, Irvington Publishers, 1990.

3.6   Reprinted with permission from the *Diagnostic and Statistical Manual of Mental Disorders,* Fourth edition, Text Revision. Washington, DC, American Psychiatric Association, 2000.

4.1   Adapted from Behrman RE, Kliegman RM: Nelson's *Essentials of Pediatrics,* 2nd ed. Philadelphia, WB Saunders, 1994, p 61.

4.2   Adapted from Behrman RE, Kliegman RM: Nelson's *Essentials of Pediatrics,* 2nd ed. Philadelphia, WB Saunders, 1994, p 199.

4.3   From American Academy of Pediatrics Committee on Nutrition: Fluoride supplementation for children: Interim policy recommendations. *Pediatrics* 95(5):777, 1995. © American Academy of Pediatrics.

4.7   Adapted from Winters RW: *Principles of Pediatric Fluid Therapy.* Boston, Little, Brown & Company, 1982. pp 75, 78.

4.9   Adapted from Feld LG, Kaskel FJ, Schoeneman MJ: The approach to fluid and electrolyte therapy in pediatrics. *Adv Pediatr* 35:497–535, 1988.

6.1   From Starfield B: Childhood morbidity: Comparisons, clusters, and trends. *Pediatrics* 88(3):519–526, 1991.

6.2   Adapted from Flores G: Culture and patient–physician relationship: Achieving cultural competency in health care. *J Pediatr* 136:14–23, 2000.

8.8   Adapted from information in Halpern R, Lee MY, Boulter PR, et al: A synthesis of nine major reports on physicians' competencies for the emerging practice environment. *Acad Med* 76(6):606–615, 2001.

12.1   From Early Intervention Program, New York State Department of Health: *Early Intervention Memorandum 1999–1992: Reporting of Children's Eligibility Status Based on Diagnosed Conditions With High Probability of Developmental Delay,* December 10, 1999, Albany, New York, New York State Department of Health.

12.2   Adapted from Capute AJ, Accardo PJ (eds): *Developmental Disabilities in Infancy and Childhood,* 2nd ed. Baltimore, Paul Brookes Publishing, 1996, pp 327–330.

12.3   Adapted from Behrman RE, Keligman RM, Jenson HB (eds): *Nelson's Textbook of Pediatrics,* 16th ed. Philadelphia, WB Saunders, 2000, p 126.

12.4   Adapted from Molnar GE, Alexander MA (eds): *Pediatric Rehabilitation,* 3rd ed. Philadelphia, Hanley & Belfus, 1999, p 194.

12.7   Reprinted with permission from the *Diagnostic and Statistical Manual of Mental Disorders,* 4th ed., Text Revision. Washington, DC, American Psychiatric Association, 2000. p 75.

14.9   Adapted from New MI, del Balzo P, Crawdford C, et al: The adrenal cortex. In *Clinical Pediatric Endocrinology,* 2nd ed. Edited by Kaplan SA. Philadelphia, WB Saunders, 1990, p 187, Table 6–1.

14.13   Adapted from Bacon GE, Spencer ML, Hopwood NJ, et al: *A Practical Approach to Pediatric Endocrinology,* 3rd ed. Chicago, Year Book Medical Publishers, 1990, p 189, Table 8–2.

14.14   Adapted from Wilson JD, Foster D: *Williams Textbook of Endocrinology,* 8th ed. Philadelphia, WB Saunders, 1992, p 333.

14.15   Adapted from Bode HH: Disorders of the posterior pituitary. In *Clinical Pediatric Endocrinology,* 2nd ed. Edited by Kaplan SA. Philadelphia, WB Saunders, 1990, p 74, Table 2–3.

14.16   Adapted from Kovacs L, Robertson GL: Syndrome of inappropriate antidiuresis. *Endocrinol Metab Clin North Am* 21(4):859–874, 1992.

14.17   Adapted from Wilson JD, Foster D: *Williams Textbook of Endocrinology,* 8th ed. Philadelphia, WB Saunders, 1992, p 343.

17.10 From Behrman R, Kliegman RM: *Nelson's Essentials of Pediatrics*, 4th ed. St. Louis, WB Saunders, 2002, p 317.

18.22 From Consensus Statement: National Institute of Health Consensus Development Conference on Infantile Apnea and Home Monitoring, Sept. 29–Oct. 1, 1986. *Pediatrics*, 79:292, 1987.

20.9 Reproduced with permission from Hellerstein S: Urinary tract infections. Old and new concepts. *Pediatr Clin North Am* 42(6):1433–1457, 1995, p 1442.

20.13 From the National High Blood Pressure Education Program Working Group on Hypertension Control in Children and Adolescents: Update on the 1987 task force report on high blood pressure in children and adolescents: A Working Group Report from the National High Blood Pressure Education Program. *Pediatrics* 98(4 Pt 1):649–658, 1996.

20.14 From the National High Blood Pressure Education Program Working Group on Hypertension Control in Children and Adolescents: Update on the 1987 task force report on high blood pressure in children and adolescents: A Working Group Report from the National High Blood Pressure Education Program. *Pediatrics* 98(4 Pt 1):649–658, 1996.

23.3 Adapted from Avner JR, Hain L: Pediatric trauma. In *Clinical Manual of Emergency Pediatrics*. Edited by Crain EF, Gershel JC, Gallagher EJ. New York, McGraw-Hill, 1992, Table 22–2.

26.4 From Shelov SP, et al: *Primary Care Pediatrics*. New York, Appleton-Century-Crofts, 1984.

26.8 Modified from Deatsch WW, Levin S: Ear, nose and throat. In *Current Diagnosis and Treatment*. Edited by Brainerd H, Krupp MA, Chatton MJ, et al. Los Altos, CA, Lange Medical Publishing, 1970.

26.11 From Cuthertson MC Jr, Manning SC: Epistaxis. In *Pediatric Otolaryngology*, 2nd ed. Edited by Blueston CD, Stool SE. Philadelphia, WB Saunders, 1990, p 674.

26.12 From Nakayama DK, Rowe MI: Inguinal hernia and the acute scrotum in infants and children. *Pediatr Rev* 11(3):90, 1989. Reproduced by permission of *Pediatrics in Review*.

APPENDICES

2.1. From American Academy of Pediatrics: The injury prevention program. Elk Grove Village, IL, American Academy of Pediatrics. Copyright 1994, updated 2001 American Academy of Pediatrics.

Index

Page numbers followed by an "f" denote figures; those followed by a "t" denote tables.